# One Health

## The Theory and Practice of Integrated Health Approaches

FSC
www.fsc.org
MIX
Paper from
responsible sources
FSC® C013604

# One Health

## The Theory and Practice of Integrated Health Approaches

---

*Edited by*

**Jakob Zinsstag**

*Swiss Tropical and Public Health Institute, Basel, Switzerland*
*University of Basel, Basel, Switzerland*

**Esther Schelling**

*Swiss Tropical and Public Health Institute, Basel, Switzerland*
*University of Basel, Basel, Switzerland*

**David Waltner-Toews**

*University of Guelph, Canada*

**Maxine Whittaker**

*University of Queensland, Australia*

*and*

**Marcel Tanner**

*Swiss Tropical and Public Health Institute, Basel, Switzerland*
*University of Basel, Basel, Switzerland*

www.cabi.org

**CABI is a trading name of CAB International**

CABI
Nosworthy Way
Wallingford
Oxfordshire OX10 8DE
UK

Tel: +44 (0)1491 832111
Fax: +44 (0)1491 833508
E-mail: info@cabi.org
Website: www.cabi.org

CABI
38 Chauncy Street
Suite 1002
Boston, MA 02111
USA

Tel: +1 800 552 3083 (toll free)
Tel: +1 (0)617 395 4051
E-mail: cabi-nao@cabi.org



A catalogue record for this book is available from the British Library, London, UK.

**Library of Congress Cataloging-in-Publication Data**

One health (Zinsstag)
One health : the theory and practice of integrated health approaches / edited by Jakob Zinsstag, Esther Schelling, David Waltner-Toews, Maxine Whittaker, Marcel Tanner.
p. ; cm.
Includes bibliographical references and index.
ISBN 978-1-78064-341-0 (alk. paper)
I. Zinsstag, Jakob, editor. II. Schelling, Esther, editor. III. Waltner-Toews, David, 1948- , editor. IV. Whittaker, Maxine, Professor, editor. V. Tanner, Marcel, editor. VI. C.A.B. International, issuing body. VII. Title.
[DNLM: 1. Communicable Diseases, Emerging--prevention & control. 2. Public Health Practice. 3. Zoonoses--prevention & control. WA 110]

RA643
616.9--dc23

2014033215

ISBN-13: 978 1 78064 341 0

Commissioning editors: Sarah Hulbert and Claire Parfitt
Editorial assistant: Alexandra Lainsbury
Production editor: Shankari Wilford

Typeset by SPi, Pondicherry, India
Printed and bound in the UK by CPI Group (UK) Ltd, Croydon, CR0 4YY

# Contents

# Contributors

**Lisa Allen-Scott**, Department of Community Health Sciences, Faculty of Medicine, University of Calgary 7th Floor, TRW Building, 3330 Hospital Drive NW, Calgary, Alberta, Canada T2N 4N1. E-mail: lallen@ucalgary.ca

**Mark W. Atkinson**, Wildlife Health & Health Policy Program, Wildlife Conservation Society, 2300 Southern Boulevard, Bronx, NY 10460, USA. E-mail: atkinsonm@me.com

**Shirley J. Atkinson**, Wildlife Health & Health Policy Program, Wildlife Conservation Society, 2300 Southern Boulevard, Bronx, NY 10460, USA. E-mail: satkinson@wcs.org

**Zolzaya Baljinnyam**, Animal Health Project, Swiss Agency for Development and Cooperation, Mongolia Swiss Agency for Development and Cooperation-Mongolia, Government Building 11, Room 601, Chingeltei District 4, J.Sambuu Street-11, Ulaanbaatar 15141, Mongolia. E-mail: zola.baljinnyam@yahoo.com

**Mahamat Béchir Mahamat**, Centre National de Nutrition et de Technologie Alimentaire du Ministère de la Santé Publique au Tchad, N'Djaména, Chad, Ministère de la Santé Publique, N'Djaména, Chad and Centre de Support en Santé Internationale, N'Djaména, Chad. E-mail: mahamatbechir@yahoo.fr

**Andrea Beetz**, Department of Special Education, University of Rostock, Germany, Department of Behavioural Biology, University of Vienna, Austria, Institut für Sonderpädagogische Entwicklungsförderung und Rehabilitation, August-Bebel-Str. 28, 18055 Rostock, Germany. E-mail: andrea.m.beetz@gmail.com

**Eric Boa**, Independent Consultant, 17 Overdale Avenue, New Malden, Surrey KT3 3UE, UK. E-mail: eric_boa@hotmail.com

**Bassirou Bonfoh**, Centre Suisse de Recherches Scientifiques en Côte d'Ivoire, Abidjan, Côte d'Ivoire. E-mail: bassirou.bonfoh@csrs.ci

**Michael Bresalier**, Department of History, King's College London, Strand, London WC2R 2LS. E-mail: michael.bresalier@kcl.ac.uk

**Martin Bunch**, Faculty of Environmental Studies, York University, 4700 Keele Street, Toronto, Ontario, Canada M3J 1P3. E-mail: bunchmj@yorku.ca

**Bonnie Buntain**, Department of Ecosystem and Public Health, Faculty of Veterinary Medicine, Department of Community Health Sciences, Faculty of Medicine, University of Calgary TRW 2D19, 3280 Hospital Dr NW, Calgary, Alberta, Canada T2N 4Z6. E-mail: bonnie.buntain@ucalgary.ca

**Aurelie Cailleau**, Centre Suisse de Recherches Scientifiques en Côte d'Ivoire, Abidjan, Côte d'Ivoire. E-mail: aurelie.cailleau@gmail.com

**Angela Cassidy**, Department of History, King's College London, Strand, London WC2R 2LS. E-mail: angela.cassidy@kcl.ac.uk; angela.cassidy@gmail.com

**Nakul Chitnis**, Swiss Tropical and Public Health Institute, Socinstrasse 57, PO Box CH-4002, Basel. University of Basel, Basel, Switzerland. E-mail: nakul.chitnis@unibas.ch

**Adnan Choudhury**, The University of Queensland School of Population Health, Herston, Queensland 4006, Australia. E-mail: a.choudhury@sph.uq.edu.au

**Sarah Cleaveland**, Institute of Biodiversity, Animal Health and Comparative Medicine, University of Glasgow College of Medical, Veterinary & Life Sciences, Graham Kerr Building, University of Glasgow, Glasgow G12 8QQ, Scotland. E-mail: Sarah.Cleaveland@glasgow.ac.uk

**Paul Coleman**, Department of Disease Control, Faculty of Infectious and Tropical Diseases, London School of Hygiene & Tropical Medicine, Keppel Street, Bloomsbury, London WC1E 7HT. E-mail: paul.coleman@h2ovp.com

**Susan Cork**, Department of Ecosystem & Public Health, Faculty of Veterinary Medicine, University of Calgary, 3280 Hospital Drive, Calgary NW, T2N 4Z6. E-mail: sccork@ucalgary.ca

**Lisa Crump**, Swiss Tropical and Public Health Institute, Socinstrasse 57, PO Box CH-4002, Basel. University of Basel, Basel, Switzerland. E-mail: lisa.crump@unibas.ch

**David H.M. Cumming**, Percy FitzPatrick Institute, DST/NRF Centre of Excellence, University of Cape Town, South Africa; Tropical Resource Ecology Programme, Department of Biological Sciences, University of Zimbabwe, PO Box MP 167, Mount Pleasant, Harare, Zimbabwe. E-mail: cummingdhm@gmail.com

**Graeme S. Cumming**, Percy FitzPatrick Institute of African Ornithology, DST/NRF Centre of Excellence, University of Cape Town, Rondebosch 7701, South Africa. E-mail: gscumming@gmail.com

**Phung Dac Cam**, National Institute of Hygiene and Epidemiology, 1 Yersin Street, Hai Ba Trung, Hanoi, Vietnam. E-mail: cam@fpt.vn

**Solveig Danielsen**, CABI, Kastanjelaan 5, 3833 AN Leusden, the Netherlands. E-mail: s.danielsen@cabi.org

**Anna Dean**, Swiss Tropical and Public Health Institute, Socinstrasse 57, PO Box CH-4002, Basel. University of Basel, Basel, Switzerland. E-mail: deanan@who.int

**Samuel Fuhrimann**, Swiss Tropical and Public Health Institute, Socinstrasse 57, PO Box CH-4002, Basel. University of Basel, Basel, Switzerland. E-mail: samuel.fuhrimann@unibas.ch

**Dorothy Geale**, Canadian Food Inspection Agency, 7494 Vimy Ridge Road, Port Hope, Ontario, L1A 3V6, Canada. E-mail: dwgeale@gmail.com

**Delia Grace**, International Livestock Research Institute, Box 30709, Nairobi, Kenya. E-mail: d.grace@cgiar.org

**Cheri T. Grigg**, One Health Office, National Center for Emerging and Zoonotic Infectious Diseases, Centers for Disease Control and Prevention, 1600 Clifton Road NE, MS A-30, Atlanta, GA 30333, USA. E-mail: cgrigg@cdc.gov

**Sophie Haesen**, Swiss Tropical and Public Health Institute, Socinstrasse 57, PO Box CH-4002, Basel. University of Basel, Basel, Switzerland. E-mail: sophie.haesen@unibas.ch

**Felix Hafner**, Faculty of Law, University of Basel, Peter Merian-Weg 8, PO Box CH-4002, Basel. E-mail: Felix.hafner@unibas.ch

**David Hall**, Department of Ecosystem & Public Health, Faculty of Veterinary Medicine, University of Calgary, 3280 Hospital Drive, Calgary NW, Canada T2N 4Z6. E-mail: dchall@ucalgary.ca

**Jennifer Hatfield**, Global Health and International Partnerships, Faculty of Medicine, University of Calgary 7th Floor, TRW Building, 3330 Hospital Drive NW, Calgary, Alberta, Canada T2N 4N1. E-mail: jennifer.hatfield@ucalgary.ca

**Jan Hattendorf**, Swiss Tropical and Public Health Institute, Socinstrasse 57, PO Box CH-4002, Basel. University of Basel, Basel, Switzerland. E-mail: jan.hattendorf@unibas.ch

**Daniel Haydon**, Institute of Biodiversity, Animal Health and Comparative Medicine, University of Glasgow College of Medical, Veterinary & Life Sciences, Graham Kerr Building, University of Glasgow, Glasgow G12 8QQ, Scotland. E-mail: Daniel.Haydon@glasgow.ac.uk

**Karin Hediger**, Swiss Tropical and Public Health Institute, University of Basel; Institute for Interdisciplinary Research on the Human–Animal Relationship (IEMT) Zurich, Socinstrasse 57, PO Box CH-4002, Basel. University of Basel, Basel, Switzerland. E-mail: karin.hediger@unibas.ch

**Karen L.F. Houle**, University of Guelph, 337 MacKinnon Building, Guelph, Ontario, Canada N1G 2W1. E-mail: khoule@uoguelph.ca

**Abderahim Ibrahim**, Université de N'Djaména, Faculté des Sciences et de la Santé, N'Djaména, Chad. E-mail: abderahimibrahim@yahoo.fr

**Fabienne N. Jaeger**, Swiss Tropical and Public Health Institute, Socinstrasse 57, PO Box CH-4002, Basel. University of Basel, Basel, Switzerland. E-mail: fabienne.jaeger@unibas.ch

**Vreni Jean-Richard**, Swiss Tropical and Public Health Institute, Socinstrasse 57, PO Box CH-4002, Basel. University of Basel, Basel, Switzerland. E-mail: vreni@jean-richard.ch

**Mike Kama**, Fiji Centre for Communicable Disease Control, Fiji Ministry of Health, Mataika House, Tamavua, The Republic of Fiji. E-mail: mnkama02@gmail.com

**Joldoshbek Kasymbekov** Swiss Tropical and Public Health Institute, Institute of Biotechnology of the National Academy of Sciences of the Kyrgyz Republic, 243 Chui Avenue, Bishkek 720071, Kyrgyzstan. E-mail: joldoshbek.kasymbekov@gmail.com

**Lonnie J. King**, College of Veterinary Medicine, Ohio State University, 1900 Coffey Road, Columbus, Ohio 43210, USA. E-mail: King.1518@osu.edu

**Rebekah M. Kunkel**, One Health Office, National Center for Emerging and Zoonotic Infectious Diseases, Centers for Disease Control and Prevention, 600 Clifton Road NE, MS A-30, Atlanta, GA 30333, USA. E-mail: rkunkel@cdc.gov

**Monique Léchenne**, Swiss Tropical and Public Health Institute, University of Basel, Socinstrasse 57, PO Box CH-4002, Basel. E-mail: monique.lechenne@unibas.ch

**Anne Lévy Goldblum**, Gesundheitsdepartement Basel-Stadt, Gerbergasse 13, PO Box CH-4001, Basel. E-mail: anne.levy@bs.ch

**Andrea Meisser**, Swiss Tropical and Public Health Institute, University of Basel, Socinstrasse 57, PO Box CH-4002, Basel. E-mail: andrea.meisser@unibas.ch

**Mary Elizabeth Miranda**, Research Institute for Tropical Medicine, Department of Health, the Philippines, 10 Aralia St, Ayala Westgrove Heights, Silang, Cavite, the Philippines 4118. E-mail: betsygmiranda2@gmail.com

**Vi Nguyen**, Centre for Public Health and Ecosystem Research, Hanoi School of Public Health, 138 Giang Vo, Hanoi, Vietnam. E-mail: vivivinguyen@gmail.com

**Hung Nguyen-Viet**, Hanoi School of Public Health, 17A, Nguyen Khang Street, Trung Hoa Ward, Cau Giay District, Hanoi, Vietnam. E-mail: h.nguyen@cgiar.org

**Michelle North**, Department of Ecosystem and Public Health, University of Calgary TRW 2D26, 3280 Hospital Dr NW, Calgary, Alberta, Canada T2N 4Z6. E-mail: manorth@ucalgary.ca

**Peter Odermatt**, Swiss Tropical and Public Health Institute, Socinstrasse 57, PO Box CH-4002, Basel. E-mail: peter.odermatt@unibas.ch

**Anna Okello**, Division of Pathway Medicine & Centre for Infectious Diseases, School of Biomedical Sciences, College of Medicine & Veterinary Medicine, The University of Edinburgh, Chancellor's Building, 49 Little France Crescent, Edinburgh, EH16 4SB, Scotland. E-mail: Anna.Okello@ed.ac.uk

**Steven A. Osofsky**, Wildlife Health & Health Policy Program, Wildlife Conservation Society, 2300 Southern Boulevard, Bronx, NY 10460, USA. E-mail: sosofsky@wcs.org

**Karim Ouattara**, Centre Suisse de Recherches Scientifiques en Côte d'Ivoire, Abidjan, Côte d'Ivoire. E-mail: karim.ouattara@csrs.ci

**Phuc Pham-Duc**, Centre for Public Health and Ecosystem Research, Hanoi School of Public Health, 138 Giang Vo, Hanoi, Vietnam. E-mail: pdp@hsph.edu.vn

**Luu Quoc Toan**, Centre for Public Health and Ecosystem Research, Hanoi School of Public Health, 138 Giang Vo, Hanoi, Vietnam. E-mail: lqt@hsph.edu.vn

**Vanessa Racloz**, Roll Back Malaria, World Health Organization, Avenue Appia 20, CH-1211, Geneva. E-mail: raclozv@who.int

**Simon Reid**, The University of Queensland School of Population Health, Herston, QLD 4006, Australia. E-mail: simon.reid@uq.edu.au

**Melanie Rock**, Department of Community Health Sciences, Faculty of Medicine, Department of Ecosystem and Public Health, University of Calgary TRW 3E13, 3280 Hospital Dr NW, Calgary, Alberta, Canada T2N 4Z6. E-mail: mrock@ucalgary.ca

**Felix Roth**, Swiss Tropical and Public Health Institute, Socinstrasse 57, PO Box CH-4002, Basel. E-mail: felix.roth@unibas.ch

**Carol Rubin**, One Health Office, National Center for Emerging and Zoonotic Infectious Diseases, Centers for Disease Control and Prevention, 1600 Clifton Road NE, MS A-30, Atlanta, GA 30333, USA. E-mail: crubin@cdc.gov

**Esther Schelling**, Swiss Tropical and Public Health Institute, Socinstrasse 57, PO Box CH-4002, Basel. E-mail: esther.schelling@unibas.ch

**Alexandra Shaw**, The University of Edinburgh, Edinburgh, UK; Upper Cottage, Abbotts Ann, Andover Hants SP11 7DA, UK. E-mail: alex@apconsultants.co.uk

**Katharina Stärk**, SAFOSO AG, Bern, Switzerland, and Royal Veterinary College, Department of Production and Population Health, Hawkshead Lane, North Mymms AL9 7TA, UK. E-mail: kstaerk@rvc.ac.uk

**Craig Stephen**, Executive Director, Canadian Cooperative Wildlife Health Centre and Professor, Western College of Veterinary Medicine, University of Saskatchewan, 52 Campus Drive, Saskatoon, Canada, S7N 5B4. E-mail: cstephen@cwhc-rcsf.ca

**Marcel Tanner**, Swiss Tropical and Public Health Institute, Socinstrasse 57, PO Box CH-4002, Basel. E-mail: marcel.tanner@unibas.ch

**Pham Thi Huong Giang**, Centre for Public Health and Ecosystem Research, Hanoi School of Public Health, 138 Giang Vo, Hanoi, Vietnam. E-mail: pthg@hsph.edu.vn

**Tran Thi Tuyet Hanh**, Centre for Public Health and Ecosystem Research, Hanoi School of Public Health, 138 Giang Vo, Hanoi, Vietnam. E-mail: tth2@hsph.edu.vn

**Abdessalam Tidjani**, University of N'Djaména, Faculty of Science and Health, Université de N'Djaména, N'Djaména, Chad. E-mail: abdelti@yahoo.fr

**Karin Tschanz Cooke**, Director of Post-Graduate Mas in Systemic Pastoral Counseling and Pastoral Psychology, University of Bern, Switzerland. E-mail: karin.tschanz@yahoo.com

**Rea Tschopp**, Armauer Hansen Research Institute, PO Box 1005, Addis Ababa, Ethiopia. E-mail: rea.tschopp@unibas.ch

**Dennis C. Turner**, IEMT, IEAP/IET, Seestrasse 254, CH-8810 Horgen, Switzerland. E-mail: dennis@turner-iet.ch

**Minh Van Hoang**, Institute of Public Health and Preventive Medicine, Hanoi Medical University, 1 Ton That Tung Street, Dong Da, Hanoi, Vietnam. E-mail: hoangvanminh@hmu.edu.vn

**Alain Vandersmissen**, European Union, European External Action Service, B-1046 Brussels, Belgium. E-mail: alain.vandersmissen@ex.europa.eu

**Le Vu Anh**, Hanoi School of Public Health, 138 Giang Vo Street, Hanoi, Vietnam. E-mail: lva@hsph.edu.vn

**Tu Vu-Van**, Centre for Public Health and Ecosystem Research, Hanoi School of Public Health, 138 Giang Vo Street, Hanoi, Vietnam. E-mail: vuvantu@gmail.com

**David Waltner-Toews**, Professor Emeritus, Department of Population Medicine, University of Guelph, Founding President, Veterinarians without Borders/Vétérinaires sans Frontières – Canada, 33 Margaret Ave, Kitchener, Ontario, Canada N2H 4H1. E-mail: dwtoews@gmail.com

**Susan C. Welburn**, Division of Infection and Pathway Medicine, School of Biomedical Sciences, College of Medicine & Veterinary Medicine, The University of Edinburgh, Chancellor's Building, 49 Little France Crescent, Edinburgh EH16 4SB, UK. E-mail: sue.welburn@ed.ac.uk

**Lenke Wettlaufer**, Faculty of Law, University of Basel, Peter Merian-Weg 8, PO Box CH-4002, Basel. E-mail: lenke.wettlaufer@unibas.ch

**Maxine Whittaker**, School of Population Health, University of Queensland, Room 123, Public Health Building, Medical School, Herston Rd, Herston, Qld 4006, Australia. E-mail: m.whittaker@uq.edu.au

**Abigail Woods**, Department of History, King's College London, Strand, London WC2R 2LS. E-mail: abigail.woods@kcl.ac.uk

**Dang Xuan Sinh**, Centre for Public Health and Ecosystem Research, Hanoi School of Public Health, 138 Giang Vo Street, Hanoi, Vietnam. E-mail: dxs@hsph.edu.vn

**Jakob Zinsstag**, Swiss Tropical and Public Health Institute, Socinstrasse 57, PO Box CH-4002, Basel. E-mail: jakob.zinsstag@unibas.ch

**Chris Zurbrügg**, Swiss Federal Institute of Aquatic Science and Technology, Department of Water and Sanitation in Developing Countries, PO Box CH-8600, Dübendorf, Switzerland. E-mail: Christian.Zurbruegg@eawag.ch

# Editors' Preface

Since the late 1990s, One Health has become a unifying concept for a wide variety of governmental and non-governmental organizations concerned with human and animal health, wildlife conservation and environmental sustainability. In the wake of the avian influenza pandemic threat, the World Health Organization (WHO), the Food and Agriculture Organization (FAO) and the World Organisation for Animal Health (OIE) joined forces in what is called the 'Tripartite' engagement at the human–animal–ecosystem interface. One Health has become the lead concept in research, capacity building and translational consortia such as the EU-funded Integrated Control of Neglected Zoonoses (ICONZ) and the Training of the One Health Next Generation (OH-NEXTGEN) as well as the Wellcome Trust-funded Afrique One consortium.

We understand One Health foremost as any added value in terms of better health and well-being for humans and animals, financial savings and improved environmental services achieved from closer cooperation between practitioners and scholars concerned with human health, animal health and related outcomes, beyond what can be achieved by working alone. This operational statement shows the need for underlying theory, practical methods and case examples.

What is the added value of another book? Our experiences in Africa, Central Asia, North America, Asia, the Pacific and Australia/New Zealand show that human and animal health professionals remain in their specific silos despite encouraging improvements. We are always surprised how little the different disciplines know about each other and how little they communicate among and between each other.

Beyond merely research, One Health should translate into policy and practice for the betterment of health of communities, their animals and the integrity of their environment. The relationship between theory, policy and practice is a recursive one. Implementing One Health activities in different cultures can lead us to question some of our fundamental ideas about what constitutes good health, which then changes how we practise, which leads to further questioning. In order to learn from our experience in this process and to keep these ideas relevant in chaotic times and diverse settings, it is important to examine more explicitly both ourselves and the central ideas on which the programmes we promote are based. We hope this book both informs its readers and stretches us to reflect and learn from our personal experiences of One Health, as well as those of the people, animals and environments with which we work.

The present interdisciplinary textbook is based on more than a decade of experiences of research and translational teams and provides a comprehensive but minimal essential overview on One Health theory and practice. It is intended for all those working for the health of communities in research and implementation, who see the need in their daily activities to liaise with other disciplines and sectors. This involves among others, human and animal health, social and cultural sciences, economics, environmental sciences and engineering and conservation. The book will benefit students in human and veterinary medicine, health and environmental sciences and biology to ground them in modern inter- and transdisciplinary methods. The book should also serve professionals in academia, technical authorities and government with its numerous practical examples and case studies on disease control, service provision, conservation and academic teaching.

The making of this book would not have been possible without the dedicated coordination of Dr Lisa Crump, whose tireless support is gratefully acknowledged. We would like to thank all lead authors and co-authors for their important contributions and hope that they will benefit from the book for their own work. Numerous external reviewers are thanked for their critical comments which greatly helped to improve the content of the book. We thank Bolor Bold, Sophie Haesen, Monique Léchenne, Rose Marie Subasic and Kurt Pfister for their support with copy-editing. Dr Borna Müller graciously contributed numerous graphical representations and figures. We would like to thank Rachel Cutts and Alexandra Lainsbury from CABI for their most helpful support.

**Jakob Zinsstag**
**Esther Schelling**
**David Waltner-Toews**
**Maxine Whittaker**
**Marcel Tanner**
May 2014

# FAO Foreword

The One Health concept, or approach, is far from new, but its rediscovery is most welcome. Hippocrates (460–370 BCE) purportedly stated 'The soul is the same in all living creatures, although the body of each is different', recognizing that at the time, the soul had a more encompassing definition than we give today with regard to intellectual, emotional intensity or energy.

Such great thinkers as Rudolf Virchow, Robert Koch, Louis Pasteur, Aldo Leopold, Rachel Carlson, Pedro Acha and Calvin Schwabe contributed to our growing understanding of humans within their environment, the cause and effect and interrelationships between microbes, pathogens, contaminants, health and disease in a biotic and abiotic realm. While most human diseases that have emerged in the last half a century can be traced to an animal source, mostly coming from wildlife, and are often the focus for One Health discussions, non-zoonotic diseases cannot be excluded from the One Health dialogue. Animal diseases – in their entirety – limit efficiencies in production and erode biodiversity. They affect public health in terms of lower availability of quality nutritious products of animal origin and negatively influence the cognitive development of children, the responsiveness of the immune system and maternal health. In addition, these diseases negatively impact livelihoods, community trade and individual and national wealth.

Undoubtedly, addressing and attaining global health is a complex endeavour. It requires more than physicians and veterinarians collaborating to address individual or communal health. The disease drivers to emergence, maintenance and spread, dynamically revolve around factors and trends in population growth, demand for more dietary protein, widespread poverty, access to goods and services from the private and public sectors, growing trade and globalization. They further include environmental encroachment and natural resource degradation, immigration and peri-urban sprawl, political and social instability and economics. To address disease prevention at the root, classic non-health discipline specialists such as economists, sociologists, wildlife biologists, communication specialists, city and global planners and financiers have much to contribute.

The Food and Agriculture Organization (FAO) brings together top leaders in economic and social development, forestry and natural resources managers, environmental scientists, specialists in aquaculture and fisheries, nutritionists and geneticists, crop production specialists and pathologists, statisticians, veterinary public health and infectious disease experts from more than 194 countries for the purpose of eliminating hunger and poverty. The production of quality and nutritious food in a resilient environment is the cornerstone to health. Without health, we and our partners will not eliminate hunger or poverty. FAO, thus, is a One Health organization.

Throughout this book numerous cases studies show that the operationalization of One Health is possible and indicators of its positive impact in health terms crystalize at the local level. International institutions such as the FAO, the World Organisation for Animal Health and the World Health Organization recognize their joint responsibility and have established common platforms to address critical issues such as antimicrobial resistance or pandemic threats. Elements for furthering the impact of the One Health approach remain elusive and will need to develop national and regional bodies to embrace the required collaborative, multisectoral and transdisciplinary approach. This book provides a valuable resource for the theoretical background, novel methods and practical examples on One Health and will be a valuable reference for all.

**Juan Lubroth**
Food and Agriculture Organization of the United Nations

# OIE Foreword

One Health seeks incremental benefits from closer cooperation of public and animal health. Such approaches have gained significant momentum in the past decades at the level of the international organizations, national governments, technical authorities and academia. From the perspective of the World Organisation of Animal Health (OIE), I particularly welcome this textbook providing a theoretical foundation, genuine One Health methods, numerous practical examples on disease control and experiences from local and national policy and academic curricula.

As a common theme the book seeks to demonstrate added value of collaborative approaches in human and animal health, social and environmental sciences and economics. After a historical overview, theoretical foundations of One Health provide a framework for the development of interconnected methods measuring quantitative and qualitative benefits using many different disciplines ranging from mathematics to molecular biology and the social sciences. One Health challenges the legal aspects of the human–animal relationship, eliciting new thinking on an intrinsic value of animals. The book documents the important role of wildlife conservation on the development of One Health by the formulation of the Manhattan principles. It suggests that sustainable conservation of wildlife requires healthy humans and animals surrounding protection areas. The social and educational sciences contribute and benefit from One Health shedding light on the human–animal bond and its ramifications far beyond infectious diseases.

One Health becomes a key approach for risk assessment and food safety. Population growth and the livestock revolution warrant novel ideas for environmental sanitation, which are addressed with examples from South-east Asia. The book shows further how health and demographic surveillance of human populations can be extended to livestock, which makes a lot of sense for pastoralist populations worldwide.

Joint animal and human health approaches for the control of zoonotic diseases like brucellosis, bovine tuberculosis, rabies, leptospirosis and trypanosomiasis provide key examples for One Health. They are complemented by a particularly compelling story on joint human and animal vaccination services to mobile pastoralists in Chad. It is based on the observation that in the pastoralist area of Lake Chad there were more cattle vaccinated than children. Several chapters show that One Health is not only applicable in developing countries but has a high potential for industrial and transition countries to address non-communicable diseases or antimicrobial resistance surveillance.

One Health academic studies provide the basis for policy and practice with examples from New Zealand, the Fiji Islands, the USA and Canada. The last part of the book outlines efforts and enabling environment for capacity building, such as joint appointments between veterinary and medical faculties and the development of new One Health research groups in Asia and Africa.

In the past decade, OIE adopted a leadership role early on and has been instrumental in putting the One Health vision into practice. This has been facilitated by a formal alliance on this topic with the World Health Organization (WHO) and the Food and Agriculture Organization of the United Nations (FAO). The three organizations have published a joint Concept Note clarifying their reciprocal responsibilities and their objectives in this field.

The OIE publishes international standards on the good governance of both the public and private sector components of veterinary services, including the initial training and continuing education of the various actors involved. Furthermore, if an OIE member country so wishes, the OIE can carry out an independent assessment of their veterinary services' compliance with OIE quality standards using the Performance of Veterinary Services (PVS) Evaluation Tool. It can also carry out further assessments that enable member countries to calculate the investments and legislative and technical reforms needed to bring their veterinary services into line with these quality standards.

These assessments, which are known collectively as the OIE 'PVS Pathway', have already benefited nearly 120 member countries. As part of the Pathway, the OIE is piloting an assessment tool that evaluates the One Health component of veterinary services; this tool has already been successfully tested in three countries. It is designed to help countries to establish closer collaboration between veterinary services and public health services, in compliance both with the quality standards of the OIE and with the International Health Regulations (IHR) of the WHO. The recent decision of the WHO to develop a tool similar to the PVS Evaluation Tool to assist its member countries to assess their compliance with the IHR (and estimate the costs of improving it) is another example of the benefits of the collaborative One Health approach. Recently, WHO and OIE developed together an operational guide for member countries explaining how PVS principles and IHR obligations can be implemented together in a parallel way in full cooperation between veterinary services and public health services.

I commend the editors for putting together this textbook, which will further strengthen the efforts of OIE and provide a comprehensive overview for all those who want to put One Health to action for the betterment of the health of humans, livestock, companion animals and wildlife.

**Bernard Vallat**
World Organisation for Animal Health (OIE)

# WHO Foreword

This book is a tribute to the advances being made in changing the paradigm to address effectively the health and well-being of people and animals within the environment that they share.

It is a significant resource not only for health and veterinary practitioners, but for the larger community that increasingly recognizes the benefits of interlinking different disciplines and sectors to solve problems at the interface of people, animals and their environment. It makes the case of complementarity and that pooling of expertise, data, knowledge, functional networks, operational systems and stakeholders translates into improved health outcomes, better livelihoods and increased effectiveness. The authors present case studies based on first experiences of how One Health policies can successfully be put into practice in a variety of settings, with a strong focus on the benefits, including the economic benefits, which can be achieved through integrated health approaches through One Health.

**Bernadette Abela-Ridder**
World Health Organization

# 1 One Health in History

**Michael Bresalier,* Angela Cassidy and Abigail Woods**
*Department of History, King's College London, UK*

## Introduction

The purpose of this chapter is to outline the history of One Health. This task immediately raises the question of how to approach the history of a subject that only became known as 'One Health' a few years ago, and is still evolving conceptually under the influence of health challenges, scientific advances, and political, economic, environmental and professional priorities. While there were many precedents to One Health, they did not go by this term, and they occurred at times when health problems, scientific ideas and the wider world were very different to today. This state of affairs makes it impossible to impose a simple structure on to past events, or to link them, in linear fashion, to present-day One Health.

It is important to highlight this problem because existing histories of One Health usually gloss over it. These accounts are structured around key historical figures and scientific advances, whose contributions to health are used to argue for the importance of pursuing a One Health approach today. The achievements of Rudolf Virchow, Robert Koch, William Osler, John McFadyean, James Steele and Calvin Schwabe are routinely celebrated, along with the health benefits of vaccination, the germ theory and zoonosis control. While the importance of these individuals and activities cannot be denied, their roles within the history of One Health require more critical consideration. The accounts in which they feature are neither politically neutral nor historically well-grounded and have been assembled not for the purpose of understanding the past but for advancing the case for One Health today. While this strategy may be useful in justifying and winning support for One Health, it has resulted in an extremely partial and selective reading of the past.

Rather than analysing history retrospectively from the perspective of present-day agendas, this chapter adopts a neutral, prospective, evidence-based approach that pays due regard to historical context.[1] Drawing on an extensive body of historical literature and source material, we aim to effect a fundamental shift in the way that the history of One Health is popularly conceived. We take as our subject matter the constellation of ideas, practices and circumstances that brought human and animal health (and to a lesser extent, the environment) into alignment, the people and institutions involved and the reasons for change over time. This chapter will demonstrate that while at certain points in history, particular individuals

*E-mail: michael.bresalier@kcl.ac.uk

made deliberate attempts to rally people and resources in support of an integrated agenda, there were often many people already working along these lines, in accordance with established scientific ideas and practices.

This account makes no claim to completeness, in part, due to space constraints. Only a brief summary is offered of very recent events as these are well described elsewhere (Lebouef, 2011; Cassidy, 2014). It also reflects the fact that many aspects of One Health history have yet to be subjected to the sort of systematic, contextualized analysis needed to make sense of individual observations. Amongst the neglected areas is the history of One Health in non-western contexts. Owing to the fragmentary state of this field, this chapter focuses overwhelmingly on western medical and veterinary traditions. However, it does acknowledge the importance of cross-cultural exchanges, which were often facilitated by international health organizations concerned with human and animal disease control.

The first section analyses intersections between human and animal health in the pre-modern era. It will reveal how deeply animals and animal health were embedded within human medicine and the importance of the environment to health ideas and practices. The second section extends from the late 18th-century foundation of the veterinary profession until the turn of the 20th century. It tracks the evolving relationship between the veterinary and medical professions, and how, as scientific ideas and practices changed, new links were forged between humans, animals and the environment. The third section extends this analysis into the 20th century, focusing particularly on the changing status of animals within medical research, and on international efforts to develop comparative medicine and veterinary public health. The conclusion reflects on the importance of these findings for history, and for One Health today.

## Pre-Modern Connections

Looking back on the pre-modern era, commentators often highlight the existence of a fundamental, well-entrenched distinction between humans and animals, which derived from the Christian belief that only humans had souls (Hardy, 2003). In fact, this divide has been overstated, for the perceived boundaries between humans and animals were often blurred and unstable (Fudge, 2000). In health and medicine there existed historically three key points of intersection: (i) animals were used to work out the anatomy and physiology of human bodies; (ii) they were studied in comparison to humans in order to work out the relations between them; and (iii) the theory and practice of animal medicine attracted the attention of human doctors, usually as an end in itself, but occasionally as a basis for comparison with human medicine. Aspects of these connections can be identified in very ancient civilizations (Gordon and Schwabe, 2004). However, as all three featured in Ancient Greek thought, which exerted a powerful influence in the west until the 17th century, this will form the starting point of our survey.

Around one-quarter of the surviving works produced by the Greek philosopher Aristotle in the 4th century BC are devoted to animals, most importantly *History of Animals*, *Parts of Animals* and *Generation of Animals*. While Aristotle distinguished humans from animals through their possession of a rational soul, he also sought to relate them, by documenting differences and similarities in the form, function and purpose of their parts and drew up a taxonomic system. The numerous dissections he conducted in the course of this work illustrated the possibility of learning about humans from animals (Clutton-Brock, 1995). Taboos on the use of human bodies led the famous Greek doctor, Galen, working in 2nd-century Rome, to follow Aristotle's lead. In an extensive and influential body of writing, he documented the results of his numerous observations and experiments on animals. The errors he made in extrapolating from animal to human anatomy were not discovered until Andreas Vesalius (1514–1564) revived human dissection at Padua University in the 16th century (Guerrini, 2003).

Vesalius, and several of his contemporaries and successors, also vivisected animals in their attempts to work out the differences between living and dead bodies and to describe and explain how body parts functioned

(Shotwell, 2013). Vivisection was problematic: debates surrounded the value of knowledge drawn from animals and the suffering involved (Guerrini, 2003). Nevertheless, it enabled Realdo Columbo (1516–1559) and Fabricius (1537–1619) to identify the pulmonary transit of the blood and the function of the venous valves, respectively. After studying under Fabricius, William Harvey took up an Aristotelian programme of research on animals that resulted in his novel and, at the time, controversial proposal that the blood circulated. Meanwhile, as part of the wider investigation of nature, medical doctors followed Aristotle in dissecting dead animals, for example at the elite Paris Academy Royale des Sciences during the 1660s and 1670s. This activity, described as 'comparative anatomy', drew on animals derived from colonial conquests that were contained within European leaders' menageries (Cunningham, 2010).

The health of humans and animals were defined by the same medical theory: humoralism. This awarded a significant role to the environment in maintaining, disturbing and restoring health status. Drawing on the ideas of Hippocrates and Galen, humoralism formed the dominant system of medical thought until the 18th century. It held that all bodies were composed of four humours, influenced by factors such as feeding, climate, ventilation, exercise and sexual behaviour. Disease of individual bodies resulted from an imbalance between the humours (Curth, 2002). In addition, the rise and fall of epidemics was attributed to changes in the wider environment, as described by the Hippocratic text, *Airs, Waters, Places* (Wilkinson, 1992; Nutton, 2004). These theories implied that similar interventions, such as bleeding, purging, lifestyle changes and improvements in air quality could restore or maintain the humoral balance in both human and animal bodies. Formally trained healers usually focused on one or the other. Physicians, surgeons and apothecaries treated humans, while animals received dedicated attention from medieval veterinarians at the Mamluk courts and from British farriers, French marechals, Spanish beitars and their equivalents in other countries (Conrad *et al.*, 1995; Shehada, 2012). However, such healers were expensive and few in number. Consequently, most humans and animals relied on self-help, clergymen, gentry and the various self-styled healers that made up the 'medical marketplace'. Here, the division between species was less well defined (Curth, 2002).

The 17th and 18th century movement away from ancient Greek thought brought humans and animals into even greater proximity. The new experimental philosophy of nature, and Rene Descartes' (1596–1650) conception of animals as 'automata' (self-operating machines), resulted in the more extensive use of animal vivisection in medical research and teaching (Guerrini, 2003). For example, Swiss physiologist Albrecht von Haller (1708–1777) used live animals to work out human neurological functions (Eichberg, 2009). At Leiden in the Netherlands, and later in Edinburgh, Scotland, anatomy lecturers vivisected dogs and dissected humans simultaneously, in order to demonstrate to students the structure and the function of body parts (Guerrini, 2006). A new scheme of classifying animals, drawn up by Swedish naturalist Carolus Linnaeus (1707–1778), placed humans, apes, monkeys and bats within the same order of primates and brought humans and orang-utans together in the genus *Homo*, thereby challenging notions of a human–animal divide (Ritvo, 1995). Subsequently, in Paris, additional classification schemes were drawn up using dissected animals from the Versailles menagerie. Here, the key figures were George Buffon (1739–1788), the medically trained comparative anatomist, Louis Daubenton (1716–1799) and Georges Cuvier (1769–1832) (Cunningham, 2010).

One of Daubenton's pupils, the physician Vicq d'Azyr (1749–1794), went beyond comparative anatomy to develop a truly comparative form of medicine. His initial concern was cattle plague or rinderpest. This disease was prevalent throughout Europe in the 18th century. It inspired much medical comment and attempts to control it by quarantine, modelled on responses to bubonic plague in humans (Wilkinson, 1992). After reporting upon this disease to the French government, d'Azyr was made secretary to a Royal Commission of Enquiry into epidemics and epizootics and steered its 1778 evolution into the Société Royale de Médicine. His investigations demonstrate the continuing importance of the environment in thinking about human and animal health and disease. Drawing on medical meteorology and topology, D'Azyr correlated human and animal epidemics with climatic and geographical conditions. D'Azyr also performed animal experiments. He believed that by understanding the functioning of organs in health, it was possible to make sense of their dysfunction in disease (Hannaway, 1994). Perceiving no dividing line between human and animal medicine, he argued that 'considerations on the diseases which attack man are applicable without any exception to those which attack animals. Medicine is one: and its general principles, once set out, are very easy to apply to different circumstances and species' (Hannaway, 1977).

A similar stance was adopted by a number of British surgeons, who became actively involved in equine health care during the second half of the 18th century. Arguing that 'physic' (conventional medicine) was the same whether practised on humans or horses, they wrote manuals of farriery and established infirmaries for the treatment of horses and tuition of pupils. For them, farriery was part of natural history or comparative anatomy. It was therefore a polite practice, suitable for a gentleman (MacKay, 2009). Comparative anatomy was consolidated as a medical practice by the surgeon John Hunter (1728–1793). He established his own menagerie and spent hours each day dissecting and experimenting upon animals. He incorporated their bodies into his museum, which numbered over 500 species with 13,000 specimens at his death in 1793 (Chaplin, 2008). Hunter's influence on the field of surgery and its growing profile kept animals at the forefront of medical research in subsequent years (Lawrence, 1996). It was one of his pupils, Edward Jenner, who showed in 1796 that cowpox inoculation could protect humans from smallpox (Fisher, 1991).

## Enter the Vets

The connections outlined above reveal that in many ways, pre-modern medicine really was 'one'. So how did the creation of the veterinary profession impact this situation? The first schools were established in Lyons (1762) and Alfort (1777). By 1791, they existed throughout much of Europe: in Dresden, Freiburg, Karlsruhe, Berlin and Munich in Germany; Turin, Padua and Parma in Italy; as well as Vienna, Budapest, Copenhagen, Sweden and London (Cotchin, 1990). Historical accounts often portray their creation as a significant break with the past, which led to a new enlightened approach to animal healing (Schwabe, 1978, 1984, 2004; Wilkinson, 1992). However, this interpretation is deeply flawed, for as shown above, animal bodies and their treatment in health and disease had already attracted substantial attention from medical doctors.

It is perhaps more accurate to view the veterinary schools as an expression of pre-existing medical interest in animals, because although circumstances varied from school to school, doctors often played important roles in driving and shaping veterinary education. The doctors' commitment to studying the health and medicine of animals is shown by the fact that they did not automatically cede this field to the new veterinary profession. Rather, as shown below, they intensified their investigations during the first half of the 19th century and drew on vets as collaborators. Therefore, although in time the connections between human and animal health lessened, this was not an immediate or inevitable consequence of the veterinary profession's formation.

In the 1780s, against the wishes of founder Claude Bourgelat, the physician Vicq d'Azyr refashioned the Alfort veterinary school into a research institution and assumed the chair of comparative anatomy. Teaching was extended to human fracture care and midwifery to enable vets to offer an extended service to rural communities. For political reasons, these changes were reversed in 1788 (Hannaway, 1977, 1994). However, from the 1790s, a number of Alfort veterinary and medical staff, including Francois Magendie in the 1820s, engaged in the systematic vivisection of horses, making this one of the first contexts for the development of experimental physiology in France (Elliott, 1987). The subsequent expansion of this field within Germany, France and, later in the century, Britain, in the face of anti-vivisectionist opposition, considerably enhanced the use of animals as experimental tools within medicine (Bynum, 1994). For proponent Claude Bernard these uses were entirely justified, for 'to learn how man and animals live, we cannot avoid seeing great numbers of them die' (Bernard, 1957).

In London, surgeons and, less commonly, physicians acted as governors for the Veterinary College (est. 1791), ran examinations for students and were well represented on the student body: 130 surgeons had qualified as veterinarians by 1830. Edward Coleman, principal of the college from 1796 to 1839, was also a surgeon, appointed on the strength of his research on animals and ability to teach learned farriery. He modelled veterinary education on that of human surgery. Veterinary students were encouraged to attend lectures in the London medical schools, while medical students had the opportunity to attend lectures on veterinary topics. However, little research was undertaken at the college. This drew criticism from the medical press, which campaigned with disaffected vets for the reform of the school. In 1844, vets replaced doctors in the control of student examinations. Concurrently, reforms in medical education restricted the courses on offer. These shifts enhanced the institutional separation of the professions.

However, as shown by the many reports on animal health issues that appeared in the medical press, doctors retained their interest in this topic to the extent that veterinary surgeons sometimes accused them of stealing their patients. Doctors also conducted numerous investigations into animal disease pathology and epidemiology. Their infrequent use of the term 'comparative' to describe such investigations suggests that they regarded them as part of mainstream medicine. Their aims were to document animal diseases, to describe their analogies with human diseases and to learn about the nature of disease in general. These investigations featured a remarkable and formerly unrecognized degree of collaboration between doctors and veterinary surgeons. Vets drew doctors' attention to interesting cases and outbreaks, facilitated their access to live animals and dead bodies and offered personal insights based on clinical experience. Less frequently, doctors assisted vets in their animal disease investigations. Grass-roots collaboration between the professions was therefore important to the development of mid-19th-century understandings of human and animal disease.

Medical interest in animals was promoted further by two key scientific developments. First, investigations during the 1830s suggested that glanders in horses, rabies in dogs and anthrax in animals were causally connected to the equivalent diseases in humans (Wilkinson, 1992). Second, there emerged a Romantic or philosophical form of comparative anatomy, which suggested that humans and animals were formed on the same general plan. In their efforts to comprehend this plan, doctors compared the anatomy and pathology of the bodies and embryos of multiple animal species (Jacyna, 1984; Hopwood, 2009). Humans and animals were thereby brought together in ways that are usually attributed to Darwinism and the germ theory, 30 years later. This finding reveals that contrary to popular belief, the latter events did not spell a complete break with the past. Rather, they formed part of an ongoing process of making and remaking links between human and animal bodies and diseases.

Veterinary education emerged later in North America than in Europe. While some of the earliest qualified vets were European émigrés, physicians were also extremely active. In the period 1820–1870 they investigated and reported on livestock diseases, campaigned for veterinary education and established and taught at early veterinary schools that were mostly short-lived (Smithcors, 1959). In 1863, Scottish vet Duncan McEachran founded the Montreal Veterinary College. Believing that veterinary medicine was a branch of human medicine, he modelled teaching on that of the McGill medical school. One of his best known collaborators was William Osler, a former student of Virchow's and lecturer in medicine at McGill, 1874–1884. Osler taught veterinary students, undertook research (mostly unpublished) into the diseases of animals and asserted the value of comparative medicine to medical audiences. Although today he is often heralded as a figurehead of One Health, he was not unusual at the time. His predecessors and successors at McGill also taught veterinary students, and several, such as J.G. Adami, produced more extensive and significant research in comparative medicine (Teigen, 1984, 1988).

The late-19th century saw a number of important developments within science and medicine that had mixed implications for the history of One Health (Wilkinson, 1992; Hardy, 2002). The 1859 publication of Darwin's *Origin of the Species* claimed that all living organisms descended by evolution from a common ancestor. It inspired some doctors to trace the evolutionary history of disease by examining its manifestations in different animal species. The most famous participant was Eli Metchnikoff, whose Nobel prize-winning theory of phagocytosis was inspired by evolutionary thinking (Tauber, 1994).

The 1860s and 1870s saw the development of the notion that diseases were caused by germs. In Britain, the acceptance of this theory was precipitated by the devastating 1865–1867 epidemic of cattle plague, whose pathology and epidemiology was subjected to scientific investigation by medical doctors (Worboys, 1991). Elsewhere, seminal insights into germs derived from studying the nature, prevention and spread of animal diseases. In France, Louis Pasteur produced vaccines against chicken cholera, anthrax and rabies. His German counterpart, Robert Koch, investigated anthrax and tuberculosis, as well as tropical animal diseases, which inspired his concept of the carrier state.

Vets made important contributions to all these investigations, which used a myriad of animals for the purposes of research, diagnosis and the production of vaccines and sera (Bynum, 1990; Wilkinson, 1992; Gradmann, 2009, 2010). Existing aetiological connections between human and animal diseases were redefined in terms of germs. A new category of diseases, the zoonoses, emerged to incorporate these and parasitic diseases like trichinellosis, whose life cycle and spread via the meat trade were worked out from the mid-1850s to 1870s by Virchow, amongst others. They formed the focus of a new field of veterinary public health (VPH).

However, while in some ways, germ theory served to promote One Health approaches, in other ways it undermined them. Up to this point in time, the environment had played a central role in explaining patterns of health and disease. However, it was marginalized by germ theories that explained disease in much narrower terms, as the straightforward product of infectious agents invading susceptible bodies (Worboys, 2000). While the appearance of VPH led many individuals, particularly veterinary surgeons, to advocate closer veterinary-medical relations, in practice, collaborative working patterns became more competitive as the two professions battled for control over research and policy (Waddington, 2006; Woods, 2014).

Medical and veterinary perspectives on zoonoses often differed because doctors prioritized human health and vets prioritized the health of animals and agriculture. In 1901, Robert Koch famously reversed his earlier opinion that human and bovine tuberculosis were not alike, adding to a climate of uncertainty about the nature, extent and even existence of transmission pathways. Doctors and vets clashed over the health threats posed by meat and milk, the regulation of these foodstuffs and how to define a healthy animal. The stakes were raised by western governments' growing assumption of responsibility for health and their increasing reliance on experts. Veterinary and medical disciplinary differences were given structural and political expression by their employment in separate government departments. Doctors generally had the upper hand, because their profession possessed a higher status and had forged a public role years before the creation of state veterinary services. Throughout Europe and North America, dissatisfied vets organized and lobbied for state recognition and legal protection.[2] They gained some ground towards the end of the century, in inspecting meat at slaughterhouses and regulating the supply of clean milk. However, the nature and extent of these roles varied considerably between and within nations (Schmaltz, 1936; Koolmees, 2000; Hardy, 2002; Jones, 2003; Orland, 2003; Brantz, 2005; Waddington, 2006; Berdah, 2014).

## Animals and Humans in 20th-Century Medicine

The 20th century was characterized by considerable ambiguity in the perceived relations between humans and animals in health and disease. This was particularly apparent in the status of animals within medical research, which underwent an important epistemological shift around the turn of the 20th century. Earlier, scientists had drawn on a diversity of species, including but not confined to earthworms, horses, birds, frogs, pets, zoo animals, horses, livestock and fish. They were usually familiar with these animals, having encountered them in farming, field sports, natural historical pursuits, zoos, and urban streets populated with horse-drawn transport, stray dogs and livestock for sale and slaughter (Kete, 2007). The sheer ubiquity of animals made it easy to acquire them for experiment in life, and dissection after death. The resulting research was truly comparative. It sought to build general truths through examination of similarities and differences between animals. Acknowledging, with a nod to evolution, that species' differences were to be expected, researchers did not assume that a finding was true of all animals until they had demonstrated it in a host of different species (Logan, 2002).

Subsequently, however, scientists moved away from demonstrating generality to presuming its existence. Animal diversity became a confounding factor rather than a research strength. It can be no coincidence that as towns grew larger, as animals disappeared from the streets and urban upbringings became the norm, scientists began to restrict their gaze to a handful of animal species that could be kept within the laboratory. Paralleling the rise of standardization and mass production within industry, scientists entered into the mass production of standardized laboratory animals whose features could be quantified or mechanically assessed. By the interwar period, with diversity reduced further through standardized husbandry and environments, these animals formed the mainstay of scientific work on cancer, genetics and drug standardization. Their uses continued to expand throughout the second half of the century. By then, however, biomedical scientists were no longer engaging with them as animals, but as functional equivalents or 'models' of the human body whose scientific legitimacy was underpinned by the theory of evolution (Clause, 1993; Logan, 2002; Löwy, 2003; Rader, 2004; Kirk, 2008).

One interesting inversion of this state of affairs occurred in the context of veterinary medicine in the late 20th century. The increasing importance of human relationships with pets, and owners' greater willingness to invest financially in this relationship, resulted in the growing veterinary use of insulin treatment, orthopaedic surgery and transplant surgery. Originally these technologies were trialled on animal models before entering human medical practice. Now, their use in animal patients was informed by clinical trials and experiences in humans, who effectively became the models (Degeling, 2009; Gardiner, 2009; Schlich *et al.*, 2009).

The increasing use of standardized animals within medical research caused some vets in Europe and North America to carve out a new role in caring for them. In the light of continuing public concerns about animal experimentation, they guided medical scientists on how to maximize experimental outcomes while minimizing animal welfare costs (Kirk, 2009). Such work was reminiscent of how vets had facilitated medical research on animal diseases during the mid-19th century, but the science, the setting and the animals were now very different. However, not all vets embraced the changing status of the laboratory animal. Starting in the 1920s, some voiced criticisms of animal models and called instead for the study of spontaneous disease events in zoo, farm, wild and pet animals (Allbutt, 1924). They argued, as in the 19th century, that diversity was important to the creation of scientific knowledge, and they perceived disease problems in different species as analogous rather than identical. They referred to this form of investigation as 'comparative medicine' (although confusingly, the use of this term today applies to the care of laboratory animal models as well).

Interwar comparative medicine advocates included O. Charnock Bradley (1871–1937),

Principal of the Royal (Dick) Veterinary College, Edinburgh, and T.W.M. Cameron, professor and director of parasitology at McGill University (Bradley, 1927; Cameron, 1938a,b). Investigation of comparative medicine gathered momentum in the decades after the Second World War. Meetings at the New York Academy of Medicine, University of Michigan, Rockefeller Foundation, University of Pennsylvania and the London Zoological Society aimed to demonstrate its practical value and to debate its incorporation within medical, veterinary and graduate school curricula (Jones, 1959). In 1958, a joint Washington meeting of medical and veterinary experts attached to the World Health Organization (WHO) and the Pan-American Sanitary Bureau (PASB) proposed the creation of a new programme in comparative medicine, with the aim of expanding the kinds of animals and animal diseases used in basic medical research (WHO, 1958a; WHO, Chronicle, 1961). W.I.B. Beveridge, director of the Institute of Animal Pathology at Cambridge University, was the lead consultant (Beveridge, 1969). Initially concentrating on cardiovascular disease and cancer, the official task of this programme expanded in the early 1960s to include comparative virology, neuropathology and mycoplasmology, as well as work on the welfare of primates in medical research centres (Kaplan, 1961; Cotchin, 1962).

From the 1920s onwards, advocates of this form of enquiry adopted an almost identical refrain. They argued that comparative medicine could tackle a wider range of diseases than could be experimentally induced and would produce fundamental insights common to all species. Although it required knowledge of species' similarities and differences, veterinary surgeons already possessed such insights. Moreover, the approach would help to bridge professional, epistemological and practical divisions between veterinary and human medicine (Bradley, 1927; Cameron, 1938a,b; Beveridge, 1972). Renewed calls for unifying veterinary and human medicine were made within this context, on the assumption that these were the two strands of 'one' medicine.

Today, the coining of the term 'One Medicine' is usually attributed to Calvin Schwabe, a vigorous proponent of comparative medicine, who employed the term frequently in the third edition of his volume *Veterinary Medicine and Human Health* (1984). However, it was used on many earlier occasions to illustrate the nature and value of comparative medicine (Bradley, 1927, p. 129; Shope, 1959; Beveridge, 1969). During the mid-20th century, it was particularly associated with authors from the University of Pennsylvania veterinary school (Schmidt, 1962; Allam, 1966; Cass, 1973) and the University of Minnesota.[3] It is likely that Schwabe adopted the term 'One Medicine' from mid-20th century currents of thinking within comparative medicine.

By the 1970s the results of comparative medical research into chronic human disease were still rather uneven. It seems that the skills required for conducting this research were rather difficult to obtain and that few scientists were convinced by its claimed superiority over other methods or by broader visions of 'One Medicine'. The failure to advance comparative medicine was indicative of the growing differences between the professions in their research orientation and in the status they awarded to animals. Such differences were consolidated by 20th-century research and development infrastructures, which allocated human and animal health to different funding streams, research institutions and international organizations.

Yet at the same time, certain individuals, working in specific settings on particular disease problems, brought human and animal health into closer alignment. One key institution was the Rockefeller Foundation, which made the study of animal pathology central to many of its medical, scientific and public health programmes (Corner, 1964). Theobald Smith, the first director of its Department of Animal Pathology at Princeton (established in 1915), had made his name at the Bureau of Animal Industry, where he applied a comparative, ecological approach to the study of Texas fever (Méthot, 2012). Both he and his successor, Richard E. Shope, who discovered the influenza virus of pigs and proposed its role in human influenza, were medically trained, yet they saw animal pathology as the necessary foundation of *all* medicine (Shope, 1959). One particularly productive line of work, begun by Peyton Rous on chickens and continued later on rabbits in collaboration with Shope, was the role of viruses in cancer causation (Rous, 1910; Shope, 1933). Elsewhere in the USA, the University of Pennsylvania, the Mayo Clinic at the University of Minnesota (incorporated in 1915) and the Hooper Foundation for Medical Research at the University of California (established in 1913), were among a cluster of institutions that supported medical-veterinary interactions in research and post-graduate education (Steele, 1991). In France and Germany, the Pasteur and Koch institutes remained committed to a comparative approach, as did other medical research centres in Europe (Gradmann, 2010). In Britain, the Medical Research Council established a programme of research into dog distemper, which helped scientists to discover the human influenza virus in 1933 (Bresalier and Worboys, 2014).

Twentieth-century relations between health and the role of the environment in ideas of human and animal health also varied by time. As noted above, the acceptance of germs as causal agents diverted attention away from the environmental factors that influenced the emergence, spread and clinical impacts of disease. This shift was accentuated by development of vaccines and antibiotics. These were so successful in the West that, despite a few opposing voices, by the 1960s and 1970s it was widely believed the conquest of infectious disease was in sight. From the 1980s, this optimism was dashed by the emergence and re-emergence of infectious diseases like AIDS, Ebola and BSE, which reinforced the connections between the health of humans, animals and the environment (Anderson, 2004). A different disease trajectory occurred in certain colonial and post-colonial settings where infectious diseases remained a problem and the role of the environment could not be ignored. Investigations were approached in a more ecological fashion, as seen in the study of trypanosomiasis during the first half of the century. A highly ecological set of investigations resulted which drew on entomology, medicine, veterinary medicine and agricultural science to generate a dynamic picture of the disease (Tilley, 2011).

The integration of human and animal health within colonial and post-colonial settings was further driven by the elevation of development as an economic and political priority (Staples, 2006). In 1948, as part of an international drive to improve human health through disease control and better nutrition, the WHO set up a Veterinary Public Health (VPH) unit within its Division of Communicable Diseases (WHO, 1958b). Headed by the American Martin Kaplan, who had degrees in veterinary medicine and public health, it developed close relations with the Food and Agriculture Organization (FAO), other UN agencies and the World Organisation for Animal Health (OIE) (Kaplan, 1953). A series of joint WHO/FAO meetings in the 1950s led to collaborative programmes on zoonoses, meat hygiene and veterinary education. It also brought a working definition of VPH as comprising 'all the community efforts influencing and influenced by the veterinary medical arts and sciences applied to the prevention of diseases, protection of life and promotion of the well-being and efficiency of man' (WHO/FAO, 1951).

In framing animal health as a crucial problem of human health and development, the FAO and WHO positioned veterinarians, trained and working within public health, as vital to realizing these goals. However, most countries lacked such personnel (WHO/FAO, 1956), therefore establishing new education and training programmes became a key focus. Through the 1950s and 1960s, WHO and FAO acted to support and fund veterinary and VPH education in the developing world (WHO/FAO, 1975). These activities relied on expertise drawn from the USA, which led the post-war development of VPH at national, state and local levels, as well as internationally through the Pan-American Health Bureau (PAHB). The leading figure in these initiatives was James H. Steele (Steele, 2008). Trained in both veterinary medicine and public health, he was a prodigy of the Swiss-American veterinary pathologist Karl F. Meyer, himself a vocal proponent of the integration of human and animal medicine. It was Meyer who established the Hooper Foundation as a world-leading research centre on zoonoses and food safety.

As is evident from the above, post-colonial and international health contexts were very important in shaping the careers and ideas of many of the key figures who aligned themselves with a 'One Medicine' agenda. Their work within developing countries also enabled them to engage in cross-cultural encounters and exchanges with pastoral and agricultural peoples, which informed their thinking about the relationship between human and animal health, disease and medicine (Kaplan, 1966; Green, 1998; Beinart and Brown, 2013). The influence of these experiences and contexts can, for example, be detected in Calvin Schwabe's frequently cited work, *Veterinary Medicine and Human Health* (Schwabe 1964, 1969, 1984). More generally, this history indicates that many of the roots of present-day One Health lie in earlier currents of veterinary thought and practice that were deeply entangled with projects of development, international health, aid and post-colonial reconstruction.

## Conclusion: From One Medicine to One Health

In analysing the changing relations between the health of humans, animals and the environment, this chapter has demonstrated the many and varied links between them. Human medicine, in particular, has a rich history of engagement with animals, their diseases and the people and institutions dedicated to animal health. Correspondingly, since the late 18th-century creation of their profession, vets have supported, collaborated and sometimes competed with this medical programme. These interconnections can be explained, in part, by reference to prevailing scientific ideas, practices and disease problems, but they can only be fully understood by examining the people involved, their institutional settings and the wider professional, political, economic and environmental contexts. The historical specificity of these factors, as well as the variability of the health activities they influenced, make it impossible to construct a simple, linear narrative linking past to present. Nor is it possible to draw direct lessons from history, or to claim – as do many existing histories – that the work of certain historical figures demonstrates the importance of pursuing One Health today.

This does not mean, however, that the past is completely irrelevant to the present. One key finding to emerge from this account is that while they varied over time and place, the historical links between the health of humans, animals and the environment were multiple and profound. Embedded within scientific concepts and practices, they shaped the way in which doctors and vets approached the problem of disease. For the most part, these individuals did not feel the need to articulate their activities, self-consciously, within a 'veterinary public health', 'comparative medicine' or 'One Medicine' agenda. These terms were only adopted at certain historical junctures by advocates who aimed to validate or win wider support for operationalizing their activities. Pushing beyond these labels and the rhetoric that surrounded them, and looking at what individuals on the ground were actually thinking and doing, reveals that integrated approaches to health were much more widespread and more significant than previously realized. It is no understatement to say that health and medicine today are heavily shaped and underpinned by the many precursors to One Health.

One Health itself, as a self-consciously labelled set of activities and agendas, has emerged very recently out of a complex and rapidly shifting coalition of international health bodies, veterinary associations, academic advocates, environmental organizations and pharmaceutical companies. While its history has been fully explored elsewhere (e.g. Lebouf, 2011; Chien, 2013; Cassidy, 2014), this chapter concludes by sketching out the broad contours of these developments in order to put the rest of this volume into context. During the 2000s, elements of the ongoing traditions of comparative medicine and VPH came together into a rearticulated vision of 'One Medicine, One Health'. This involved the alliance or convergence of veterinary and human medical research and/or clinical practice, including collaborative research, and shared clinics, vaccination strategies, equipment and drug development (e.g. King *et al.*, 2008).

In parallel, a different (albeit overlapping) set of actors and agendas came together around the term 'One World, One Health'™ (OWOH). In contrast to the veterinary-medical focus of One Medicine, OWOH tended to address a broader range of disciplines across the life and environmental sciences while maintaining a relatively tight focus on issues such as zoonotic diseases. The idea of 'One World' (OW) has its origins in mid-20th-century debates about international relations and the formation of UNESCO (Sluga, 2010). It was taken up by health actors during the 1990s, when the global scale and potential wildlife origins of the HIV/AIDS pandemic were recognized (Whiteside, 1996; King, 2004), alongside the emergence and re-emergence of many other infectious diseases (Anderson, 2004). In 2004, the first of a series of meetings between human public health, conservation and infectious disease experts was organized by the US-based Wildlife Conservation Society on the theme of OWOH. The idea then found strong purchase in international responses to the outbreak of highly pathogenic avian influenza (HPAI), and was adopted by WHO, FAO, OIE and others in a shared statement of cooperative intent (FAO *et al.*, 2008) following the HPAI crisis (Scoones and Forster, 2008). These disease events, alongside reconfigurations of the organizations which deal with them, have contributed to a renewed awareness of the environmental causes of disease. This has taken on new forms, combining with late-20th-century understandings of 'the environment', to be rearticulated in (for example) arguments for understanding and preserving 'ecosystem health' (Zinsstag *et al.*, 2012).

Over this decade the 'One Medicine' and 'One World' agendas have become more and more intertwined, increasingly sharing the broader, snappier and more widely used banner of One Health (e.g. Zinsstag *et al.*, 2005; FAO *et al.*, 2010). The recent adoption of the language of One Health by key organizations across the worlds of veterinary and human medicine, international health, national governments and research funding bodies, represents the integration of these various agendas. Advocates based particularly in the USA and Switzerland have organized workshops, conferences, reports, websites and journal publications to promote it. As an organizing concept, it has proved flexible enough to encompass very different languages, ideas and working practices, yet coherent enough to enable communication across disciplinary and organizational divides (Lebouef, 2011; Chien, 2013). However, questions remain about the long-term viability and practical utility of One Health (Lee and Brumme, 2013; Cassidy, 2014), as well as how it can engage productively with questions of colonial and post-colonial legacies, power, and ongoing tensions between local and 'global' approaches to health (Scoones and Forster, 2008; Bonfoh *et al.*, 2011; Beinart and Brown, 2013; Green, 2012).

Like its predecessors, the rise of One Health cannot be explained solely by advocacy, internal scientific logic, or as the natural and inevitable outcome of long-standing efforts to bring humans, animals and the environment closer together. A product of 21st-century concerns, it forms part of a wider cluster of research and policy agendas, including 'food security', 'biosecurity', 'global health' and 'translational medicine', which also aim to break down barriers between disciplines. Rather than competing for resources or legitimacy, arguments for these agendas tend to be mutually reinforcing. Jointly, they could be described as part of a collective response to a (re)emerging set of highly complex concerns which extend across traditional disciplinary boundaries – over environmental damage, scarce resources, food availability and disease/health (Rushton, 2011; Cassidy, 2014). This is the arena in which the future of One Health will be forged. However, in looking ahead, we must also remember to look back, in order to understand how today's rapidly changing situation has been shaped by its past.

## Notes

[1] For another balanced historical perspective on this topic, see Kirk and Worboys (2011).

[2] Numerous papers on this topic were delivered to the 2012 Congress of the World Association for the History of Veterinary Medicine. For a summary see Woods (2012).

[3] Today Pennsylvania Vet School has its own trademarked slogan, 'Many Species, One Medicine'™, attributed broadly to another 19th-century 'founding father', Benjamin Rush MD (Hendricks *et al.*, 2009).

## References


Allam, M.W. (1966) The M.D. and the V.M.D. *Pennsylvania Medicine* 69(8), 57–60.

Allbutt, C. (1924) The integration of medicine. *Proceedings of the Royal Society of Medicine* (Section of Comparative Medicine) 17, 1–3.

Anderson, W. (2004) Natural histories of infectious disease: ecological vision in 20th century biomedical science. *Osiris* 19, 39–61.

Beinart, W. and Brown, K. (2013) *African Local Knowledge and Livestock Health: Diseases and Treatments in South Africa*. Boydell & Brewer Ltd, Woodbridge, UK.

Berdah, D. (2014) Meat, public health and veterinary expertise: eating beef from tuberculous bovines in France, late 19th century (in preparation).

Bernard, C. (1957) *An Introduction to the Study of Experimental Medicine* (English translation of 1865 text). Courier Dover Publications, 1957.

Beveridge, W.I.B. (1969) Comparative medicine in theory and practice. *WHO Chronicle* 23(12), 547–553

Beveridge, W.I.B. (1972) *Frontiers in Comparative Medicine*. Oxford University Press, London.

Bonfoh, B., Raso, G., Koné, I., Dao, D., Girardin, O., Cissé, G., Zinsstag, J., Utzinger, J. and Tanner, M. (2011) Research in a war zone. *Nature* 474(7353), 569–571.

Bradley, O.C. (1927) What is Comparative Medicine? *Proceedings of the Royal Society of Medicine* 21(1), 129–134.

Brantz, D. (2005) Animal bodies, human health, and the reform of slaughterhouses in 19th century Berlin. *Food and History* 3, 193–215.

Bresalier, M. and Worboys, M. (2014) 'Saving the lives of our dogs': the development of canine distemper vaccine in interwar Britain. *British Journal for the History of Science* 47(173 Pt 2), 305–334.

Bynum, W. (1990) 'C'est un malade': animal models and concepts of human diseases. *Journal of the History of Medicine* 45, 397–413.

Bynum, W. (1994) *Science and the Practice of Medicine in the 19th Century*. Cambridge University Press, Cambridge.

Cameron, T.W.M. (1938a) Veterinarians and medicine. *Canadian Journal of Comparative Medicine* 2, 119–120.

Cameron, T.W.M. (1938b) Diseases common to animals and man. *Canadian Journal of Comparative Medicine* 2, 121–128.

Cass, J. (1973) One Medicine - human and veterinary. *Perspectives in Biology and Medicine* 16(3), 418–426.

Cassidy, A. (2014) One Medicine? Cross-disciplinary advocacy for animal and human health (in preparation).

Chaplin, S. (2008) Nature dissected, or dissection naturalized? The case of John Hunter's museum. *Museum and Society* 6, 135–151.

Chien, Y.-J. (2013) How did international agencies perceive the avian influenza problem? The adoption and manufacture of the 'One World, One Health' framework. *Sociology of Health & Illness* 35(2), 213–226.

Clause, B. (1993) The Wistar rat as a right choice: establishing mammalian standards and the ideal of a standardized mammal. *Journal of the History of Biology* 26, 329–349.

Clutton-Brock, J. (1995) Aristotle, the scale of nature, and modern attitudes to animals. *Social Research* 62, 421–440.

Conrad, L., Neve, M., Nutton, V., Porter, R. and Wear, A. (1995) *The Western Medical Tradition, 800BC to AD1800*. Cambridge University Press, Cambridge.

Corner, G.W. (1964) *The Rockefeller Institute: Origins and Growth, 1901–1953*. Rockefeller Institute Press, New York.

Cotchin, E. (1962) The problems of comparative oncology. *Bulletin of the World Health Organisation* 26, 633–648.

Cotchin, E. (1990) *The Royal Veterinary College London: A Bicentenary History*. Barracuda, Buckingham, UK.

Cunningham, A. (2010) *The Anatomist Anatomis'd: An Experimental Discipline in Enlightenment Europe*. Ashgate, Farnham, UK.

Curth, L. (2002) The care of the brute beast: animals and the 17th century marketplace. *Social History of Medicine* 15, 375–392.

Degeling, C. (2009) Negotiating value. Comparing human and animal fracture care in industrial societies. *Science, Technology and Human Values* 34, 77–101.

Eichberg, S. (2009) Constituting the human via the animal in eighteenth-century experimental neurophysiology: Albrecht von Haller's sensibility trials'. *Medizinhistorisches Journal* 44(3–4), 274–295.

Elliott, P. (1987) Vivisection and the emergence of experimental physiology in 19th century France. In: Rupke, N. (ed.) *Vivisection in Historical Perspective*. Croom Helm, London.
FAO, OIE, WHO, UN System Influenza Coordination, World Bank & UNICEF (2008) Contributing to One World, One Health: A Strategic Framework for Reducing Risks of Infectious Diseases at the Animal-Human-Ecosystems Interface. Available at: http://www.fao.org/docrep/011/aj137e/aj137e00.htm (accessed 18 July 2014 ).
FAO, OIE and WHO (2010) The FAO-OIE-WHO Collaboration. Sharing Responsibilities and Coordinating Global Activities to Address Health Risks at the Animal-Human-Ecosystems Interfaces. A Tripartite Concept Note. Geneva: World Health Organization. Available at: http://www.who.int/influenza/resources/documents/tripartite_concept_note_hanoi/en (accessed 18 July 2014).
Fisher, R.B. (1991) *Edward Jenner 1749–1823*. André Deutsch, London.
Fudge, E. (2000) *Perceiving Animals: Humans and Beasts in Early Modern English Culture*. Macmillan/St Martin's Press, Basingstoke, UK.
Gardiner, A. (2009) The animal as surgical patient: a historical perspective on the 20th century. *History and Philosophy of the Life Sciences* 31, 355–378.
Gordon, A.H. and Schwabe, C.W. (2004) *The Quick and the Dead: Biomedical Theory in Ancient Egypt*. Brill, Leiden.
Gradmann, C. (2009) *Laboratory Disease: Robert Koch's Medical Bacteriology*. Johns Hopkins University Press, Baltimore, Maryland.
Gradmann, C. (2010) Robert Koch and the invention of the carrier state: tropical medicine, veterinary infections and epidemiology around 1900. *Studies in History and Philosophy of Biological and Biomedical Sciences* 41, 232–240.
Green, E.C. (1998) Etiology in human and animal ethnomedicine. *Agriculture and Human Values* 15, 127–131.
Green, J. (2012) 'One health, one medicine' and critical public health. *Critical Public Health* 22(4), 377–381.
Guerrini, A. (2003) *Experimenting with Humans and Animals: From Galen to Animal Rights*. John Hopkins University Press, Baltimore, Maryland.
Guerrini, A. (2006) Alexander Monro primus and the moral theatre of anatomy. *The Eighteenth Century* 47, 1–18.
Hannaway, C. (1977) Veterinary medicine and rural health care in pre-Revolutionary France. *Bulletin of the History of Medicine* 51, 431–447.
Hannaway, C. (1994) Vicq d'Azyr, anatomy and a vision of medicine. In: La Berge, A. and Feingold, M. (eds) *French Medical Culture in the 19th Century*. Rodopi, Clio Medica 25, Amsterdam, the Netherlands.
Hardy, A. (2002) Pioneers in the Victorian provinces: veterinarians, public health and the urban animal economy. *Urban History* 29(3), 372–387.
Hardy, A. (2003) Animals, disease and man: making connections. *Perspectives in Biology and Medicine* 46, 200–215.
Hendricks, J., Newton, C.D. and Rubenstein, A. (2009) 'One Medicine - One Health' at the School of Veterinary Medicine of the University of Pennsylvania - the first 125 years. *Veterinaria Italiana* 45(1), 183–194.
Hopwood, N. (2009) Embryology. In: Bowler, P.J. and Pickstone, J.V. (eds) *The Cambridge History of Science,* vol. 6: *The Modern Biological and Earth Sciences*. Cambridge University Press, pp. 285–315.
Jacyna, S. (1984) The Romantic programme and the reception of cell theory in Britain. *Journal of the History of Biology* 17, 13–48.
Jones, S.D. (2003) *Valuing Animals: Veterinarians and Their Patients in Modern America*. Johns Hopkins University Press, Baltimore, Maryland.
Jones, T.L. (1959) Comparative medicine - the half-open door. *Canadian Journal of Comparative Medicine and Veterinary Science* 22(12), 416–419.
Kaplan, M.M. (1953) The concept of veterinary public health and its application in the World Health Organization. *Bulletin of the World Health Organization* 7(9), 227–236.
Kaplan, M.M. (1961) Comparative medical studies of chronic degenerative diseases as a veterinary public health activity. *Journal of the American Medical Women's Association* 16, 296–299.
Kaplan, M.M. (1966) Social effects of animal diseases in developing countries. *Bulletin of the Atomic Scientists* 22(9), 15–21.
Kete, K. (2007) Introduction: animals and human empire. In: Kete, K. (ed.) *A Cultural History of Animals in the Age of Empire, 1800–1920*, Vol. 5. Berg, Oxford/New York.
King, L.J., Anderson, L.R., Blackmore, C.G., Blackwell, M.J., Lautner, E.A., Marcus, L.C., *et al.* (2008) Executive summary of the AVMA One Health Initiative Task Force report. *Journal of the American Veterinary Medical Association* 233(2), 259–261.

King, N.B. (2004) The scale politics of emerging diseases. *Osiris* 19, 62–76.
Kirk, R.G.W. (2008) 'Wanted – standard guinea pigs': standardisation and the experimental animal market in Britain ca. 1919–1947. *Studies in the History and Philosophy of the Biological and Biomedical Sciences* 39, 280–291.
Kirk, R.G.W. (2009) Between the clinic and the laboratory: ethology and pharmacology in the work of Michael Robin Alexander Chance, c.1946–1964. *Medical History* 53, 513–536.
Kirk, R.G.W. and Worboys, M. (2011) Medicine and species: one medicine, one history? In: Jackson, M. (ed.) *The Oxford Handbook of the History of Medicine*. Oxford University Press, Oxford.
Koolmees, P. (2000) Veterinary inspection and food hygiene in the twentieth century. In: Smith, D. and Phillips, J. (eds) *Food Science, Policy and Regulation in the Twentieth Century*. Routledge, London, pp. 53–68.
Lawrence, S. (1996) *Charitable Knowledge: Hospital Pupils and Practitioners in 18th Century London*. Cambridge University Press, Cambridge.
Leboeuf, A. (2011) Making Sense of One Health. Cooperating at the Human-Animal-Ecosystem Health Interface. Institut Français des relations internationales (Ifri), Paris. IFRI Health and Environment Reports 7.
Lee, K. and Brumme, Z.L. (2013) Operationalizing the One Health approach: the global governance challenges. *Health Policy and Planning* 28(7), 778–785.
Logan, C. (2002) Before there were standards: the role of test animals in the production of empirical generality in physiology. *Journal of the History of Biology* 35, 329–363.
Löwy, I. (2003) Experimental bodies. In: Cooter, R. and Pickstone, J.V. (eds) *Companion to Medicine in the Twentieth Century*. Routledge, London, pp. 435–450.
MacKay, M. (2009) The rise of a medical speciality: the medicalization of elite equine medical care, 1680–1800. PhD thesis, University of York, chapters 1,4.
Méthot, P.-O. (2012) Why do parasites harm their hosts? On the origin and legacy of Theobald Smith's 'law of declining virulence' - 1900–1980. *History and Philosophy of the Life Sciences* 34(4), 561–601.
Nutton, V. (2004) *Ancient Medicine*. Routledge, London.
Orland, B. (2003) Cow's milk and human disease: bovine tuberculosis and the difficulties involved in combating animal diseases. *Food and History* 1, 179–202.
Rader, K. (2004) *Making Mice: Standardizing Animals for American Biomedical Research, 1900–1955*. Princeton University Press, Princeton, New Jersey.
Ritvo, H. (1995) Border trouble: shifting the line between people and other animals. *Social Research* 62, 481–500.
Rous, P. (1910) A transmissible avian neoplasm (sarcoma of the common fowl). *Journal of Experimental Medicine* 12, 697–705.
Rushton, S. (2011) Global health security: security for whom? Security from what? *Political Studies* 59(4), 779–796.
Schlich, T., Mykhalovsky, E. and Rock, M. (2009) Animals in surgery – surgery in animals: nature and culture in animal-human relationship and modern surgery. *History and Philosophy of the Life Sciences* 31, 321–354.
Schmaltz, R. (1936) *Entwicklungsgeschichte des tierärztlichen Berufes und Standes in Deutschland*. Verlagsbuchhandlung von Richard Schoetz, Berlin.
Schmidt, C.F. (1962) Editorial: One Medicine for more than one world. *Circulation Research* 11(6), 901–903.
Schwabe, C.W. (1964, 1969, 1984) *Veterinary Medicine and Human Health*. Williams and Wilkins, Baltimore, Maryland.
Schwabe, C.W. (1978) *Cattle, Priests and Progress in Medicine*. University of Minnesota Press, Minneapolis.
Schwabe, C.W. (2004) Keynote address: The calculus of disease – importance of an integrating mindset. *Preventive Veterinary Medicine* 62, 193–205.
Scoones, I. and Forster, P. (2008) The International Response to Highly Pathogenic Avian Influenza: Science, Policy and Politics (STEPS Working Paper No. 10). Available at: http://steps-centre.org/publication/the-international-response-to-highly-pathogenic-avian-influenza-science-policy-and-politics (accessed 18 July 2014).
Shehada, H.A. (2012) *Mamluks and Animals: Veterinary Medicine in Medieval Islam*. Brill, Leiden.
Shope, R.E. (1933) Infectious papillomatosis in rabbits. *Journal of Experimental Medicine* 58, 607–624.
Shope, R.E. (1959) *Comparative Medicine*. Rockefeller Institute, New York.
Shotwell, R.A. (2013) The revival of vivisection in the sixteenth century. *Journal of the History of Biology* 46, 171–197.
Sluga, G. (2010) UNESCO and the (One) World of Julian Huxley. *Journal of World History* 21(3), 1–18.
Smithcors, J. (1959) Medical men and the beginnings of veterinary medicine in America. *Bulletin of the History of Medicine* 33, 330–341.

Staples, A.L.S. (2006) *The Birth of Development: How the World Bank, Food and Agriculture Organization, and World Health Organization Changed the World, 1945–1965*. Kent State University Press, Kent, Ohio.

Steele, J. (1991) History of veterinary public health in the United States of America. *Rev. Sci. Tech. Off. Int Epiz. [Scientific and Technical Review of the OIE]* 10(4), 951–983.

Steele, J. (2008) Veterinary public health: past success, new opportunities. *Preventive Veterinary Medicine* 86, 224–243.

Swabe, J. (1998) *Animals, Disease and Human Society*. Routledge, London.

Tauber, A. (1994) *The Immune Self: Theory or Metaphor?* Cambridge University Press, Cambridge.

Teigen, P. (1984) William Osler and comparative medicine. *Canadian Veterinary Journal* 25, 400–405.

Teigen, P. (1988) The establishment of the Montreal Veterinary College 1866/67-1874/75. *Canadian Veterinary Journal* 29, 185–189.

Tilley, H. (2011) *Africa as a Living Laboratory: Empire, Development and the Problem of Scientific Knowledge 1870–1850*. University of Chicago Press, Chicago, Illinois.

Waddington, K. (2006) *The Bovine Scourge: Meat, Tuberculosis and Public Health, 1850–1914*. Boydell Press, Woodbridge, UK.

Whiteside, A. (1996) Vancouver AIDS conference: special report. A verdict on the conference: sadly, not one world or one hope. *AIDS Analysis Africa* 6(4), 2.

WHO (1958a) WHO Document MHO/PA/71.59 (unpublished).

WHO (1958b) *The First Ten Years of the World Health Organization*. World Health Organization, Geneva, pp. 211–227.

WHO Chronicle (1961) *Comparative Medicine*, vol. 15. No. 11 (November), pp. 399–405.

WHO/FAO (1951) Joint WHO/FAO Expert Committee on Zoonoses. *WHO Technical Report Series*, No. 40. World Health Organization, Geneva.

WHO/FAO (1956) Advisory group on veterinary public health. *WHO Technical Report Series*, No. 111. World Health Organization, Geneva.

WHO/FAO (1975) The Veterinary Contribution to Public Health Practice, Report of a Joint FAO/WHO Expert Committee on Veterinary Public Health. *WHO Technical Report Series*, No. 573. World Health Organization, Geneva.

Wilkinson, L. (1992) *Animals and Disease: An Introduction to the History of Comparative Medicine*. Cambridge University Press, Cambridge.

Woods, A. (2012) Vets and historians gain from joint approach to international subjects. *Veterinary Times* 15 October, 14.

Woods, A. (2014) Animals and their doctors in Victorian Britain (in preparation).

Worboys, M. (1991) Germ theories of disease and British veterinary medicine, 1860–1890. *Medical History* 35, 308–327.

Worboys, M. (2000) *Spreading Germs: Disease Theories and Medical Practice in Britain, 1865–1900*. Cambridge University Press, Cambridge.

Zinsstag, J., Schelling, E., Wyss, K. and Mahamat, M.B. (2005) Potential of cooperation between human and animal health to strengthen health systems. *Lancet* 366(9503), 2142–2145.

Zinsstag, J., Meisser, A., Schelling, E., Bonfoh, B. and Tanner, M. (2012) From 'two medicines' to 'One Health' and beyond. *Onderstepoort Journal of Veterinary Research* 79(2), 1–5.

# 2 Theoretical Issues of One Health

**Jakob Zinsstag,[1,2]* David Waltner-Toews[3] and Marcel Tanner[1,2]**
[1]*Swiss Tropical and Public Health Institute, Basel, Switzerland;*
[2]*University of Basel, Basel, Switzerland;* [3]*Ontario Veterinary College, University of Guelph, Canada*

## One Health: An Empirical Working Definition

The convergence of interests in human and animal health, based on careful observation and scientific study, has been recognized and promoted by luminaries in the field of health sciences (Box 2.1). Much of it is based on inferences and analogies from empirical observations of specific diseases and comparative anatomy rather than on broader definitions of health (Bresalier *et al.*, Chapter 1, this volume). Rudolf Virchow, the founder of cellular pathology at the end of the 19th century and Calvin Schwabe (Box 2.2), an internationally renowned veterinary epidemiologist and pioneer of veterinary public health in the 20th century, were among the first to articulate key points that have motivated elaboration of the premise of the 'One Health'. Dealing with bovine tuberculosis (Tschopp, Chapter 15, this volume) at a hearing in the Prussian senate, Virchow stated: 'There is no scientific barrier between veterinary and human medicine, nor should there be. The experiences of one must be used for the development of the other'[1] (Saunders, 2000). Influenced by his experience of working with Dinka pastoralists in Sudan, Schwabe coined the term of 'one medicine' to make the point that 'There is no difference of paradigm between human and veterinary medicine. Both sciences share a common body of knowledge in anatomy, physiology, pathology, on the origins of diseases in all species' (Schwabe, 1984).

Indeed, the methods of comparative medicine used in both, human and veterinary medicines, respectively, are closely related and have produced – and continue to produce – enormous mutual benefits. Most therapeutic interventions in human medicine have been developed and tested in animals. Under the increasing influence of specialization, however, human and veterinary medicine have diverged, and too often fail to communicate, even when they share interests in the same disease. For example, during a recent outbreak of Q-fever in the Netherlands, public health authorities were not informed by veterinary authorities about a wave of abortions in goats (Enserink, 2010). Similarly, outbreaks of Rift Valley fever in humans in Mauritania were mistakenly identified as yellow fever. The correct diagnosis was made only after public health services contacted livestock services and learned about the occurrence of abortions in cattle (Digoutte, 1999; Zinsstag *et al.*, 2007).

*E-mail: jakob.zinsstag@unibas.ch

**Box 2.1.** Selected luminaries in the field of health sciences relevant to one health (adapted from Zinsstag and Sackmann, 2007; Zinsstag *et al.*, 2011).

Giovanni Filippo Ingrassias (Venice, 1568) is quoted as saying that veterinary medicine is basically united with human medicine: 'Quod veterinaria medicina formaliter una, eademque cum nobiliore hominis medicina sit'. A Chinese text by Xu Dachun ('On the origin and development of medicine') from the 18th century states that: 'The foundations of veterinary medicine are as comprehensive and subtle as those of human medicine and it is not possible to place one above the other'. Claude Bourgelat, the founder of the first veterinary school in Lyon in 1762, was heavily criticized when he recommended human clinical training for the veterinary curriculum. However, in the 19th century, with the advent of cellular pathology, scientists like Rudolf Virchow developed a strong interest in linking human and veterinary medicine as a form of comparative medicine based on the discovery of similar disease processes in humans and animals. Integrated medical thinking was conveyed to North America by William Osler, a student of Virchow. He is credited for having coined the term 'one medicine', although no direct written evidence for this has been found (Cardiff, R.D., personal communication). Karl F. Meyer, a veterinarian from Basel, Switzerland, director of the Hooper Institute (1921–1951), discoverer of the horse encephalitis virus, founded the first American Public Health Course.

**Box 2.2.** Calvin Schwabe 15 March 1927–27 July 2006 (Zinsstag and Sackmann, 2007).

Calvin Schwabe graduated first in zoology in 1948 and obtained his doctorate in veterinary medicine in 1954. At Harvard he obtained a master in public health and a PhD in parasitology and tropical medicine (1956). During 10 years Schwabe worked at the American University in Beirut. His main interests were parasitic diseases, mainly echinococcosis. He initiated control programmes and led the WHO expert committee on veterinary public health in Geneva. In 1966 he became a full professor in veterinary epidemiology in Davis (California). Schwabe's interests reached far beyond health issues towards more integrated approaches to science. His overarching views on health of all species have influenced modern concepts of veterinary public health, One Health and ecosystem health. His vast bibliography is accessible at http://www. nlm.nih.gov/hmd/manuscripts/ead/schwabe.html.

Collaboration between veterinarians and physicians should produce benefits that are much more than merely additive. The beyond-additive value-added benefits are related to direct positive outcomes not just in reduced risks and improved health and well-being of animals and humans, but also in financial savings, reduced time to detection of disease outbreaks and subsequent public health actions as well as improved environmental services (Zinsstag *et al.*, Chapter 5, this volume). For example, a mixed team of doctors and veterinarians examining human and animal health in mobile pastoralist communities in Chad found that more cattle were vaccinated than children. None of the children were fully vaccinated against childhood diseases. Recognition of this fact enabled synergistic subsequent joint human and animal vaccination campaigns providing preventive vaccination to children who would otherwise not have had access to health services. Clearly a closer cooperation of veterinarians and doctors has generated a better health status than what could have been achieved by working in isolation (Schelling *et al.*, 2007a; Schelling *et al.*, Chapter 20, this volume). Such joint services are scalable to national and regional level by adopting a systems strengthening perspective leading to an extension of Calvin Schwabe's concept of 'One Medicine' to 'One Health' (Zinsstag *et al.*, 2005), which has been further and clearly validated as a public health concept in different areas of the world ranging from Africa to Asia (Zinsstag *et al.*, 2011).

Today, One Health has become a broad international movement supported by the World Health Organization (WHO), the Food and Agriculture Organization of the United Nations (FAO) and the World Organisation for Animal Health (OIE). The World Bank has produced a first account of economic aspects of One Health (World Bank, 2010). One Health is a movement that has its origins in the management of disease threats to humans and animals (Zinsstag, 2013). Theoretical reflections on One Health are induced from case examples and empirical results. Hence we attempt to inductively define and generalize One Health as a problem-solving concept combining research and public health action in an iterative process.

To fully understand the range of potential benefits implies a deeper and comprehensive recognition and understanding of how humans and animals and their environment are interrelated. Equally important, it requires a demonstration and documentation of the benefits and added values resulting from the cross-talk and closer cooperation between human and animal health. *One Health can thus be defined as any added value in terms of health of humans and animals, financial savings or environmental services achievable by the cooperation of human and veterinary medicine when compared to the two medicines working separately.*

The equal focus on the health of people and the animals is one of the characteristics that has differentiated the organization, strategy and practice of One Health from several other related fields, such as veterinary public health, resilience and ecohealth. The latter two consider ecological resilience and sustainability more prominently (see more discussion on this below).

Based on these characteristics, the challenge is to show how, through highly iterative processes and actions, doctors directly and indirectly serve animal health and veterinarians serve public health. We need methods that are capable to quantitatively and qualitatively measure interactions at the interface of human and animal health. Such methods have been developed for survey design (Schelling and Hattendorf, Chapter 10, this volume), health services (Schelling *et al.*, Chapter 20, this volume) and animal to human transmission of infectious diseases (Zinsstag *et al.*, Chapters 12 and 13, this volume).

## Cultural Differences in Human–Animal Relations and their Implications

Dealing with human and animal health as One Health inevitably sheds light on the human–animal relationship and bond. Domestication of wild animals has been one of the fundamental cultural achievements of humans and the use of animals for hunting and as livestock was critical for human development and culture. One Health, even in a more restricted definition as offered here, faces challenging questions regarding cultural differences in view of animals and how they are valued. Thus One Health should reflect on the normative aspects (values) of the human–animal relationship with emphasis on improving animal protection and welfare. Second, even if ecological resilience or health is not the primary outcome of concern, One Health implies an interface of humans and animals and the environment, which can be highly complex requiring systemic approaches to the physical and social environment. They relate human and environmental systems and are also called social-ecological systems (SES). SES relate to theory of complexity (Ostrom, 2007). Third, One Health empirical experience involves not only human and animal health professionals but also reaches out to many other academic domains as well as to non-academic actors like public and private institutions, authorities, civil societies, communities and households. It engages with the public in a transdisciplinary way, considering all forms of academic and non-academic knowledge for practical problem solving at the animal–human interface (Schelling *et al.*, Chapter 30, this volume). The strongest leverage of One Health is observed when it is applied to practical societal problem solving.

### Normative aspects of the human–animal relationship

Similarly to the human–human relationship, the human–animal relationship is governed by norms and values determined by culture and religion. Animals are regarded as intimate companions with a high emotional value or as simple prey with a financial value for their meat. Humans are also valued as a prey by animals under certain circumstances. This is certainly one of the reasons for deep-seated fears against wildlife, which have led to the extinction or threat of extinction of predators in large parts of the world

(Cumming and Cumming, Chapter 4 and Cumming *et al.*, Chapter 21, this volume). There is no biological reason why humans should not consider their surrounding domesticated animals and wildlife as close relatives and treat them with utmost care. Currently, on one hand, globalized livestock production maximizes profits with little regard for humane standards towards animals. At the same time, moderate intensification of livestock production is a way out of the poverty trap for millions of smallholder farmers. On the other hand, we observe very close relationships with companion animals, to the point of humanizing them and considering them as family members. Although not adhering to any of the more dogmatic and naturalist-populist moves, with the promotion of person rights to primates and whales, we must recognize that animals cannot be considered as commodities without certain rights. We refer the reader to the growing literature on the moral status of animals and animal welfare (Wettlaufer *et al.*, Chapter 3, this volume).

Ancient Egyptians saw humans and animals as 'one flock of God', and contemporary Fulani express similar views in their creation myths in West Africa (Sow, 1966). Medical knowledge in India is influenced by beliefs about metempsychosis and reincarnation between animals and humans. According to various schools of Hinduism spirituality, there is no distinction between human beings and other life forms. All life forms, including plants and animals, possess souls. This means that humans can be reborn as animals and vice versa. Such thinking greatly influences the way animals are perceived and handled. Comparable to Hinduism[2] and Jainism, in Buddhism as little harm as possible is done to animals. Buddhists treat the lives of human and non-human animals with equal respect (Ryder, 1964; Cowell, 1973; Sangave, 1991). A brief historical and cultural evolutionary look is most enlightening in this respect. Biblical texts report that humans and terrestrial animals were created on the same day, and the Sabbath regulations also imply the resting of livestock, indicating a strong co-creational attitude in the Judeo-Christian Bible. In the Qur'an, animals are considered close to humans. Modern animal welfare has roots in Southern German pietism; here we can cite Albert Schweitzer, who was inspired for his philosophical idea of 'reverence for life' or in the original German language, 'Ehrfurcht vor dem Leben'. In summary, the contemporary human–animal relationship is polarized between merciless exploitation of livestock and humanizing of pets. Within the dilemma of aspirations of a globalized economy, social development and animal welfare, culture and religion as well as economic considerations largely influence the human–animal relationship and subsequently the potential of a closer cooperation of human and animal health.

Working in different cultures to achieve One Health outcomes implies adopting the view that there are multiple legitimate perspectives, and that practices must be adapted to local contexts. We need to clarify both our own perspective and point of view, respectively. Adopting a *self-reflexive attitude* we may ask: What is the personal cultural/religious background driving my animal–human relationship? Our own attitude towards animals influences how we value animal life economically or emotionally. For example, the dogs in Plate 1a have a market value for consumption of approximately US$12 on a local market in West Africa, whereas the pet cat in Plate 1b is part of a household in Europe, which is prepared to spend a considerable amount of money for its veterinary care. Consequently, when we report about our research from One Health studies we also need to explain the *perspective*, i.e. the social, cultural and religious background, from which the animal–human relationship is seen as it strongly determines the valuing in economic frameworks and societal contexts (Zinsstag and Weiss, 2001; Narrod *et al.*, 2012). The overarching approach in practising One Health, however, clearly ought not to be driven by any specific perspective but rather by the pragmatic approach that effectively brings together resources from the different disciplines and resources to address the priorities of the human and animal populations concerned.

## One Health and animal ethical and welfare issues

A One Health perspective also encompasses reflections on human and animal well-being per se. Humans have rights and are seeking to maximize their well-being; similarly, one might ask, whether and if animals have rights, how we consider their well-being (Wettlaufer *et al.*, Chapter 3, this volume). Despite an overall protective attitude in most cultures and religions, as described above, the reality is appalling. Worldwide and across different cultures and religions, animals are reared, transported and slaughtered in the millions under terrible and non-humane conditions, which urgently calls for a much stronger engagement for animal protection and welfare.

Animal biodiversity contributes to stable ecosystem services and extensive livestock rearing maintains carbon sequestration in semi-arid areas. Animal diseases threaten human health and food security, for example by the transmission of zoonotic diseases or by the loss of animals for ploughing. Large parts of the world could not be inhabited without the use of livestock in a moderate way. Consequently, we can no longer close our eyes on the close linkage, interrelations and interdependencies of human and animal health without considering simultaneously the maintenance of stable ecosystem services, some of which are seriously threatened by livestock rearing methods and/or excessive human exploitive activities.

Peter Rabinowitz, an occupational physician from Yale University, proposes that humans should change their point of view towards animals from an 'us versus them' towards a 'shared risk' attitude between humans and animals (Rabinowitz *et al.*, 2008; Rabinowitz and Conti, 2010). As an example we can consider the high cancer rate of Beluga whales in the Saguenay fiord in Canada. Belugas are continuously exposed to waste water of industries and of mostly human origin. The Beluga cancer incidence has become an indicator of environmental quality. Therefore, humans have an interest in preserving the quality of the environment in a state that dos not adversely affect both whale and human health.

Hence, from an integrative One Health, conservation biology and/or an ecosystem perspective, animals should be much better valued and treated as part of an overall effort to maintain and sustain ecosystem integrity and, thus, comprehensive well-being. This involves among others, animal husbandry and rearing, animal transport, slaughter practices, animal traction and wildlife conservation (see Wettlaufer *et al.*, Chapter 3, Cumming and Cumming, Chapter 4 and Cumming *et al.*, Chapter 21, this volume).

Globally, most livestock holders treat their animals well. In Plate 2 we can observe an almost unrestrained husbandry. The horse being milked by the Kyrgyz woman is just standing still without being tied. Similarly, the Fulani cattle and horses in Chad are quiet and obviously well treated. However, animal welfare is clearly insufficient in semi-intensive and intensive production systems. Livestock holders should be continuously trained on best animal welfare practices in their rearing system. From an animal welfare perspective, the current practice of transporting livestock on foot, say from Ireland to France for slaughter, is not acceptable. Similarly, in developing countries, small ruminants and poultry are often transported for hundreds of kilometres under congested conditions, without water and being beaten severely. Slaughtering practices should aim at reducing stress during animal handling. As part of economic growth, meat consumption has grown massively in the last decades. From a One Health point of view we do not want to advocate vegetarianism. Livestock plays an important role especially in the livelihoods of hundreds of millions of small-scale farmers.

Animals are also (one might say mostly) used in agriculture in developing countries for ploughing, transport and traction of carriages. While cattle and camels used for ploughing or transport are usually well treated, there is undeniably a huge suffering of horses and donkeys used for transport. Donkeys are probably among the worst treated animals worldwide and urgently need better treatment and husbandry. There is increasing research on livestock, companion animals and wildlife in developing countries. However, there is almost a complete lack of legislation on animal testing. Care should be taken that animal testing is not exported from industrialized countries to evade stringent regulations. We should not forget the welfare standards for pets, which may similarly undergo huge suffering. For example, dogs and cats are often abandoned at the beginning of the summer holidays, so that owners do not have to care for them.

From a One Health perspective the notion of burden of disease should be extended to animals to reflect the toll of life and suffering of humans and animals for example in road traffic accidents, which cause the death of hundreds of thousands of wildlife. Road safety should then be expressed as causing this number of human and this number of animal casualties. Modern highway planning effectively protects animal life by protective fencing, bridges and tunnels for safe animal movement. While animal life can be counted, estimating animal suffering and disability, similar to the human burden measures like the disability adjusted live years (DALYs) is hardly possible because of the variation of norms and values across cultures and production systems. For example, how would expected years of life of male calves or fattening pigs be adequately assessed. There is an ongoing and controversial debate but still not enough research undertaken in the development for a combined metric of human and animal disease burden. Improving animal welfare remains a permanent challenge to any effort and ethical aspiration of One Health (Wettlaufer *et al.*, Chapter 3, this volume).

### One Health as embedded in landscapes

One Health as presented here is not an isolated idea. There are earlier more limited but also broader concepts. We should mention Evgeny Pavlovsky's (1884–1965) concept of disease nidality. He considered pathogens from an ecological perspective having their own ecological niche. This can be a specific space in an ecosystem but also an animal or organ to which they are most adapted. For example marmots in Mongolia carry *Yersinia pestis*, the agent of plague, without symptoms. Occasionally marmot hunters become ill with plague after handling marmot carcasses. Calvin Schwabe met Evgeny Pavlovsky in Leningrad in 1965 and writes in his memoirs:

> The only noteworthy work-related event in Leningrad was my meeting with Eugene Pavlovsky, the dean of the Soviet descriptive epidemiologists, formal developer of medical ecological notions like 'landscape epidemiology' and 'natural foci of infections'. . . He had read Veterinary Medicine and Human Health [(Schwabe, 1984) reference added] already and said he was pleased to see an American author write on the 'Ecological Study of Disease', which was my title of the 1st edition chapter introducing epidemiology.[3]

One of the most prominent interactions of human and animal health is Veterinary Public Health (VPH), which is defined as the contribution of veterinary medicine to public health. VPH is well established in international organizations, governmental administrations and academia. VPH was originally conceived at the Centers for Disease Control in Atlanta by James H. Steele. Schwabe refers to it as 'the innovative Veterinary Public Health Unit founded by Jim Steele,. . . helping to demonstrate the value of an organized and systematic capability for disease intelligence'.[4]

Compared to One Health, VPH is mainly serving public health. Conceptually it does not consider a mutual benefit from public health for animal health.

A much broader concept is an 'ecosystem approach to health' or 'ecohealth'. Ecohealth considers inextricable linkages between ecosystems, society and health (Rapport *et al.*, 1999). It seeks in-depth understanding of ecological processes and their relation to human and animal health. For example, using an ecohealth approach it could be demonstrated that mercury poisoning of fish and impeding health risks for humans in the Amazon were not due to upstream gold mining but due to soil erosion following deforestation (Forget and Lebel, 2001). Ecohealth has become an internationally scholarly movement organized by the International Association for Ecology and Health.[5] Ecohealth is a systemic approach, tackling complex problems as embedded in non-linear systems dynamics quantitatively and qualitatively. It involves transdisciplinary approaches, connecting academic and non-academic knowledge in a mutual learning process. It includes all stakeholders from communities to authorities as actors in the research process, pays particular attention to gender and social equity and thrives to put knowledge into action through policy change, interventions and improvement of practices (Charron, 2012). Hence, One Health is embedded in and an integral part of the ecohealth concept (Zinsstag, 2013).

Knowledge and information in veterinary and medical sciences are growing continuously with the consequence that we know more and more about progressively narrowing subjects. The ongoing and accelerated fragmentation of veterinary and medical science is not conducive to complex problem solving and we face an increasing risk for misinterpretation, for example in comparative diagnosis and pathology (Cardiff *et al.*, 2008; Zinsstag *et al.*, 2009). Mainstream reductionist research seeks to explain phenomena at an increasingly smaller scale. On the other hand, major current challenges, like the development of antimicrobial resistance in a complex environment, call for a rethinking of the modern theory of health of animals and humans: One Health provides the respective conceptual grounding and operational outlook.

There are signs of convergence in various fields in systems biology, the social sciences and networks of ecological scholars such as resilience alliance (Zinsstag *et al.*, 2011). The interactions of humans, animals and the environment are not straightforward. They are part of human–environment systems or social-ecological systems (SES). SES are, in the words of economist Elinor Ostrom, complex, multivariable, nonlinear, cross-scale and changing (Ostrom, 2007). Humans and animals are inextricably linked to ecological systems, be they natural or man-made; called cultural and social systems. Biomedical health sciences need to interact with all scholarly pursuits related to social systems, like sociology, economy, political sciences, anthropology and religion. Similarly they need to interact with ecology, geography and all environment-related sciences. All these processes span across scales such as from molecules to populations. Health can be considered as an outcome of SES and hence we speak about Health in Social-Ecological Systems (HSES) (Fig. 2.1). HSES clearly transcends One Health conceptual thinking as defined above. Considering health as an outcome of SES relates to theory of complexity and systems theory (von Bertalanffy, 1951). Attempts to understand health in complex systems can be regarded as processes; generating unexpected and new phenomena (Emergence)[6] (Houle, Chapter 33, this volume). Currently we are exposed to several unintended and poorly understood damages to natural resources and life support systems, such as climate change or nuclear catastrophes, which cannot be tackled by normal reductionist scientific approaches. Normal expert knowledge is no longer sufficient in situations of high uncertainty as we have experienced in the recent past and as it is well postulated in the writing about

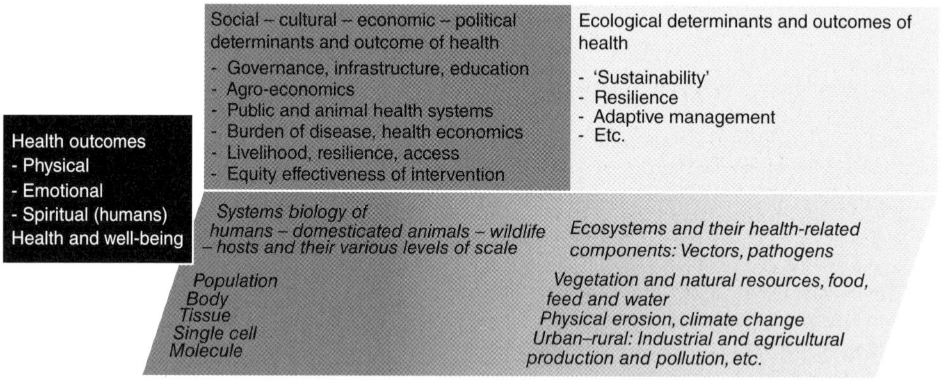


**Fig. 2.1.** Generalized framework of health of humans and animals as outcomes of a social-ecological system across scales from molecules to populations (inclined plane) and the socially (dark grey) and ecologically (light grey) related concepts (Zinsstag *et al.*, 2011).

'post-normal science' (Bunch and Waltner-Toews, Chapter 34, this volume).

## One Health and transdisciplinarity

As developed in the previous section, One Health is a scientifically established and validated concept that created also a movement with its origins in the management of disease threats to humans and animals (Zinsstag, 2013). During the development of health services and zoonoses control in developing countries scientists engaged intuitively with communities, authorities and other stakeholders (Léchenne *et al.*, Chapter 16, Schelling *et al.*, Chapters 20 and 30, this volume). Periodic communication of research findings by scientists to all stakeholders, such as local communities, peripheral health workers and public health and VPH practitioners as well as authorities, has led to more integrated research processes, assuring validity, social relevance and translation for impact. As a consequence, mutual trust has gradually built up. Progress in One Health research can clearly benefit from combining academic and non-academic knowledge in the search for improving health and access to health care for humans and animals in pastoralist communities (Schelling *et al.*, 2007b). Engagement of science with non-academic stakeholders and knowledge is a form of 'transdisciplinary' research, as a further development of 'interdisciplinary' approaches usually combining different academic disciplines, i.e. medicine and social science, and not reaching out to non-academic stakeholders. Mittelstrass defines 'transdisciplinarity' as a form of research that transcends disciplinary boundaries to address and solve problems related to the life-world (Hirsch Hadorn *et al.*, 2008). Transdisciplinarity clearly matches the concept of 'post-normal' science as discussed above (Hirsch Hadorn *et al.*, 2008; Bunch and Waltner-Toews, Chapter 34, this volume).

In conclusion, One Health represents a harmonic development of the traditional VPH within the context of transdisciplinarity and post-normal science, challenged by the situation of our planet that is threatened by the almost overwhelming demands of populations of people and livestock (Box 2.3). As such, it raises questions that encompass conventional understandings of comparative medicine, but go far beyond this into the intense, unstable and complex interactions among culture, economic aspirations and ecological sustainability.

## Acknowledgment

Mitchell Weiss and Giorgios Pavlakos are acknowledged for critical comments to the manuscript and references to Asian literature. Gwendolyn Schwabe is acknowledged for access to Calvin Schwabe's unpublished memoirs.

**Box 2.3.** Summary of theoretical issues of One Health.

One Health can be defined as any added value in terms of health of humans and animals, financial savings or environmental services achievable by the cooperation of human and veterinary medicine when compared to the concepts of approaches of the two medicines working separately.

- One Health inevitably sheds light on the human–animal relationship and bond. It should reflect on the normative aspects (values) of the human–animal relationship with emphasis on improving animal protection and welfare in an inter-cultural context.
- One Health studies declare the perspective, i.e. the social, cultural and religious background, from which the human–animal relationship is seen. Improving animal welfare remains a permanent challenge to any effort and ethical aspiration of One Health.
- One Health engages with the public in a transdisciplinary way, considering all forms of academic and non-academic knowledge for practical problem solving at the animal–human interface. The strongest leverage of One Health can actually be observed when it is applied to practical societal problem solving.
- One Health approaches are embedded into ecohealth conceptual thinking, which are further expanded to 'Health in Social-Ecological Systems' (HSES) addressing complex issues of human–environment systems.

## Notes

[1] Original citation in German 'Es gibt keine wissenschaftliche Barriere zwischen Veterinär- und Humanmedizin, noch sollte es eine geben; die Erfahrung der einen muss gebraucht werden für die Entwicklung der anderen' (Saunders, 2000).
[2] Protocol for handling animal welfare cases in cooperation with the Hindu community. Available at: http://archive.defra.gov.uk/foodfarm/farmanimal/welfare/documents/hindu-protocol-0812.pdf (accessed 14 October 2014).
[3] Calvin Schwabe, Hoofprints of Cheiron, Book two, p. 262 unpublished memoirs.
[4] Calvin Schwabe, Hoofprints of Cheiron, Book two, p. 223 unpublished memoirs.
[5] http://www.ecohealth.net
[6] Such thoughts can be traced to process philosophy (Alfred North Whitehead). Causal inference is limited and processes appear as random events. At best we can understand partial processes.

## References


Bertalanffy, L. von (1951) General system theory - A new approach to unity of science (Symposium). In: *Human Biology*, pp. 303–361.

Cardiff, R.D., Ward, J.M. and Barthold, S.W. (2008) 'One medicine – one pathology': are veterinary and human pathology prepared? *Laboratory Investigation* 88(1), 18–26.

Charron, D.F. (2012) Ecosystem approaches to health for a global sustainability agenda. *EcoHealth* 9(3), 256–266.

Cowell, E.B. (ed.) (1973) *The Jataka: or, Stories of the Buddha's Former Births*. Translated from the Pali by various hands under the editorship of E.B. Cowell. Cosmos Publications, Delhi.

Digoutte, J.P. (1999) [Present status of an arbovirus infection: yellow fever, its natural history of hemorrhagic fever, Rift Valley fever]. *Le Bulletin de la Société de Pathologie Exotique* 92(5), 343–348.

Enserink, M. (2010) Infectious diseases. Humans, animals – it's one health. Or is it? *Science* 327(5963), 266–267.

Forget, G. and Lebel, J. (2001) An ecosystem approach to human health. *International Journal of Occupational Medicine and Environmental Health* 7(2 Suppl.), S3–38.

Hirsch Hadorn, G., Hoffmann-Reim, H., Biber-Klemm, S., Grossenbacher, W., Joye, D., Pohl, C., Wiesmann, U. and Zemp, E. (2008) *Handbook of Transdisciplinary Research*. Springer, Dordrecht, the Netherlands.

Narrod, C., Zinsstag, J. and Tiongco, M. (2012) A one health framework for estimating the economic costs of zoonotic diseases on society. *EcoHealth* 9(12), 150–162.

Ostrom, E. (2007) A diagnostic approach going beyond panaceas. *Proceedings of the National Academy of Sciences* 104(39), 15181–15187.

Rabinowitz, P.M. and Conti, L.A. (2010) *Human–Animal Medicine. Clinical Approaches to Zoonoses, Toxicants and Other Shared Health Risks*. Saunders, Elsevier, Maryland Heights, Missouri.

Rabinowitz, P.M., Odofin, L. and Dein, F.J. (2008) From 'us vs. them' to 'shared risk': can animals help link environmental factors to human health? *EcoHealth* 5(2), 224–229.

Rapport, D., Böhm, G., Buckinghamn, D., Cairns, J., Costanza, R., Karr, J.R., de Kruijf, H.A.M., Levins, R., McMichael, A.J., Nielson, N.O. and Whitford, W.G. (1999) Ecosystem health: the concept, the ISEH, and the important tasks ahead. *Ecosystem Health* 5(2), 82–90.

Ryder A.W. (1964) (Translation) *The Panchatantra*. Translated from the Sanskrit by Arthur W. Ryder. University of Chicago Press, Chicago, Illinois.

Sangave, Vilas Adinath (1991) *The Jaina Path of Ahimsa/Vilas Sangave*, 1st edn. Bhagawan Mahavir Research Centre, Solapur.

Saunders, L.Z. (2000) Virchow's contributions to veterinary medicine: celebrated then, forgotten now. *Veterinary Pathology* 37(3), 199–207.

Schelling, E., Bechir, M., Ahmed, M.A., Wyss, K., Randolph, T.F. and Zinsstag, J. (2007a) Human and animal vaccination delivery to remote nomadic families, Chad. *Emerging Infectious Diseases* 13(3), 373–379.

Schelling, E., Wyss, K., Diguimbaye, C., Bechir, M., Taleb, M.O., Bonfoh, B., Tanner, M. and Zinsstag, J. (2007b) Toward integrated and adapted health services for nomadic pastoralists and their animals: a North-South partnership. In: Hirsch Hadorn, G., Hoffmann-Reim, H., Biber-Klemm, S., Grossenbacher, W., Joye, D., Pohl, C., Wiesmann, U. and Zemp, E. (eds) *Handbook of Transdisciplinary Research. A Proposition by the Swiss Academies of Arts and Sciences*. Springer, Heidelberg, pp. 277–291.

Schwabe, C.W. (1984) *Veterinary Medicine and Human Health*. Williams & Wilkins, Baltimore, Maryland.
Sow, A.I. (1966) Louanges... la femme/'Dieu a des richesses, j'ai des vaches!' In: Sow, A.I. (ed.) *La Femme, la Vache, la Foi - Ecrivains & Poètes du Fo–ta-Djalon*. Julliard, pp. 285–335.
World Bank (2010) People, pathogens and our planet: Vol. 1: Towards a One Health approach for controlling zoonotic diseases. *Report No. 50833-GLB*, 56 pp.
Zinsstag, J. (2013) Convergence of Ecohealth and One Health. *EcoHealth* 9(4), 371–373.
Zinsstag, J. and Sackmann, W. (2007) Calvin Walter Schwabe (15 March 1927–27 July 2006). *Schweizer Archiv für Tierheilkunde Gesellschaft Schweizerischer Tierärzte* 149(1), 36–36.
Zinsstag, J. and Weiss, M. (2001) Livestock diseases and human health. *Science* 294, 477.
Zinsstag, J., Schelling, E., Wyss, K. and Bechir, M. (2005) Potential of cooperation between human and animal health to strengthen health systems. *Lancet* 2005, 2142–2145.
Zinsstag, J., Schelling, E., Roth, F., Bonfoh, B., de Savigny, D. and Tanner, M. (2007) Human benefits of animal interventions for zoonosis control. *Emerging Infectious Diseases* 13(4), 527–531.
Zinsstag, J., Schelling, E., Bonfoh, B., Fooks, A.R., Kasymbekov, J., Waltner-Toews, D. and Tanner, M. (2009) Towards a One Health research and application tool box. *Veterinaria Italiana* 45(2, 1), 121–133.
Zinsstag, J., Schelling, E., Waltner-Toews, D. and Tanner, M. (2011) From 'one medicine' to One Health and systemic approaches to health and well-being. *Preventive Veterinary Medicine* 101, 148–156.

# 3 The Human–Animal Relationship in the Law

**Lenke Wettlaufer,[1]* Felix Hafner[1] and Jakob Zinsstag[2,3]**
[1]*Faculty of Law, University of Basel, Basel, Switzerland;* [2]*Swiss Tropical and Public Health Institute, Basel, Switzerland;* [3]*University of Basel, Basel, Switzerland*

## Introduction

By postulating a closer cooperation of human and veterinary medicine, the One Health concept overtakes the general prevailing human–animal relationship in the law. Corresponding to the historical development of human and animal health into segregated disciplines on academic, governance and application levels (Zinsstag *et al.*, 2012), the law does not apply a cohesive understanding. Accordingly, the law differs between humans and animals in every aspect, including health. This chapter provides an overall introduction to the human–animal relationship in the law, as the prevailing distinction between human and animal health is grounded within the general legal distinction between animals and humans.

The chapter begins with an overview of national provisions concerning animals in constitutional law, private law and animal welfare law. The Swiss legal system serves as a model. Reference to the Swiss norms may, however, also be of service for readers in other legal systems, as most do not vary substantially regarding the general human–animal relationship (Stucki, 2012). None the less, there exist great differences with regard to the levels of animal welfare. Overall, the law distinguishes between subjects of law and objects of law. Humans are, as subjects of law, holders of subjective rights and duties. Animals – objects alike – do not have rights; they are subject to the execution of rights ascribed to humans. This distinction allows humans to use animals for their own purposes. Animal protection law, which entails health regulations, accordingly addresses humans in their use of animals. The different legal statuses result from the conviction that humans are superior to animals due to their abilities – to speak, to reason and to reflect upon their own existence. However, since the uniqueness of humans is increasingly questioned, the legal treatment of animals has become a topic of debate (Michel *et al.*, 2012). At present, individuals and numerous organizations worldwide do not concur with the current handling of animals, and seek to enhance their well-being or end their use for human purposes in general (Favre, 2012).

The chapter then introduces a selection of international agreements and organizations that affect animal welfare. Outside of some exceptions within the European Union (EU), an international animal welfare standard to judge the legislative efforts within one country does not exist. Some countries have adopted provisions strengthening animal welfare, others

*E-mail: lenke.wettlaufer@unibas.ch

have enacted welfare laws but lack enforcement resources or political will to enforce their laws, and still others have not expressed an interest in animal welfare at all (Favre, 2012). None the less, international efforts for standardization are progressing. The section will explore these efforts by looking at the following five examples: European regulations, World Trade Organization (WTO) agreements, World Organisation on Animal Health (OIE) recommendations, the International Health Regulations (IHR) by the World Health Organization (WHO), and the Convention on International Trade in Endangered Species (CITES) (see also Okello *et al.*, Chapter 24, this volume).

In the conclusion we submit that greater importance should be attached to animal welfare issues as part of the One Health concept. The One Health approach is a compelling reason to strengthen animal welfare laws with the purpose of enhancing both animal and, consequently, human health. It will be concluded that, although the aim to recognize the linkage between human and animal health does not inevitably question the overall legal boundary between animals and humans, the One Health concept does challenge current legislation. We propose that a juridification on a national level would require, at a minimum, the legal recognition of the linkage between human and animal health, as well as regulated cooperation of state institutions for human and animal health and systematized cooperation with international institutions. On an international level, efforts for standardization and faithful implementation of animal welfare laws are to be fostered, using EU legislation and recommendations of the OIE as examples. In particular, the surveillance of diseases transmissible between humans and animals should be governed by international standards matching with the IHR.

## National Regulations

National regulations that concern the human–animal relationship will be introduced on the basis of the Swiss legal system. The national Swiss law concerning animals can be divided into constitutional law, private law and animal welfare law. Penalty law will not be addressed. Similar to most legal systems, Swiss constitutional law is superior to any other law and codifies the national state organization, defines national state objectives and guarantees fundamental human rights. Constitutional law hence carries great authority and indicates social values and policies. In the words of Wagman and Liebman (2011), 'a constitution sets down basic parameters for the ordering of the daily lives of a governing body's citizens; [it is] a sort of template for common behaviours'. The constitution principally defines the legal relationship between the state and its citizens, and does not – due to its character as a general legal framework – provide meticulous rules concerning the human–animal relationship, but rather establishes fundamental positions. In contrast, private law regulations govern the legal relationship between the citizens among one another, as they, for example, sell and buy animals for business. Animal welfare law restrains the public law on the basis of the constitution, dealing with all handling of animals, their keeping and their use.

### Constitutional law

The Swiss constitution includes four articles that affect the human–animal relationship: Articles 78, 79, 80 and 120 Bundesverfassung (BV). Article 78 BV (Protection of natural and cultural heritage) and Article 79 BV (Fishing and Hunting) protect animals as species. Article 78 (4) BV states: 'It [the responsible canton] shall legislate on the protection of animal and plant life and on the preservation of their natural habitats and their diversity. It shall protect endangered species from extinction.'[1] In contrast, Article 80 BV (Protection of animals) protects the individual animal – not the particular species (Marti, 2008). Article 80 BV therefore awards the individual animal protection with a constitutional status, meaning that it must be taken into consideration within the entire Swiss regulation system (Federal Supreme Court, 2009). Accordingly, Article 80 (1) BV demands the confederation to legislate on the protection of animals. Pursuant to para. 2 lit. a–f, it shall in particular regulate:

(a) the keeping and care;
(b) experiments and procedures carried out on living animals;
(c) the use of animals;
(d) the import of animals and animal products;
(e) the trade and the transport; and
(f) the slaughter of animals.

Article 120 (2) BV (Non-human gene technology) additionally protects the dignity of the creature. It is to be noted that Switzerland was the first, and remains the only, state to insert this new subject of protection into the constitution (Goetschel, 2002; Richter, 2007). Although the dignity of the creature was established in the context of legal provisions concerning genetic engineering and reproduction medicine, it is accepted that the term is not only applicable within the named field, but rather establishes a general constitutional principle that must be adhered to throughout the entire legal system (Steiger and Schweizer, 2008). The term 'dignity of the creature' is not defined within the constitution. Scholars understand the dignity of the creature as the acknowledgement of the existence of an inherent value of the individual animal (Schweizer, 2008). Animals are to be understood as creatures that have their own individual worth, that follow their own goals, and that constitute organic integrity (Balzer *et al.*, 1997).

Although an analogy seems apparent at first sight, the legal term 'dignity of the creature' must not be equated with the legal term 'human dignity' (Errass, 2013). The inherent dignity of human beings, as for example referred to in the preamble to the United Nations Declaration on Human Rights, is understood to be inherent to all human beings and cannot be lost or acquired (Balzer *et al.*, 1997). In contrast, the dignity of the creature merely establishes a legally protected position within the balancing procedure (Krepper, 2010). Animals shall only be made of use insofar as that use can be justified within the balancing procedure between the interests of humans and the intrinsic value of the creature (Mastronardi, 2008). Accordingly, the dignity of the creature – unlike human dignity – does not guarantee the individual animal an absolute right to live (Mastronardi, 2008). None the less, several authors argue that the dignity of the creature has an impact on other articles of the constitution, and that it relativizes the anthropocentric viewpoint of the law (Errass, 2006; Schweizer, 2008).

Overall, the constitution is written from an anthropocentric perspective, that is: the human person stands in the centre of all legal relations and has subjective rights. The non-human animal does not have rights as do humans; it is merely granted legal protection. Animal protection addresses both animals in their species and the individual animal. Article 120 BV, as a Swiss particularity, includes the dignity of the creature as a subject of legal protection, which calls for the respectful handling of the animal in acknowledgement of an intrinsic value.

### Private law

Unlike constitutional law, the private law governs the legal relations of the citizens with one another. It distinguishes between subjects of law and objects of law. Subjects of law are natural persons and legal entities. The latter, also called legal persons, denote corporate bodies governed by the private law, for example joint-stock or limited liability companies. As subjects of law, these legal and natural persons are holders of subjective rights and duties (Article 11 (2), Article 53 Schweizerisches Zivilgesetzbuch, ZGB).

In contrast, objects of law are so-called things, which persons can claim to have rights over. Objects of law are generally subordinated to the power of disposition of the owner (Art. 641 (1) ZGB). Until 2003, animals were assigned to the category of objects of law under the Swiss Civil Code. This absolute object-status however stood in stark contrast to the constitutional protection of the dignity of the creature, which was already implemented in 1992 (see above section on constitutional law).

Furthermore, the classification of animals as things was seen as outdated pursuant to the public opinion (Kommission für Rechtsfragen des Ständerats, 2002; Goetschel and Bolliger, 2003). Accordingly, the Federal Supreme Court argued in 1989 that the general attitude of humans towards animals has changed with time to an 'ethical animal welfare', which respects the animal as a living and feeling creature (Federal Supreme Court, 1989). In 1990, the Federal Supreme Court affirmed that animals have more than mere property value, and they should be awarded an intrinsic value (Federal Supreme Court, 1990). Based upon this development, the law was changed.

Since 2003, the Swiss Civil Code (Art. 641a (1) ZGB) states explicitly that animals are not things. The alteration aimed to improve the legal position of animals and the special relations that humans have developed with their pets (Arnet and Belser, 2012). The bisection of persons and things was altered into a trisection of natural and legal persons, things and animals. However, the new category 'animal' did not bring about a new defined legal status of animals (Goetschel and Bolliger, 2003; Gruber, 2006; Wiegand, 2011). Under Article 641a (2) ZGB, animals are treated generally analogous to things under the reformed private law. Variances exist, for example, in the law of inheritance (Art. 482 (IV) ZGB) and bankruptcy (Art. 92 (Ia) Bundesgesetz über Schuldbetreibung und Konkurs). The alteration of the law, however, remains to be of mostly declaratory character (Wolf, 2011; Arnet and Belser, 2012). In short, animals are no longer treated as things, but rather like things (Wiegand, 2011).

### Animal welfare law

The general right to use animals for one's own purposes is restricted by the animal welfare law, which provides norms for the use of animals. These regulations are enacted on the grounds of the constitution, and are therefore consistent with the above outlined constitutional foundations. As a consequence, animals can be treated like things as long as the treatment fulfils the requirements of the animal welfare laws, and respectively the constitution (Gruber, 2006). For example, an animal can be sold and shipped like a table as long as it is packed in a way suitable for the animal and transported no longer than 6 h without interruption.

As with most European animal welfare laws, Swiss animal welfare law is based on the concept of ethical animal protection (Goetschel and Bolliger, 2003). The concept of ethical protection safeguards the animal for the animal's own sake. Because the animal is respected as a living and sentient fellow creature, its needs set the reference for legal protection (von Loeper, 2002; Michel, 2012). Ethical animal welfare can further be divided into pathocentric animal welfare, which focuses on the capacity of suffering of animals, and biocentric animal welfare, which concentrates on the mere existence of the living creature as the motive for protection (Michel, 2012). In contrast, the anthropocentric concept of animal protection merely guards animals indirectly, for the sake of human beneficiary interests. During the 19th century, animal welfare came into focus to prevent cruelty to animals (Wiegand, 1979; von Loeper, 2002). Subsequently, animal welfare provisions only applied if mistreatment was conducted in public; acts committed in private remained unpunished (Michel, 2012).

In Switzerland, animal welfare is regulated by both the Animal Welfare Law (Tierschutzgesetz, TSchG) and the Animal Welfare Order (Tierschutzverordnung, TSchVO). The animal welfare norms govern the handling of animals, their keeping and their usage and intrusions by humans (Art. 1 TSchV). Animal welfare law is primarily applicable to vertebrates. Invertebrates are only protected where the Federal Council of Switzerland has explicitly ordered an application of the animal welfare law due to scientific results concerning the capacity of sensitivity of the species (Art. 2 (1) TSchG). In compliance with the constitution, the animal welfare law does not establish subjective rights for animals, but rather sets rules of conduct for humans. Animal welfare law stands in a field of stark tension between human beneficiary and animal protection interests. As a consequence, animal welfare constitutes a mere legal position that is to be considered within the specific balancing of legally protected interests (Michel, 2012).

Article 1 TSchG sets out the purpose of protecting the dignity and the well-being of the animal. Consequently, the dignity of the creature is further defined within the animal welfare law, whereas the constitution does not provide any definition. Pursuant to Article 3 lit. a TSchG, dignity defines the intrinsic value of the animal that has to be respected. The dignity of the animal is injured when an intrusion of the animal cannot be justified with outweighing legitimate interests. An intrusion is especially given when the animal suffers pain, fear, damages, humiliation, its appearance is decisively altered, its physical abilities are decisively disturbed or it suffers excessive exploitation. Well-being is considered given when the following occur: (i) the keeping and feeding of the animal does not disturb its bodily functions and behaviour in a way to which the animal cannot adapt; (ii) the usual species behaviour within its biological capacity of adaptation is possible; and (iii) the animals are of clinical health, and pain, suffering and damages are avoided (Art. 3 lit. b TSchG). Pursuant to Article 4 (1) TSchG, everyone who uses and handles animals must take account of their needs as best as possible and must care for their well-being as far as the purpose of the intended usage allows to do so. It is forbidden to unjustifiably inflict pain, suffering, fear, damage or the violation of the dignity in another way (Art. 4 (2) TSchG).

Due to political pressure, Switzerland enacted animal welfare laws that ensure a high standard of protection when compared to other states' legislations (Goetschel, 2002; Goetschel and Bolliger, 2003).

## International Regulations and Organizations

As a consequence of the constantly progressing political and economic international linkage, states have severe difficulties to exercise animal protection efficiently on their own. Issues involving international animal transportation and the question of admissibility of animal testing conducted abroad exemplify the necessity for international corresponding regulations (Goetschel and Bolliger, 2003). The need for standardization is likewise reflected in several non-binding international declarations of intent, such as the Universal Declaration on Animals Rights, which was announced in 1978 under the patronage of UNESCO (for further information see Neumann, 2012). International law is, however – in comparison to national law – less precise, harder to enforce and wider in scope (Wagman and Liebman, 2011). With the exception of the law of the EU, even binding international law cannot be ruled upon by a particular national court, nor can it be altered by a national parliament, nor can there exist coercive mechanisms such as fines and imprisonment. Notwithstanding, many participants in international agreements accept the governance of a central institution entitled to control actions of the agreement's member countries, and respectively that of the citizens of the member states. Also, international law is regularly inserted into national law.

### European Regulations

European recommendations and regulations have been developed within both the Council of Europe (COE) and the European Union (EU) since the 1970s. The COE is an international organization comprising 47 European countries set up to promote democracy, and to protect human rights and the rule of law. It has adopted the following conventions to control the use of animals:[2]

- European Convention for the protection of animals kept for farming purposes, ETS No. 87, March 1976;
- European Convention for the protection of animals for slaughter, ETS No. 102, May 1979;
- European Convention for conservation of European wildlife and natural habitats, ETS No. 104, September 1979;
- European Convention for the protection of vertebrate animals used for experimental and other scientific purposes, ETS No. 123, March 1986 and the Protocol of Amendment to the European Convention for the protection of vertebrate animals used for experimental and other scientific purposes, ETS No. 170, June 1998;
- European Convention for the protection of pet animals, ETS No. 125, November 1987;

- Revised European Convention for the protection of animals during international transport, ETS No. 193, November 2003.

The EU is an economic and political partnership with 28 member states that have delegated some of their state sovereignty to the union. As decisions on specific matters of joint interest can be made democratically on a European level, the EU differs significantly from other intergovernmental organizations. All member states of the EU are member states to the COE.

Until 2009, animal welfare had not been a contract objective of the EU; therefore EU competence was originally limited to fields where national regulations on animal welfare touched economic issues of the common market. For this reason, issues of pet and wild animal treatment were reserved for national member states to decide (Goetschel and Bolliger, 2003). Regarding farm animals that influence the common market, the EU enacted several directives and regulations with set requirements for housing and treatment of food animals (Blokhuis, 2004). The most relevant directives and decisions concerning farm animals[3] are:

- Council Directive 98/58/EC, July 1998, concerning the protection of animals kept for farming purposes;
- Council Directive 1999/74/EC, July 1999, concerning minimum standards for the protection of laying hens;
- Council Regulation No 1/2005 EC, December 2004, concerning the protection of animals during transport and related operations;
- Council Directive 2007/43, June 2007, concerning minimum rules for the protection of chickens kept for meat production;
- Council Directive 2008/119/EC, December 2008, concerning minimum standards for the protection of calves;
- Council Directive 2008/120/EC, December 2008, concerning minimum standards for the protection of pigs;
- Council Regulation No 1099/2009 EC, September 2009, concerning the protection of animals at the time of killing.

Regarding the protection of animals used for scientific purposes the following directive was enacted:

- Directive 2010/63/EU of the European Parliament and of the Council, September 2010, concerning the protection of animals used for scientific purposes.

Since the enactment of the Treaty of Lisbon in 2009, the EU member states explicitly recognize that animals are sentient beings, and they commit to thorough animal protection. Article 13 of the Treaty on the Functioning of the EU accordingly states:

> In formulating and implementing the Union's agriculture, fisheries, transport, internal market, research and technological development and space policies, the Union and the Member States shall, since animals are sentient beings, pay full regard to the welfare requirements of animals, while respecting the legislative or administrative provisions and customs of the Member States relating in particular to religious rites, cultural traditions and regional heritage.

According to the official website of the European Commission, the general aim is now to ensure that animals do not endure avoidable pain or suffering, and to oblige the owner and the keeper of animals to respect minimum welfare requirements. In respect to animal health, it is the objective to protect and raise the health status and condition of animals in the community, in particular food-producing animals, whilst permitting intra-community trade and imports of animals and animal products in accordance with the appropriate health standards and international obligations (European Commission, 2013, official website). Further, intentions are fostered to establish general principles in a consolidated revised EU legislative framework concerning the protection and welfare of animals (European Commission, 2012). According to Kelch (2011):

> it can probably be said with confidence that the EU is at the forefront of international efforts to improve the welfare of animals. Nonetheless, for those who wish to see the abolition of the use of animals in

> agriculture, experimentation and other areas, there is continuing frustration with the general underlying premise in all of these efforts that these uses of animals are morally justified and that our focus should be on making the lives of the animals used more pleasant, not on ending their use.

## General Agreement on Tariffs and Trade

In 1948, twenty-three countries committed to the General Agreement on Tariffs and Trade (GATT) with the purpose of encouraging trade liberalization and international economic cooperation in the area of making trade fair, profitable and subject to consistent rules (Wagman and Liebman, 2011). Because every country treated animals as legal property, the GATT regulations applied to any international trade involving animals or animal products. In 1995 the World Trade Organization (WTO) was founded as a successor to the GATT. The original GATT text is still in effect under the WTO framework with the modifications of GATT 1994. According to its official website, the WTO currently counts 159 member states. Therefore, the WTO includes more states as signatories than any other economic treaty. Furthermore, it is known for its relatively effective enforcement mechanisms and conflict settlement processes (Kelch, 2011; Wagman and Liebman, 2011).

The WTO agreements comprise three core principles for trade obligations and rights: The Most-Favoured-Nation Treatment, the National Treatment Regulation and the Prohibition on Quantitative Restrictions. The Most-Favoured-Nation Treatment prohibits discrimination of like products from different countries (Article I GATT), signifying that all similar products must be given an equal opportunity to enter a country's marketplace. If two products are alike, then a country may not differentiate between them without violating the GATT. The question of what constitutes a 'like' product is the focus of animal protectionists (Kelch, 2011; Wagman and Liebman, 2011). It remains under discussion whether a trade restriction can be undertaken based on the level of animal welfare applied during the breeding, keeping and killing of the animal. Wagman and Liebman (2011) exemplify the difficulty as follows:

> In short, some say an egg is an egg, and despite what might be a national policy against mistreatment of chickens, Country A cannot currently make a differentiation that resulted in discrimination in trade based on its opinion that chickens from country B were being cruelly treated in order to produce eggs.

The second core principle, the National Treatment Regulation, prohibits a nation from favouring its own domestic goods over similar imported goods (Article III GATT). The third core principle, the Prohibition on Quantitative Restrictions, generally forbids quotas, licences or other measure on exported and imported goods (Article XI GATT). In compliance with the major intention of the WTO – to ensure efficient and fair passage of goods across international borders – the purpose of this principle is to provide a general sense of fairness and uniformity (Wagman and Liebman, 2011). The WTO also stated the goal to protect and to preserve natural resources and the environment (Preamble to the Agreement establishing the WTO, 15 April 1994). None the less, in the light of the above-introduced rules, the WTO regulations may result in the contrary, since the WTO member states are limited in their rights to restrict imported goods (Hunter *et al.*, 1998; Kelch, 2011; Wagman and Liebman, 2011). This dilemma can be illustrated by cases brought before the WTO Tribunal that held a member country's measures to protect threatened species violated the WTO regulations (Tuna-Dolphin I Case, 3 September 1991; Tuna-Dolphin II Case, 16 June 1994; Shrimp-Turtle Case I, 12 October 1998; Shrimp-Turtle Case II, 22 October 2001; the facts of these cases are set out in Wagman and Liebman, 2011).

However, the WTO does also adhere to animal health and welfare regulations. Under the Agreement on the Application of Sanitary and Phytosanitary Measures, the WTO members are bound to the standards for animal health established by the World Organisation for Animal Health (OIE). As a result, the situation may not be as dire as it appears at first glance (Kelch, 2011). Furthermore, Article XX GATT lays out several instances in which

WTO member states may be exempted from GATT principles for free trade. A WTO member country may enact measures that are 'necessary to protect public morals' (lit. a), 'necessary to protect human, animal or plant life or health' (lit. b) or that relate 'to the conservation of exhaustible natural resources if such measures are made effective in conjunction with restrictions on domestic production or consumption' (lit. g). Thereby, rules must not be applied as a means of 'arbitrary or unjustifiable discrimination between countries where the same conditions prevail' and must not be 'a disguised restriction on international trade'. Still, member states must provide conclusive proof that the taken measures fall under the GATT exceptions.

## World Organisation for Animal Health

The World Organisation for Animal Health (OIE) is the direct successor of the Office International des Epizooties, founded in 1924 in order to fight animal diseases at a global level. In 2003 the Office International des Epizooties became the World Organisation for Animal Health, keeping the historical acronym OIE. The OIE is a reference organization to the WTO with a total of 178 member states. The organization is under the authority and control of the World Assembly of Delegates consisting of Delegates designated by the governments of all member states. Under the Agreement on the Application of Sanitary and Phytosanitary Measures (SPS Agreement), which entered into force with the establishment of the WTO on 1 January 1995, the OIE is charged with creating standards for animal health. Historically, the OIE has focused on disease prevention and sanitary standards for animals and animal products in international trade (Kelch, 2011). The World Organisation for Animal Health (2011–2015) Fifth Strategic Plan perpetuates scientifically based standards and guidelines for animal health, animal welfare and animal production food safety.[4] The Terrestrial Animal Health Code of the OIE, which was adopted in its 21st edition by the World Assembly of the Delegates of the OIE members in May 2012, includes several provisions concerning animal welfare in Volume 1 Section 7. All of the provisions are phrased as recommendations. Article 7.1.2 (1–8) provides the following guiding principles for animal welfare:

**1.** That there is a critical relationship between animal health and animal welfare.
**2.** That the internationally recognized 'five freedoms' (freedom from hunger, thirst and malnutrition; freedom from fear and distress; freedom from physical and thermal discomfort; freedom from pain, injury and disease; and freedom to express normal patterns of behaviour) provide valuable guidance in animal welfare.
**3.** That the internationally recognized 'three Rs' (reduction in numbers of animals, refinement of experimental methods and replacement of animals with non-animal techniques) provide valuable guidance for the use of animals in science.
**4.** That the scientific assessment of animal welfare involves diverse elements which need to be considered together, and that selecting and weighing these elements often involves value-based assumptions which should be made as explicit as possible.
**5.** That the use of animals in agriculture, education and research, and for companionship, recreation and entertainment, makes a major contribution to the well-being of people.
**6.** That the use of animals carries with it an ethical responsibility to ensure the welfare of such animals to the greatest extent practicable.
**7.** That improvement in farm animal welfare can often improve productivity and food safety, and hence lead to economic benefits.
**8.** That equivalent outcome based on performance criteria, rather than identical systems based on design criteria, be the basis for comparison of animal welfare standards and recommendations.

Subsequent, more specific sections pertaining to, for example, transport of farmed fish (7.2) and slaughter of animals for disease control (7.6) are also specified as mere recommendations. None the less, as put forward by Kelch (2011), the OIE has begun a fledgling effort to create international standards of animal welfare relating to trade of animals. It is further to be noted that as a new major element of its work, the OIE has implemented the application of the One Health concept for the reduction of risks of high impact diseases at the animal–human–ecosystems interface. According to the Fifth Strategic Plan, this will require consideration of work in certain non-traditional areas, such as infectious diseases in wildlife, working animals, and competition and companion animals, in addition to food-producing animals.[4]

### International Health Regulations by the World Health Organization

A central responsibility of the WHO is the management of a global regime for control of the international spread of disease. The International Health Regulations (IHR) of the WHO were drafted to meet this purpose, and were first adopted by the Health Assembly in 1969, having been preceded by the International Sanitary Regulations adopted by the World Health Assembly in 1951 (WHO, 2008). Because the IHR were considered nonresponsive to the major challenges of emerging infectious diseases and bioterrorism, the WHO engaged in a process to modernize the IHR (Gostin, 2004). As a result, the IHR 2005 were adopted by the World Health Assembly in May 2005, and entered into force in June 2007 as a legally binding agreement. Among other improvements, the IHR 2005 contain a scope not limited to any specific disease or manner of transmission. They also state: party obligations to develop certain minimum core public health capacities in disease surveillance and response; party obligations to notify the WHO of events that may constitute a public health emergency according to defined criteria; provisions authorizing WHO to take unofficial reports into consideration; and protection of the human rights of persons and travellers (WHO, 2008). According to the WTO's official website, the WHO's work in support of Global Capacities, Alert and Response, under IHR (2005, Article 2 IHR) aims at, first:

> further developing and maintaining an effective international system that is able to continuously assess the global context of public health risks and is prepared to respond rapidly to unexpected, internationally-spreading events and to contain specific public health threats. The second aim is to provide guidance and support to countries to build strong national public health systems that can maintain active surveillance of diseases and public health events; rapidly investigate detected events; report and assess public health risk; share information; and implement public health control measures.

Currently, 196 member states are parties to the IHR 2005.

The IHR do not specifically focus on fighting animal diseases. None the less, animals are included in the scope of application of the IHR. For example, 'contamination' is defined as the presence of an infectious or toxic agent or matter on a human or animal body surface, 'goods' mean tangible products, including animals and plants, and 'infection' means the entry and development or multiplication of an infectious agent in the body of humans and animals (Article 1 IHR). Pursuant to Article 22 (1) lit. e IHR, the competent authorities shall be responsible for the supervision of the removal and safe disposal of any contaminated water or food and human or animal dejecta. Further, for responding to events that may constitute a public health emergency of international concern, designated airports, ports and ground crossings must provide assessment of and care for affected travellers or animals, by establishing arrangements with local medical and veterinary facilities for their isolation, treatment and other support services (Annex 1. B. 2. lit. b).

In general, the IHR 2005 provides a remarkable new legal framework to promote international public health. An especially unique aspect is the collective commitment requiring close intersectoral cooperation between the WTO and the state parties, as well as within the states themselves, which includes cooperation among different administrative or governmental levels, and horizontally across ministries and disciplines (Rodier *et al.*, 2006). As public health emergencies do not respect international boundaries, a common interest exists for all countries to possess the capacities and capabilities identified in the IHR 2005 to detect, assess, report and respond to public health threats (Katz *et al.*, 2010).

### Convention on International Trade in Endangered Species of Wild Fauna and Flora

The Convention on International Trade in Endangered Species of Wild Fauna and Flora (CITES) from 3 March 1973 is an international agreement that aims at protecting plant and animal species in danger of depredation or extinction. The 175 member nations to the convention submit, through mutual agreement, to the regulation or prohibition of international trade in the specified species (see for further information: Kelch, 2011; Wagman and Liebman, 2011). One of the difficulties with the convention is the fact that enforcement is essentially left to the member states. Several countries have enacted corresponding national regulations, such as the Endangered Species Act of 1973 in the USA and the Environment Protection and Biodiversity Conservation Act of 2000 in Australia.

## Prospects

The One Health approach is a compelling reason to enact further animal welfare legislation, as strengthened animal welfare laws will improve animal health and successively lead to enhanced human health. Since the aim to recognize the linkage between human and animal health remains human-centred, the concept will not inevitably question the overall set legal boundary between animals and humans. Nevertheless, the One Health concept does challenge prevailing legislation. Initial, indefinite thoughts on a legal implementation of the One Health concept regarding the aspect of unified human–animal medicine lead to the following considerations:

On a national level, a juridification of the One Health concept would require at least three alterations.

**1.** The correlation of human and animal health must be explicitly recognized in the law. An explicit legal recognition of the linkage would set the foundation for a juridification of the One Health concept regarding the aspect of unified human–animal medicine.

**2.** Regulated cooperation of state departments and institutions for human and animal health would have to be achieved. Type and scope of the regulated cooperation of the distinct departments and institutions would need to be implemented in the law. In most countries, there are different departments and institutions competent to deal with either human health issues or animal health issues (such as the Bundesamt für Gesundtheit and the Bundesamt für Lebensmittelsicherheit und Veterinärwesen in Switzerland). Differentiation between competencies follows the differentiation in the law.

**3.** Regulated cooperation with international institutions and other states would have to be realized.

On an international level, animal welfare law would have to be expanded and faithfully implemented. Excluding certain exceptions in the EU, no agreement exists that ensures the welfare of animals, nor is there any international standard that regulates and defines acceptable treatment (Favre, 2012). The consequence is diverse standards regarding animal protection – and successively, animal health. Some countries have adopted comprehensive laws on animal welfare issues, others have enacted welfare laws but lack enforcement resources or political will to enforce their laws, while still others have not expressed any interest in animal welfare at all (Favre, 2012).

Health threats cannot be ameliorated by states acting on their own. Present global health challenges instead require a multisectoral approach in which health is a fundamental value within global governance and international law (Garcia and Gostin, 2012). Existing international efforts for standardization, such as the introduced EU legislation and recommendations of the OIE, are consequently to be fostered and extended. In particular, the surveillance of diseases transmissible between humans and animals should be governed by global cross-sectoral standards matching with the IHR.

Clearly, we do not advocate new unified institutions for human and animal health, but rather a legal basis for a closer cooperation of human and veterinary medicine within the One Health concept. One Health not only influences thinking on legal provisions for the interaction of humans and animals, but in addition it requires future legal considerations for the cross-sector cooperation between human and animal health.

## Notes

[1] All translations of the Swiss legal texts are taken from the official website of the Federal Authorities of the Swiss Confederation: http://www.admin.ch (accessed 18 March 2014).

[2] All texts can be found at: http://coe.int/t/e/legal_affairs/legal_cooperation/biological_safety_and_use_of_animals/Conventions.asp (accessed 18 March 2014).

[3] All texts can be found at: http://ec.europa.eu/food/animal/welfare/references_en.htm (accessed 18 March 2014).

[4] OIE Fifth Strategic Plan, 2011–2015. Available at: http://www.oie.int/doc/en_document.php?numrec=4103803 (accessed 18 March 2014).

## References


Arnet, R. and Belser, E.M. (2012) Handkommentar zum Schweizer Privatrecht – Sachenrecht – Article 641-977 ZGB. In: Breitschmid, P. and Rumo-Jungo, A. (eds) *Handkommentar zum Schweizer Privatrecht*, 2nd edn. Schulthess, Zürich, Switzerland, pp. 15–16.

Balzer, P., Rippe, K.P. and Schaber, P. (1997) Was heisst Würde der Kreatur? *Schriftenreihe Umwelt* 294, 1–55.

Blokhuis, H.J. (2004) Recent developments in European and international welfare regulations. *World's Poultry Science Journal* 60, 469–477.

Errass, C. (2006) *Öffentliches Recht der Gentechnologie im Ausserhumanbereich*. Stämpfli, Bern, Switzerland.

Errass, C. (2013) 20 Jahre Würde der Kreatur. *Zeitschrift des bernischen Juristenvereins* 149, 187–232.

European Commission (2012) Communication from the Commission to the European Parliament, the Council and the European Economic and Social Committee on the European Union Strategy for the Protection and Welfare of Animals 2012–2015. Available at: http://ec.europa.eu/food/animal/welfare/index_en.htm (accessed 18 March 2014).

European Commission (2013) Animal Health and Animal Welfare. Available at: http://ec.europa.eu/food/animal/index_en.htm (accessed 18 March 2014).

Favre, D.S. (2012) An international treaty for animal welfare. *Journal of Animal & Natural Resource Law* 8, 237–280.

Federal Supreme Court (1989) BGE 115 IV, 248–255.

Federal Supreme Court (1990) BGE 116 IV, 364–370.

Federal Supreme Court (2009) BGE 135 II, 384–405.

Garcia, K.K. and Gostin, L.O. (2012) One Health, One World – the intersecting legal regimes of trade, climate change, food security, humanitarian crises, and migration. *Laws* 1, 4–38.

Goetschel, A.F. (2002) Würde der Kreatur als Rechtsbegriff und Rechtspolitische Postulate daraus. In: Liechti, M. (ed.) *Die Würde des Tieres*. Harald Fischer, Erlangen, Germany, pp. 141–180.

Goetschel, A.F. and Bolliger, G. (2003) *Das Tier im Recht. 99 Facetten der Mensch-Tier-Beziehung von A bis Z*. Orell Füssli, Zürich, Switzerland.

Gostin, L.O. (2004) International infectious disease law. Revision of the World Health Organization's international health regulations. *Journal of the American Medical Association* 21, 2623–2627.

Gruber, M. (2006) *Rechtsschutz für nichtmenschliches Leben. Der moralische Status des Lebendigen und seine Implementierung in Tierschutz-, Naturschutz- und Umweltrecht*. Nomos, Baden-Baden, Germany.

Hunter, D., Salzman, J. and Zaelke, D. (1998) *International Law and Policy*. Foundation Press, New York.

Katz, R.L., Fernandez, J.A. and McNabb, S.J.N. (2010) Disease surveillance, capacity building and implementation of the International Health Regulations (IHR 2005). *BMC Public Health* 10, (Suppl. 1). Available at: http://www.biomedcentral.com/1471-2458/10/S1/S1 (accessed 18 March 2014).

Kelch, T.G. (2011) *Globalization and Animal Law. Comparative Law, International Law and International Trade*. Kluwer Law International, Alphen aan den Rijn, the Netherlands.

Kommission für Rechtsfragen des Ständerats (2002) Parlamentarische Initiative. Die Tiere in der schweizerischen Rechtsordnung. *Bundesblatt* 23, 4164–4174.

Krepper, P. (2010) Tierwürde im Recht – am Beispiel von Tierversuchen. *Aktuelle Juristische Praxis*, 303–312.
Marti, A. (2008) Kommentar zu Article 79 BV. In: Ehrenzeller, B., Mastronardi, P., Schweizer, R.J. and Vallender, K.A. (eds) *Die schweizerische Bundesverfassung, Kommentar*, 2nd edn. Dike/Schulthess, Zürich, St Gallen, Switzerland, pp. 1402–1409.
Mastronardi, P. (2008) Kommentar zu Article 7 BV. In: Ehrenzeller, B., Mastronardi, P., Schweizer, R.J. and Vallender, K.A. (eds) *Die schweizerische Bundesverfassung, Kommentar*, 2nd edn. Dike/Schulthess, Zürich, St Gallen, Switzerland, pp. 164–178.
Michel, M. (2012) Tierschutzgesetzgebung im Rechtsvergleich: Konzepte und Entwicklungstendenzen. In: Michel, M., Kühne, D. and Hänni, J. (eds) *Tier und Recht, Entwicklungen und Perspektiven im 21. Jahrhundert [Animal Law – Developments and Perspectives in the 21st Century]*. Dike, Zürich, St Gallen, Switzerland, pp. 593–624.
Michel, M., Kühne, D. and Hänni, J. (eds) (2012) *Tier und Recht, Entwicklungen und Perspektiven im 21. Jahrhundert [Animal Law – Developments and Perspectives in the 21st Century]*. Dike, Zürich, St Gallen, Switzerland.
Neumann, J.M. (2012) La Déclaration Universelle des Droits de l'Animal ou l'égalité des espèces face à la vie. In: Ehrenzeller, B., Mastronardi, P., Schweizer, R.J. and Vallender, K.A. (eds) *Die schweizerische Bundesverfassung, Kommentar*, 2nd edn. Dike/Schulthess, Zürich, St Gallen, Switzerland, pp. 361–395.
Richter, D. (2007) Die Würde der Kreatur. Rechtsvergleichende Betrachtungen. *Zeitschrift für ausländisches öffentliches Recht und Völkerrecht* 67, 319–349.
Rodier, G., Hardiman, M., Plotkin, B. and Ganter, B. (2006) Implementing the International Health Regulations (2005) in Europe. *Eurosurveillance* 11 (12). Available at: http://eurosurveilllance.org/ViewArticle.aspx?Articled=664 (accessed 18 March 2014).
Schweizer, R.J. (2008) Kommentar zu Article 120 BV. In: Ehrenzeller, B., Mastronardi, P., Schweizer, R.J. and Vallender, K.A. (eds) *Die schweizerische Bundesverfassung, Kommentar*, 2nd edn. Dike/Schulthess, Zürich, St Gallen, Switzerland, pp. 1861–1873.
Steiger, A. and Schweizer, R.J. (2008) Kommentar zu Article 80 BV. In: Ehrenzeller, B., Mastronardi, P., Schweizer, R.J. and Vallender, K.A. (eds) *Die schweizerische Bundesverfassung, Kommentar*, 2nd edn. Dike/Schulthess, Zürich, St Gallen, Switzerland, pp. 1410–1421.
Stucki, S. (2012) Rechtstheorethische Reflexionen zur Begründung eines tierlichen Rechtssubjekts. In: Michel, M., Kühne, D. and Hänni, J. (eds) *Tier und Recht, Entwicklungen und Perspektiven im 21. Jahrhundert [Animal Law – Developments and Perspectives in the 21st Century]*. Dike, Zürich, St Gallen, Switzerland, pp. 143–172.
von Loeper, E. (2002) Einführung in das Recht der Mensch-Tier-Beziehung. In: Kluge, H. (ed.) *Tierschutzgesetz*. Kohlhammer, Stuttgart, Germany, pp. 27–85.
Wagman, B.A. and Liebman, M. (2011) *A Worldview of Animal Law*. Carolina Academic Press, Durham, North Carolina.
Wiegand, K.D. (1979) Die Tierquälerei. Ein Beitrag zur historischen, strafrechtlichen und kriminologischen Problematik der Verstöße gegen § 17 Tierschutzgesetz. In: Geerds, F. (ed.) *Kriminalwissenschaftliche Abhandlungen*, Vol. 11. Schmidt-Römhild, Lübeck, Germany, pp. 1–152.
Wiegand, W. (2011) Article 641a ZGB. In: Honsell, H., Vogt, P.N. and Geiser, T. (eds) *Basler Kommentar. Zivilgesetzbuch II*, 4th edn. Helbing Lichtenhahn, Basel, Switzerland, pp. 836–837.
Wolf, S. (2011) Article 641a ZGB. In: Kostkiewicz, J.K., Nobel, P., Schwander, I. and Wolf, S. (eds) *ZGB Kommentar – Schweizerisches Zivilgesetzbuch*, 2nd edn. Orell Füssli, Zürich, Switzerland, pp. 920–921.
World Health Organization (2008) International Health Regulations (2005). Available at: http://www.who.int/ihr/publications/9789241596664/en (accessed 18 March 2014).
World Organisation for Animal Health (2011–2015) Fifth Strategic Plan. Available at: http://www.oie.int/about-us/director-general-office/strategic-plan (accessed 21 March 2014).
Zinsstag, J., Mackenzie, J.S., Jeggo, M., Heymann, D.L., Patz, J.A. and Daszak, P. (2012) Mainstreaming One Health. *EcoHealth* 9, 107–110.

# 4 One Health: an Ecological and Conservation Perspective

**David H.M. Cumming[1,2]* and Graeme S. Cumming[1]**
[1]*Percy FitzPatrick Institute, DST/NRF Centre of Excellence, University of Cape Town, South Africa;* [2]*Tropical Resource Ecology Programme, University of Zimbabwe, Harare, Zimbabwe*

## Introduction

As our planet becomes increasingly dominated by human activities and impacts we find ourselves living in a world in which natural areas are being broken into smaller and smaller parts. On the other hand, technological advances are leading to increased connectivity and creating new linkages between people, ecosystems and landscapes across the globe (Helping, 2013). The consequences for health, whether of humans, domestic and wild animals, cultivated and wild plants, or of social and ecological systems and processes, are enormous and unprecedented. There are both spatial and temporal dimensions to the changes that humans have set in motion, and the rate of change continues to escalate. It is within this context that a One Health paradigm, which fully includes the environment, and ecosystem and social-ecological systems approaches, becomes increasingly important (e.g. Walker and Salt, 2006; Waltner-Toews *et al.*, 2008).

Over the course of the 20th century the concept of 'health' gradually became more inclusive. It progressed from an early focus on human health to include the health of domestic animals and cultivated plants, to wild animals and plants, to ecological systems and the environment. It has now extended to a global scale, as witnessed, for example, in the Global Geosphere-Biosphere Program with its focus on global climate change.

As the One Health concept linked human and veterinary medicine, conservationists and environmentalists developed 'conservation medicine' and 'ecosystem health' (Meffe, 1999; Osofsky *et al.*, 2000). These advances were foreshadowed by the earlier writings of Aldo Leopold (Berkes *et al.*, 2012), Rachel Carson's *Silent Spring* (Carson, 1962) and the contribution of medical anthropology in linking health to cultural and social systems (Singer and Baer, 2012). A greater involvement of veterinarians during the 1990s in conservation agencies and conservation practice, beyond the immobilization and translocation of wild animals and care of captive animals, resulted in the generation of the Pilanesburg Resolution in 2001 at a joint meeting of the Society for Tropical Veterinary Medicine and the Wildlife Disease Association (Karesh *et al.*, 2002). This was followed in 2004 by the Manhattan Principles (see Box 4.1), which served to catalyse a resurgence of integrative thinking within the biomedical community. The inclusion of environmental health in the equation is a relatively new development as reflected, for example,

*E-mail: cummingdhm@gmail.com

**Box 4.1.** The Manhattan Principles on 'One World, One Health'.

As defined during the meeting titled 'One World, One Health: Building Interdisciplinary Bridges to Health in a "Globalized World"' held in 2004 (Cook *et al.*, 2004).

Recent outbreaks of West Nile virus, Ebola hemorrhagic fever, SARS, monkeypox, mad cow disease and avian influenza remind us that human and animal health are intimately connected. A broader understanding of health and disease demands a unity of approach achievable only through a consilience of human, domestic animal and wildlife health – One Health. Phenomena such as species loss, habitat degradation, pollution, invasive alien species and global climate change are fundamentally altering life on our planet from terrestrial wilderness and ocean depths to the most densely populated cities. The rise of emerging and resurging infectious diseases threatens not only humans (and their food supplies and economies), but also the fauna and flora comprising the critically needed biodiversity that supports the living infrastructure of our world. The earnestness and effectiveness of humankind's environmental stewardship and our future health have never been more clearly linked. To win the disease battles of the 21st century while ensuring the biological integrity of the Earth for future generations requires interdisciplinary and cross-sectoral approaches to disease prevention, surveillance, monitoring, control and mitigation as well as to environmental conservation more broadly.

We urge the world's leaders, civil society, the global health community and institutions of science to:

**1.** Recognize the essential link between human, domestic animal and wildlife health and the threat disease poses to people, their food supplies and economies, and the biodiversity essential to maintaining the healthy environments and functioning ecosystems we all require.
**2.** Recognize that decisions regarding land and water use have real implications for health. Alterations in the resilience of ecosystems and shifts in patterns of disease emergence and spread manifest themselves when we fail to recognize this relationship.
**3.** Include wildlife health science as an essential component of global disease prevention, surveillance, monitoring, control and mitigation.
**4.** Recognize that human health programmes can greatly contribute to conservation efforts.
**5.** Devise adaptive, holistic and forward-looking approaches to the prevention, surveillance, monitoring, control and mitigation of emerging and resurging diseases that take the complex interconnections among species into full account.
**6.** Seek opportunities to fully integrate biodiversity conservation perspectives and human needs (including those related to domestic animal health) when developing solutions to infectious disease threats.
**7.** Reduce the demand for and better regulate the international live wildlife and bushmeat trade not only to protect wildlife populations but to lessen the risks of disease movement, cross-species transmission, and the development of novel pathogen–host relationships. The costs of this worldwide trade in terms of impacts on public health, agriculture and conservation are enormous, and the global community must address this trade as the real threat it is to global socio-economic security.
**8.** Restrict the mass culling of free-ranging wildlife species for disease control to situations where there is a multidisciplinary, international scientific consensus that a wildlife population poses an urgent, significant threat to human health, food security, or wildlife health more broadly.
**9.** Increase investment in the global human and animal health infrastructure commensurate with the serious nature of emerging and resurging disease threats to people, domestic animals and wildlife. Enhanced capacity for global human and animal health surveillance and for clear, timely information-sharing (that takes language barriers into account) can only help improve coordination of responses among governmental and non-governmental agencies, public and animal health institutions, vaccine/pharmaceutical manufacturers and other stakeholders.
**10.** Form collaborative relationships among governments, local people and the private and public (i.e. non-profit) sectors to meet the challenges of global health and biodiversity conservation.
**11.** Provide adequate resources and support for global wildlife health surveillance networks that exchange disease information with the public health and agricultural animal health communities as part of early warning systems for the emergence and resurgence of disease threats.
**12.** Invest in educating and raising awareness among the world's people and in influencing the policy process to increase recognition that we must better understand the relationships between health and ecosystem integrity to succeed in improving prospects for a healthier planet.

*Continued*

**Box 4.1.** Continued.

It is clear that no one discipline or sector of society has enough knowledge and resources to prevent the emergence or resurgence of diseases in today's globalized world. No one nation can reverse the patterns of habitat loss and extinction that can and do undermine the health of people and animals. Only by breaking down the barriers among agencies, individuals, specialities and sectors can we unleash the innovation and expertise needed to meet the many serious challenges to the health of people, domestic animals and wildlife and to the integrity of ecosystems. Solving today's threats and tomorrow's problems cannot be accomplished with yesterday's approaches. We are in an era of 'One World, One Health' and we must devise adaptive, forward-looking and multi-disciplinary solutions to the challenges that undoubtedly lie ahead.

in the launch of the journal *EcoHealth* in 2004. These initiatives have been followed by more recent attempts to establish a broader One Health paradigm (Zinsstag *et al.*, 2011; Zinsstag, 2012). The inclusion of biodiversity conservation perspectives in the control and management of both infectious and non-infectious diseases is also a recent development. They are now bringing health research and policy into the mainstream, through an increasingly holistic approach to the control and management of animal, plant and human diseases, and the environments in which they are embedded.

Given earlier pioneering work and writing on 'One Medicine' (see Bresalier *et al.*, Chapter 1 and Zinsstag *et al.*, Chapter 2, this volume), why did it take so long for a broader, more inclusive One Health paradigm to be more widely adopted? Why only now in the early 21st century? The answers lie partly in the slowly changing paradigms of the disparate disciplines (e.g. human and veterinary medicine, public health, epidemiology, ecology, parasitology) involved in disease issues. They also lie in recent technical developments and the shocks delivered by recent emerging diseases such as HIV-AIDS, SARS, and the potential for an avian influenza pandemic that may have triggered a paradigm shift (Kuhn, 1970; Lakatos, 1978). It is thus instructive to examine the shifting paradigms in human and animal medicine, epidemiology (and its branches), ecology and conservation biology, and emerging concepts of ecosystem and environmental health. It is important to do so because, in many parts of the world, earlier paradigms and practices persist and even predominate. The necessary revolutions in science, and their influence on policy and practice in relation to One Health, are far from complete, in both the developed and developing worlds (Bonds *et al.*, 2009, 2012).

This chapter initially outlines paradigm shifts in epidemiology and ecology and their converging approaches to health and disease during the 20th century. We then examine the problem of defining and measuring ecosystem health, ecosystem integrity and environmental health. Both infectious and non-infectious diseases of plants and animals (including humans) are embedded in, and interact with, the environments in which they occur. We use examples to illustrate the complexity of these interactions and the important role of conservation in a developing One Health paradigm, introducing the concepts of adaptive capacity, resilience and transformability in social-ecological systems. These concepts enrich the One Health paradigm and align it more closely with global concerns about sustainability (Rockstrom *et al.*, 2009).

## Global Change and Converging Paradigms in the 20th Century

Epidemiology as a quantitative discipline had its roots in 17th-century writings on the social distribution of ill health and death in cities, such as London. According to Susser and Susser (1996a,b), these early developments gave rise to the Sanitary Movement in the early 19th century. Three periods in epidemiology followed. The first was an era of sanitary statistics based on the belief that ill health was caused by miasmas. With the advent of the microscope and the discovery of microbes, this era gave way to a second ('germ theory') era of infectious disease epidemiology (c. 1850 to 1950), which focused on single infectious agents and treatment. The third era, during the second half of the 20th century, focused on chronic disease epidemiology and the 'black box' paradigm in which exposure and risk factors relating to non-communicable diseases (e.g. tobacco smoking and lung cancer) were investigated in large cohorts of subjects but direct causal factors were generally unknown. Susser and Susser (1996a) and Schwartz *et al.* (1999) argued that changing global health patterns (e.g. the emergence of new infectious diseases and previously rare 'lifestyle diseases') and new technologies were providing the basis for the emergence of a new paradigm in epidemiology that they characterized as eco-epidemiology (Susser and Susser, 1996b). Changes in approaches to the science of human health through the 20th century were also characterized by the adoption of an evidence-based and more rigorous approach to understanding causality (Plowright *et al.*, 2008).

Parasitology focused primarily on describing the intricate life cycles of parasites until Anderson and May (1978) and May and Anderson (1978) took the important step of integrating parasitology with population ecology as a special case of prey–predator interactions. Population dynamics theory was applied to the study of HIV-AIDS and Anderson (1991), in his Tansley lecture to the British Ecological Society ('Populations and infectious diseases: ecology or epidemiology?'), emphasized the links between the two disciplines. Anderson and May, through a series of papers during the 1970s, effectively led the new discipline of ecological epidemiology. They also introduced the useful distinction between micro- and macro-parasites.

Ecology emerged as a discipline in the early 20th century with an initial focus on describing the distribution of plants and plant communities, and successional change (reviewed by Sheail, 1987). The development of animal ecology soon followed (Elton, 1927). Three overarching and contested paradigms in ecology are concerned with the extent to which ecosystems are: (i) characterized by equilibrial or non-equilibrial dynamics; (ii) controlled by unidirectional or reciprocal forces or drivers, particularly in the interaction between abiotic and biotic components; and (iii) dominated by single or multiple (non-linear) causes. The view that a 'balance of nature' existed originated in early Greek philosophy and dominated views of natural systems and their management until recently (Botkin, 1990). Its underlying assumptions have, however, been found to be untenable (Pickett *et al.*, 2007). The idea that ecosystems are controlled by the abiotic environment (Gleason, 1939) also dominated ecology but it has now been well established that plants and animals can modify abiotic drivers and that reciprocal, multiple drivers and feedbacks predominate. Non-equilibrial, reciprocal and multiple causation paradigms lead into complexity theory and a view of ecosystems as complex adaptive systems (Norberg and Cumming, 2008).

The belief that intact 'natural' systems, untouched by any human influence, exist is also no longer tenable. Human domination of the Earth is well established (Vitousek *et al.*, 1997; Foley *et al.*, 2005; Nekola *et al.*, 2013). Major geochemical cycles, such as those of water, carbon and nitrogen cycles, have been greatly altered when compared with pre-industrial levels. The impacts of persistent synthetic organic compounds on ecosystems are profound and have impacted on the incidence of both non-communicable and infectious diseases in humans, other animals and plants. Associated with these health and environmental changes has been the rapid development of molecular tools, data processing capacity and analytical tools that have facilitated the emergence of new sub-disciplines in the investigation of human, animal and environmental health. Notable amongst these is the emergence of molecular epidemiology and the ability to distinguish and trace the origins of rapidly evolving pathogen strains (Morand *et al.*, 2012).

The view in the latter half of the 20th century that infectious diseases were being brought under control has been shattered by the recent increasing incidence of new and re-emerging diseases (Fauci *et al.*, 2005). These include avian influenza, serious acute respiratory syndrome (SARS), multi-drug resistant tuberculosis (Kant *et al.*, 2010), dengue fever (Guha-Sapir and Schimmer, 2005; Bhatt *et al.*, 2013), and the emergence of fungal threats to both animals and plants (Gurr *et al.*, 2011; Fisher *et al.*, 2012).

The converging paradigms in disease-related disciplines, conservation medicine (Osofsky *et al.*, 2000; Lafferty and Gerber, 2002), ecology and the developing field of One Health have now, nearly a decade later, taken us beyond the Manhattan Principles to a broader perspective on environmental and systems health (Cumming, 2010 and below). However, definitions and measurement of system 'health', and particularly ecosystem health, remain under debate.

## Philosophical Issues in Defining and Measuring 'Ecosystem Health'

The terms 'ecosystem health', 'ecosystem integrity', 'environmental health' and 'global health' are widely used.[1] They are, however, normative terms, in the sense that they include, or imply, imparted values to the criteria used to measure health. In this sense the health of an ecosystem, or an environment, is not an independent, objective, property in the same way that the health of an individual can be measured by, for example, body temperature. As a result, it is argued (Lackey, 2001, 2003, 2007) that ecosystem health can only be measured in terms of particular criteria that reflect the values of those interested in measuring, for whatever reason, the 'health' of a selected system. Lackey (2004) considers ecosystem health to be a value-driven policy construct and not science, as the following conundrum from his chapter illustrates:

> One person's 'damaged' ecosystem is another person's 'improved' ecosystem. A 'healthy' ecosystem can be either a malarial infested swamp or the same land converted to an intensively managed rice paddy. Neither condition can be seen as 'healthy' except through the lens of an individual's values and policy preferences.

However, the debate is partly clouded by a failure to distinguish between the different ways in which the term 'ecosystem' is used. Tansley (1935) defined an ecosystem as 'a biotic community or assemblage and its associated physical environment in a specific place'. Pickett and Cadenasso (2002) argued that the ecosystem is a multidimensional concept, and that it is important to distinguish between the differing contexts in which it is used: meaning, model, and metaphor. Fundamentally, ecosystem 'health' is a reflection of some element of either 'structure' or 'function', or some combination of the two; assessments of the integrity of either attribute must be undertaken in relation to a reference system or reference state (Jax, 2010). Similarly, Callicott (1992) provides a helpful discussion of Leopold's concept of 'land health' and the relationship between objective and value-based (normative) components of conservation as both a scientific discipline and a value-driven pursuit.

Even if we accept that some kinds of ecosystem change will result in departures from 'healthy' reference systems, and that such changes can be labelled as 'unhealthy' if they result in decreased levels of biodiversity and/or specified ecosystem functions, questions still remain about the normative values of environmental change and decisions relating to trade-offs between different ecosystem services. For example, construction of impoundments may be 'unhealthy' for a freshwater ecosystem, but may be of prime importance to supply water to a nearby human community. The legal and regulatory problems that arise from the difficulties in defining ecosystem health and integrity are highlighted in the debate surrounding the introduction of genetically modified crops in Europe[2] (Heink *et al.*, 2012). Woodward *et al.* (2012) examined the effects of nutrient pollution on leaf litter breakdown, a fundamental ecosystem process, in 100 streams across a 1000-fold nutrient gradient. The work was stimulated by the introduction of far-reaching legislation to redress human impacts on aquatic ecosystems in Europe that lacked an understanding of ecosystem functional responses (such as litter breakdown) to nutrient loading. Their study raised 'fundamental questions about how to determine ecosystem health' and highlighted 'the need for differential diagnoses in environmental assessment, as is standard practice in medicine'.

One of Lackey's concerns was that advocacy would result in top down, command and control, implementation of policy, based on normative, flawed science (Lackey, 2001, 2007). While this may be a danger at higher levels of policy formulation relating to regional and national environmental management, participatory approaches to explicitly link peoples' values in resource management have been developed. One of these approaches is the Holistic Ecosystem Health Indicator (HEHI) framework that facilitates the inclusion of information from ecological, social, economic and interactive indicators (Muñoz-Erickson *et al.*, 2007). The HEHI approach basically involves building and managing a human designed ecosystem, or even a social-ecological system. The approach has elements of ecological engineering, in which Costanza (2012) characterizes ecosystem health as a 'comprehensive, multiscale, measure of system vigor, organization and resilience' that is closely linked to the concept of sustainability.

Wiegand *et al.* (2010) applied the HEHI approach to the Ythan estuary in Scotland using a 50-year time series data set. The authors found that HEHI provided different insights to those provided by traditional biophysical methods for managing the estuary. Biophysical methods indicated that ecological health declined slightly over the 50-year period, but showed a slight increase during the final decade while HEHI indicated opposite trends for the period. Wiegand *et al.* (2010) concluded that the application of ecosystem health to the Ythan revealed major gaps in data and that mismatches occurred between ecological and social research boundaries, presumably because stakeholders were not involved in the early stages.

In exploring the disconnect between human and ecosystem health, Palmer and Febria (2012), in their aptly titled paper 'Heartbeat of ecosystems', emphasize the enormous amount of research still needed to devise effective, scientifically objective and agreed measures of ecosystem health. However, the normative element of whose values decide what health entails is likely to remain problematic. Despite the difficulties in defining and measuring ecosystem health and One Health, the concepts provide useful metaphors upon which to base greater integrated management of the environment in ways that may improve the health of plants and animals, conserve biodiversity and ecosystem function, and maintain ecosystem services. It may ultimately make better sense to restrict the use of health concepts to system elements of particular concern, such as populations and habitats, rather than trying to apply them to an entire ecosystem or social-ecological system.

## One Health, Biodiversity and Ecosystems

There appear to be strong links between environmental change and both infectious and non-communicable diseases of humans, wild and domestic animals and plants. The health of animals and plants is influenced by the environment in which they exist, through both direct and indirect effects (Woolhouse and Gowtage-Sequeria, 2005). Direct effects refer to contacts between organisms and pathogens; their frequency and intensity may be influenced by changes in the biophysical and/or biotic environments. For example, environmental factors such as carcinogenic pollutants (e.g. pesticides, PCBs), endocrine-disrupting substances and geochemical variables (Davies, 2013) can directly affect the health of animals, plants and people. Indirect effects refer to those that influence aspects of pathogen transmission that are not directly linked to the target (host, reservoir) population. For example, land clearing for agriculture may favour mosquitoes and result in an increase in cases of human malaria (Patz *et al.*, 2004). Here we examine three aspects of the interrelationship between health and the environment: the influence of biodiversity on disease transmission, the potential influence of environmental and landscape homogenization on disease dynamics and food security, and the impacts of changing biogeochemical cycles on human and system health. Each has both direct and indirect elements, emphasizing the complexity of the relationships between pathogens and their environments.

## Biodiversity and Infectious Disease Transmission

Charles Elton (1957) drew attention to the greater frequency of outbreaks of pests and diseases in simplified ecological systems such as fields of crops, orchards and plantations in contrast to tropical forests with their high species and structural diversity where outbreaks seldom occurred. The relationship between host diversity and risk of infection in humans has been intensively studied in the case of Lyme disease, which is caused by a tick-borne spirochaete *Borrelia burgdorferi* and transmitted by an ixodid tick. Research in the USA on Lyme disease indicated that a greater diversity of hosts might lower transmission risks to humans (Van Buskirk and Ostfeld, 1995; Ostfeld and Keesing, 2000). The results further suggested that a dilution effect resulting from higher biodiversity in host populations may be a more general phenomenon. Its direct corollary (logical consequence of the theory), that a loss of biodiversity would likely result in an increase of infectious disease transmission to humans, was widely quoted. Biodiversity was thus seen as an ecosystem service that should be maintained to lower the risk of infectious diseases. However, Begon (2008), for example, used analytical models and empirical studies to investigate the effects of host diversity on disease dynamics and found little support for the probability of a dilution effect resulting from the presence of multiple host species. Wood and Lafferty (2013) found 'strong evidence for a positive link between biodiversity and Lyme disease at broad spatial scales (urban to suburban to rural) and equivocal evidence for a negative link between biodiversity and Lyme disease at varying levels of biodiversity within forests'. They concluded that, 'This finding suggests that, across zoonotic disease agents, the biodiversity–disease relationship is scale dependent and complex.' Li *et al.* (2012) explored the relationships between habitat fragmentation and Lyme disease using cellular automata models (i.e. grid-based, rule-driven spatial simulations) and found a strong relationship between Lyme disease risk, patch size and spatial configuration of patches of forest-grassland-bare ground in the landscape.

Although the links between disease risk from Lyme disease and biodiversity are complex and equivocal, evidence of dilution and/or amplification effects as a result of increasing host diversity has been found in several other studies of the relationship between disease and biodiversity. Pongsiri *et al.* (2009, in table 2) reviewed case studies linking biodiversity change to health effects in humans. These include an outbreak of hantavirus pulmonary syndrome in Panama that was associated with less diverse rodent assemblages, reduced West Nile virus infection rates in humans associated with high avian diversity, and increased incidence of human schistosomiasis in parts of Lake Malawi where the fish predators of intermediate snail hosts had been depleted. The concept of dilution in the transmission of vector-borne diseases remains controversial, however (Randolph and Dobson, 2012), because several different mechanisms can create a relationship between biodiversity and parasite or pathogen prevalence and these mechanisms do not uniformly lead to a negative relationship between prevalence and diversity. For example, Kilpatrick *et al.* (2006) found that robins in the south-west USA are particularly good reservoir hosts for West Nile virus, acting as 'super-spreaders' that can inflate infection rates and ultimately pathogen prevalence. In a randomly assembled community, the likelihood of including a super-spreader increases with the number of species that occur within the community, providing a potential mechanism by which biodiversity might increase rather than decrease pathogen prevalence within the system.

## Globalization, Emerging Diseases, Biodiversity and Food Security

Plants provide the basic support system for life on earth. Despite their pivotal importance, the health of both wild and domestic plants receives little attention beyond diseases of important agricultural crops and timber plantations, and remarkably little attention in the conservation literature.

Fisher *et al.* (2012) have highlighted the importance of emerging fungal diseases and their threats to animal, plant and ecosystem health. For example, fungi were found to be responsible for 72% of disease-related animal–host regional extirpations and extinctions, and 62% of plant–host regional extirpations and extinctions. There has also been a very sharp rise in the number of extirpation and extinction events post-2000 (Fisher *et al.*, 2012). The authors point out several key biological features of fungi that can result in host extinctions, such as high virulence to naive hosts, long-lived dormant or quiescent environmental stages, broad host ranges, rapid phenological responses to climate and habitat change and the ease with which spores can be transported around the globe.

Gurr *et al.* (2011) highlight the impacts of three fungal diseases (rice blast, wheat stem rust and late blight of potato) on global food security and two recently emerging diseases of animals with devastating effects, one on amphibians (chytridiomycosis) and one on bats (white nose syndrome). In an epidemiological analysis based on the disease triangle (Scholthof, 2007), Gurr *et al.* (2011) identified important gaps in the information required to control emerging fungal diseases. The Irish potato famine represents a classic example of the link between disease, food security and social disruption (Fraser, 2003). Invasive species that carry pathogens to which they are immune, but that can cause major declines or extinctions of naive species, emphasize the complexity of interactions between invasive species and diseases in ecosystems (Reynolds, 2013).

Disease dynamics are influenced by processes at several scales, from those of infectious agents to the landscapes in which they occur. Lambin *et al.* (2010) used eight case studies to explore the dynamic interaction between disease and landscape elements (see Fig. 4.1). Their study emphasizes the importance of adopting a more dynamic view of the spatial and temporal interaction between scales and between infectious agents, vectors, infected organisms and the range of biotic and abiotic factors that influence disease.

## Biogeochemical Cycles, Health and Planetary Boundaries

The last 60 years have witnessed a rapid acceleration in a wide range of environmental

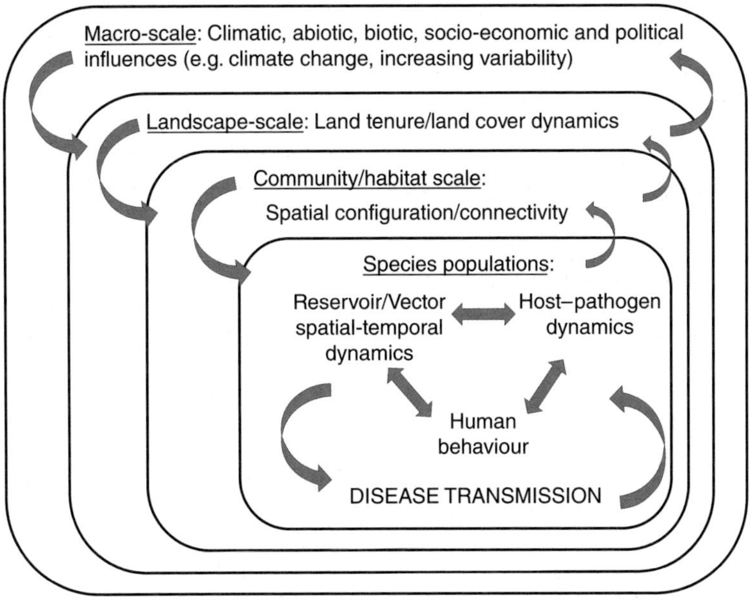


**Fig. 4.1.** Cross-scale landscape determinants of disease transmission with both top-down influences and bottom-up feedbacks between and across scales (simplified from Lambin *et al.*, 2010).

and social indicators of global change, such as human population growth, urban population growth, number of motor vehicles, increases in atmospheric $CO_2$, $N_2O$ and $CH_4$ concentrations, fertilizer consumption, water use, and loss of tropical forests (Syvitski, 2012). Associated with these rapid changes have been major increases in nutrient loading to ecosystems and fluxes of carbon, nitrogen and phosphorus, resulting in changes in ecosystem dynamics, function, and species loss (Rockstrom *et al.*, 2009). These changes have affected occurrences of infectious and non-infectious diseases (Johnson *et al.*, 2010). The increasing occurrence of harmful algal blooms, that release a range of hepatic, neural and gastro-intestinal toxins (O'Neil *et al.*, 2012), with wide-ranging ecosystem and health impacts in both freshwater and marine systems as a result of nutrient loading is one example (Vitousek *et al.*, 1997; Gachon *et al.*, 2010). Increasing environmental circulation of cadmium, lead and mercury that have directly harmful effects on humans and wildlife and the release into the environment of an increasing array of novel chemicals, such as pesticides, provides additional examples (Vitousek *et al.*, 1997).

## One Health and Social-ecological System (SES) Resilience

It is clear that many of the One Health-related concepts that have been developed in ecological contexts apply equally to the human community, and vice versa. For example, the importance of asymptomatic disease carriers is widely recognized in both human and animal epidemiology (Latorre-Margalef *et al.*, 2009; Gaidet *et al.*, 2010). The parallels between human and animal health go beyond parallels, however, with the realization that pathogens exist within a linked system of people and ecosystems in which changes in the health status of either the human community or the community of other animals can have knock-on effects through the entire system. For example, in the well-documented case of Indian vultures, diclofenac that was used to treat cattle depleted vulture numbers; declines in vulture numbers led to increases in populations of rats and feral dogs, which are vectors for a wide range of human pathogens; and the prevalence of related human diseases, such as rabies, increased. Increases in the numbers of rotting carcasses also had effects on water quality with direct impacts on human health.

Once the connections between social, economic and ecological systems are appreciated, and the likelihood that humans will respond to disease epidemics is recognized as part of the dynamics of the system, it becomes apparent that One Health is more than just a metaphor. It explicitly includes the issue of health in social-ecological systems (Zinsstag *et al.*, 2011). Social-ecological systems theory, which has arisen from the interplay of systems theory and complexity theory, offers one set of approaches for thinking about the ways in which the One Health concept might be further developed. Among its fundamental constructs are ideas about feedbacks, thresholds, adaptation and resilience (Folke *et al.*, 2004; Walker and Salt, 2006).

Feedbacks may be stabilizing (also termed 'negative', although not in a normative sense) or destabilizing (self-reinforcing, or 'positive'). Stabilizing feedbacks are responses within the system that tend to reduce the severity of fluctuations and push the system back towards a steady state. In human physiology, for example, sweat provides a stabilizing feedback in response to overheating. By contrast, destabilizing feedbacks amplify perturbations and often result in changes in the state of the system. For example, blood platelet clotting leads to further clotting. Most social-ecological systems that exist in a state of relative stability are maintained by a set of stabilizing feedbacks, such as the responses of health care services to disease epidemic events; by treating sick individuals, the potential for further pathogen transmission is reduced. By contrast, disease outbreaks become epidemics via destabilizing feedbacks, as occur when the number of infections increases exponentially in a naive population.

Perturbations, in combination with destabilizing feedbacks, may (if strong enough) push social-ecological systems into new domains or attractors in which their structure and function differ from what they were prior to the perturbation. This may involve the system taking on a new identity (Cumming and Collier, 2005). For example, the economic risks posed by outbreaks of H5N2 avian influenza on ostrich farms in Oudtshoorn, South Africa, have resulted in some farmers abandoning ostrich production and returning to more conventional farming systems. In these instances the nature of the farms has been transformed. Other farms appear to have been more resilient to avian influenza outbreaks and have continued with ostrich production despite suffering significant losses during recent H5N2 outbreaks.

Social-ecological systems respond to change through transformation, as in the ostrich example above, or by adaptation. In both cases, their ability to maintain their identity through a crisis is an indication of their resilience to that kind of shock. Resilience has also been defined as: (i) the amount of change that the system can undergo (hence, the extrinsic force that it can sustain) while still remaining within the same domain of attraction and retaining the same controls on structure and function; (ii) the degree to which the system is capable of self-organization (versus lack of organization, or organization forced by external factors); and (iii) the degree to which the system can build the capacity to learn and adapt (Carpenter *et al.*, 2001).

The emerging science of resilience management (Allen *et al.*, 2011) has high relevance to the One Health agenda. Rather than focusing on maximizing offtake (or other quantities) as the criterion for management success, resilience management focuses on building and enhancing the capacity of linked social-ecological systems to cope with perturbations (Holling and Meffe, 1996; Walker *et al.*, 2002; Allen *et al.*, 2011). Resilience approaches shift the domain of interest from a single system quantity to a more general, holistic overview that acknowledges the potential for unforeseen perturbations and surprises (Holling, 1986). In so doing, they have the potential to introduce subtle but important shifts in the ways that we approach problems. For instance, the potential relationships between biodiversity and disease regulation are not limited to effects that can be described by prevalence alone. In many cases the fundamental composition of the community has already been shaped by pathogens that have altered the species that are present. A resilience perspective provides a credible alternative in this instance, focusing less on the absolute levels of disease within the system and instead asking whether a higher biodiversity system is better able to withstand disease-related shocks (e.g. the emergence of novel pathogens or the introduction of new environmental contaminants) while maintaining basic elements of system structure and function. For example, high species diversity does not appear to have limited the spread of rinderpest in southern Africa or avian malaria in Hawaii; but in both cases, key ecological functions appear to have been retained. By contrast, the chestnut blight fungus in North America reduced forest cover by 25%, had significant impacts on populations of a wide range of vertebrates, and drove seven moth species to extinction. In comparing these and other examples of pathogen impacts, adopting a resilience perspective suggests a range of new and interesting questions, hypotheses and approaches that we might not have previously considered. For example, there should be predictable relationships between the food web position of the organisms that are affected by the pathogen and the eventual impact of the pathogen on ecosystem structure and function.

Social-ecological systems approaches recognize important roles for spatial and temporal variation and differences in the scales at which patterns and processes occur (Obrist *et al.*, 2010; Cumming, 2011). Shifts in complex systems occur when a limiting but slowly changing variable shrinks the domain of the attractor to a point at which the system can no longer remain in the same regime (Holling, 2001). In other words, something fundamental changes gradually, with profound consequences for the way that the system works. Standard examples include the accumulation of phosphorus in a clear-water shallow lake, or the age of spruce stands in a boreal forest (Holling, 1988; Carpenter, 2003). Once the phosphorus level in the lake is high enough to support algal growth, or the tree canopy of the forest is sufficiently dense to inhibit the regulation of spruce budworm populations by birds, a threshold may be crossed and the system can be propelled into a new state (with lower water quality or forest die-back, respectively). In a One Health context, potentially important slow variables include: the gradual increase in the human population (which might now sustain a global epidemic of a fast-moving, highly virulent pathogen); the huge changes over the last century in transport technologies and volumes, which permit greater mixing and dispersal of pathogens of both humans and livestock than ever before; the gradual depletion of biodiversity, with its legacy of simplified and potentially unstable ecosystems (e.g. those lacking upper trophic levels), which may have left many social-ecological systems more vulnerable to certain kinds of pathogen; and the gradual increases in production of contaminants and nutrients that are increasingly testing the coping abilities of ecosystems (MA, 2005a,b).

Although we have considered slow variables in relation to temporal dynamics, the examples discussed above also have important spatial scaling and cross-scale components (Cumming, 2011). Cross-scale feedbacks occur when A influences B and B influences A, and A and B occur at different scales. Sometimes processes that occur at smaller spatial scales, such as deforestation or pathogen transmission cycles, can be scaled up through contagious or mass effects. The removal of a single tree has little effect on the global environment, but if each person cuts a tree a week, the effect can be massive. Similarly, local disease dynamics can be up-scaled through dispersal and contagion. For example, ostrich production systems in southern Africa have been vulnerable to outbreaks of high pathogenicity avian influenza (HPAI). The spread of HPAI between ostrich farms has been facilitated by the deliberate movements of ostriches of successive life stages between different farms. Network analysis suggests that expanding the ostrich movement network over time resulted in a loss of resilience in the ostrich production system prior to the last major HPAI outbreak in 2011 (Moore *et al.*, 2014). Deliberately creating different 'compartments' and then permitting farmers to exchange birds within compartments but not between compartments could enhance resilience in this system. It is precisely because of these effects that the world watches each new local outbreak of highly pathogenic avian influenza anxiously to see whether it might become an epidemic or a pandemic (Pickles, 2006; Morens *et al.*, 2008; Krauss and Webster, 2010). Despite their importance for global health, however, cross-scale epidemiological interactions are poorly understood and there has been relatively little research on the scaling of infectious disease dynamics in ecological communities.

## Conclusion

In the next decade we can expect increasingly detailed insights into the complexity of relationships between changing environmental factors and disease. These developments will be further accelerated by the emergence of larger data sets and advances in analytical and statistical techniques. The likely result is the rapid development of new paradigms in epidemiology and ecology of both infectious and non-infectious diseases.

The roles of biodiversity, biodiversity loss and the likely pervasive effects of altered biogeochemical cycles together with increasing numbers of new manufactured chemical compounds on the environment, the dynamics of human, wild and domestic animals, and plant diseases and health is clearly a priority research area for One Health. Further, there is now an increasing appreciation that we are dealing with health issues within a complex adaptive systems framework. Approaching the management of health (animal, plant and environmental) through the lens of resilience and the sustainability of social-ecological systems, as outlined briefly here, promises to bring new insights into, and strengthen, the developing One Health paradigm.

## Notes

[1] A Google search for 'ecosystem health' will turn up >900,000 hits, and Google Scholar >60,000.

[2] In July 2013 Monsanto withdrew from attempts to introduce GM crops in Europe citing interminable delays in the decision making and regulatory process. 'The decision covered five EU approval requests to grow genetically modified maize, plus one soybean and one sugar beet.' Reuters 25/07/13.

## References

Allen, C.R., Cumming, G.S., Garmestani, A., Taylor, P.D. and Walker, B.H. (2011) Managing for resilience. *Wildlife Biology* 17, 337–349.

Anderson, R.M. (1991) The eighth Tansley Lecture. Populations and infectious diseases: ecology or epidemiology? *Journal of Animal Ecology* 60, 1–50.

Anderson, R.M. and May, R.M. (1978) Regulation and stability of host-parasite population interactions, I. Regulatory processes. *Journal of Animal Ecology* 47, 219–247.

Begon, M. (2008) Effects of host diversity on disease dynamics. In: Ostfeld, R.S., Keesing, F. and Eviner, V.T. (eds) *Infectious Disease Ecology: Effects of Ecosystems on Disease and of Disease on Ecosystems*. Princeton University Press, Princeton, New Jersey, pp. 12–29.

Berkes, F., Doubleday, N.C. and Cumming, G.S. (2012) Aldo Leopold's land health from a resilience point of view: self-renewal capacity of social–ecological systems. *EcoHealth* 9, 278–287.

Bhatt, S., Gething, P.W., Brady, O.J., Messina, J.P., Farlow, A.W., Moyes, C.L., Drake, J.M., Brownstein, J.S., Hoen, A.G., Sankoh, O., Myers, M.F., George, D.B., Jaenisch, T., Wint, G.R.W., Simmons, C.P., Scott, T.W., Farrar, J.J. and Hay, S.I. (2013) The global distribution and burden of dengue. *Nature* 496, 504–507.

Bonds, M.H., Keenan, D.C., Rohani, P. and Sachs, J.D. (2009) Poverty trap formed by the ecology of infectious diseases. *Proceedings of the Royal Society B: Biological Sciences* 277, 1185–1192.

Bonds, M.H., Dobson, A.P. and Keenan, D.C. (2012) Disease ecology, biodiversity, and the latitudinal gradient in income. *PLoS Biol* 10(12): e1001456. doi:10.1371/journal.pbio.1001456

Botkin, D.B. (1990) *Discordant Harmonies: A New Ecology for the Twenty-First Century*. Oxford University Press, New York.

Callicott, J.B. (1992) Aldo Leopold's metaphor. In: Costanza R., Norton, B.G. and Haskell, B.D. (eds) *Ecosystem Health: New Goals for Environmental Management*. Island Press, Washington, DC, pp. 42–56.

Carpenter, S. (2003) *Regime Shifts in Lake Ecosystems: Patterns and Variation*. Excellence in Ecology Series Number 15, Ecology Institute, Oldendorf/Luhe, Germany.

Carpenter, S., Walker, B., Anderies, J.M. and Abel, N. (2001) From metaphor to measurement: resilience of what to what? *Ecosystems* 4, 765–781.

Carson, R. (1962) *Silent Spring*. Houghton Mifflin, Boston, Massachusetts.

Cook, R.A., Karesh, W.B. and Osofsky, S.A. (2004) The Manhattan Principles on 'One World, One Health.' New York: Wildlife Conservation Society. Available at: http://www.oneworldonehealth.org (accessed 1 August 2013).

Costanza, R. (2012) Ecosystem health and ecological engineering. *Ecological Engineering* 45, 24–29.

Cumming, G.S. (2010) Risk mapping for avian influenza: a social–ecological problem. *Ecology and Society* 15(3), 32.

Cumming, G.S. (2011) *Spatial Resilience in Social-Ecological Systems*. Springer, Dordrecht, the Netherlands.

Cumming, G.S. and Collier, J. (2005) Change and identity in complex systems. *Ecology and Society* 10, 29.

Davies, T.C. (2013) Geochemical variables as plausible aetiological cofactors in the incidence of some common environmental diseases in Africa. *Journal of African Earth Sciences* 79, 24–49.

Elton, C. (1927) *Animal Ecology*. Sedgwick & Jackson, London.

Elton, C. (1957) *The Ecology of Invasions by Animals and Plants*. Methuen, London.

Fauci, A.S., Touchette, N.A. and Folkers, G.K. (2005) Emerging infectious diseases: a 10-year perspective from the National Institute of Allergy and Infectious Diseases. *Emerging Infectious Diseases* 11, 519–525.

Fisher, M.C., Henk, D.A., Briggs, C.J., Brownstein, J.S., Madoff, L.C., McCraw, S.L. and Gurr, S.J. (2012) Emerging fungal threats to animal, plant and ecosystem health. *Nature* 484, 186–194.

Foley, J.A., DeFries, R., Asner, G.P., Barford, C., Bonan, G., Carpenter, S.R., Chapin, F.S., Coe, M.T., Daily, G.C., Gibbs, H.K., Helkowski, J.H., Holloway, T., Howard, E.A., Kucharik, C.J., Monfreda, C., Patz, J.A., Prentice, I.C., Ramankutty, N. and Snyder, P.K. (2005) Global consequences of land use. *Science* 309, 570–574.

Folke, C., Carpenter, S., Walker, B., Scheffer, M., Elmqvist, T., Gunderson, L. and Holling, C.S. (2004) Regime shifts, resilience, and biodiversity in ecosystem management. *Annual Review of Ecology, Evolution, and Systematics* 35, 557–581.

Fraser, E. (2003) Social vulnerability and ecological fragility: building bridges between social and natural sciences using the Irish potato famine as a case study. *Conservation Ecology* 7(2), 9.

Gachon, C.M.M., Sime-Ngando, T., Strittmatter, M., Chambouvet, A. and Kim, G.H. (2010) Algal diseases: spotlight on a black box. *Trends in Plant Science* 15, 633–640.

Gaidet, N., Cappelle, J., Takekawa, J.Y., Prosser, D.J., Iverson, S.A., Douglas, D.C., Perry, W.M., Mundkur, T. and Newman, S.H. (2010) Potential spread of highly pathogenic avian influenza H5N1 by wildfowl: dispersal ranges and rates determined from large-scale satellite telemetry. *Journal of Applied Ecology* 47, 1147–1157.

Gleason, H.A. (1939) The individualistic concept of plant association. *American Midland Naturalist* 21, 92–110.
Guha-Sapir, D. and Schimmer, B. (2005) New paradigms for a changing epidemiology. *Emerging Themes in Epidemiology* 2, 1 doi:10.1186/1742-7622-2-1.
Gurr, S., Samalova, M. and Fisher, M. (2011) The rise and rise of emerging infectious fungi challenges food security and ecosystem health. *Fungal Biology Reviews* 25, 181–188.
Heink, U., Bartz, R. and Kowarik, I. (2012) How useful are the concepts of familiarity, biological integrity, and ecosystem health for evaluating damages by GM crops? *Journal of Agricultural and Environmental Ethics* 25, 3–17.
Helping, D. (2013) Globally networked risks and how to respond. *Nature* 497, 51–59.
Holling, C.S. (1986) The resilience of terrestrial ecosystems: local surprise and global change. In: Clark, W.C. and Munn, R.E. (eds) *Sustainable Development of the Biosphere*. Cambridge University Press, Cambridge, pp. 292–317.
Holling, C.S. (1988) Temperate forest insect outbreaks, tropical deforestation and migratory birds. *Memoirs of the Entomological Society of Canada* 146, 22–32.
Holling, C.S. (2001) Understanding the complexity of economic, ecological, and social systems. *Ecosystems* 4, 390–405.
Holling, C.S. and Meffe, G.K. (1996) Command and control and the pathology of natural resource management. *Conservation Biology* 10, 328–337.
Jax, K. (2010) *Ecosystem Functioning*. Cambridge University Press, Cambridge, UK.
Johnson, P.T.J., Townsend, A.R., Cleveland, C.C., Glibert, P.M., Howarth, R.W., McKenzie, V.J., Rejmankova, E. and Ward, M.H. (2010) Linking environmental nutrient enrichment and disease emergence in humans and wildlife. *Ecological Applications* 20, 16–29.
Kant, S., Maurya, A.K., Kushwaha, R.A.S., Nag, V.L. and Prasad, R. (2010) Multi-drug resistant tuberculosis: an iatrogenic problem. *Bioscience Trends* 4, 48–55.
Karesh, W.B., Osofsky, S.A., Rocke, T.E. and Barrows, P.L. (2002) Joining forces to improve our world. *Conservation Biology* 16, 1432–1434.
Kilpatrick, M., Daszak, P., Jones, M.J., Marra, P.P., Ishii, N. and Fujii, N. (2006) Host heterogeneity dominates West Nile virus transmission. *Proceedings of the Royal Society of London, B, Biological Sciences* 276, 2327–2333.
Krauss, S. and Webster, R.G. (2010) Avian influenza virus surveillance and wild birds: past and present. *Avian Diseases* 54, 394–398.
Kuhn, T.S. (1970) *The Structure of Scientific Revolutions*, 2nd edn. University of Chicago Press, Chicago, Illinois.
Lackey, R.T. (2001) Scientific objectivity, value systems, and policymaking. *BioScience* 51, 437–443.
Lackey, R.T. (2003) Appropriate use of ecosystem health and normative science in ecological policy. In: Rapport, D.J., Lasley, W.L., Rolston, D.E., Nielsen, N.O., Qualset, C.Q. and Damania, A.B. (eds) *Managing for Healthy Ecosystems*. Lewis Publishers, Boca Raton, Florida, pp. 175–186.
Lackey, R.T. (2004) Normative science. *Fisheries* 29, 38–39.
Lackey, R.T. (2007) Science, scientists and policy advocacy. *Conservation Biology* 21, 12–17.
Lafferty, K.D. and Gerber, L.R. (2002) Good medicine for conservation biology: the intersection of epidemiology and conservation theory. *Conservation Biology* 16, 593–604.
Lakatos, I. (1978) *The Methodology of Scientific Research Programmes*. Cambridge University Press, Cambridge, UK.
Lambin, E.F., Tran, A., Vanwambeke, S.O., Linard, C. and Soti, V. (2010) Pathogenic landscapes: interactions between land, people, disease vectors, and their animal hosts. *International Journal of Health Geographics* 9, 54.
Latorre-Margalef, N., Gunnarsson, G., Munster, V.J., Fouchier, R.A.M., Osterhaus, A., Elmberg, J., Olsen, B., Wallensten, A., Haemig, P.D., Fransson, T., Brudin, L. and Waldenstrom, J. (2009) Effects of influenza A virus infection on migrating mallard ducks. *Proceedings of the Royal Society B, Biological Sciences* 276, 1029–1036.
Li, S., Hartemink, N., Speybroeck, N. and Vanwambeke, S.O. (2012) Consequences of landscape fragmentation on Lyme disease risk: a cellular automata approach. *PLoS One* 7, e39612, 1–12.
MA (2005a) (Millennium Assessment) *Ecosystems and Human Well-being: Biodiversity Synthesis*. Island Press, Washington, DC.
MA (2005b) (Millennium Assessment) *Ecosystems and Human Well-being: Scenarios. Findings of the Scenarios Working Group*. Island Press, Washington, DC.
May, R.M. and Anderson, R.M. (1978) Regulation and stability of host-parasite population interactions, II. Destabilising processes. *Journal of Animal Ecology* 47, 249–267.
Meffe, G.K. (1999) Conservation medicine. *Conservation Biology* 13, 953–954.

Moore, C., Cumming, G.S., Slingsby, J. and Grewar, J. (2014) Tracking socioeconomic vulnerability using network analysis: insights from an avian influenza outbreak in an ostrich production network. *PLoS ONE* 9(1), e86973. doi:10.1371/journal.pone.0086973
Morand, S., Beaudeau, F. and Cabaret, J. (2012) *New Frontiers of Molecular Epidemiology of Infectious Diseases*. Springer, Dordrecht, the Netherlands.
Morens, D.M., Folkers, G.K. and Fauci, A.S. (2008) Emerging infections: a perpetual challenge. *Lancet Infectious Diseases* 8, 710–719.
Muñoz-Erickson, T.A., Aguilar-González, B. and Sisk, T.D. (2007) Linking ecosystem health indicators and collaborative management: a systematic framework to evaluate ecological and social outcomes. *Ecology and Society* 12(2), 6.
Nekola, J.C., Allen, C.D., Brown, J.H., Burger, J.R., Davidson, A.D., Fristoe, T.S., Hamilton, M.J., Hammond, S.T., Kodric-Brown, A., Mercado-Silva, N. and Okie, J.G. (2013) The Malthusian–Darwinian dynamic and the trajectory of civilization. *Trends in Ecology and Evolution* 28, 127–130.
Norberg, J. and Cumming, G.S. (2008) *Complexity Theory for a Sustainable Future*. Columbia University Press, New York.
Obrist, B., Pfeiffer, C. and Henley, R. (2010) Multi-layered social resilience: a new approach in mitigation research. *Progress in Development Studies* 10, 283–293.
O'Neil, J.M., Davis, T.W., Burford, M.A. and Gobler, C.J. (2012) The rise of harmful cyanobacteria blooms: the potential roles of eutrophication and climate change. *Harmful Algae* 14, 313–334.
Osofsky, S.A., Karesh, W.B. and Deem, S.L. (2000) Conservation Medicine: a veterinary perspective. *Conservation Biology* 14, 336–337.
Ostfeld, R.S. and Keesing, F. (2000) Biodiversity and disease risk: the case of Lyme disease. *Conservation Biology* 14, 722–728.
Palmer, M.A. and Febria, C.M. (2012) The heartbeat of ecosystems. *Science* 336, 1393–1394.
Patz, J.A., Daszak, P., Tabor, G.M., Aguirre, A.A., Pearl, M., Epstein, J., Wolfe, N.D., Kilpatrick, A.M., Foufopoulos, J., Molyneux, D. and Bradley, D.J. (2004) Unhealthy landscapes: policy recommendations on land use change and infectious disease emergence. *Environmental Health Perspectives* 112, 1092–1098.
Pickett, S.T.A. and Cadenasso, M.L. (2002) The ecosystem as a multidimensional concept: meaning, model, and metaphor. *Ecosystems* 5, 1–10.
Pickett, S.T.A., Jones, C. and Kolasa, J. (2007) *Ecological Understanding: the Nature of Theory and the Theory of Nature*. Academic Press, New York.
Pickles, H. (2006) Avian influenza - preparing for the pandemic - using lessons from the past to plan for pandemic flu. *British Medical Journal* 332, 783–786.
Plowright, R.K., Sokolow, S.H., Gorman, M.E., Daszak, P. and Foley, J.E. (2008) Causal inference in disease ecology: investigating ecological drivers of disease emergence. *Frontiers in Ecology and Environment* 6, 420–429.
Pongsiri, M.J., Roman, J., Ezenwa, V.O., Goldberg, T.L., Koren, H.S., Newbold, S.C., Ostfeld, R.S., Pattanayak, S.K. and Salkeld, D.J. (2009) Biodiversity loss affects global disease ecology. *BioScience* 59, 945–954.
Randolph, S.E. and Dobson, A.D.M. (2012) Pangloss revisited: a critique of the dilution effect and the biodiversity-buffers-disease paradigm. *Parasitology-Cambridge* 139, 847–864.
Reynolds, S.E. (2013) Immunity and invasive success. *Science* 340, 816–817.
Rockstrom, J., Steffen, W., Noone, K., Persson, A., Chapin, F.S., Lambin, E., Lenton, T.M., Scheffer, M., Folke, C., Schellnhuber, H., Nykvist, B., De Wit, C.A., Hughes, T., van der Leeuw, S., Rodhe, H., Sörlin, S., Snyder, P.K., Costanza, R., Svedin, U., Falkenmark, M., Karlberg, L., Corell, R.W., Fabry, V.J., Hansen, J., Walker, B.H., Liverman, D., Richardson, K., Crutzen, C. and Foley, J. (2009) A safe operating space for humanity. *Nature* 461, 472–475.
Scholthof, K.-B.G. (2007) The disease triangle: pathogens, the environment and society. *Nature Reviews: Microbiology* 5, 152–156.
Schwartz, S., Susser, E. and Susser, M. (1999) A future for epidemiology. *Annual Review of Public Health* 20, 15–33.
Sheail, J. (1987) *Seventy-five Years in Ecology: the British Ecological Society*. Blackwell Scientific Publications, Oxford, UK.
Singer, M. and Baer, H. (2012) *Introducing Medical Anthropology: A Discipline in Action*. AltaMira Press, Plymouth, UK.
Susser, M. and Susser, E. (1996a) Choosing a future for epidemiology: I. Eras and paradigms. *American Journal of Public Health* 86, 668–673.

Susser, M. and Susser, E. (1996b) Choosing a future for epidemiology: II. From black box to Chinese boxes and eco-epidemiology. *American Journal of Public Health* 86, 674–677.
Syvitski, J. (2012) Anthropocene: an epoch of our making. *Global Change*, Issue 78, 12–15.
Tansley, A.G. (1935) The use and abuse of vegetational concepts and terms. *Ecology* 16, 284–307.
Van Buskirk, J. and Ostfeld, R.S. (1995) Controlling Lyme disease by modifying the density and species composition of tick hosts. *Ecological Applications* 5, 1133–1140.
Vitousek, P.M., Mooney, H.A., Lubchenco, J. and Melillo, J. (1997) Human domination of earth's ecosystems. *Science* 277, 494–499.
Walker, B. and Salt, D. (2006) *Resilience Thinking: Sustaining Ecosystems and People in a Changing World.* Island Press, Washington, DC.
Walker, B., Carpenter, S., Anderies, J., Abel, N., Cumming, G.S., Janssen, M., Lebel, L., Norberg, J., Peterson, G.D. and Pritchard, R. (2002) Resilience management in social-ecological systems: a working hypothesis for a participatory approach. *Conservation Ecology* 6, 14.
Waltner-Toews, D., Kay, J.J. and Lister, N.-M.E. (2008) *The Ecosystem Approach: Complexity, Uncertainty, and Managing for Sustainability*. Columbia University Press, New York.
Wiegand, J., Raffaelli, D., Smart, J.C.R. and White, P.C.L. (2010) Assessment of temporal trends in ecosystem health using an holistic indicator. *Journal of Environmental Management* 91, 1446–1455.
Wood, C.L. and Lafferty, K.D. (2013) Biodiversity and disease: a synthesis of ecological perspectives on Lyme disease transmission. *Trends in Ecology and Evolution* 28, 239–247.
Woodward, G., Gessner, M.O., Giller, P.S., Gulis, V., Hladyz, S., Lecerf, A., Malmqvist, B., McKie, B.G., Tiegs, S.D., Cariss, H., Dobson, M., Elosegi, A., Ferreira, V., Graça, M.A.S., Fleituch, T., Lacoursière, J.O., Nistorescu, M., Pozo, J., Risnoveanu, G., Schindler, M., Vadineanu, A., Vought, L.B.-M. and Chauvet, E. (2012) Continental-scale effects of nutrient pollution on stream ecosystem functioning. *Science* 336, 1438–1440.
Woolhouse, M.E.J. and Gowtage-Sequeria, S. (2005) Host range and emerging and reemerging pathogens. *Emerging Infectious Diseases* 11, 1842–1847.
Zinsstag, J. (2012) Convergence of Ecohealth and One Health. *EcoHealth* 9, 371–373.
Zinsstag, J., Schelling, E., Waltner-Toews, D. and Tanner, M. (2011) From 'one medicine' to One Health and systemic approaches to health and well-being. *Preventive Veterinary Medicine* 101, 148–156.

# 5 Measuring Added Value from Integrated Methods

**Jakob Zinsstag,[1,2]* Mahamat Béchir Mahamat[2] and Esther Schelling[1,2]**
*[1]Swiss Tropical and Public Health Institute, Basel, Switzerland; [2]University of Basel, Basel, Switzerland; [2]Ministère de Santé Publique, and Centre de Support en Santé Internationale, N'Djaména, Chad*

## Introduction

In Chapter 2 (this volume) we have proposed a working definition of One Health as any added value in terms of health of humans and animals, financial savings or environmental services, which is achievable by the cooperation of human and veterinary medicine when compared to the two medicines working alone (Zinsstag *et al.*, Chapter 2, this volume). Cooperation between different disciplines should lead to an added value or synergistic effect. Otherwise such cooperation can be hardly justified, especially if it requires investment in time, financial resources and intellectual effort of connecting research and implementation methods. We should mention here that many issues in human and veterinary medicine, like fundamental research, drug and surgery development, are closely connected. Others are so highly specialized that they cannot and need not be interconnected. The modern concept of One Health aims at identifying areas in both medicines and their related sciences, such as public health, which have the potential to generate further added value. In Fig. 5.1, we list some areas where both medicines collaborate already closely or appropriately concentrate on their specialist field. Priority activities of One Health are presented as part of an intersecting set within a social-ecological system.

This chapter concentrates on the question of 'added value' as a constituent part of modern One Health conceptual thinking. Why this is needed has already been outlined in Chapter 2 with the example of poor early communication between public and animal health authorities that contributed to the recent Q-fever outbreak in the Netherlands leading to thousands of avoidable human cases (Enserink, 2010). However, added value through fostered communication leading to earlier detection may be difficult to quantify in some instances, because alternative scenarios do not mean nothing would be done. For example, joint surveillance can be described qualitatively resulting in a shortened decision pathway.

What does an 'added value' really mean and how can it be measured? Depending on the type of added value, new methods are required to quantify or qualify the benefits of such a closer cooperation. Added value of closer cooperation may appear at different levels within a web of causation (Fig. 5.2). The most proximal added values are *saved human and animal lives, reduced human and animal suffering, financial savings and improved ecosystem*

*E-mail: jakob.zinsstag@unibas.ch

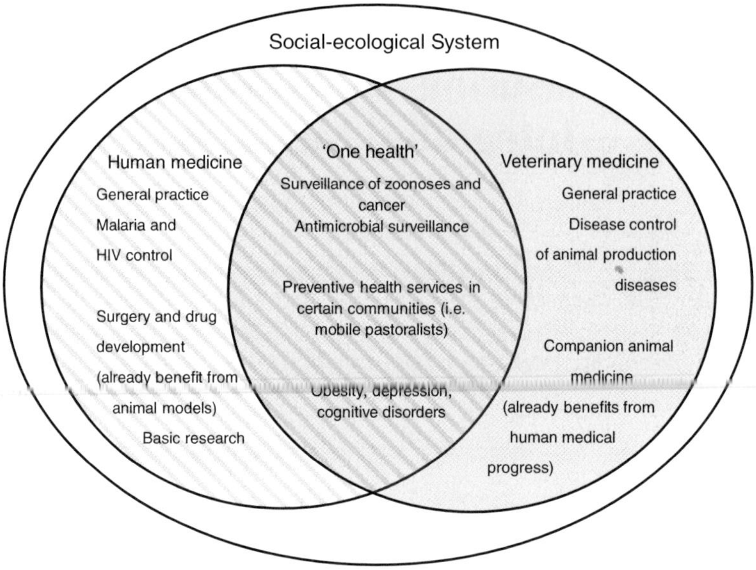


**Fig. 5.1.** Examples of 'stand alone' activities of human and veterinary medicine versus priority One Health activities that would generate an added value through closer cooperation.

*services* (such as pasture management, reforestation and safe water). Such a web is open and can be extended further as new evidence becomes available. It can happen that a suggested animal–human linkage is actually only of marginal importance and an integrated approach is therefore not necessary. For example, although bovine tuberculosis is an important animal disease in Ethiopia, we found only very few human cases and consequently did not include a public health economic assessment of its cost, but stayed with a restricted cost estimate for the Ethiopian livestock production (Tschopp *et al.*, 2013; Tschopp, Chapter 15, this volume).

## Reduced Time to Detection of Disease

Cross-sectional animal–human disease frequency studies on brucellosis and Q-fever may identify the animal source of human disease more quickly (Schelling *et al.*, 2003; Bonfoh *et al.*, 2012). This requires methods that are able to relate animal and human disease frequency in space and time (see also Schelling and Hattendorf, Chapter 10, this volume). Another example is the recording of the number of dog-bite victims for every rabies-suspected dog diagnosed in a veterinary laboratory (Kayali *et al.*, 2003; Léchenne *et al.*, Chapter 16, this volume). This approach should be connected with studies on dog-bite victims in health centres and hospitals to obtain a more complete view on the effective incidence of suspected dog bites and human exposure (Cleaveland *et al.*, 2002; Frey *et al.*, 2013; Léchenne *et al.*, Chapter 16, this volume). Ecological studies identify the linkage and importance of animal–human nutrition flows. In mobile pastoralist women in Chad we could show that human serum retinol levels depended on the milk retinol and beta-carotene content of their cattle (Zinsstag *et al.*, 2002; Béchir *et al.*, Chapter 23, this volume). Such studies can be extended to assessing the source of hygiene-related pathogens and contaminants like heavy metals (Forget and Lebel, 2001). At this point One Health is extended to ecosystem health (http://www.ecohealth.net), including ecosystem services (see below and Zinsstag *et al.*, Chapter 2, this volume). The above examples result in *reduced time to detection and earlier intervention at the source*. A similar effect could be expected from interconnected

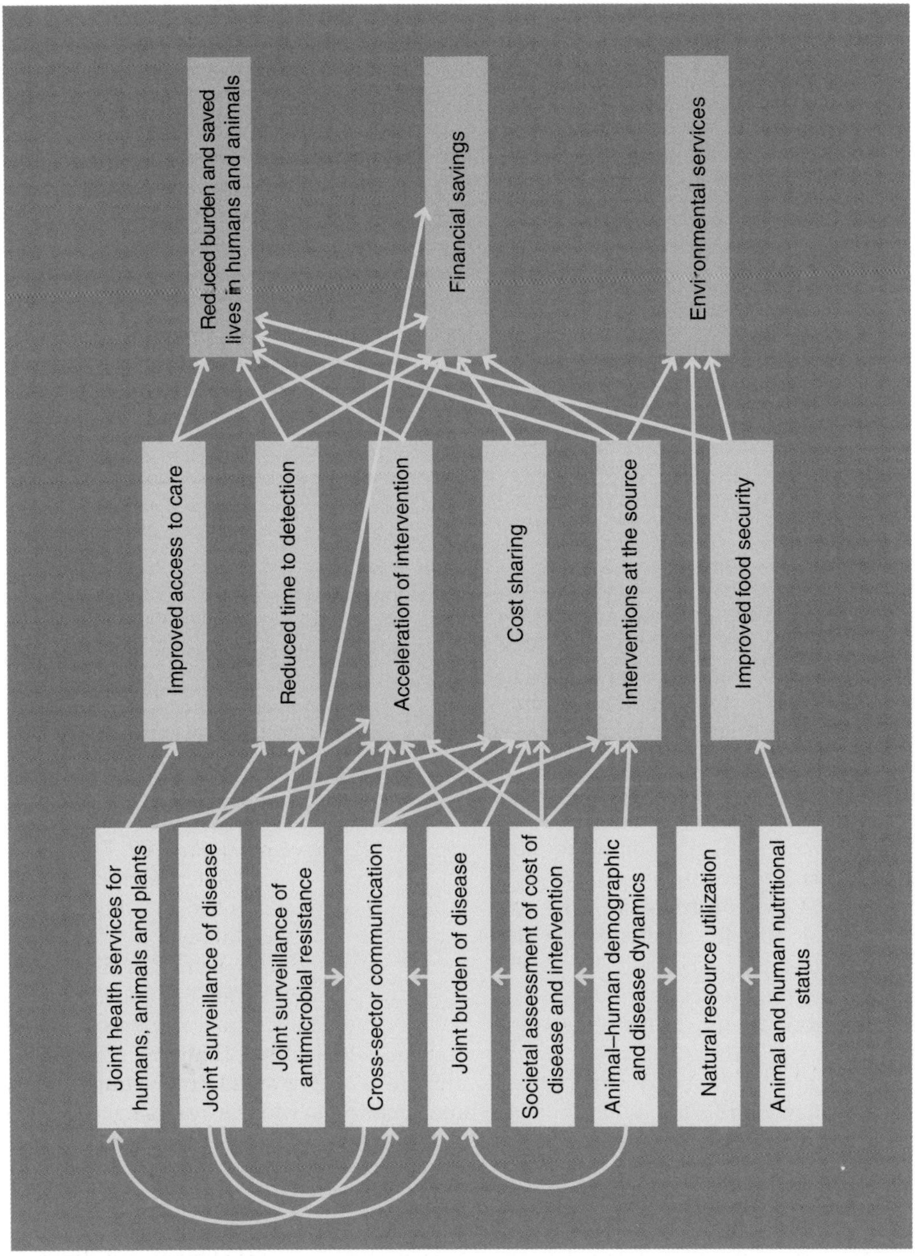


**Fig. 5.2.** Web of causation of distal and proximal added value of One Health.

surveillance of zoonoses in humans and animals, or of antimicrobial resistance. For example, the Canadian integrated programme for antimicrobial resistance surveillance oversees the occurrence of antimicrobial resistance in humans, animals and the environment simultaneously (http://www.phac-aspc.gc.ca/cipars-picra/index-eng.php). This integrated surveillance involves not only the technical capacity, sharing of equipment and human resources, but most importantly *cross-sector communication* and decision pathways.

## Joint Burden of Disease

Often diseases and health risks not only affect human lives but also animal lives. The assessment of the burden of disease in humans and animals is important for ethical, ecological and economic reasons. For example, road traffic does not only kill humans but many more wild animals (Erritzoe *et al.*, 2003).

We do not recommend extending the methods for the measurement of the burden of disease in humans (disability adjusted life years (DALYs)) to animals but rather financial valuing of losses to animal production in a given context (Zinsstag *et al.*, Chapter 12, this volume). In turn, this does not consider the emotional value of companion animals that goes beyond a financial value of livestock. Similarly, the expression of the value of human life as valued statistical life (VSL) is controversial. The use of DALY has a broader acceptance in the health economic literature and in public health, because the former bears the risk of maximizing good health rather than minimizing ill-health burden (Shwiff *et al.*, 2013). For example, brucellosis transmission causes human suffering, which can be expressed as loss in DALYs and a financial loss to livestock production (Roth *et al.*, 2003). In most cases the added value of a One Health approach is thus presented as an array of outputs composed of saved lives, financial savings and possibly qualitative gain. Assessing the *joint impact of disease in humans and animals* is thus an important added value for decision making.

## Societal Cost of Disease and Sharing of Costs

Cross-sector economic studies address cost of disease to the sectors of public health, livestock production and other sectors such as markets and tourism. Interventions in one sector may result in benefits in the other sectors, thus providing a more comprehensive view of *the societal cost of disease and benefits of disease control*. This clearly adds value when compared to benefits of a single sector (Roth *et al.*, 2003; Zinsstag *et al.*, 2007; Zinsstag *et al.*, Chapter 12, this volume). Understanding the societal and ecological effects of a disease or risk provides the economic argument to negotiate the *sharing of intervention cost* between sectors, which reduces the cost to individual sectors, albeit not to society. In joint disease surveillance systems, further cost savings can be obtained from sharing of laboratory resources, expensive equipment and manpower. For example, the currently only tuberculosis laboratory in Chad handles human and livestock samples and hence saves financial and human resources of running two mycobacteria laboratories, one for public health and one for the veterinary services (Diguimbaye *et al.*, 2006; Diguimbaye-Djaibe *et al.*, 2006). The Canadian Science Centre in Winnipeg is a high security laboratory for human and animal diseases under one roof. Savings on operations are estimated at 26% when compared to two fully separated laboratories (World Bank, 2012).

## Interventions with Highest Leverage

Transmission of disease between animals and humans is often dynamic, requiring mathematical models to address non-linear processes (Zinsstag *et al.*, Chapter 11, this volume). Such models allow simulating interventions in different sectors and together with economic analyses. In this way *interventions with the highest leverage, profitability and best cost-effectiveness* can be identified between all involved sectors. For example, a dog–human model of rabies transmission in an African city clearly showed that dog mass vaccination became more profitable and cost-effective after 6 years, when compared to human post-exposure prophylaxis alone. These results could not be obtained from separate studies in dogs and humans (Zinsstag *et al.*, 2009). The best intervention for a zoonosis may be outside the health sectors. For example, neurocysticercosis in people can be effectively controlled by reducing open defecation in people.

## Access to Care

Lack of access to health care for human and animals is one of the main reasons for the poor community effectiveness of health interventions (Obrist *et al.*, 2007). A better understanding of the factors determining access to health care and subsequent implementation may have even a higher leverage on the improvement of health status than a new drug or vaccine (Zinsstag *et al.*, 2011a). One such example emanated from a joint study of the vaccination status in humans and animals among mobile pastoralists in Chad. Livestock were vaccinated during compulsory veterinary campaigns, but no child was vaccinated. Negotiations with the Chadian health and livestock authorities led to joint preventive health services to humans and animals. This led to *improved access to care* for communities who were previously not served (Schelling *et al.*, 2007; Schelling *et al.*, Chapter 20, this volume). In many developing but also industrialized countries, there is a permanent human resource crisis in the health and veterinary sectors. Service provision to humans, animals and plants (Boa *et al.*, Chapter 22, this volume) is an open field for innovation. Scarce resources for transport are another critical aspect that may lead to new forms of cost sharing and cross-sector communication.

## Food Security

Despite all the technical progress in food production, food security remains a painful shortfall of decades of international development cooperation. Its causes are a complex interplay of social, economic and ecological factors to which a One Health approach can contribute. Animal source food and livestock production directly affect populations such as mobile pastoralists (Béchir, 2010; Béchir *et al.*, 2012a,b) but also a large part of the estimated 800 million small-scale farmers for which their livelihoods depend essentially or partially from livestock production (Béchir *et al.*, Chapter 23, this volume). Cross-sector studies of human and animal food security may lead to improved emergency planning for destocking and restocking of livestock in pastoralist production systems, saving human lives but also reducing animal suffering. For example, during the drought period in 2006 in the Sahelian countries, early destocking and conservation of animal source food on the spot could have saved substantial resources and human lives (Plate 3).

## Ecosystem Services

Addressing health issues at the human–animal interface depends on ecosystem services such as clean water, pasture for grazing and others. Work on brucellosis in Mongolia involving livestock demographic simulation revealed dramatic effects of political change and climate variability. The end of the socialist period led to a rapid increase of livestock populations, especially goats, because of the high market value of cashmere. In the same time consecutive snowstorm catastrophes (dzud) killed several tens of millions of animals. Overall the Mongolian livestock population has increased to a level causing substantial degradation of pasture (Shabb *et al.*, 2013). Future Mongolian livestock development policy should consider stabilizing livestock population size to maintain pasture availability. Future livestock production will depend on mitigation of pasture degradation. Animal disease control and elimination (i.e. foot and mouth disease) plays an important role for future livestock and meat exports by reducing stocking density. This example shows how health and ecosystem services are intimately connected. This field of research is specifically addressed by so called 'ecosystem approaches to health' in which One Health is embedded (Charron, 2012; Zinsstag, 2012).

Sustained or restored environmental services can be an important added value but their assessment requires advanced study design capable of measuring a causal relationship between health in humans and animals and ecosystem services. Future systemic study designs to human and animal health will quantify causal linkages to social-ecological systems resulting in an array of additional added value (Ostrom, 2007; Zinsstag *et al.*, 2011b).

## Conclusion

In this chapter we concentrated on those examples of added value for which we have empirical evidence. Additional added value can be expected from numerous other aspects and types of collaboration between human and animal health. Joining of cancer registries for dogs and humans could possibly lead to an accelerated detection of environmental cancer risks. Living with dogs may reduce obesity and depression (Turner, Chapter 19, this volume). Cognitive capacity may be improved from regular contact with dogs (Hediger and Beetz, Chapter 7, this volume). Joint human and animal health services could also be linked with plant health and improve access to plant health services (Boa *et al.*, Chapter 22, this volume). Joint contingency plans for epidemic diseases can improve management of outbreaks and decrease human and animal morbidity and deaths. In the case of elimination programmes for zoonotic diseases joint efforts are essential for success, as shown for rabies (Léchenne *et al.*, Chapter 16, this volume). Insect repellents can decrease livestock infection with blood parasites and human malaria. Healthy animals and humans are a prerequisite for sustainable wildlife conservation (Cumming *et al.*, Chapter 21, this volume). In conclusion, the presented examples support the understanding of One Health as a measurable qualitative or quantitative added value of closer cooperation between human and animal health and other related disciplines and approaches.

## References

Béchir, M. (2010) Food quality, nutrition and food security in relation to milk production among nomadic pastoralists in Chad. Unpublished PhD thesis, University of Dakar.

Béchir, M., Schelling, E., Hamit, M.A., Tanner, M. and Zinsstag, J. (2012a) Parasitic infections, anemia and malnutrition among rural settled and mobile pastoralist mothers and their children in Chad. *EcoHealth* 9(2), 122–131.

Béchir, M., Schelling, E., Kraemer, K., Schweigert, F., Bonfoh, B., Crump, L., Tanner, M. and Zinsstag, J. (2012b) Retinol assessment among women and children in Sahelian mobile pastoralists. *EcoHealth* 9(2), 113–121.

Bonfoh, B., Kasymbekov, J., Durr, S., Toktobaev, N., Doherr, M.G., Schueth, T., Zinsstag, J. and Schelling, E. (2012) Representative seroprevalences of brucellosis in humans and livestock in Kyrgyzstan. *EcoHealth* 9(2), 132–138.

Charron, D.F. (2012) Ecosystem approaches to health for a global sustainability agenda. *EcoHealth* 9(3), 256–266.

Cleaveland, S., Fevre, E.M., Kaare, M. and Coleman, P.G. (2002) Estimating human rabies mortality in the United Republic of Tanzania from dog bite injuries. *Bulletin of the World Health Organization* 80(4), 304–310.

Diguimbaye, C., Hilty, M., Ngandolo, R., Mahamat, H.H., Pfyffer, G.E., Baggi, F., Tanner, M., Schelling, E. and Zinsstag, J. (2006) Molecular characterization and drug resistance testing of Mycobacterium tuberculosis isolates from Chad. *Journal of Clinical Microbiology* 44(4), 1575–1577.

Diguimbaye-Djaibe, C., Hilty, M., Ngandolo, R., Mahamat, H.H., Pfyffer, G.E., Baggi, F., Hewinson, G., Tanner, M., Zinsstag, J. and Schelling, E. (2006) Mycobacterium bovis isolates from tuberculous lesions in Chadian zebu carcasses. *Emerging Infectious Diseases* 12(5), 769–771.

Enserink, M. (2010) Infectious diseases. Humans, animals – it's one health. Or is it? *Science* 327(5963), 266–267.

Erritzoe, J., Mazgajski, T.D. and Rejt, L. (2003) Bird casualties on European roads - a review. *Acta Ornithologica* 38(2), 77–93.

Forget, G. and Lebel, J. (2001) An ecosystem approach to human health. *International Journal of Occupational Medicine and Environmental Health* 7(2 Suppl.), S3–38.

Frey, J., Mindekem, R., Kessely, H., Doumagoum Moto, D., Naissengar, S., Zinsstag, J. and Schelling, E. (2013) Survey of animal bite injuries and their management for an estimate of human rabies deaths in N'Djamena, Chad. *Tropical Medicine & International Health* 18(12), 1555–1562.

Kayali, U., Mindekem, R., Yemadji, N., Oussiguere, A., Naissengar, S., Ndoutamia, A.G. and Zinsstag, J. (2003) Incidence of canine rabies in N'Djamena, Chad. *Preventive Veterinary Medicine* 61(3), 227–233.

Obrist, B., Iteba, N., Lengeler, C., Makemba, A., Mshana, C., Nathan, R., Alba, S., Dillip, A., Hetzel, M.W., Mayumana, I., Schulze, A. and Mshinda, H. (2007) Access to health care in contexts of livelihood insecurity: a framework for analysis and action. *PLoS Medicine* 2007, 1584–1588.

Ostrom, E. (2007) A diagnostic approach going beyond panaceas. *Proceedings of the National Academy of Sciences* 104(39), 15181–15187.

Roth, F., Zinsstag, J., Orkhon, D., Chimed-Ochir, G., Hutton, G., Cosivi, O., Carrin, G. and Otte, J. (2003) Human health benefits from livestock vaccination for brucellosis: case study. *Bulletin of the World Health Organization* 81(12), 867–876.

Schelling, E., Diguimbaye, C., Daoud, S., Nicolet, J., Boerlin, P., Tanner, M. and Zinsstag, J. (2003) Brucellosis and Q-fever seroprevalences of nomadic pastoralists and their livestock in Chad. *Preventive Veterinary Medicine* 61(4), 279–293.

Schelling, E., Béchir, M., Ahmed, M.A., Wyss, K., Randolph, T.F. and Zinsstag, J. (2007) Human and animal vaccination delivery to remote nomadic families, Chad. *Emerging Infectious Diseases* 13(3), 373–379.

Shabb, D., Chitnis, N., Baljinnyam, Z., Saagii, S. and Zinsstag, J. (2013) A mathematical model of the dynamics of Mongolian livestock populations. *Livestock Science* 157, 280–288.

Shwiff, S., Hampson, K. and Anderson, A. (2013) Potential economic benefits of eliminating canine rabies. *Antiviral Research* 98(2), 352–356.

Tschopp, R., Hattendorf, J., Roth, F., Choudhoury, A., Shaw, A., Aseffa, A. and Zinsstag, J. (2013) Cost estimate of bovine tuberculosis to Ethiopia. *Current Topics in Microbiology and Immunology* 365, 249–368.

World Bank (2012) People, pathogens and our planet: Vol. 2: The economics of One Health. *Report No. 69145-GLB*, 50 pp.

Zinsstag, J. (2012) Convergence of EcoHealth and One Health. *EcoHealth* 9(4), 371–373.

Zinsstag, J., Schelling, E., Daoud, S., Schierle, J., Hofmann, P., Diguimbaye, C., Daugla, D.M., Ndoutamia, G., Knopf, L., Vounatsou, P. and Tanner, M. (2002) Serum retinol of Chadian nomadic pastoralist women in relation to their livestocks' milk retinol and beta-carotene content. *International Journal for Vitamin and Nutrition Research* 72(4), 221–228.

Zinsstag, J., Schelling, E., Roth, F., Bonfoh, B., de Savigny, D. and Tanner, M. (2007) Human benefits of animal interventions for zoonosis control. *Emerging Infectious Diseases* 13(4), 527–531.

Zinsstag, J., Durr, S., Penny, M.A., Mindekem, R., Roth, F., Menendez Gonzalez, S., Naissengar, S. and Hattendorf, J. (2009) Transmission dynamics and economics of rabies control in dogs and humans in an African city. *Proceedings of the National Academy of Sciences* 106(35), 14996–15001.

Zinsstag, J., Bonfoh, B., Cissé, G., Nguyen, V.H., Silué, B., N'Guessan, T.S., *et al.* (2011a) Towards equity effectiveness in health interventions. In: Weismann, U. and Hurni, H. (eds) *Research for Sustainable Development: Foundations, Experiences, and Perspectives*. Perspectives of the Swiss National Centre of Competence in Research (NCCR) North-South, Geographica Bernensis, Berne, Switzerland, 6, 623–640.

Zinsstag, J., Schelling, E., Waltner-Toews, D. and Tanner, M. (2011b) From 'one medicine' to 'one health' and systemic approaches to health and well-being. *Preventive Veterinary Medicine* 101, 148–156.

# 6 The Role of Social Sciences in One Health – Reciprocal Benefits

**Maxine Whittaker***
*School of Population Health, University of Queensland, Herston, Australia*

## Introduction

This chapter will discuss the role of social sciences in understanding individual and community perspectives of health and illness in animals and humans. Social science is the 'study of society and the manner people behave and impact on the world around them' (International Health Group, 2007). It encompasses a range of scholarly or scientific disciplines such as sociology, psychology, anthropology, economics, political science and history. These perspectives, and the social, economic and cultural determinants of people's lives and ability to take action, affect health-seeking behaviour and capacity to utilize preventative measures for human and animal health. The complex relationships between animals, humans and the environment, how people may perceive risk, and their ability to respond to risks and to health promotion will be explored. The chapter will briefly describe some social science approaches to collect data on social, cultural and community perspectives of infectious diseases, risks and strategies. Key points will be illustrated with examples from Africa, Asia, Australia and the Pacific. In this chapter I discuss both broadening of the One Health approach by exploring the role of adding in social science perspectives and expanding the social science frameworks used in exploring the various aspects of the human animal–non-human animal–environment–health interactions. This expanded approach adds further value to social sciences' contribution to One Health and One Health's contribution to social science.

## Background

> Human behavior may be the key that unlocks the proverbial Pandora's Box, allowing infectious diseases to emerge.
>
> (Alexander and McNutt, 2010)

In their paper Alexander and McNutt illustrate this statement by reviewing the relationships between culturally different domestic stock grazing practices among pastoralists in Botswana and Kenya, their domestic dogs that work with them and the African wild dog, and the infectious diseases in this environment. This paper along with others (Gillett, 1985; Brown, 2002; Macpherson, 2005; Sukthana, 2006; Parrish *et al.*, 2008) identify the importance of understanding human behaviour (such as social and demographic, farming and animal husbandry

*E-mail: m.whittaker@uq.edu.au

practices, belief and cultural systems) when trying to understand infectious diseases, especially zoonoses and human health and human responses to prevent and manage the health problems arising from those infectious diseases.

Gillett (1985), an entomologist, discussed the forgotten factor – human behaviour – and the complex relationships that exist between human behaviours and public works, urbanization, packaging, agricultural practices – and the transmission of vector-borne diseases. Although he did not discuss it in his paper, the appreciation of how animals live and interact in those environments with humans is another dimension that a One Health approach brings to the analysis. Elaborating upon this aspect of human behaviour Macpherson (2005) discusses the importance of understanding human attitudes towards domesticated animals as well as the complexities affecting those behaviours such as culture, religion, social environment, age group, ownership of the animals, gender and occupation (see Zinsstag *et al.*, Chapter 2 and Wettlaufer *et al.*, Chapter 3, this volume). The importance of a social science approach to assist in the prevention, management and education of owners of domesticated animals (dogs and cats) for managing enteric parasitic zoonoses in humans and their animals was described by Robertson and Thompson (2002). These social science understandings have been highlighted as important by Wolfe *et al.* (2005) when considering the risks associated with bush-meat hunting, trade and consumption, especially related to indigenous theories of infectious diseases and rules associated with eating bush meat and rituals that may be attached to such consumption. The changes in intensification of aquaculture, the variations in use of animal and human manure as fertilizers and the increases in fish consumption in Vietnam and in global markets and cultural preferences in many countries for raw fish can be examined by using social science approaches to help understand the dynamics and points of intervention (Do Trung Dung *et al.*, 2007). Alexander and McNutt (2010) identified several points in the continuum of pathogen emergence from animals (domestic or wildlife) into the human-animal environment where human behaviour is an important variable to understand and study (see Fig. 6.1).

The Institute of Medicine and National Research Council (IOM and NRC, 2009) further discussed the drivers of pathogen interactions for emerging zoonotic infections and cited Treadwell's model (Fig. 6.2). All of these drivers have a human behavioural and/or attitudinal element that requires exploration in order to prevent or manage these illnesses. It also requires understanding the context of human lives and behaviours. Furthermore, understanding how people perceive the risks and respond to them and the social sciences can bring this knowledge to health programmes (FAO/OIE/WHO, 2011). Sadique *et al.* (2007), using psychological measures, noted the cultural basis of differences in perceptions of the risk and responses to SARS. They noted that a risk must be perceived by a targeted population if one is to achieve some behaviour change. Weiss (2001) has developed an approach entitled cultural epidemiology that merges the identification of the 'locally valid representations of illness and their distributions in a cultural context. These representations are specified by variables, descriptions and narrative accounts of illness experience, its meaning, and associated illness behavior' (see below).

## Blending Various Social Science Approaches and Theories to Understand One Health

There are various social science approaches to understanding the interactions between humans and their environment that provide insights into how these interactions may affect the health of human and non-human animals and shape the responses to health and illnesses in both groups.

### Syndemics

Social scientists using a syndemics concept view the physical and social environments and their intersections with humans and animals and the range of social, political and economic contexts that affect and impact upon those

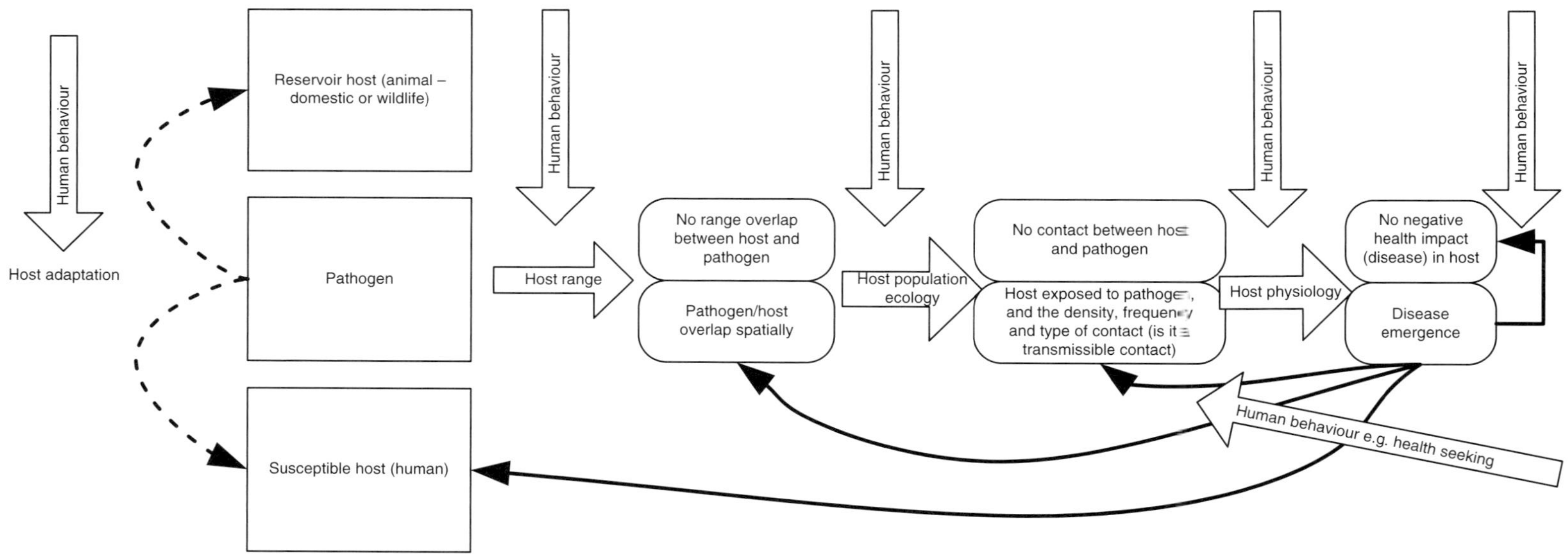


**Fig. 6.1.** A conceptual model of the potential influence of human behaviour on the emergence and transmission of infectious pathogens at the human–animal–environment interface (adapted from Alexander and McNutt, 2010).

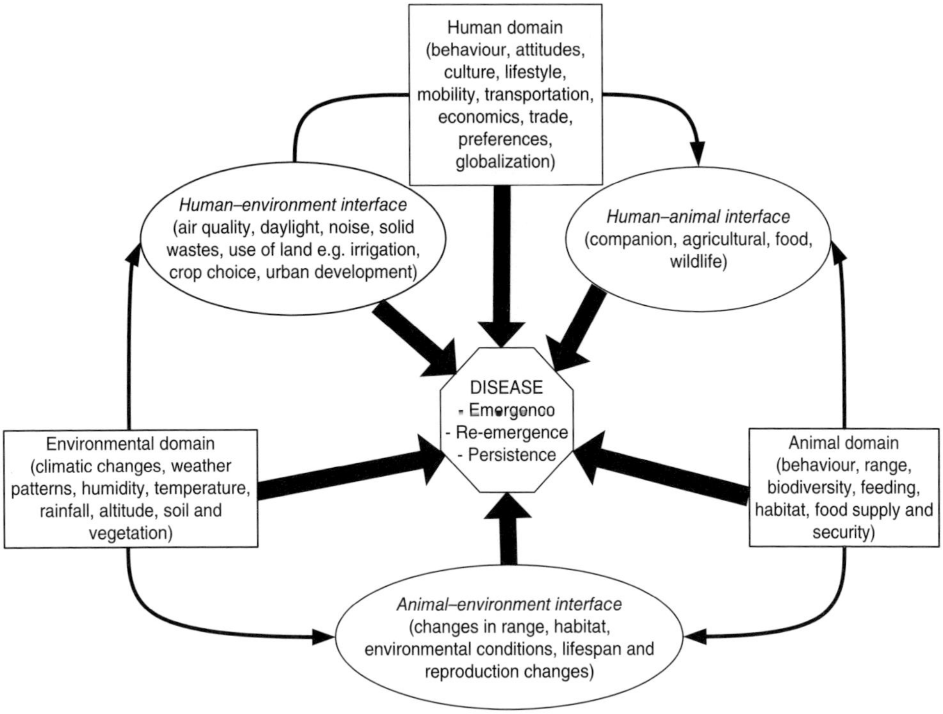


**Fig. 6.2.** Treadwell's model of drivers of pathogen interactions for emerging zoonotic infections (adapted from IOM and NRC, 2009).

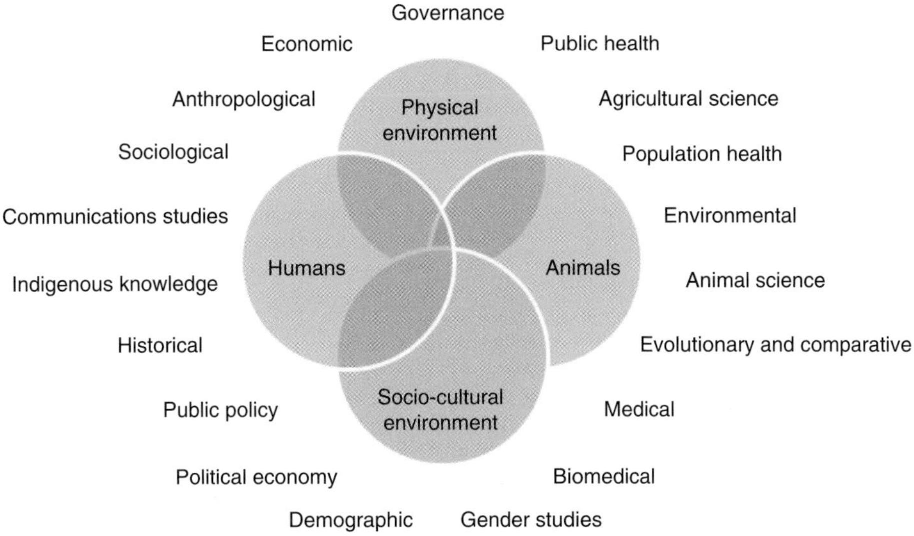


**Fig. 6.3.** Perspectives used to inform a syndemic approach (adapted from Rock *et al.*, 2009).

(Fig. 6.3). Singer (2009) defined the syndemic approach as:

> the concentration and deleterious interaction of two or more diseases or other health conditions in a population, especially as a consequence of social inequity and unjust exercise of power … (which) does not stop with a consideration of the biological connections … Because human diseases

> within us are greatly impacted by the conditions that comprise the built and interactive social worlds of disease sufferers.

Proponents of syndemic approaches, including Singer (2009) and Rock *et al.* (2009), have noted that there is a tension between biological scientists, who are ambivalent about the legitimacy of social science (Albert *et al.*, 2008), and social scientists, who question the power of biomedicine (as a construct and industry). This has meant that even as the 'one medicine' and One Health approaches have been developed there has been limited attention to social science research on animal–human connections in health, diseases and health systems. Proponents of syndemics have furthered its application to understanding and providing One Health responses to human health conditions, especially infectious diseases, by including ecological and other environmental factors and socio-political environments in their analyses. Rock *et al.* (2009) illustrated the various 'lenses' one could use to examine these interactions in their work on syndemics. They expanded syndemics to include 'two or more afflictions that interact synergistically within the context of specific physical and social environments, especially as a result of inequality within and between human populations, to produce excess disease burdens in a human population, an animal population or multiple such populations'. They further used syndemics to improve understanding ways to prevent diseases. An expansion of One Health to specifically address systemic ecological and social dimensions has led to the new term 'health in social-ecological systems' (Zinsstag *et al.*, 2011).

### Multispecies ethnography

The complexity of the systems in which animal, human and wildlife health and well-being, and the interfaces between these, operate as well as the diversity in social, economic, cultural, environmental and biological dimensions of these interfaces means that one disciplinary approach to understanding these will be inadequate (Jones *et al.*, 2013; Bunch and Waltner-Toews, Chapter 34, this volume). Thus, a range of social science methods will be required. An emerging field is multispecies ethnography (Kirksey and Helmreich, 2010), defined as 'studying a host of organisms whose lives and deaths are linked to human social worlds … Centres on how a multitude of organisms' livelihoods shape and are shaped by political, economic and cultural forces'. One example is the work of Lowe (2010), who undertook a multispecies ethnography (domestic poultry, wild birds, Indonesian citizens – including general population, consumers, cockfighters and other animal species) when exploring H5N1. Another such multispecies ethnography was described by Fuentes (2010), examining monkeys, tourists, temple workers and local citizens in Bali and the risks of rabies and bite-related injuries.

### Food anthropologies

Reviewing the relationships between food and its production, humans and health has been another area where integrated social sciences approaches have been used to explore a health issue in a more holistic One Health manner. Broglia and Kapal (2011) discuss the role of change in dietary habits and the emergence of parasitic zoonotic illnesses that are food borne. Food habits, global trade and availability of food, changes in food production systems, population growth and movement and climatic changes are affecting the foods that are available, affordable, demanded and how and where these foods are produced. Like the syndemic concept above, they discuss the complex system of interconnected biologicals, economic, social and cultural variables on the development and management of food-borne parasitic diseases, and how these illnesses should be addressed 'by considering the interface between animals (domestic and wildlife), humans and the ecosystems (natural and agricultural)'. Ayele *et al.* (2004) explored the various relationships between humans and cattle and the spread of *Mycobacterium bovis*. They noted that behaviours such as consumption of raw or undercooked meat, close contact with animals due to living conditions and nomadic lifestyles and dependency, and drinking and cultural preferences for unpasteurized (and infected) milk contribute toward the transmission of this disease. These attitudes and behaviours need to be explored to find solutions to prevent the disease – a role for social science.

## Ecological anthropology and ethnoecology

There are other social science frameworks that can supplement or deepen these analyses. The way humans think about animals – wild, domestic or sylvatic – affects the types of exposures and risks that humans and animals may have from each other in sharing infectious and even other non-communicable risks. Shanklin (1985) described the roles of ecological anthropology to understand animals as sustenance and symbols. He discussed the role of cultural ecology to understand the functions of animals to human groups and of social anthropology to investigate adaptation of humans to animals. He further discusses ethnoecology as playing a role in how the relevant environmental factors may affect the way the local culture ascribes importance to animals.

## Economics

The economic value of animals to a family and a community also affects the way they interact with their animals, the way they view symptoms in their animals and their adherence (or non-adherence) to management strategies prescribed. One example discussed in Breiman *et al.* (2007) using economics as a social science discipline, relates to the culling of poultry in Nigeria in response to avian influenza. This strategy affected rural and semi-urban communities – especially backyard and small-scale farmers – who were at the same time the most impoverished. At a higher national economic level, they noted that the poultry industry is worth 10% of the gross domestic product of the country. Zinsstag *et al.* (2007) further elaborated on the importance of understanding the value assigned to animals and the cultural perceptions of economic benefits from interventions proposed (Zinsstag *et al.*, Chapter 2, this volume).

## Psychology

The role of different personalities and societal values has also been shown to influence risk of exposure to diseases. These include behavioural dispositions such as gregariousness and openness (Thornhill *et al.*, 2010). Human adaptation to situations such as protection of food sources may lead to rituals and norms that protect them from food-borne illnesses. Thornhill *et al.* (2010) suggested that zoonotic parasite prevalence is strongly negatively associated with individualism as a societal value and positively linked to collectivism.

## Health systems

Some researchers have used social science methods to understand how populations access health services for human or non-human animals. They have explored the accessibility, acceptability and affordability of integrating the health services. For example, amongst pastoralists in Chad, Zinsstag *et al.* (2005) studied ways of integrating childhood immunization services with outreach veterinary services (Schelling *et al.*, Chapter 20, this volume).

## Veterinary anthropology

Some social scientists have reviewed animal behaviours in an attempt to gain an understanding of human behaviours, responses to stress and mental health (Hediger and Beetz, Chapter 7 and Turner, Chapter 19, this volume). Several authors used evolutionary biological theories and principles to try to understand human behaviours and their coping mechanisms such as depression panic, depression and sexual behaviours (Gladue, 1989).

## Indigenous knowledge

The recent introduction of indigenous knowledge sciences into the discussions of human, animal and environmental interactions has provided further concepts of implementation of the social-ecological system approaches.

For example, considering ways to manage feral animals, which may be a risk for human and wildlife well-being, can be informed by understanding indigenous approaches to natural resource management (Robinson and Wellington, 2012). Environmental scientists have used indigenous perspectives to reconsider the value of culling feral pigs in Australia. These perspectives included a consideration of the importance of feral pig meat as a source of protein, the cultural importance of social interactions for sharing of food, and the importance of feral pigs as a source of income through tourism (viewing wildlife) and hunting. Working with indigenous groups, environmental scientists were made aware of the importance of preserving other food sources such as yam sites and freshwater turtle habitats. Social science qualitative methods such as transect walks and narratives were a foundation of this work.

Other examples of indigenous knowledge sciences include understanding the reasons why agro-ecological farming techniques are taken up and the linkages of the territorial delineation of agricultural land between groups (using critical geography) and social determinants of health and well-being of these agricultural communities (Rosset and Martinez-Torres, 2012). This emerging field of indigenous knowledge science provides further tools in the social science toolbox to use in One Health interventions. An important aspect of this is the engagement of science with non-academic actors for practical societal problem solving, called transdisciplinary research (Schelling and Zinsstag, Chapter 30, this volume).

Table 6.1 illustrates some of the many and varied social, human political contexts that can affect human and animal interactions and effects upon health, and some of the social science disciplinary approaches that have been used to examine aspects of these.

## Applying Integrated Social Science Approaches to Address One Health Problems

The application of a more holistic social science approach linked to a One Health thinking is illustrated in the following two case studies. The first case study reviews how social science perspectives help to address different contexts of henipavirus infections in humans and in animals. The second case study presents the approach taken by the Fijian Ministry of Health to develop its leptospirosis strategic plan by including social science perspectives in the deliberations and how these have contributed value to the strategy. It has helped identify different risk behaviours and settings, social factors that may affect preventive message uptake and human–animal interactions that also affect risk and responses to those risks.

### Case study: nipah and hendra virus: elaborating a One Health social science perspective to the emergence and management of these infections

Nipah virus in Bangladesh, Malaysia and Singapore and hendra virus in Australia illustrate a human–animal–environment interface issue that has become a health problem for some non-human and human animals. A One Health approach has been suggested by many to address this issue – both in research on various models of transmission, for instance, palm sugar and bat urine in Bangladesh (Luby *et al.*, 2006; Khan *et al.*, 2011, 2012; Rahman *et al.*, 2011) and in finding management solutions to the problem, as done by using skirts on date palm trees (Nahar *et al.*, 2010), and vaccinations of horses and humans, flying fox colony management and improved infection control of sick horses in Australia (Mackenzie *et al.*, 2003; Mahalingam *et al.*, 2012).

Anthropogenic changes in the physical environment, as well as some natural events, have led to a reduction in available flowering and fruiting tress in clusters or forests, which has led to bats (*Pteropus*) encroaching on cultivation areas and urban areas in search of food (Degeling and Kerridge, 2013). Horses, pigs, dogs and humans, either via direct contact with sick animals or through food products, can be exposed. Environmental changes, including intensive cultivation practices and urbanization, affect the forest structure and extent. Some also suggest that stress on the flying foxes and

**Table 6.1.** Examples of the social science frameworks used to examine One Health.

| Contexts | Variables that may affect the human and/or animal health impacts | Examples of social science approaches |
|---|---|---|
| Economics | How evenly wealth is distributed throughout society<br>'Wealthiness' of group<br>Sufficiency of income – basics, discretionary<br>Cultural values associated with wealth, poverty, employment, unemployment, benefits<br>Basic economic unit (individual, family, collective)<br>Patterns of labour<br>Control of land and technology<br>Distribution and exchange of money/commodities<br>Savings from closer cooperation between human and animal health (Zinsstag *et al*., Chapter 12, this volume) | Economic anthropology<br>Critical anthropology<br>Political economics<br>Cross-sector economics |
| Family and household structures | Functions of and within families and households<br>Types of family formation: nuclear, extended, joint, one-parent<br>Household organization<br>Interaction, cohesion and mutual support among family members<br>Emphasis: individual or familial<br>Responsibility for child rearing, animal (baby animal) rearing, provision of food, care of the elderly, sick and dying (human and animal) and how shared in family<br>Role of animals in family | Cultural anthropology<br>Sociology<br>Demography<br>Veterinary anthropology |
| Patterns of subsistence | Food foraging<br>Food producing (and what type): horticulture, pastoralism and what role (rearing, preparing for market, production, marketing, 'fork' ready) | Veterinary anthropology<br>Agricultural anthropology<br>Biological anthropology<br>Ethnobiology |
| Environment | Relationships to land, water, etc. may be affected by at least: religion, ownership, inheritance, identity, male and female, indigenous populations | Ecological anthropology<br>Biological anthropology<br>Ethnobiology<br>Indigenous studies |
| Culture and communications | Who, in various cultural contexts, is the main communication channel: respected persons (whom), segmentation difference (e.g. gender, age), mandated | Cultural anthropology<br>Organizational and evolutionary psychology<br>Indigenous studies |
| Cultural change | Mechanisms of change: e.g. innovation, diffusion, loss, forced (e.g. acculturation, directed genocide), modernization<br>Reactions to change (adoption, revitalization, rebellion) | Cultural anthropology<br>Political anthropology<br>Critical anthropology |
| Political organization and social change | Political systems<br>Leadership<br>Social control mechanisms (internal, external)<br>Religion<br>Gender | Cultural anthropology<br>Political anthropology<br>Critical anthropology<br>Evolutionary psychology |
| Gender roles | Division of labour: work, stay at home, prepare food, care for children, care for animals, collect water etc.<br>Social rights, obligations and expectations associated with gender roles<br>Cultural beliefs about appropriate behaviour for each gender<br>Threshold of consultation for each gender | Feminist anthropology<br>Evolutionary psychology |

*Continued*

**Table 6.1.** Continued.

| Contexts | Variables that may affect the human and/or animal health impacts | Examples of social science approaches |
|---|---|---|
| Diet and food | How food gathered/bought, prepared, stored and preserved<br>Gender bias in amounts of food allocated<br>Does food routinely contain contaminants<br>Whether food is symbolically classified or linked to cultural meanings and events<br>Special diets during life stages e.g. pregnancy, ill health<br>Use of western food products<br>Changing dietary habits and preferences – for a range of cultural, economic and global change reasons<br>Religious or cultural preferences for food preparation | Nutritional anthropology<br>Cultural anthropology<br>Evolutionary psychology<br>Ethnobiology |
| Personal hygiene | Is personal hygiene neglected/encouraged<br>Rituals with washing and sanitation<br>Bathing arrangements (private, communal) | Cultural anthropology |
| Housing arrangements | Construction, siting and internal division of living space<br>Who/what occupies the space (same family, language group, animals)<br>Number of occupants (human and animal) per room/house/hut)<br>Allocation of space (age/gender/marital status)<br>Other buildings attached and roles and use | Cultural anthropology<br>Veterinary anthropology<br>Ecological anthropology |
| Sanitation arrangements | Modes of disposal: any differences in human (infant/adult) and animal (infant/adult/species)<br>Who carries out disposal<br>How are wastes disposed of and where disposed of or are they used for other functions | Cultural anthropology<br>Religious studies |
| Religion/philosophy | World view attached to religion, e.g. karma, sorcery, animism, stoicism<br>Religious practices, e.g. food taboos, feasts, mass pilgrimages | Cultural anthropology<br>Religious studies |
| Occupations | Of men/women/youth<br>Certain occupations reserved for particular individuals, groups, castes<br>Prestige attached to occupations<br>Techniques used in occupations, e.g. traditional, modern | Cultural anthropology<br>Gender studies<br>Critical anthropology<br>Economics |
| Domestic animals and birds | Nature and number of domestic livestock and pets<br>Where housed<br>Degree of physical contact between animals and humans<br>Animal husbandry systems<br>Religious/cultural classification of cleanliness of animals<br>Slaughtering practices | Biological anthropology<br>Veterinary anthropology<br>Ethnobiology |

bats may increase their viral shedding (Parrish *et al.*, 2008). Additional complexities arose in managing this issue when accounting for human perceptions of bats, either as a 'nuisance' in Australia (Degeling and Kerridge, 2013) or as of other significance (Wood *et al.*, 2012). These perceptions altered and/or reinforced the community response and political reaction to the problem. In Australia, this view of bats as a nuisance, identified and characterized through social science research, has made it difficult for the communities and politicians to understand why the flying foxes (although many species are listed as vulnerable) are protected whereas humans are at risk. This view has threatened the implementation of the management strategies (Degeling and Kerridge, 2013). In Bangladesh there was also evidence of human-to-human transmission through nosocomial exposure, although this was not seen in Singapore or Malaysia. Using social science methods to review the quality of services in health settings could support the proposal that the quality of infection control in hospital settings was a factor and that this is influenced by health care policy and financing (Gurly *et al.*, 2007). The uncertainty about henipavirus transmission has fuelled concern among the general population about it, and may lead to mistrust of the expert advice being provided and the policy decisions being made (Degeling and Kerridge, 2013).

In this case, there is a need to understand the social factors resulting in changes to the physical environment, the economic and agricultural/land uses by the human populations and what is driving those decisions and behaviours, the human behavioural responses to threat and to expert and political advice, and any perceptions already held about bats/flying foxes and their good or 'evil' and their uses. Understanding how communities affected by the viruses will respond to management protocols will require social science perspectives, e.g. vaccination of horses, allowing bat colonies to remain in their district. Bringing together social science insights into the situation will strengthen the effectiveness, acceptability and efficiency of the One Health approach.

### Case study: leptospirosis in Fiji – the One Health social science approach

The development of the policy and research framework for leptospirosis, as described by Reid and Kama (Chapter 17, this volume), was informed by considering the human–animal–environment contexts and how human behaviours may impact upon and be impacted by these other contexts. At the described workshop, the participants were challenged to consider the following interactions and influences and how these may affect approaches, responses, acceptability and effectiveness of the programmatic and policy approaches employed especially with response to influencing human behaviour. Some examples are provided in Table 6.2.

**Table 6.2.** Human behaviour/leptospirosis interface in Fiji.

| Human behaviour issues to consider with respect to health outcomes | Leptospirosis characteristics | Human characteristics |
|---|---|---|
| Exposure to reservoirs | Animal reservoirs (rats, cattle, local fauna, dogs) but may be different in different populations (farms, domestic), seasons (wet, dry), geographies (flood plains, highlands), land use (urban, sugarcane, cattle) | Access to water<br>Cultural/religious uses of water<br>Ethnicity: different relationships with animals (totems, beliefs about cleanliness)<br>Gender: agricultural exposure, water related work/housework exposures<br>Poverty, e.g. housing quality, location of house to land use or flood prone<br>Mobility of animals/humans and how it affects exposure |
| Prevention practices<br>Early presentation helps clinical outcome | Non-specific symptoms associated with leptospirosis<br>Common/familiar symptoms so accepted as 'normal' or misdiagnosed | Gender: male/female use of health services<br>Poverty: ability to seek care (costs of care – direct and indirect, opportunity costs), affordability of prevention<br>Occupation, e.g. sugarcane worker, beef or dairy industry worker<br>Age group: children playing in water, adults in occupations |

By broadening the view of determinants of leptospirosis, the strategy included stronger focus on gaining evidence through social science research, strengthened and refined health promotion programmes to account for different ages, occupational and social groups, and different timing of interventions (flood times versus routine occupational risks). Measuring the effectiveness of the strategy also included behavioural and coverage indicators, which will require social science methods as part of the transdisciplinary approach (Schelling and Zinsstag, Chapter 30, this volume).

## Conclusion

As outlined in this chapter, social science adds value in the identification, design and implementation of One Health interventions and has been used to provide insights into:

- the human behaviours that may be driving environmental changes that affect animal–human contact;
- human behaviours and attitudes towards animals – as companion animals, as food producers, as agricultural work animals, as food sources;
- human behaviours and beliefs regarding the value of and meaning of animals, both culturally and religiously;
- human uses of health services for themselves and their animals – what affects their use, factors that affect acceptability, affordability and accessibility, and any factors that may affect that such as gender, age group, poverty;
- historical perspectives of what has shaped and is shaping human behaviours and responses to change; and
- local contexts including economic and socio-cultural factors.

The One Health approach also brings together a broad range of social science disciplines to examine these issues, as well as theoretical and integrative innovations in understanding culture, economics, gender, ecology, behaviours, political contexts and indigenous knowledge.

## References


Albert, M., Laberge, S., Hodges, B., Regehr, G. and Lingard, L. (2008) Biomedical scientists' perception of the social science in health research. *Social Science and Medicine* 66, 2520–2531.

Alexander, K. and McNutt, W. (2010) Human behavior influences infectious disease emergence at the human–animal interface. *Frontiers in Ecology and the Environment* 8, 522–526.

Ayele, W.Y., Neill, S.D., Zinsstag, J., Weiss, M.G. and Pavlik, I. (2004) Bovine tuberculosis: an old disease but a new threat to Africa. *The International Journal of Tuberculosis and Lung Disease* 8(8), 924–937.

Breiman, R., Nandi, A., Katz, M., Njenga, M. and Vertefeuille, J. (2007) Preparedness for highly pathogenic avian influenza pandemics in Africa. *Emerging Infectious Diseases* 13, 1453–1455.

Broglia, A. and Kapal, C. (2011) Changing dietary habits in a changing world: emerging drivers for the transmission of food borne parasitic zoonoses. *Veterinary Parasitology* 182, 2–13.

Brown, F. (2002) Animal husbandry practices and risk factors with particular reference to bovine spongiform encephalopathy. In: IOM (eds) *The Emergence of Zoonotic Diseases: understanding the impact on animal and human health: workshop summary.* National Academies Press, Washington, DC, pp. 59-61.

Degeling, C. and Kerridge, I. (2013) Hendra in the news: public policy meets public morality in times of zoonotic uncertainty. *Social Science and Medicine* 82, 156–163.

Do Trung Dung, Nguyen Can Del, Walcagul, J., Dalsgaard, A., Jong-Yil Chai, Woon-Mok Sohn and Murrell, K. (2007) Fishborne zoonotic intestinal trematodes in Vietnam. *Emerging Infectious Diseases* 13, 1828–1833.

FAO/OIE/WHO Joint Scientific Consultation Writing Committee (2011) Influenza and other emerging diseases at the human-animal interface. *Proceedings of the FAO/OIE/WHO Joint Scientific Consultation 27–29 April 2010, Verona.* FAO Animal Production and Health Proceedings No. 13, FAO, Rome.

Fuentes, A. (2010) Natural cultural encounters in Bali: monkeys, temples, tourists and ethnoprimatology. *Cultural Anthropology* 25, 600–624.

Gillett, J. (1985) The behaviour of *Homo sapiens*, the forgotten factor in the transmission of tropical diseases. *Transactions of the Royal Society of Tropical Medicine and Hygiene* 79, 12–20.

Gladue, B. (1989) Evolutionary controversy and psychobiology. *Journal of Social Biological Structure* 12, 251–258.

Gurly, E., Montgomery, J., Hossain, M., Bell, M., Azas, A., Islam, M., Molla, M., Carroll, D., Ksiazek, T., Rota, P., Lowe, L., Comer, J., Rollin, P., Czub, M., Grolla, A., Feldmann, H., Luby, S., Woodward, J. and Breiman, R. (2007) Person to person transmission of Nipah virus in a Bangladeshi community. *Emerging Infectious Diseases* 13, 1031–1037.

International Health Group of the Centre for Public Health Research, Brunel University (2007) *Applied social sciences for public health (ASSPH)*. WHO, Geneva.

IOM (Institute of Medicine) and NRC (National Research Council) (2009) *Sustaining Global Surveillance and Response to Emerging Zoonotic Diseases*. The National Academies Press, Washington, DC.

Jones, B., Grace, D., Kock, R., Alonso, B., Rushton, J., Said, M., McKeever, D., Mutua, F., Young, J., McDermott, J. and Pfeiffer, D. (2013) Zoonoses emergence linked to agricultural intensification and environmental change. *Proceedings of the National Academy of Sciences of the United States of America* 110, 8399–8404.

Khan, M.S., Hossain, J., Gurley, E.S., Nahar, N., Sultana, R. and Luby, S. (2011) Use of infrared camera to understand bats' access to date palm sap: implications for preventing Nipah virus transmission. *EcoHealth* DOI: 10.1007/s10393-010-0366-2.

Khan, S.U., Gurley, E.S., Hossain, M.J., Nahar, N., Sharker, M.A.Y., *et al.* (2012) A randomized controlled trial of interventions to impede date palm sap contamination by bats to prevent Nipah virus transmission in Bangladesh. *PLoS ONE* 7(8): e42689. doi:10.1371/journal.pone.0042689.

Kirksey, S. and Helmreich, S. (2010) The emergence of multispecies ethnography. *Cultural Anthropology* 25, 545–576.

Lowe, C. (2010) Viral clouds: becoming H5N1 in Indonesia. *Cultural Anthropology* 25, 625–649.

Luby, S.P., Rahman, M., Hossain, M.J., Blum, L.S., Husain, M.M., *et al.* (2006) Foodborne transmission of Nipah virus, Bangladesh. *Emerging Infectious Diseases* 12, 1888–1894.

Mackenzie, J.S., Field, H. and Guyatt, K. (2003) Managing emerging diseases borne by fruit bats (flying foxes), with particular reference to henipaviruses and Australian bat lyssavirus. *Journal of Applied Microbiology* 94, 59S–69S.

Macpherson, C. (2005) Human behaviour and the epidemiology of parasitic zoonoses. *International Journal for Parasitology* 35, 1319–1331.

Mahalingam, S., Herrero, L., Playford, E.G., Spann, K., Herring, B., Rolph, M., Middleton, D., McCall, B., Field, H. and Lin-Fa Wang (2012) Hendra virus: an emerging paramyxovirus in Australia. *Lancet Infectious Diseases* 12, 799–807.

Nahar, N., Sultana, R., Gurley, E.S., Hossain, M.J. and Luby, S.P. (2010) Date palm sap collection: exploring opportunities to prevent Nipah transmission. *EcoHealth* 7, 196–203.

Parrish, C., Homes, E., Morens, D., Park, E., Burke, D., Calister, C., Laughlin, C., Sarf, L. and Daszak, P. (2008) Cross species virus transmission and the emergence of new epidemic diseases. *Microbiology and Molecular Biology Reviews* 72, 457–470.

Rahman, M.A., Hossain, M.J., Sultana, S., Homaira, N., Khan, S.U., Rahman, M., Gurley, E., Rollin, P., Lo, M., Comer, J., Lowe, L., Rota, P., Ksiazek, T., Kenah, E., Sharker, Y. and Luby, S. (2011) Date palm sap linked to Nipah virus outbreak in Bangladesh, 2008. *Vector-Borne and Zoonotic Diseases*. In: Choffnes, E., Relman, D., Olsen, L., Hutton, R. and Mack, A. (eds) 2012 *Improving Food Safety Through A One Health Approach Workshop Summary. Forum on Microbial Threats Board On Global Health*. The National Academies Press, Washington, DC, pp. 283–297.

Robertson, I. and Thompson, R. (2002) Enteric parasitic zoonoses of domesticated dogs and cats. *Microbes and Infection* 4, 867–873.

Robinson, C. and Wellington, T. (2012) Boundary work: engaging knowledge systems in co-management of feral animals in indigenous lands. *Ecology and Society* 17, 16–24.

Rock, M., Buntain, B., Halfeld, J. and Hallgrimssson, B. (2009) Animal-human connections, One Health and the syndemic approach to prevention. *Social Science and Medicine* 68, 991–995.

Rosset, P. and Martinez-Torres, M. (2012) Rural social movements and agroecology: context, theory and process. *Ecology and Society* 17(3), 17–23.

Sadique, M., Edmunds, W., Smith, R., Meerding, W., de Zwart, D., Brug, J. and Beutels, P. (2007) Precautionary behaviour in response to perceived threat of pandemic influenza. *Emerging Infectious Diseases* 13, 1307–1313.

Shanklin, E. (1985) Sustenance and symbol: anthropological studies of domesticated animals. *Annual Review of Anthropology* 14, 375–403.

Singer, M. (2009) Doorways in nature: syndemics, zoonotics and public health. A commentary on Rock, Buntain, Hatfield and Hallgrimsson. *Social Science and Medicine* 68, 996–999.

Sukthana, Y. (2006) Toxoplasmosis: beyond animals and humans. *Trends in Parasitology* 22, 137–142.

Thornhill, R., Fincher, V.C., Murray, D. and Schaller, M. (2010) Zoonotic and non-zoonotic diseases in relation to human personality and societal value: support for the parasite-stress model. *Evolutionary Psychology* 8, 151–169.

Weiss, M. (2001) Cultural epidemiology: an introduction and overview. *Anthropology & Medicine* 8, 5–29.

Wolfe, N., Daszak, P., Kilpatrick, A. and Burke, S.D. (2005) Bushmeat hunting, deforestation and prediction of zoonotic disease emergence. *Emerging Infectious Diseases* 11, 1822–1827.

Wood, J., Leach, M., Waldman, L., MacGregor, H., Fooks, A., Jones, K., Restif, O., Dechmann, D., Hayman, D., Baker, K., Peel, A., Kamins, A., Fahr, J., Ntiamoa-Baidu, Y., Breiman, R., Epstein, J., Field, H. and Cunningham, A. (2012) A framework for the study of zoonotic disease emergence and its drivers: spill-over of bat pathogens as a case study. *Philosophical Transactions of the Royal Society, Biological Sciences* 367, 2881–2892.

Zinsstag, J., Schelling, E., Wyss, K. and Mahomet, M. (2005) Potential of cooperation between human and animal health to strengthen health systems. *Lancet* 366, 2142–2145.

Zinsstag, J., Schelling, E., Roth, F., Bonfoh, B., de Savingny, D. and Tanner, M. (2007) Human benefits of animal interventions for zoonoses control. *Emerging Infectious Diseases* 13, 527–531.

Zinsstag, J., Schelling, E., Waltner-Toews, D. and Tanner, M. (2011) From 'one medicine' to 'One Health' and systemic approaches to health and well-being. *Preventive Veterinary Medicine* 101, 148–156.

# 7 The Role of Human–Animal Interactions in Education

**Karin Hediger[1,2]* and Andrea Beetz[2]**
[1]*Institute for Interdisciplinary Research on the Human–Animal Relationship (IEMT), Basel, Switzerland;* [2]*Swiss Tropical and Public Health Institute, Basel, Switzerland;* [3]*University of Basel, Basel, Switzerland;* [4]*Department of Special Education, University of Rostock, Germany and Department of Behavioural Biology, University of Vienna, Austria*

## Introduction

In the last decade, research has demonstrated a multitude of positive effects of human–animal interactions on human health and well-being, and pointed to underlying mechanisms that explain why using animals can sometimes be more effective than interventions by humans alone. These effects represent an important aspect of One Health, which will be reviewed in this chapter.

Animals can play a significant role in the education of children, within the family as well as at school, and have the potential to promote children's socio-emotional and probably also cognitive development. The positive effects of human–animal interaction are used in animal-assisted interventions in educational contexts, such as special training programmes for social competence, reading skills or via introducing animals, particularly dogs, into the classroom.

Education is one central factor that influences children's development and, therefore, their health. Looking at human health from a biopsychosocial perspective, the psychological, social, or educational effects of animals clearly are highly relevant.

First, we will give a short overview of the general known positive effects from contact with animals. Subsequently, we will provide an overview of the specific effects on children and their education and illustrate these on the basis of recent studies. Finally, possible psychophysiological mechanisms will be discussed.

## General Positive Effects from Contact with Animals

Most studies investigating effects from contact with animals have been conducted with adults. Although this chapter focuses on children, it is worth noting the profound impact that animals can have on humans in general. The research available on effects of interaction with animals on children will be discussed in the next section.

The research findings will be integrated in a biopsychosocial health model, since all three aspects are relevant for 'human health'. This chapter can only provide a rough categorization of effects among the labels 'bio', 'psycho' and 'social', but many overlaps exist, and interrelations between

*E-mail: karin.hediger@unibas.ch

the presented effects as well as between the three different areas occur.

## Psychological Effects

In addition to the positive effects of interactions with animals on children's empathy and learning, which will be discussed in the next section, several positive effects on the psychological aspect of the biopsychosocial health model have been documented by research.

### Promotion of positive mood and reduction of depression and feelings of loneliness

Interaction with and ownership of an animal can be significantly associated with improved mood, and reduction of depression and loneliness (Jessen *et al.*, 1996; Holcomb *et al.*, 1997; Banks and Banks, 2002, 2005; Turner *et al.*, 2003; Colombo *et al.*, 2006). In their meta-analysis, Souter and Miller (2007) concluded that animal-assisted therapy can lead to a significant reduction of depressive symptoms.

The effect of improved mood seems to occur also in children and adults with physical or mental problems, e.g. chronic schizophrenia patients (Nathans-Barel *et al.*, 2005) and hospitalized children (Kaminski *et al.*, 2002). Moreover, children in psychotherapy profited from animal-assisted interventions with regard to their intra-emotional balance (Prothmann *et al.*, 2006).

### Reduction of fear and anxiety and promotion of calmness

Several studies provide evidence that the presence of and interacting with an animal can reduce self-reported anxiety and fear when exposed to a stressor (Barker *et al.*, 2003; Shiloha *et al.*, 2003; Cole *et al.*, 2007). This effect can also be observed in psychotherapy sessions (Barker and Dawson, 1998) and intervention programmes for psychiatric patients (Berget *et al.*, 2011). In addition, interaction with a dog was shown to reduce tension and confusion in elderly residents of a nursing home (Crowley-Robinson *et al.*, 1996) as well as restlessness in patients with dementia (Filan and Llewellyn-Jones, 2006; Perkins *et al.*, 2008).

### Improved pain management

First field reports suggest a reduced use of pain medication in nursing homes and homes for the elderly when an animal is present (Darrah, 1996). However, well-designed and controlled studies on the effect of human–animal interaction on pain management are still lacking.

## Social Effects

### Increased positive social attention from others and stimulation of social behaviour

A relatively large body of research has focused on the effect of the presence of an animal on the perception of the human in its company, on the one hand, and on the stimulation of social behaviour, on the other hand. This latter effect is usually referred to as the 'social catalyst effect' and research demonstrating this will be discussed in more detail in the next section.

Several studies demonstrated that people indeed receive more positive attention from others in the presence of a friendly animal, e.g. individuals in wheelchairs in the company of a service dog (Hart *et al.*, 1987). Strangers also smiled more at adults in wheelchairs and started more and longer conversations with them when a service dog was present (Eddy *et al.*, 2001). Similar effects were found in children with visible disabilities, in a mall or at a playground (Mader *et al.*, 1989). Additionally, people without disabilities received more positive attention from strangers in public when they were accompanied by dogs (Wells, 2004). These results were found in a cultural context of Western civilization, and cannot be generalized to cultures with different perceptions of animals (see Zinsstag *et al.*, Chapter 2, this volume).

### Increased trust and trustworthiness

Moreover, the presence of animals affects the trust the accompanied person receives from strangers as well as this person's trustworthiness in the eyes of others. Specifically, Schneider and Harley (2006) demonstrated that students who watched a video of a psychotherapist depicted with a friendly dog were more willing to disclose personal information to this psychotherapist than when he was depicted without a dog. In a study by Gueguen and Ciccotti (2008), the company of a dog was associated with a significantly higher rate of helping behaviour and a significantly higher compliance with the requests for a phone number from strangers on the street.

### More positive perception of people and environment

In photographs, people are perceived as more friendly, less threatening, and happier in the company of an animal (Lockwood, 1983). This is particularly true for the company of dogs, which also increases the ratings of the depicted person's relaxation and happiness (Rossbach and Wilson, 1992).

Moreover, the presence of an animal can even positively influence the perception of someone's environment or of a person who is not depicted with the animal (Wells and Perrine, 2001). Students in an experiment perceived the office of a professor as more comfortable and the professor as more friendly when there was a dog in the office, in comparison with the presence of a cat or when no animal was present. In addition, the presence of a cat made the professor appear less busy than a professor who has a dog or no animal in the office (Wells and Perrine, 2001).

### Social support, attachment, and consequences of loss

Companion animal owners frequently report that their animals can effectively provide social support (Bonas *et al.*, 2000; Doherty and Feeney, 2004; McNicholas and Collis, 2006) and contribute to their feelings of safety, especially in the case of dogs (Endenburg, 1995). Therefore, in times of stress, anxiety, grief, or pain, adult and child owners seek proximity to their pets and even prefer their presence to the presence of a family member or friend (Melson and Schwarz, 1994; Rost and Hartmann, 1994; Kurdek, 2009a,b).

Parallel to the positive feelings due to the interaction and relationship with the companion animal, the loss of a pet can lead to strong emotional reactions (Archer and Winchester, 1994). It is often perceived as the loss of a family member (Gerwolls and Labott, 1994) and linked to depressive symptoms (Stallones, 1994; Hunt *et al.*, 2008).

## Biological Effects

A large body of scientific research in the area of human–animal interactions addresses effects on physiological parameters or human health in general (see Turner, Chapter 19, this volume).

### General and cardiovascular health effects

In several surveys with large and representative samples, dog and cat owners reported fewer visits to health-care providers and taking less medication for sleeping problems than non-pet owners (Headey, 1999). Also, dog owners slept better, exercised more frequently and took fewer days off from work than comparable non-dog owners (Headey *et al.*, 2008). In Australia and Germany, people who continuously owned a pet over several years were the healthiest in contrast to those who had either lost or just acquired a pet. Even when controlling for age, marital status, gender, income and other variables associated with health, the dog owners reported 15% fewer annual doctor visits than non-owners (Headey and Grabka, 2007).

Several studies indicated that pet ownership also improves cardiovascular health (Levine *et al.*, 2013). This may be mediated by more physical activity (especially walking) of the dog-owners. Friedmann and colleagues (1980) found that high social support and owning a dog, but not a cat, enhanced chances for 1-year survival in patients after an acute myocardial infarction.

### Stress buffering effects

Studies on the effect that interacting with animals has on stress have focused either on endocrinological or cardiovascular parameters. There is evidence that interaction with a friendly animal, in particular a dog, positively affects endocrine stress responses, as indicated by changes in the levels of cortisol, epinephrine and norepinephrine (Cole *et al.*, 2007), suggesting an attenuation of stress responses via human–animal interactions.

Interacting with a dog per se can lead to a reduction in plasma and salivary cortisol (Odendaal, 2000; Odendaal and Meintjes, 2003; Barker *et al.*, 2005). In particular, in stressful situations, social support by a dog can more effectively buffer the cortisol reaction in children with insecure attachment representations than support by a friendly human (Beetz *et al.*, 2011, 2012a). This stress-buffering effect was stronger with increasing time the children spent in physical contact with the dog during the experiment.

A number of well-designed studies found that interacting with a dog also leads to lower blood pressure (Friedmann *et al.*, 1983; Grossberg and Alf, 1985; Vormbrock and Grossberg, 1988) and heart rate (Kaminski *et al.*, 2002; Cole *et al.*, 2007; Handlin *et al.*, 2011) in the absence of a specific stressor. Similar cardiovascular effects were also found with unfamiliar pets during a stress-inducing task (Nagengast *et al.*, 1997; DeMello, 1999; Allen *et al.*, 2001). Allen and colleagues, for example, reported that during a stressful task, the presence of a dog reduces pulse rate, blood pressure and skin conductance even more than the presence of a friend (Allen *et al.*, 1991, 2002).

That animals can buffer stress and promote relaxation was also demonstrated on a behavioural level. Specifically, children displayed less behavioural distress in the company of a friendly dog than in the company of other humans (Nagengast *et al.*, 1997; Hansen *et al.*, 1999).

### Effect on the immune system and oxytocin

Relatively few studies investigated parameters of the immune system and found a significant effect. However, Charnetski and colleagues (2004) demonstrated that stroking a live dog significantly increased salivary immunoglobulin A, compared to stroking a stuffed toy dog or sitting quietly on a couch.

Other research has investigated the influence of human–animal interaction on the human oxytocin system. Several studies found that especially physical contact with a subject's own dog but also interactions with unfamiliar dogs lead to increased levels of the hormone oxytocin (Odendaal, 2000; Odendaal and Meintjes, 2003; Miller *et al.*, 2009; Nagasawa *et al.*, 2009; Handlin *et al.*, 2011). Some authors argue that the activation of the oxytocin system may be a key mechanism in explaining many of the positive effects of human–animal interaction, such as the modulation of stress responses, improved health parameters, improved mood and trust, as well as social attention and interaction (Beetz *et al.*, 2012b). This aspect will be discussed in more detail in the later section on psychophysiological mechanisms.

## Specific Effects on Children and their Education

The mental, physical and socio-emotional health of children largely depends on interactions with primary caregivers, most of all, the parents and direct family. Over the course of development, secondary caregivers in educational facilities such as day-care, kindergarten and school also start to play a more important role. First and foremost, the quality of the social interactions between child and caregiver is strongly associated with the quality of children's development, not only in the social domain but probably also with regard to cognitive learning (Hattie, 2009; Julius *et al.*, 2013). However, interactions and relationships with companion animals also may affect children's development and quality of life. For example, many children regard their pets as close friends and family members, to whom they turn in times of distress

(Kurdek, 2009a,b). Additionally, animal interactions are currently even part of education and therapeutic interventions. In central Europe an increasing number of teachers take dogs into the classroom on a regular basis or keep animals in the classroom (Agsten, 2009; Beetz, 2012). In special education, therapeutic riding or dog-assisted interventions are also gaining in popularity. In the following, we provide a short overview of research demonstrating positive effects of human–animal interaction on child development.

## Human–Animal Interaction and Child Development

In this section, the influence of interacting with animals on the development of social competence, empathy and self-esteem will be discussed, based on the available research.

### Social competence and behaviour

Studies addressing facilitation of interpersonal interaction indicate that the presence of, or interaction with, an animal can improve social behaviour and competence. Regarding children with psychiatric diagnoses, a study shows that therapeutic riding increased the social motivation of children with autism (Bass *et al.*, 2009). In a group of children with autism, occupational therapy with a dog resulted in an increased use of language and more social interaction among the children, compared to sessions without a dog (Sams *et al.*, 2006). In line with these results, children with various psychiatric diagnoses reported higher social extraversion after psychotherapy sessions involving a dog compared to sessions without a dog (Prothmann *et al.*, 2006). Similar effects were found in adults with psychiatric disorders or dementia, as well as in the elderly and prison inmates (Haughie *et al.*, 1992; Fick, 1993; Marr *et al.*, 2000; Filan and Llewellyn-Jones, 2006; Fournier *et al.*, 2007; Perkins *et al.*, 2008; Villalta-Gil *et al.*, 2009). Generally, the data suggest that animal assistance can enhance effects of conventional interventions (Bernstein *et al.*, 2000; Marr *et al.*, 2000; Kramer *et al.*, 2009; Wesley *et al.*, 2009).

The presence of a dog also leads to better social integration of children in their class, and to decreased aggressive behaviour in the classroom (Hergovich *et al.*, 2002; Kotrschal and Ortbauer, 2003). Moreover, children who obtained a new dog were more often visited by friends, and their families engaged in more leisure activities together 1 month after obtaining the dog (Paul and Serpell, 1996).

### Confidence and self-esteem

Growing up with an animal seems to be associated with significantly higher self-confidence (Covert *et al.*, 1985). Also Bergesen (1989) found that the presence of an animal in a classroom significantly increased self-confidence of children over a period of 9 months; children with low confidence profited the most. While in the family environment a direct effect of the companion animal cannot be easily derived from the correlation, the results point to a potential positive effect of human–animal interaction on confidence and self-esteem.

### Empathy

Although studies investigating effects of pet ownership on empathy often face methodological problems that do not allow conclusions on cause and effect, several studies point to a potential positive effect of animal contact on empathy (Daly and Morton, 2003, 2006, 2009). Poresky and Hendrix (1990), for example, found that the bond with a pet was positively related to the level of empathy and social competence in young children, as assessed via reports by their mothers.

Hergovich *et al.* (2002) investigated the effects of the presence of a dog in a class of first-graders in comparison to a control class. Over a period of 3 months, empathy increased in the dog-class while aggression declined. Additionally, the dog-class received higher scores in field independence, indicating a better segregation of self from non-self as a basis of the sensitivity towards other's needs, and therefore an indicator of empathic competences (Hergovich *et al.*, 2002). In summary, these data point to the positive effect of interaction with a dog on empathy in children.

## Learning, Attention and Concentration

The fact that growing up with a pet can positively influence children's development may be one of the reasons why teachers take dogs or other animals to school and integrate them in their lessons. Another reason may be that, even though not always based on data but rather personal experience from practice, several authors report the presence of animals helps promote human attention towards the environment (Katcher and Wilkins, 1994; Wilson and Turner, 1998; Leser, 2008). In particular, dogs are frequently used successfully in practice to stimulate communication and memory in residents of nursing homes, as well as stimulating their attention and concentration.

Teachers who bring their dogs or other animals to class often report a variety of positive effects on children's social behaviour and the climate in the classroom. Animals contribute to a good environment for learning, a positive atmosphere, friendly communication, attention and relaxation (Agsten, 2009; Beetz, 2012). This is contrary to the fear of some headmasters or parents that the animals could distract the children and prevent them from learning.

Gee and colleagues conducted several studies on the effect of the presence of a dog while children performed different tasks (Gee *et al.*, 2007, 2009, 2010a,b). In a motor skill task, a group of developmentally delayed and a group of normally developing children performed faster, with the same level of accuracy, in the presence of a dog than when no dog was present (Gee *et al.*, 2007). The authors speculated that the dog served as an effective motivator or that the dog's presence led to increased relaxation and a reduction of stress during execution of the task, which in turn increased the speed of performance. Additionally, pre-schoolers with and without language impairments adhered better to instructions during an imitation task when a dog was present, in contrast to the presence of a human or a toy dog (Gee *et al.*, 2009). Furthermore, children needed fewer prompts in a memory task when a dog was present and required the most prompts in the presence of another human (Gee *et al.*, 2010a). This finding may be taken as an indicator for better concentration. Similarly, preschool children made fewer errors, i.e. irrelevant choices, in a match-to-sample task when a dog accompanied them (Gee *et al.*, 2010b).

In line with these results, Kotrschal and Ortbauer (2003) demonstrated that the presence of a dog in a classroom reduced overt activity and withdrawal as well as aggressive interactions but enhanced group activities and thus positive social interaction. The children also paid more attention to the teacher when the dog was in the classroom. The authors concluded that 'the presence of a dog in a classroom could positively stimulate social cohesion in children and provide a relatively cheap and easy means of improving teaching conditions' (Kotrschal and Ortbauer, 2003).

In a study with eight children with Down's syndrome, Limond *et al.* (1997) found that children were more attentive to a real dog in contrast to a toy dog and were also more responsive to the adults in the room when the real dog was present. Children in a psychiatric facility rated themselves as significantly more attentive, concentrated, well-adjusted and less distractible after interacting with a live dog for 30 min (Prothmann, 2008). While the reported findings point to enhanced concentration and attention only via indirect variables (e.g. children's behaviour), the only study addressing effects on directly measurable attention performance found no result (Prothmann, 2008).

A recent study provides the first evidence for positive effects of a dog on children's attention, concentration and learning performance (Hediger, 2014). Twenty-four healthy children between 10 and 14 years participated in a randomized controlled cross-over trial. The children completed a memory task (subtest 'digit span' from the intelligence test HAWIK-IV (Petermann and Petermann, 2010)) and three neuropsychological attention tests ('cancellation screen', 'continuous performance test' and 'divided attention test bimodal' (Candit, 2001)). The testing was performed twice, with a week between testing sessions. During the tests, a biological correlate of attention was assessed via passive infrared hemoencephalography (pIR-HEG). In the dog condition, the children could interact with a trained therapy dog for 15 min. While performing the tasks, the dog was lying beside the child's chair.

In the control condition, the robot dog AIBO (Sony, ERS-210), which interacts and obeys to commands, was present.

While children generally improved from session one to session two, this improvement was significantly larger when the dog was present in the second session, showing that the presence of the dog enhanced the learning effect. Regarding the pIR-HEG measure, frontal activity decreased significantly when AIBO was present during the last and most challenging task (divided attention), whereas in the presence of the dog this reduction was not found. This study demonstrated that the presence of a dog did not distract the children, but rather could enhance attention, concentration and memory. In addition to this, the presence of a dog seemed to prevent the decrease of frontal brain activity which occurred in the presence of AIBO after a certain time.

In summary, a growing body of research underlines the potential positive effects of animals on children's development and mental health in the form of pet ownership or in the frame of animal-assisted interventions. Education, in the family as well as at school, is a central element for children's development, well-being and health. Executive functions such as attention and concentration, or rather problems with these, pose an increasing problem in Western societies. Depending on the diagnostic criteria, from 5 to 7% of children are affected by attention deficit hyperactivity disorder (ADHD) (Polanczyk *et al.*, 2007; Willcutt, 2012), which seems to be one of the most common diagnoses in school-aged children. Alternative interventions enhancing concentration and attention, besides pharmacological approaches, could indeed profit significantly from animal involvement. However, more research directly investigating these parameters, especially also in clinical samples, is needed.

## Possible Psychophysiological Mechanisms Underlying Positive Effects of Animals on Children's Development and Education

Health promotion as well as many of the other described effects of human–animal interactions seem to be mediated via the activation of the oxytocin system. There is a considerable overlap of demonstrated effects of human–animal interaction and effects related to increase of oxytocin levels, as demonstrated by experimental research in humans and animals (see Beetz *et al.*, 2012b). Oxytocin buffers the activity of the stress systems, reduces cortisol levels, heart rate and blood pressure. It increases trust and positive social interaction, improves mood and decreases depression and anxiety (Uvnäs-Moberg, 2003; Heinrichs and Domes, 2008).

This direct and indirect evidence of the activation of the oxytocin system via animal contact can be understood as a main factor in explaining positive biological (physiological), psychological and social effects of animals on humans (Julius *et al.*, 2013).

A suboptimal regulation of the stress systems, i.e. frequently or continuously high levels of stress, not only has direct negative health effects on a physiological level but also has a negative impact on learning and thus affects education (Howland and Wang, 2008). Under physiological stress, executive functions (Miyake *et al.*, 2000; Diamond and Lee, 2011) such as concentration, impulse control, self-motivation or higher cognitive/deductive processes are impaired in comparison to active but non-stressful states. Additionally, a positive atmosphere with good social interactions supports optimal executive functions (Diamond and Lee, 2011). Therefore, via positively affecting stress regulation, social interactions and direct effects on concentration, animals have the potential to promote learning or preconditions of learning, both in the cognitive and the socio-emotional domains (Beetz, 2012; Beetz *et al.*, 2012b; Julius *et al.*, 2013).

On a psychosocial level, several more mechanisms combine to explain the presented effects with respect to education. Animals communicate non-verbally, and for many children, as well as adults with impairments, this more direct and authentic communication is easier to understand and accept (Prothmann, 2008). Moreover, motivational effects may play a significant role. In general, children seem interested in animals and highly motivated to interact with them. The presence of an animal can therefore increase children's intrinsic motivation to learn, as well as their curiosity and attention. This not only concerns learning directly about the animal, but also learning and performing tasks unrelated to the animal while in its presence.

A biopsychosocial approach can explain most of the demonstrated positive effects of human–animal interaction: promotion of health, mood, mental and physiological relaxation, trust and social interaction.

## Implications

Animals have the potential to positively affect children's development, to support effective education and therefore to contribute to better biopsychosocial health of children and juveniles.

The presented mechanisms address important issues and problems in Western societies. Stress-related diseases and mental health problems are increasing and will become one of the biggest health challenges in the Western world. In Switzerland, mental disorders and cardiovascular diseases are currently the most expensive diseases, with annual costs of approximately CHF20 billion (Maercker *et al.*, 2013).

In this respect, interactions with animals seem to have a great preventive as well as therapeutic potential. However, it is not simply companion animal ownership or prescribed contact with the animal which is the key. More precisely, it seems as if a positive regard for the animal, positive interaction, and maybe even an emotionally relevant relationship might be prerequisites for the positive effects (Julius *et al.*, 2013).

To perceive the animal as a social partner is the crucial basis of all the effects. Animals represent an important part of our social environment and can provide a relevant complement to human relationships. Since one of the most important health-related factors lies in our social relationships and social support by others (Coan, 2011), it is not surprising that companion animals have such a significant impact on human health (Headey and Grabka, 2007).

Animals cannot and should not replace human relationships. However, due to their special qualities such as unconditional acceptance (Olbrich, 2009) and non-verbal communication, animals may be more effective than human therapists, teachers, or just friends and family alone in certain situations or for a given group of patients or students. Furthermore, animals can provide close physical contact that teachers or therapists cannot provide to the same extent, due to social norms and the therapeutic relationship. The presence of an animal can lead to a joint focus of the therapist and patient as well as to a change of roles. The patient suddenly is no longer only one who is in need, but also one who is also able to care for another living being.

It also should be kept in mind that only healthy and mentally stable animals can provide these positive effects, ideally those from a domesticated species and well socialized with their own species as well as humans (Julius *et al.*, 2013). Only an animal that likes to work in such educational or therapeutic settings and does so without high levels of stress will contribute in the ways described above. In the thinking of One Health, this aspect of the animal's well-being in animal-assisted interventions and companion animal ownership is of utmost importance.

## References

Agsten, L. (2009) *HuPäSch: Hunde in die Schulen - und alles wird gut!?* Books on Demand, Norderstedt.

Allen, K., Blascovich, J., Tomaka, J. and Kelsey, R.M. (1991) Presence of human friends and pet dogs as moderators of autonomic responses to stress in women. *Journal of Personality and Social Psychology* 61, 582–589.

Allen, K., Shykoff, B.E. and Izzo, J.L. (2001) Pet ownership, but not ACE inhibitor therapy, blunts home blood pressure responses to mental stress. *Hypertension* 38, 815–820.

Allen, K., Blascovich, J. and Mendes, W.B. (2002) Cardiovascular reactivity and the presence of pets, friends, and spouses: the truth about cats and dogs. *Psychosomatic Medicine* 64, 727–739.

Archer, J. and Winchester, G. (1994) Bereavement following death of a pet. *British Journal of Psychology* 85, 259–271.

Banks, M.R. and Banks, W.A. (2002) The effects of animal-assisted therapy on loneliness in an elderly population in long-term care facilities. *Journals of Gerontology. Series A, Biolocigal Sciences and Medical Sciences* 57, M428–M432.

Banks, M.R. and Banks, W.A. (2005) The effects of animal-assisted therapy on loneliness in an elderly population in long-term care facilities. *Anthrozoös* 18, 396–408.

Barker, S.B. and Dawson, K.S. (1998) The effects of animal-assisted therapy on anxiety ratings of hospitalized psychiatric patients. *Psychiatric Services* 49, 797–801.

Barker, S.B., Pandurangi, A.K. and Best, A.M. (2003) Effects of animal-assisted therapy on patients' anxiety, fear, and depression before ECT. *Journal of Electroconvulsive Therapy* 19, 38–44.

Barker, S.B., Knisely, J.S., McCain, N.L. and Best, A.M. (2005) Measuring stress and immune response in healthcare professionals following interaction with a therapy dog: a pilot study. *Psychological Reports* 96, 713–729.

Bass, M.M., Duchowny, C.A. and Llabre, M.M. (2009) The effect of therapeutic horseback riding on social functioning in children with autism. *Journal of Autism and Developmental Disorders* 39, 1261–1267.

Beetz, A. (2012) *Hunde im Schulalltag: Grundlagen und Praxis*. Ernst Reinhardt Verlag, München.

Beetz, A., Kotrschal, K., Turner, D.C., Hediger, K., Uvnäs-Moberg, K. and Julius, H. (2011) The effect of a real dog, toy dog and friendly person on insecurely attached children during a stressful task: an exploratory study. *Anthrozoös* 24, 349–368.

Beetz, A., Julius, H., Turner, D.C. and Kotrschal, K. (2012a) Effects of social support by a dog on stress modulation in male children with insecure attachment. *Frontiers in Psychology* 3, 352.

Beetz, A., Uvnäs-Moberg, K., Julius, H. and Kotrschal, K. (2012b) Psychosocial and psychophysiological effects of human-animal interactions: the possible role of oxytocin. *Frontiers in Psychology* 3, 234.

Bergesen, F.J. (1989) The effects of pet facilitated therapy on the self-esteem and socialisation of primary school children. Paper presented at the 5th International Conference on the Relationship between Human and Animals. Monaco, 1989.

Berget, B., Ekeberg, O., Pedersen, I. and Braastad, B.O. (2011) Animal-assisted therapy with farm animals for persons with psychiatric disorders: effects on anxiety and depression, a randomized controlled trial. *Occupational Therapy in Mental Health* 27, 50–64.

Bernstein, P.L., Friedmann, E. and Malaspina, A. (2000) Animal-assisted therapy enhances resident social interaction and initiation in long-term care facilities. *Anthrozoös* 13, 213–224.

Bonas, S., McNicholas, J. and Collis, G.M. (2000) Pets in the network of family relationships: an empirical study. In: Podberscek, A.L., Paul, E.S. and Serpell, J.A. (eds) *Companion Animals and Us: Exploring the relationships between people and pets*. Cambridge University Press, Cambridge, UK, pp. 209–236.

Candit (2001) Computergestützte Diagnostik. Manual.

Charnetski, C.J., Riggers, S. and Brennan, F.X. (2004) Effect of petting a dog on immune system function. *Psychological Reports* 95, 1087–1091.

Coan, J.A. (2011) Social regulation of emotion. In: Decety, J. and Cacioppo, J. (eds) *Handbook of Social Neuroscience*. Oxford University Press, New York, pp. 614–623.

Cole, K.M., Gawlinski, A., Steers, N. and Kotlerman, J. (2007) Animal-assisted therapy in patients hospitalized with heart failure. *American Journal of Critical Care* 16, 575–585; quiz 586; discussion 587–578.

Colombo, G., Buono, M.D., Smania, K., Raviola, R. and De Leo, D. (2006) Pet therapy and institutionalized elderly: a study on 144 cognitively unimpaired subjects. *Archives of Gerontology and Geriatrics* 42, 207–216.

Covert, A.M., Whiren, A.P., Keith, J. and Nelson, C. (1985) Pets, early adolescents and families. *Marriage and Family Review* 8, 95–108.

Crowley-Robinson, P., Fenwick, D.C. and Blackshaw, J.K. (1996) A long-term study of elderly people in nursing homes with visiting and resident dogs. *Applied Animal Behaviour Science* 47, 137–148.

Daly, B. and Morton, L.L. (2003) Children with pets do not show higher empathy: a challenge to current views. *Anthrozoös* 16, 298–314.

Daly, B. and Morton, L.L. (2006) An investigation of human-animal interactions and empathy as related to pet preference, ownership, attachment, and attitudes in children. *Anthrozoös* 19, 113–127.

Daly, B. and Morton, L.L. (2009) Empathic difference in adults as a function of childhood and adult pet ownership and pet type. *Anthrozoös* 22, 371–382.

Darrah, J.P. (1996) A pilot survey of animal-facilitated therapy in Southern California and South Dakota nursing homes. *Occupational Therapy International* 3, 105–121.

DeMello, L.R. (1999) The effect of the presence of a companion-animal on physiological changes following the termination of cognitive stressors. *Psychology and Health* 14, 859–868.

Diamond, A. and Lee, K. (2011) Interventions shown to aid executive function development in children 4 to 12 years old. *Science* 333, 959–964.
Doherty, N.A. and Feeney, J.A. (2004) The composition of attachment networks throughout the adult years. *Personal Relationships* 11, 469–488.
Eddy, J., Hart, L.A. and Boltz, R.P. (2001) The effects of service dogs on social aknowledgements of people in wheelchairs. *Journal of Psychology* 122, 39–45.
Endenburg, N. (1995) The attachment of people to companion animals. *Anthrozoös* 8, 83–89.
Fick, K.M. (1993) The influence of an animal on social interactions of nursing home residents in a group setting. *American Journal of Occupational Therapy* 47, 529–534.
Filan, S.L. and Llewellyn-Jones, R.H. (2006) Animal-assisted therapy for dementia: a review of the literature. *International Psychogeriatrics* 18, 597–611.
Fournier, A.K., Geller, E.S. and Fortney, E.V. (2007) Human-animal interaction in a prison setting: impact on criminal behavior, treatment progress, and social skills. *Behavior and Social Issues* 16, 89–105.
Friedmann, E., Katcher, A.H., Lynch, J.J. and Thomas, S.A. (1980) Animal companions and one-year survival of patients after discharge from a coronary care unit. *Public Health Reports* 95, 307–312.
Friedmann, E., Katcher, A.H., Thomas, S.A., Lynch, J.J. and Messent, P.R. (1983) Social interaction and blood pressure. Influence of animal companions. *Journal of Nervous and Mental Disease* 171, 461–465.
Gee, N.R., Harris, S.L. and Johnson, K.L. (2007) The role of therapy dogs in speed and accuracy to complete motor skills tasks for preschool children. *Anthrozoös* 20, 375–386.
Gee, N.R., Sherlock, T.R., Bennett, E.A. and Harris, S.L. (2009) Preschoolers' adherence to instructions as a function of presence of a dog and motor skill tasks. *Anthrozoös* 22, 267–276.
Gee, N.R., Christ, E.M. and Carr, D.N. (2010a) Preschool children require fewer instructional prompts to perform a memory task in the presence of a dog. *Anthrozoös* 23, 173–184.
Gee, N.R., Church, M.T. and Altobelli, C.L. (2010b) Preschoolers make fewer errors on an object categorization task in the presence of a dog. *Anthrozoös* 23, 223–230.
Gerwolls, M.K. and Labott, S.M. (1994) Adjustment to the death of a companion animal. *Anthrozoös* 7, 172–187.
Grossberg, J.M. and Alf, E.F. (1985) Interaction with pet dogs: effects on human cardiovascular response. *Journal of the Delta Society* 2, 20–27.
Gueguen, N. and Ciccotti, S. (2008) Domestic dogs as facilitators in social interaction: an evaluation of helping and courtship behaviors. *Anthrozoös* 21, 339–349.
Handlin, L., Hydbring-Sandberg, E., Nilsson, A., Ejdebäck, M., Jansson, A. and Uvnäs-Moberg, K. (2011) Short-term interaction between dogs and their owners: effects on oxytocin, cortisol, insulin and heart rate – An exploratory study. *Anthrozoös* 24, 301–315.
Hansen, K.M., Messinger, C.J., Baun, M.M. and Megel, M. (1999) Companion animals alleviating distress in children. *Anthrozoös* 12, 142–148.
Hart, L.A., Hart, B.L. and Bergin, B. (1987) Socializing effects of service dogs for people with disabilities. *Anthrozoös* 1, 41–44.
Hattie, J. (2009) *Visible Learning: a synthesis of meta-analyses relating to achievement.* Routledge, Abingdon, UK.
Haughie, E., Milne, D. and Elliott, V. (1992) An evaluation of companion pets with elderly psychiatric patients. *Behavioural Psychotherapy* 20, 367–372.
Headey, B. (1999) Health benefits and health costs savings due to pets: preliminary estimates from an Australian national survey. *Social Indicators Research* 47, 233–243.
Headey, B. and Grabka, M.M. (2007) Pets and human health in Germany and Australia: national longitudinal results. *Social Indicators Research* 80, 297–311.
Headey, B., Na, F. and Zheng, R. (2008) Pet dogs benefit owners' health: a 'natural experiment' in China. *Social Indicators Research* 84, 481–493.
Hediger, K. (2014) Can dogs enhance children's attention performance? A randomized controlled cross-over trial. *Human–Animal Interaction Bulletin* 2, 21–39.
Heinrichs, M. and Domes, G. (2008) Neuropeptides and social behaviour: effects of oxytocin and vasopressin in humans. *Progress in Brain Research* 170, 337–350.
Hergovich, A., Monshi, B., Semmler, G. and Zieglmayer, V. (2002) The effects of the presence of a dog in the classroom. *Anthrozoös* 15, 37–50.
Holcomb, R., Jendro, C., Weber, B. and Nahan, U. (1997) Use of an aviary to relieve depression in elderly males *Anthrozoös* 10, 32–36.
Howland, J.G. and Wang, Y.T. (2008) Synaptic plasticity in learning and memory: stress effects in the hippocampus. *Progress in Brain Research* 169, 145–158.

Hunt, M., Al-Awadi, H. and Johnson, M. (2008) Psychological sequelae of pet loss following Hurricane Katrina. *Anthrozoös* 21, 109–121.
Jessen, J., Cardiello, F. and Baun, M.M. (1996) Avian companionship in alleviation of depression, loneliness, and low morale of older adults in skilled rehabilitation units. *Psychological Reports* 78, 339–348.
Julius, H., Beetz, A., Kotrschal, K., Turner, D.C. and Uvnäs-Moberg, K. (2013) *Attachment to Pets. An Integrative View of Human-Animal Relationships with Implications for Therapeutic Practice*. Hogrefe, Göttingen.
Kaminski, M., Pellino, T. and Wish, J. (2002) Play and pets: the physical and emotional impact of child-life and pet therapy on hospitalized children. *Children's Health Care* 31, 321–335.
Katcher, A. and Wilkins, G.G. (1994) Helping children with attention-deficit hyperactive and conduct disorders through animal-assisted therapy and education. *InterActions* 12, 5–10.
Kotrschal, K. and Ortbauer, B. (2003) Behavioral effects of the presence of a dog in a classroom. *Anthrozoös* 16, 147–159.
Kramer, S.C., Friedmann, E. and Bernstein, P.L. (2009) Comparison of the effect of human interaction, animal-assisted therapy, and AIBO-assisted therapy on long-term care residents with dementia. *Anthrozoös* 22, 43–57.
Kurdek, L.A. (2009a) Pet dogs as attachment figures for adult owners. *Journal of Family Psychology* 23, 439–446.
Kurdek, L.A. (2009b) Young adults' attachment to pet dogs: findings from open-ended methods. *Anthrozoös* 22, 359–369.
Leser, M. (2008) Tiere und ihre Wirkungen auf den Menschen. In: Leser, M. (ed.) *Mensch-Tier-Beziehungen. Tiereinsätze im Heimbereich*. CURAVIVA Schweiz, Bern.
Levine, G.N., Allen, K., Braun, L.T., Christian, H.E., Friedmann, E., Taubert, K.A., Thomas, S.A., Wells, D.L. and Lange, R.A. (2013) Pet ownership and cardiovascular risk: a scientific statement from the American Heart Association. *Circulation* 127, 2353–2363.
Limond, J.A., Bradshaw, J.W.S. and Cormack, K.F.M. (1997) Behavior of children with learning disabilities interacting with a therapy dog. *Anthrozoös* 10, 84–89.
Lockwood, R. (1983) The influence of animals on social perception. In: Katcher, A.H. and Beck, A.M. (eds) *New Perspectives on Our Lives with Companion Animals*. University of Pennsylvania Press, Philadelphia, pp. 64–71.
Mader, B., Hart, L.A. and Bergin, B. (1989) Social acknowledgements for children with disabilities: effects of service dogs. *Child Development* 60, 1529–1534.
Maercker, A., Perkonigg, A., Preisig, M., Schaller, K. and Weller, M. (2013) The costs of disorders of the brain in Switzerland: an update from the European Brain Council Study for 2010. *Swiss Medical Weekly* 143:w13751.
Marr, C.A., French, L., Thompson, D., Drum, L., Greening, G., Mormon, J., *et al.* (2000) Animal-assisted therapy in psychiatric rehabilitation. *Anthrozoös* 13, 43–47.
McNicholas, J. and Collis, G.M. (2006) Animal as social supports: insights for understanding animal-assisted therapy. Theoretical foundations and guidelines for practice. In: Fine, A.H. (ed.) *Handbook on Animal-Assisted Therapy. Theoretical Foundations and Guidelines for Practice*, 2nd edn. Elsevier, San Diego, California, pp. 49–71.
Melson, G.F. and Schwarz, R. (1994) Pets as social support for families of young children. Paper presented at the annual meeting of the Delta Society, New York.
Miller, S.C., Kennedy, C., DeVoe, D., Hickey, M., Nelson, T. and Kogan, L. (2009) An examination of changes in oxytocin levels in men and women before and after interaction with a bonded dog. *Anthrozoös* 22, 31–42.
Miyake, A., Friedman, N.P., Emerson, M.J., Witzki, A.H., Howerter, A. and Wager, T.D. (2000) The unity and diversity of executive functions and their contributions to complex 'Frontal Lobe' tasks: a latent variable analysis. [Research Support, U.S. Gov't, Non-P.H.S.]. *Cognitive Psychology* 41, 49–100.
Nagasawa, M., Kikusui, T., Onaka, T. and Ohta, M. (2009) Dog's gaze at its owner increases owner's urinary oxytocin during social interaction. *Hormones and Behavior* 55, 434–441.
Nagengast, S.L., Baun, M.M., Megel, M. and Leibowitz, J.M. (1997) The effects of the presence of a companion animal on physiological arousal and behavioral distress in children during a physical examination. *Journal of Pediatric Nursing* 12, 323–330.
Nathans-Barel, I., Feldman, P., Berger, B., Modai, I. and Silver, H. (2005) Animal-assisted therapy ameliorates anhedonia in schizophrenia patients. A controlled pilot study. *Psychotherapy and Psychosomatics* 74, 31–35.
Odendaal, J.S. (2000) Animal-assisted therapy - magic or medicine? *Journal of Psychosomatic Research* 49, 275–280.

Odendaal, J.S. and Meintjes, R.A. (2003) Neurophysiological correlates of affiliative behaviour between humans and dogs. *Veterinary Journal* 165, 296–301.

Olbrich, E. (2009) Bausteine einer Theorie der Mensch-Tier-Beziehung. In: Otterstedt, C. and Rosenberger, M. (eds) *Gefährten, Konkurrenten, Verwandte. Die Mensch-Tier-Beziehung im wissenschaftlichen Diskurs.* Vandenhoeck & Ruprecht, Göttingen, pp. 111–132.

Paul, E.S. and Serpell, J.A. (1996) Obtaining a new pet dog: effects on middle childhood children and their families. *Applied Animal Behaviour Science* 47, 17–29.

Perkins, J., Bartlett, H., Travers, C. and Rand, J. (2008) Dog-assisted therapy for older people with dementia: a review. *Australasian Journal on Ageing* 27, 177–182.

Petermann, F. and Petermann, U. (2010) *HAWIK-IV*. Verlag Hans Huber, Bern.

Polanczyk, G., de Lima, M.S., Horta, B.L., Biederman, J. and Rohde, L.A. (2007) The worldwide prevalence of ADHD: a systematic review and metaregression analysis. *American Journal of Psychiatry* 164, 942–948.

Poresky, R.H. and Hendrix, C. (1990) Differential effects of pet presence and pet-bonding on young children. *Psychological Reports* 67, 51–54.

Prothmann, A. (2008) *Tiergestützte Kinderpsychotherapie. Theorie und Praxis der tiergestützen Psychotherapie bei Kindern und Jugendlichen*, 2nd edn. Peter Lang, Frankfurt am Main.

Prothmann, A., Bienert, M. and Ettrich, C. (2006) Dogs in child psychotherapy: effects on state of mind. *Anthrozoös* 19, 265–277.

Rossbach, K.A. and Wilson, J.P. (1992) Does a dog's presence make a person appear more likeable? *Anthrozoös* 5, 40–51.

Rost, D.H. and Hartmann, A. (1994) Children and their pets. *Anthrozoös* 7, 242–254.

Sams, M.J., Fortney, E.V. and Willenbring, S. (2006) Occupational therapy incorporating animals for children with autism: a pilot investigation. *American Journal of Occupational Therapy* 60, 268–274.

Schneider, M.S. and Harley, L.P. (2006) How dogs influence the evaluation of psychotherapists. *Anthrozoös* 19, 128–142.

Shiloha, S., Sorek, G. and Terkel, J. (2003) Reduction of state-anxiety by petting animals in a controlled laboratory experiment. *Anxiety, Stress and Coping* 16, 387–395.

Souter, M.A. and Miller, M.D. (2007) Do animal-assisted activities effectively treat depression: a meta-analysis. *Anthrozoös* 20, 167–180.

Stallones, L. (1994) Pet loss and mental-health. *Anthrozoös* 7, 43–54.

Turner, D.C., Rieger, G. and Gygax, L. (2003) Spouses and cats and their effects on human mood. *Anthrozoös* 16, 213–228.

Uvnäs-Moberg, K. (2003) *The Oxytocin Factor. Tapping the Hormone of Calm, Love, and Healing.* Da Capo Press, Cambridge.

Villalta-Gil, V., Roca, M., Gonzalez, N., Domenec, E., *et al.* (2009) Dog-assisted therapy in the treatment of chronic schizophrenia inpatients. *Anthrozoös* 22, 149–159.

Vormbrock, J.K. and Grossberg, J.M. (1988) Cardiovascular effects of human pet dog interactions. *Journal of Behavioral Medicine* 11, 509–517.

Wells, D.L. (2004) The facilitation of social interactions by domestic dogs. *Anthrozoös* 17, 340–352.

Wells, M. and Perrine, R. (2001) Pets go to college: the influence of pets on students' perceptions of faculty and their offices. *Anthrozoös* 14, 161–168.

Wesley, M.C., Minatrea, N.B. and Watson, J.C. (2009) Animal-assisted therapy in the treatment of substance dependence. *Anthrozoös* 22, 137–148.

Willcutt, E.G. (2012) The prevalence of DSM-IV attention-deficit/hyperactivity disorder: a meta-analytic review. *Neurotherapeutics* 9, 490–499.

Wilson, C.C. and Turner, D.C. (eds) (1998) *Companion Animals in Human Health*. Sage Publications, Thousand Oaks, California.

# 8 Integrated Risk Assessment – Foodborne Diseases

**Vanessa Racloz,[1]* David Waltner-Toews[2] and Katharina D.C. Stärk[3,4]**

*[1]The Roll Back Malaria Partnership Secretariat, hosted by the World Health Organization, Geneva, Switzerland; [2]Department of Population Medicine, University of Guelph, Canada; [3]Royal Veterinary College, Hertfordshire, UK; [4]SAFOSO AG, Bern, Switzerland*

## Introduction

### Foodborne disease risk assessments: a brief history

One Health as currently defined has emerged from several major streams of research and practice. One of the areas that has informed One Health is the broad area of risk analysis associated with foodborne infections and intoxications. Foodborne diseases arise from the consumption of food or associated products contaminated with viruses, parasites, bacteria (including their toxins) or chemicals. Cases can occur sporadically or, if linked by a common source, as outbreaks. Foodborne disease outbreaks are acute yet relatively short lived with regional impacts and commonly involve *Salmonella*, *Escherichia coli*, *Staphylococci*, *Listeria* or Norovirus. Yet incidents can also be prolonged due to lengthier incubation periods or long-term exposure as seen in the bovine spongiform encephalopathy epidemic (Hueston, 2013) or the more recent melamine-contaminated milk products (Nie *et al.*, 2013), both of which had economic and public health impacts on a global scale. Protracted outbreaks are often due to a failure in identifying the causative hazard or due to the inability to trace its source. Through increased urbanization and the internationalization of food production chains, the need for global surveillance of foodborne pathogens has been prioritized by national governments as well as worldwide organizations such as the Food and Agriculture Organization (FAO), the World Health Organization (WHO) and the World Organisation for Animal Health (OIE).

Improvements in surveillance along with the globalization and industrialization of agrifood systems have contributed to uncovering the magnitude of foodborne hazards currently circulating, with the result that methods for disease prevention and risk management are being sought by all stakeholders. Policy and management measures commonly include setting tolerance levels for various contaminants based on experimental evidence and forced recalls of foods where contaminant levels are found to exceed legally acceptable levels. Yet due to the nature of the response, hazards often cause dramatic effects in the consumer market and, therefore, measures have been taken to identify, prevent and manage risks of contamination before they occur. The Hazard Analysis Critical Control Points analysis

*E-mail: raclozv@who.int

(HACCP) has been useful for identifying hazards and controlling them within the confines of institutions and factories, whilst risk analysis, initially designed to manage chemical risks in the food chain, has been adapted by public health practitioners and researchers to address the broader risks of foodborne and waterborne diseases (National Research Council, 1983, 1993; Waltner-Toews and McEwen, 1994a; Pintar *et al.*, 2010). Although the primary concern of those designing and implementing risk analyses has been the health of consumers in industrialized countries, the applications have been broadened to include public health, and animal and environmental issues as well as various overlapping contexts.

Risk analysis is a framework used widely in order to identify, discuss and manage risks in a broad range of circumstances, including chemical risks and the public health context as described above. Risk assessments are the technical component of risk analyses, typically including activities for hazard characterization, exposure and consequence assessments (Fig. 8.1). Risk assessment has become the accepted standard for determining risks to consumers, particularly those related to international trade

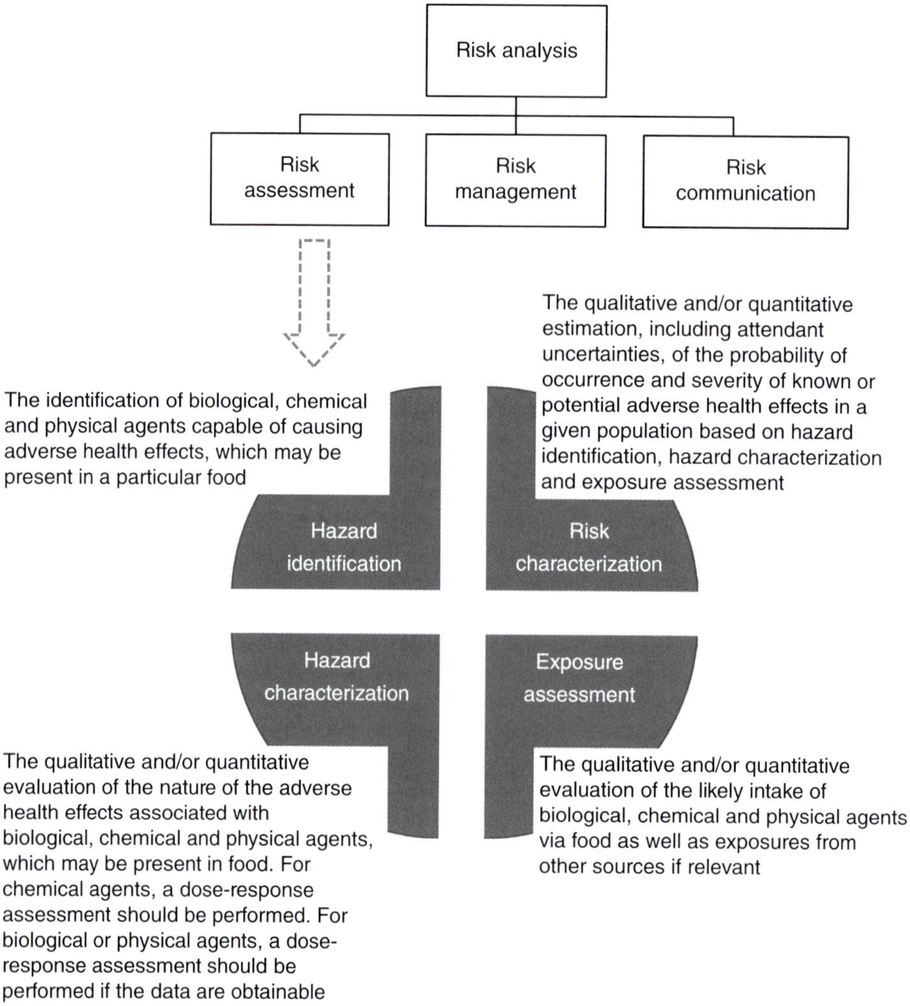


**Fig. 8.1.** Components of a risk assessment (adapted from FAO/WHO, 2005).

that are referred to in the Sanitary and Phytosanitary Agreement (CAC, 1999). The Codex Alimentarius Commission (CAC) initiated the development of a standardized framework for the application of risk assessments in relation to food through a joint FAO/WHO meeting in 1995 (FAO/WHO, 1995). The World Organisation for Animal Health (OIE) also developed standards for assessing risks related to animal health (OIE, 1999). Food safety risk assessments have been conducted for a variety of diseases (Schlundt, 2000) such as bovine spongiform encephalopathy (Kadohira *et al.*, 2012), different bacterial hazards such as *E. coli*, *Salmonella* and *Campylobacter* (Cassin *et al.*, 1998) and chemical residues (Bietlot and Kolakowski, 2012). In 2002, the European Union created the European Food Safety Authority (EFSA), an agency specifically designed to conduct risk assessments and risk communication regarding food and feed safety (EFSA, 2002).

Risk assessments are data-driven and therefore require inputs from monitoring and surveillance activities as well as from a range of experiments in animal and laboratory models. Additionally, risk assessments can also be used to inform the design of surveillance programmes. The latter approach has become known as 'risk-based surveillance' (Stark *et al.*, 2006). This has been increasingly used, particularly for the surveillance of rare events (see also Schelling and Hattendorf, Chapter 10, this volume).

## Overview of current risk assessment methods

The OIE defines a risk assessment as 'the evaluation of the likelihood and the biological and economic consequences of entry, establishment or spread of a pathogenic agent within the territory of an importing country' (OIE, 1999). It represents the process by which various pathways, involved in identification, description and analysis, associated with the transmission of a given hazard/threat are evaluated. The process should lead to a qualitative, semi-quantitative or quantitative output representing the risk that a certain hazard poses to the specified population. The amount of detail can range from a simple assessment assessed qualitatively, i.e. low versus high risk, to a full quantitative probabilistic model.

For food safety risk assessments, the framework used by the CAC is often used. Either way, such assessments are typically conducted 'from stable to table', i.e. integrating processes occurring in primary production for animal and plant source food, and also processes during harvest, processing, storage, handling and preparation. In the case of a One Health approach, the assessment should include the exposure of human and animal consumers. This typically involves consumption considerations, dietary differences among consumers and consequential exposure dosage.

Risk assessments have been useful for characterizing the types of hazards that enter food chains at various points and how these hazards are modified throughout the food handling process from 'farm to fork'. Hazards are not only categorized as microbiological but can also be attributed to include behavioural and practical aspects, and hence risk assessments which are able to encompass such a range of factors make useful contributions to a One Health approach. The purpose of a risk assessment can be related to a practical question regarding the need and choice of risk management. Risk assessment can also be used to answer research questions on disease estimates or to prioritize alternative transmission pathways. Each assessment is unique, and methodologies have to take into account this heterogeneity. Efforts need to be made to include not only end-point consumers but also the risk to producers, distributors and communities, in addition to the ecosystems in which they are embedded. Ideally, risk assessments should be able to handle interactions and trade-offs among multiple, multi-scalar impacts of different food production and distribution programmes. In order to include aspects affecting public, animal and ecosystem health, multiple outcomes should include: impact on farmers (health, sustainability, income, social well-being); water resources; other natural resources (protein inputs to animal feeds, fossil fuels); land use (and its effect on wild populations, both in terms of conservation and the likelihood of infectious hazards, such as H5N1 or Nipah virus, entering the human food chain);

micro- and global climate change. Food security should be valid and consistent (Schlundt, 2000; Ross and Sumner, 2002), whereby a probability figure or rating is given to a certain event or outcome.

Risk assessment results can be present in both qualitative and quantitative format, with associated advantages and disadvantages for both methods. Qualitative methods, as described in the OIE Code, are usually expressed as 'high', 'medium', 'low' or 'negligible' (OIE, 2004). Quantitative methods vary from spreadsheet calculations (Vose *et al.*, 2001) to probabilistic modelling or scenario tree models (Morley *et al.*, 2003). Quantitative risk assessments have certain advantages, particularly in quantifying the uncertainty and variability of parameters as well as the overall risk output. The choice of methods depends on the risk question, the availability of data and the available resources, such as access to human and veterinary health data. The choice also refers to both the available time as well as the competencies of the staff involved. To date, the majority of risk assessments conducted in relation to food safety have remained qualitative, with a few notable examples mentioned below.

## Examples of Added Value through Integrated Risk Assessments in Food Safety Issues

The following risk assessments have been specifically chosen to illustrate the different hazards relevant in the food chain, including heterogeneous spatial and temporal settings as well as source, reservoir, exposure pathway, treatment and type of incident. The characterization of these hazards and their contexts is important in its own right. Within a One Health framework, these represent nodes in more complex sets of interactions.

### Variant Creutzfeld-Jakob disease and bovine spongiform encephalopathy

Variant Creutzfeld-Jakob disease (vCJD), a fatal neurodegenerative disorder, is caused by prions and belongs to the group of transmissible spongiform encephalopathies (TSE). This hazard can serve as an example for a foodborne disease with a very long incubation period, with recent arguments stating that the disease can exceed 50 years of incubation (Collinge *et al.*, 2006). The origin of bovine spongiform encephalopathy (BSE), mad cow disease in cattle and described in humans as vCJD, is hypothesized to date back to the contamination of processed animal protein and meat-and-bone meal (MBM) with material from animals with naturally occurring TSE in the UK in the 1970s (CDC, 2014).

Primary control measures for vCJD, based on an understanding of transmission routes, have included culling of cattle based on testing or age cohorts in infected herds and feed bans. Due to its status as a rare disease in both people and cattle, active surveillance and detection is challenging. Although transmission is also possible through red blood cell and fresh frozen plasma transfusion (Bennett and Daraktchiev, 2013), the main public health risk of vCJD remains the alimentary route. In the UK alone, an estimated 3 million infected cattle entered the human food chain before massive surveillance and control measures were implemented (Smith and Bradley, 2003).

The complete list of animals that suffer from prion disease remains unresolved, and theories even include marine mammals, although to date the main impact of this type of disease has been noted in sheep and cattle. This represents a problem for decision makers who need to justify the risks posed to human health versus impacts on farmers' livelihoods as well as the export industry. One Health issues highlighted by risk assessments include the links of dietary exposure of cattle, economic incentives to both farmers (for more efficient use of feeds) and processors (to minimize energy and chemical use) and societal patterns of meat consumption (Nathanson *et al.*, 1997; Cooper and Bird, 2003). Several risk assessments are available in terms of quantifying the risk of infection within cattle across countries (Animal and Plant Health Inspection Service, 2007; Salman *et al.*, 2012), as well as comprehensive reports for human risks (Glatzel *et al.*, 2003) including a simulation for human dietary exposure intensities to BSE (Cooper and Bird, 2003).

Upon request from the European Commission, a geographical BSE risk assessment was conducted to quantify the presence of BSE-positive cattle in a geographical area or country. The obtained risk levels have also been incorporated into risk assessments with regard to human medicinal (EC, 2011) and beauty products that use animal ingredients.

As mentioned, the trade disruption caused by BSE, given the assessed human health risks, has been huge and is still preventing market access for beef from many countries. The total economic losses caused by BSE have been estimated to be several billion euros for heavily affected countries such as the UK and Germany. Due to the uncertain and public nature of this disease, substantial precautionary measures for BSE intervention were taken by policy makers. The analysis by Benedictus *et al.* (2009) has shown that under declining BSE prevalence and incidence, cost-effectiveness of such measures becomes unfavourable and the measures difficult to justify. In the Netherlands, figures ranged from €4.3 million per human life year saved in 2002 to €17.7 million in 2005. Precaution-based legislation should incorporate checks on cost-effectiveness (Zinsstag *et al.*, Chapter 12, this volume), in order to not let control strategies deviate from regular health economics thresholds as uncertainties disappear and risks become quantifiable.

Risk assessments involving the transmission of BSE have identified the complex relationships among the prion agent, environmental, public health and veterinary systems, agricultural production infrastructure, import and export routes, economic incentives, consumption issues and slaughtering processes. Characterization of these multiple impacts and relationships has provided an excellent basis for re-conceptualizing this as a One Health issue and identifying who the key stakeholders should be in negotiating long-term strategies to prevent future occurrences of similar diseases. Risk assessors are increasingly reaching out to broader assessment approaches and are flexible as new information becomes available (Berthe *et al.*, 2013).

## Salmonellosis

The epidemiology of foodborne *Salmonella* infections is very different from BSE. The incubation time is short, hours, resulting in dynamic outbreak situations. *Salmonella enteritidis* can be spread through eggs and poultry as well as other food sources, and its distribution can be accentuated by the trade of contaminated sources at an international level. Person-to-person spread is, however, rare. During the investigation of an outbreak, source tracing involves categorizing the different risks found at each production and management level, starting with the differences between farms (for example, between layers and broiler chicken), slaughterhouse infrastructure, regional or international consumption field, as well as required freshness of product (frozen versus live market).

The USDA Food Safety and Inspection Service (FSIS) demonstrated how inclusive a full risk assessment can be through a study concerning the risk of *S. enteritidis* entering human consumption through shell eggs. This process included measuring the risk at each stage of preparation, processing as well as shipment and storage of the food products (FSIS, USDA Food Safety and Inspection Service, 1998). The results of the assessment were compared with the national records of human *Salmonella* sp. cases, whereby a significant overlap was observed between consumption data and the number of human cases attributed to *S. enteritidis*-infected eggs. The main purpose of this risk assessment was to determine the discrepancies between modelled forecast of disease and live surveillance. Similar modular assessments are available for assessing the risk of *Salmonella* in sheep.

Typical components of food risk assessments along the production chain are: animal feed, primary production, transport of animals, slaughter, cutting and boning of carcasses, chilling, transport of meat, processing (on-farm or industrial), wholesale, retail, storage and home/commercial cooking (NZ Gov, 2000). In the latter risk assessment, after testing for possible contamination at each stage involving animal slaughter and processing, a human case-control study was carried out to complete the 'farm to fork' concept of food safety.

The strength of the risk assessment approach is that it allows for mapping the production chain as it is relevant in the industry of concern. The main challenges are then to parameterize the model so that the risk along the chain can be estimated. When data are lacking, expert opinion is an accepted alternative information source. More cross-sector expert knowledge and data exchange is needed to validate the risk assessments along the food chain with the disease occurrence in people.

In order to provide a comprehensive assessment of the multidimensional risks related to food, additional relevant issues should be included such as interactions between microbial ecology, economic incentives to poultry farmers, competition among vertically integrated large-scale poultry producers, consumer expectations of 'cheap' and microbiologically safe chicken in the store, fossil fuel prices, antibiotic use in poultry (which can alter microbial ecology in both the chickens and the consumers) and the effect of other disease-control programmes. For instance, some researchers have suggested that *S. enteritidis*, as a pathogen in people but not poultry, has moved its ecological niche into one vacated by *S. gallinarum*, a pathogen of poultry but not people, as the result of veterinary programmes to eradicate fowl plague (Rabsch *et al.*, 2000).

## Chemicals and pollutants

Another example of risk assessments involving food safety is seen in the management of chemical residues, organic pollutants and heavy metals, which was the origin of much of the risk assessment literature (Waltner-Toews and McEwen, 1994a). Due to the persistent nature of some chemicals and their role as environmental contaminants, this category of hazards affects the agricultural, tourist, veterinary, public health, marine and environmental sectors, and a complete risk assessment needs to take this into account. Such hazards may thus represent not only the origins of risk assessments, but also suggest some strategies for their future in a context of One Health. Recently, an integrated framework for human and animal risk assessment was published (Lavelle *et al.*, 2012).

Antibiotics, despite being a force for improved health, have also become a major chemical hazard, sometimes as residues, but often acting to select for resistant bacteria. The outcomes selected as being relevant by particular stakeholder groups (efficient animal growth for livestock producers, effective treatment for medical and veterinary practitioners) are sometimes in conflict, which makes risk assessments challenging. In most cases, effective treatment has, with good reason, trumped efficient feed utilization. Antimicrobials are widely used in human and animal medicine to prevent and combat bacterial infections. Resistance against antimicrobials is a natural and ancient phenomenon, but there is evidence that the current global levels of resistance are, in part, due to the use of antimicrobials in livestock. Defining boundaries between the use of antimicrobials in humans and their use in animals proves extremely challenging. Any use of antimicrobials in animals can ultimately affect humans, and vice versa, due to the connectedness of microorganism populations. Resistant bacteria and resistance genes carried by commensal bacteria in food-producing animals can reach people, mainly directly via the food chain. Resistant bacteria can also spread through the environment (e.g. via contaminated water) or through direct animal contact on farms or at home with pets (Wegener, 2012).

Risk assessment approaches similar to the ones described above have been used to assess the risk of antimicrobial resistance. The inclusion of various pathways at the slaughterhouse level alone, are well demonstrated in a semi-quantitative risk assessment (Presi *et al.*, 2009) for the analysis of resistant bacteria. Exposure risk was conducted through different animal sources (pigs, cattle, chicken) as well as different product categories ranging from fresh, frozen and raw, identifying the high-risk procedures involved in the contamination phase. Certain challenges remain in being able to fully assess complex relationships such as specific agent–bacterium–animal species combinations. Studies have been limited by the lack of knowledge of dose–response relationship, i.e. the health consequences of exposure of the human microbiome to resistance genes in food

(Alban *et al.*, 2008). Much more research is needed to better parameterize risk assessments. This gap is currently being addressed in a new multi-country research project on antimicrobial resistance in the food chain (see for example the EU-funded programme EFFORT, http://www.effort-against-amr.eu).

Even if all the hazards related to antimicrobial use can be parameterized, however, their use and perceived abuse involves so many conflicting pressures, demands and aspirations that a transdisciplinary One Health approach, bringing together a broad range of scientists from different field and lay groups, will likely be necessary to arrive at acceptable public policies and programmes.

Heavy metal contamination in the food chain illustrates some of the complex interactions affecting both food safety and proposed solutions. While risk assessments have been conducted and provide useful information, they are limited by the fact that interactions in cause and impact are recursive and context-dependent, both geographically and culturally. Mercury offers one example from a list of many such as cadmium, lead and arsenic. Mercury contamination in fish has been associated with many factors such as hydroelectric power generation (Bodaly *et al.*, 2007), paper production and other industrial development (Waltner-Toews and McEwen, 1994b; Wheatley, 1997), or often to provide land for new settlers or to provide other kinds of food for export (Roulet *et al.*, 1999; Da Silva *et al.*, 2005; Deutsch and Folke, 2005). A powerful example of the power of risk assessment was provided in the Amazon region. While goldmining had accounted for a high percentage of atmospheric mercury, mercury content in terrestrial and aquatic ecosystems was caused by deforestation in Amazonian watersheds (Roulet *et al.*, 1999). Through identifying the main mercury-contaminated fish source, researchers and Amazonian villagers were able to develop modified fishing and culinary practices to minimize this type of mercury exposure pathway (Forget and Lebel, 2001; Guimarães and Mergel, 2012).

Solutions in each sector and context will be different and require engagement with different stakeholders, some with legitimately differing perspectives. In Canada, aboriginal concepts of human and environmental health were not the same as those of industry and government regulators, and the social and cultural impacts of mercury pollution were far greater than direct clinical impacts (Wheatley, 1997). This underlines the need for a deeper and more complex understanding of health such as that proposed by Houle (Chapter 33, this volume).

## Risk assessment in the One Health domain

In an integrated approach for food safety risk assessment, hazards occurring in animals or plants used for food production are linked to public health outcomes. This requires knowledge of the impact of production, transportation and processing steps as well as dose–response relationships. In the past few decades, considerable effort has been directed at quantifying the hazards and exposures based on a set of linear food-chain assumptions.

For various reasons, including underreporting, the real burden of foodborne diseases is still unclear. The CDC estimated between 28.7 and 71.1 million cases per year of foodborne diseases in the USA alone, although with wide confidence intervals (CDC, 2012). Efforts are being made to quantify this burden, including the incorporation of secondary effects such as severity, duration and cost of illness as addressed by the WHO Foodborne Disease Burden Epidemiology Reference Group (FERG) rather than only the two generic morbidity and mortality measures.

When assessing risks related to food, the volume of consumption of a specific food will have direct impact on risk as it quantifies exposure. Therefore, efforts to quantify food consumptions are important to allow for valid assessments. In recent years, the EFSA has developed the Concise European Food Consumption Database, which includes a list of foods of animal origin for human consumption. This list is an example of how agricultural and veterinary information can be used for tracking and health purposes in risk assessments (EFSA, 2009). The database is being developed further and will provide better data in the future. However, food consumption data will also be required in other regions, and efforts are needed to develop the knowledge base to inform risk assessments.

In order to follow the One Health approach, multi-outcome risk assessments will be required. A One Health approach would also incorporate an understanding of the feedback loops between the livelihoods of farmers, economic and trade policies, consumer preferences, energy prices, wildlife habitats, human health and land use. This in turn will require greater communication between scientists and scholars from a variety of fields, as well as between scholars, politicians and the actual consumers themselves. Outcomes relevant to public, animal and ecosystem health should include: impact on farmers (e.g. health, sustainability, income, social well-being); water resources; other natural resources (e.g. protein inputs to animal feeds, fossil fuels); land use and its effect on wild populations, both in terms of conservation and the likelihood of infectious hazards; micro- and global climate change and food security (Schlundt, 2000; Ross and Sumner, 2002). This expansion of the scope would allow for an integrated assessment of risk related to food, with the term 'food safety' being widened to include not only the aspects of public health but also safety and sustainability for the entire food system. As this is a major development, a process of discussion and debate including all relevant stakeholders is required to enter this next phase of food safety risk assessments.

Such a broadening of scope would have to include the assessment of consequences in several relevant populations including animal, human and ecosystem health. This approach adds significant complexity and requires additional data to inform the assessment. One Health risk assessments cross boundaries between sectors and populations and, as such, will need more diverse input data. The lack of data already poses a serious challenge for more limited risk questions. It is to be expected that such comprehensive assessments will be even more challenged. A key source of risk assessment data is surveillance programmes, and therefore the demand for surveillance is likely to increase. The use of efficiently designed surveillance across the human and animal health sectors is of utmost importance (Benedictus *et al.*, 2009). Economic aspects need to be integrated in surveillance planning. Häsler *et al.* (2011) suggested that when aiming for hazard mitigation (e.g. elimination of a certain foodborne hazard from a livestock population), both costs and benefits of interventions and related surveillance activities need to be considered jointly to establish the overall value of a programme. This concept is currently being expanded to address economic aspects of surveillance in a One Health context (Babo Martins *et al.*, 2013). In this approach, depending on the status of the hazard (i.e. emerging versus endemic), information collected from animal populations may inform interventions for public health and achieve economic benefits that are distant from the original intervention.

At the international level, there has been a strong encouragement to integrate surveillance activities along the food chain to make optimal use of information collected in all relevant populations to inform interventions for both animal and public health. The OIE dedicated a recent issue of their periodical to this topic (OIE, 2012). An excellent example illustrating the benefits of cross-sectoral surveillance in a One Health context is the Canadian Integrated Program for Antimicrobial Resistance Surveillance (CIPARS) (Zinsstag *et al.*, 2011). Integrating surveillance activities across sectors has very clear advantages including faster communication, standardized protocols and financial savings through increased efficiency of laboratory work.

The risk analysis framework has recently been reviewed in general, and the suggested evolution is relevant for One Health risk assessments. The report published by the Council of Canadian Academies (2011) recommends that risk analysis should become a more multidimensional and integrated approach. This means that a much broader range of consequences should be considered, including ecological consequences. This indicates a need for formal integration of a One Health approach. Also, a much wider range of stakeholders should be consulted during the risk analysis process.

## Conclusion: the Future

In the early 1990s, Funtowicz and Ravetz (1990, 1991), reviewing risk assessments for the European Commission, identified the need for a different kind of science to inform policy decisions on risk where the information was both scarce and of uncertain quality, combined with disputed ethics and values where rapid decisions were imperative. They referred to this science as being 'post-normal' (Bunch and Waltner-Toews, Chapter 34, this volume). Similar challenges have been identified in food safety concerning hazards such as genetically modified organisms, BSE, chemical residues and bacterial contamination in the food chain. Approaches are needed for incorporating risk assessments into One Health programmes without requiring vast amounts of new data, which will be expensive and time consuming given the volatility of markets, politics, economic activities, climate and ecosystems.

Ideally, a One Health approach to the assessment of food safety risks needs to operate across multiple scales, sectors and stakeholders. Risk assessments need to take into account regional and cultural diversity of communities. Additionally, food safety risk assessments need to consider multiple outcomes reflecting the health of plants, animals and people while observing sustainable markets and marketing strategies which remain flexible in the context of changing climates and economics. This process should reach across all levels of risk management decision-making. As risk assessments are highly influential in trade economics, strong international leadership is required to make progress in this direction.

## References


Animal and Plant Health Inspection Service (2007) Peer Review of the Assessment of BSE Risk Associated with the Importation of Certain Additional Commodities from BSE Minimal Risk Regions (Canada) Available at: http://www.aphis.usda.gov/peer_review/downloads/MRR2-RA_peer-review9-2007.pdf (accessed 5 August 2013).

Alban, L., Nielson, E.O. and Dahl, J. (2008) A human health risk assessment for macrolide-resistant Campylobacter associated with the use of macrolides in Danish pig production. *Preventive Veterinary Medicine* 83(2), 115–129.

Babo Martins, S., Rushton, J. and Stärk, K.D.C. (2013) Economic assessment of surveillance in a One Health context: a research project on the impact of zoonotic disease surveillance. *Proceedings of the MedVet-Net Conference*, Copenhagen, Denmark, ES04:37

Benedictus, A., Hogeveen, H. and Berends, B.R. (2009) The price of the precautionary principle: cost-effectiveness of BSE intervention strategies in the Netherlands. *Preventive Veterinary Medicine* 89(3–4), 212–222.

Bennett, P. and Daraktchiev, M. (2013) vCJD and transfusion of blood components: an updated risk assessment. Available at: https://www.gov.uk/government/uploads/system/uploads/attachment_data/file/186959/risk_assessment_Feb_2013.pdf (accessed 5 August 2013).

Berthe, F., Hugas, M. and Makela, P. (2013) Integrating surveillance of animal health, food pathogens and foodborne disease in the European Union. *Revue Scientifique et Technique OIE* 32, 521–528.

Bietlot, H.P. and Kolakowski, B. (2012) Risk assessment and risk management at the Canadian Food Inspection Agency (CFIA): a perspective on the monitoring of foods for chemical residues. *Drug Testing and Analysis* 4(Suppl 1), 50–58.

Bodaly, R.A., Jansen, W.A., Majewski, A.R., Fudge, R.J.P., Strange, N.E., Derksen, A.J. and Green, D.J. (2007) Postimpoundment time course of increased mercury concentrations in fish in hydroelectric reservoirs of northern Manitoba, Canada. *Archives of Environmental Contamination and Toxicology* 53, 379–389.

CAC (1999) *Principles and Guidelines for the Conduct of Microbiological Risk Assessment*. CAC/GL 30 – 1999.

Cassin, M.H., Lammerding, A.M., Todd, E.C., Ross, W. and McColl, R.S. (1998) Quantitative risk assessment for *Escherichia coli* O157:H7 in ground beef hamburgers. *International Journal of Food Microbiology* 41(1), 21–44.

CDC (2012) CDC Estimates of Foodborne Illness in the United States: Findings, CDC 2011 Estimates. Available at: http://www.cdc.gov/foodborneburden/2011-foodborne-estimates.html (accessed 5 August 2013).

CDC (2014) BSE (Bovine Spongiform Encephalopathy, or Mad Cow Disease). Available at: http://www.cdc.gov/ncidod/dvrd/bse (accessed March 2014).

Collinge, J., Whitfield, J., McKintosh, E., Beck, J., Mead, S., Thomas, D.J. and Alpers, M.P. (2006) Kuru in the 21st century – an acquired human prion disease with very long incubation periods. *Lancet* 367, 2068–2074.

Cooper, J.D. and Bird, S.M. (2003) Predicting incidence of variant Creutzfeldt-Jakob disease from UK dietary exposure to bovine spongiform encephalopathy for the 1940 to 1969 and post-1969 birth cohorts. *International Journal of Epidemiology* 32, 784–791.

Council of Canadian Academies (2011) Healthy Animals, Health Canada: The Expert Panel on Approaches to Animal Health Risk Assessment. Available at: http://www.scienceadvice.ca/uploads/eng/assessments%20and%20publications%20and%20news%20releases/animal%20health/final_ah_web_report_eng.pdf (accessed 5 August 2013).

Da Silva, D.S., Lucotte, M., Roulet, M., Poirier, H., Mergler, D., Oliveira Santos, E. and Crossa, M. (2005) Trophic structure and bioaccumulation of mercury in fish of three natural lakes of the Brazilian Amazon. *Water, Air, and Soil Pollution* 165, 77–94.

Deutsch, L. and Folke, C. (2005) Ecosystem subsidies to Swedish food consumption from 1962 to 1994. *Ecosystems* 8, 512–528.

EC (2011) Note for guidance on minimising the risk of transmitting animal spongiform encephalopathy agents via human and veterinary medicinal products EMA/410/01 rev.3. Available at: http://eur-lex.europa.eu/LexUriServ/LexUriServ.do?uri=OJ:C:2011:073:0001:0018:EN:PDF (accessed 5 August 2013).

EFSA (2002) EFSA, European Food Safety Authority, Regulation (EC) No 178/2002. *Official Journal* L 031, 001/02/2002 pp. 01–24.

EFSA (2009) European Food Safety Authority; General principles for the collection of national food consumption data in the view of a pan-European dietary survey. *EFSA Journal* 7(12), 1435. [51 pp.]

FAO/WHO (1995) *Application of Risk Analysis to Food Standards Issues*. Report of the Joint FAO/WHO Expert Consultation.

FAO/WHO (2005) Food Safety Risk Analysis, PART I. An Overview and Framework Manual, Provisional Edition. Available at: http://www.fsc.go.jp/sonota/foodsafety_riskanalysis.pdf (accessed 5 August 2013).

FSIS, USDA Food Safety and Inspection Service (1998) *Salmonella Enteritidis* Risk Assessment: Shell Eggs and Egg Products. Available at: http://www.fsis.usda.gov/OPHS/risk/index.htm (accessed 5 August 2013).

Forget, G. and Lebel, J. (2001) An ecosystem approach to human health. *International Journal of Occupational Medicine and Environmental Health* 7(2 Suppl), S3–38.

Funtowicz, S. and Ravetz, J. (1990) *Uncertainty and Quality in Science for Policy*. Kluwer, Dordrecht, the Netherlands.

Funtowicz, S. and Ravetz, J. (1991) Three types of risk assessment and the emergence of post-normal science. In: Goldiung, D. and Krimsky, S. (eds) *Social Theories of Risk*. Greenwood, New York, pp. 251–273.

Glatzel, M., Abela, E., Maissen, M. and Aguzzi, A. (2003) Extraneural pathologic prion protein in sporadic Creutzfeldt-Jakob disease. *New England Journal of Medicine* 349, 1812–1820.

Guimarães, J.R.D. and Mergel, D. (2012) A virtuous cycle in the Amazon: reducing mercury exposure from fish consumption requires sustainable agriculture. In: Charron D.F. (ed.) *Ecohealth Research in Practice: Innovative Applications of an Ecosystem Approach to Health*. Springer and International Development Research Centre, Ottawa.

Häsler, B., Howe, K.S. and Stark, K.D. (2011) Conceptualising the technical relationship of animal disease surveillance to intervention and mitigation as a basis for economic analysis. *BMC Health Services Research* 11, 225.

Hueston, W.D. (2013) BSE and variant CJD: emerging science, public pressure and the vagaries of policy-making. *Preventive Veterinary Medicine* 109(3–4), 179–184.

Kadohira, M., Stevenson, M.A., Hogasen, H.R. and de Koeijer, A. (2012) A quantitative risk assessment for bovine spongiform encephalopathy in Japan. *Risk analysis: an official publication of the Society for Risk Analysis* 32(12), 2198–2208.

Lavelle, K.S., Robert, S.A., Travis, K.Z., Swaen, G.M., Pallapies, D., Money, C., Priem, P. and Vrijhof, H. (2012) Framework for integrating human and animal data in chemical risk assessment. *Regulatory Toxicology and Pharmacology* 62, 302–312.

Morley, R.S., Chen, S. and Rheault, N. (2003) Assessment of the risk factors related to bovine spongiform encephalopathy. *Revue Scientifique et Technique* 22(1), 157–178.

Nathanson, N., Wilesmith, J. and Griot, C. (1997) Bovine Spongiform Encephalopathy (BSE): causes and consequences of a common source epidemic. *American Journal of Epidemiology* 145, 959–969.

National Research Council (1983) *Risk Assessment in the Federal Government: Managing the Process*. National Academy Press, Washington, DC, 191 pp.

National Research Council (1993) *Issues in Risk Assessment.* National Academy Press, Washington, DC, 356 pp.
Nie, F., Li, X.J., Shang, P.F. and Wang, Y. (2013) Melamine-induced urinary calculi infants – sonographic manifestations and outcomes 1 year after exposure. *Pediatric Radiology* 43(4), 474–478.
NZ Gov (2000) Project Report: Quantitative risk assessment of *Salmonella* in sheep meat produced in New Zealand. Available at: http://www.foodsafety.govt.nz/elibrary/industry/quantitative-risk-assessment-research-projects/salmonella-in-sheep.pdf (accessed 5 August 2013).
OIE (1999) *Import Risk Analysis, International Animal Health Code. OIE International Animal Health Code*, 9th edn, 2000.
OIE (2004) Terrestrial Animal Health Code, Vol. 1, General provisions. Available at: http://www.oie.int/doc/ged/D10905.PDF (accessed 5 August 2013).
OIE (2012) Final Report, 80th General Session, Paris, 20–25 May 2012. Available at: http://www.oie.int/fileadmin/Home/eng/About_us/.../A_FR_2012_Public.pdf (accessed 5 August 2013).
Pintar, K., Fazil, A., Pollari, F., Charron, D., Waltner-Toews, D. and McEwen, S. (2010) A risk assessment model to evaluate the role of fecal contamination in recreational water on the incidence of Crypstosporidiosis at the community level in Ontario. *Risk Analysis* 30, 49–64.
Presi, P., Stark, K.D., Stephan, R., Breidenbach, E., Frey, J. and Regula, G. (2009) Risk scoring for setting priorities in a monitoring of antimicrobial resistance in meat and meat products. *International Journal of Food Microbiology* 130(2), 94–100.
Rabsch, W., Hargis, B.M., Tsolis, R.M., Kingsley, R.A., Hinz, K.-H., Tschäpe, H., *et al.* (2000) Competitive Exclusion of *Salmonella* Enteritidis by *Salmonella* Gallinarum in Poultry. *Emerging Infectious Diseases* [serial on the Internet]. Available at: http://wwwnc.cdc.gov/eid/article/6/5/00-0501.htm (accessed August 2013).
Ross, T. and Sumner, J. (2002) A simple, spreadsheet-based, food safety risk assessment tool. *International Journal of Food Microbiology* 77(1–2), 39–53.
Roulet, M., Lucotte, N., Farella, G., Serique, H., Coelho, C.J., Sousa Passos, E., de Jesus da Silva, P., Scavone de Andrade, D., Mergler, J.-R., Guimarães, D. and Amorim, M. (1999) Effects of recent human colonization on the presence of mercury in Amazonian ecosystems. *Water, Air, and Soil Pollution* 112, 297–313.
Salman, M., Silano, V., Heim, D. and Kreysa, J. (2012) Geographical BSE risk assessment and its impact on disease detection and dissemination. *Preventive Veterinary Medicine* 105(4), 255–264.
Schlundt, J. (2000) Comparison of microbiological risk assessment studies published. *International Journal of Food Microbiology* 58(3), 197–202.
Smith, P.G. and Bradley, R. (2003) Bovine spongiform encephalopathy (BSE) and its epidemiology. *British Medical Bulletin* 66, 185–198.
Stark, K.D., Regula, G., Hernandez, J., Knopf, L., Fuchs, K., Morris, R.S. and Davies, P. (2006) Concepts for risk-based surveillance in the field of veterinary medicine and veterinary public health: review of current approaches. *BMC Health Services Research* 6, 20.
Vose, D., Acar, J., Anthony, F., Franklin, A., Gupta, R., Nicholls, T., Tamura, Y., Thompson, S., Threlfall, E.J., Vuuren, M. van, White, D.G., Wegener, H.C. and Costarrica, M.L. (2001) Antimicrobial resistance: risk analysis methodology for the potential impact on public health of antimicrobial resistant bacteria of animal origin. *Revue Scientifique et Technique* 20(3), 811–827.
Waltner-Toews, D. and McEwen, S.A. (1994a) Chemical contaminants in foods of animal origin: an overview and risk assessment. *Preventive Veterinary Medicine* 20, 161–178.
Waltner-Toews, D. and McEwen, S.A. (1994b) Residues of industrial chemical and metallic compounds in foods of animal origin: a risk assessment. *Preventive Veterinary Medicine* 20, 210–218.
Wegener, H.C. (2012) Antibiotic Resistance - Linking human and animal health. *Improving Food Safety Through a One Health Approach: Workshop Summary.*
Wheatley, M.A. (1997) Social and cultural impacts of mercury pollution on aboriginal peoples in Canada. *Water, Air and Soil Pollution* 97, 85–90.
Zinsstag, J., Schelling, E., Waltner-Toews, D. and Tanner, M. (2011) From 'one medicine' to 'one health' and systemic approaches to health and well-being. *Preventive Veterinary Medicine* 101, 148–156.

# 9 A One Health Perspective for Integrated Human and Animal Sanitation and Nutrient Recycling

**Hung Nguyen-Viet,[1,2,3,6]* Phuc Pham-Duc,[1] Vi Nguyen,[1] Marcel Tanner,[2,3] Peter Odermatt,[2,3] Tu Vu-Van,[1] Hoang Van Minh,[4] Christian Zurbrügg,[5] Esther Schelling[2,3] and Jakob Zinsstag[2,3]**

*[1]Centre for Public Health and Ecosystem Research, Hanoi School of Public Health, Hanoi, Vietnam; [2]Swiss Tropical and Public Health Institute, Basel, Switzerland; [3]University of Basel, Basel, Switzerland; [4]Institute of Public Health and Preventive Medicine, Hanoi Medical University, Hanoi, Vietnam; [5]Eawag: Swiss Federal Institute of Aquatic Science and Technology, Department of Water and Sanitation in Developing Countries (Sandec), Dübendorf, Switzerland; [6]International Livestock Research Institute (ILRI), Hanoi, Vietnam*

## Introduction

Improving health status and conserving natural resources for sustainable development are part of the Millennium Development Goals (MDGs) (United Nations, 2006). Environmental sanitation is an important factor influencing human health status. With 2.4 billion people worldwide lacking adequate means of sanitation and 1.1 billion people living without a safe water supply, a great deal of work remains to be done to improve environmental sanitation (WHO/UNICEF, 2013). With the extensive use and depletion of natural resources, the question of how to effectively use natural and environmental resources such as those in excreta is of highest priority (Waltner-Toews, 2013). Studies have highlighted a number of issues regarding recovery and reuse of resources from waste and their impact on health (Nhapi *et al.*, 2003; Miller, 2006). It is also evident that social, economic and cultural factors play a crucial role in achieving health improvements (Marmot, 1998; Anderson *et al.*, 2003). Numerous studies have examined the impact of physical, socio-economic and cultural environments on health and on how to reduce health risks by improving these environments. However, the assessments of the impact as well as the approaches to improving health and environment have often been conducted in relative isolation, with the danger that health programmes might put environmental sustainability at risk, and vice versa. For example, Morris *et al.* (2006) assessed the combination of health and physical environments without sufficiently considering social, economic and cultural factors. In other studies, the links between health and society were addressed without adequately taking the physical environment into account (Yen and Syme, 1999; Marmot, 2005). A review of

*E-mail: h.nguyen@cgiar.org

the literature shows a dearth of assessments offering approaches that effectively integrate health and environmental factors. This is particularly relevant in discussions on development of urban and peri-urban areas, where vulnerable populations bear the brunt of the resulting health risks from poor environmental sanitation and uncontrolled urbanization (McMichael, 2000; Moore *et al.*, 2003; Montgomery and Elimelech, 2007).

In developing countries, the management of human excreta is significantly hampered by a lack of appropriate sanitation technologies, posing a significant challenge to human and environmental health. This is compounded by a similar challenge posed by animal waste. In Vietnam, large volumes of waste from livestock such as poultry, ruminants and especially pigs, raised to meet Vietnam's high pork consumption, are reused as fertilizers and feed in agriculture and aquaculture, respectively. Both human and livestock waste contribute to family livelihoods, replacing the need for expensive and potentially hazardous chemical fertilizers. Unfortunately, animal waste is usually not managed properly, which consequently becomes a source of pathogens affecting health and the environment.

As an approach being increasingly used for health and environmental assessment, quantitative microbial risk assessment (QMRA) estimates the infection risk from an exposure and can also estimate disease risk, which allows for the assessment of critical control points (CCPs) in food chains (production, transformation and consumption) and sanitation systems (Haas *et al.*, 1999). Over the last decade, it has been used to assess the health risks in drinking water (Howard *et al.*, 2006; van Lieverloo *et al.*, 2007) and in wastewater management (Westrell *et al.*, 2004; Eisenberg *et al.*, 2008). From an environmental health perspective, QMRA has been used to assess the infection risk and, subsequently, high disease risk for the population in contact with wastewater (An *et al.*, 2007; Mara *et al.*, 2007; Diallo *et al.*, 2008; Seidu *et al.*, 2008).

Another useful tool for environmental assessment is material flow analysis (MFA), which examines the flows of resources and how they change as they pass through a system. It has been applied as a tool to identify environmental and resource management problems and development of appropriate measures (Baccini and Brunner, 1991; Brunner and Rechberger, 2004). One of its interesting applications has been in optimizing water and nutrient management in environmental sanitation systems in Vietnam and China (Belevi, 2002; Huang *et al.*, 2007; Montangero *et al.*, 2007). Despite its potentials, what is lacking from this tool in providing useful information for the safe use of natural resources and reuse of waste products is potential health risks and CCPs.

For both MFA and QMRA, both quantitative and qualitative knowledge are required to comprehensively assess public health risks; specifically information on the human behavioural dimensions. Quantitative epidemiological studies can identify possible health risks within food chains and environmental sanitation systems (Beaglehole *et al.*, 2005). Cultural epidemiological studies on how health and risk are perceived by different populations through experiences, meaning and behaviour related to a particular risk also offer important insights (Weiss, 2001). However, even such comprehensive approaches do not address the issues of resource flows or cycles. In addition, social anthropological approaches focus on people and their responses to health risk as processes leading to negative outcomes (vulnerability) or positive outcomes (resilience), without consideration of the larger social-ecological systemic context (Obrist, 2006). Thus, an important consideration to address these includes access to livelihood assets and to health, environmental and social services (Obrist *et al.*, 2007).

Given these challenges, a more integrated approach to human and animal waste assessment and management may be more effective for tackling complex problems than employing a single or multidisciplinary approach. A One Health approach emerges as a good candidate for this as it addresses the complex interactions of human, animals and environment. One Health can be defined as the added value in terms of animal and human lives saved, financial savings and improved ecosystem services from a closer cooperation of human and animal health as compared to single sector approaches (Zinsstag *et al.*, 2012).

In this chapter, we present our experience of developing a conceptual framework for integrated health and environmental assessment, combining health status, physical, socio-economic and cultural environments to improve health and minimize environmental impact. We will focus on how the framework was used to manage human and animal excreta in Vietnam and the added value offered from an integrated assessment.

## Conceptual Framework Development

The details of the conceptual framework have been published previously (Nguyen-Viet *et al.*, 2009). The framework (Fig. 9.1) starts with an analysis of health status, as well as the status of the physical, social, cultural and economic environments. Starting with an analysis of the routine databases, health status can be further assessed through specifically designed epidemiological surveys. Similarly, the status of environmental sanitation – that comprises excreta, wastewater and solid waste management, and drainage and water supply management – can be evaluated through surveys, observation and mapping of water supply, excreta, wastewater, solid waste management and drainage infrastructures and services, while taking into account the technical, economic, institutional and organizational factors. Furthermore, interactions between waste management and the food chain (Zinsstag *et al.*, Chapter 12, this volume), crops and livestock can also be included (Bonfoh *et al.*, 2006). Combined, this information allows description of the current status of environmental sanitation systems, health and well-being of the local population and the key interrelations. They provide the basis for understanding the key issues for the improvement of health and environment in a given area or setting.

### Physical environment

The physical environment describes the status of the environmental sanitation system. The MFA is straightforward to apply and proven to be effective in developing country contexts with limited data availability (Montangero, 2007; Montangero *et al.*, 2007). The main steps of MFA are the conceptual representations of processes, their interaction with flows of goods (system analysis), as well as the quantification of mass flow of goods and substances. This tool provides useful information for the identification of key factors determining material flows ('CCPs') and the planning of interventions aimed at reducing resource consumption and pollutant loads into the environment. In our context of environmental sanitation in developing countries, the focus rests on the 'goods' (e.g. faeces and human and animal waste) that play an important role with regard to human health and ecological impact and the 'substances' these goods contain.

### Social, economic and cultural environment

This component entails the approaches of medical anthropology, cultural epidemiology and social economics, grouped broadly as social science analyses (SSA). A main focus of the approach lies in considering the vulnerability and resilience of the populations (Obrist, 2006) and their risk perceptions gained through experiences, meaning and behaviour related to particular illness entities (Kleinman, 1981; Weiss, 2001). Furthermore, economic appraisal is used to assess the costs and cost-effectiveness of proposed interventions. Combining economic appraisal with epidemiological, social and cultural data allows for analysis on how a more equitable access to resources and services can be achieved and to what degree (Gold *et al.*, 1996; Hutton, 2000).

### Health status

In this framework, classical epidemiology (Beaglehole *et al.*, 2005), cultural epidemiology (Weiss, 2001) and QMRA are proposed as the key methodologies to assess health and identify the determinants of disease burdens. While the basic approaches of epidemiology are well known and have been validated and applied (Beaglehole *et al.*, 2005), QMRA has been more recently applied in health status

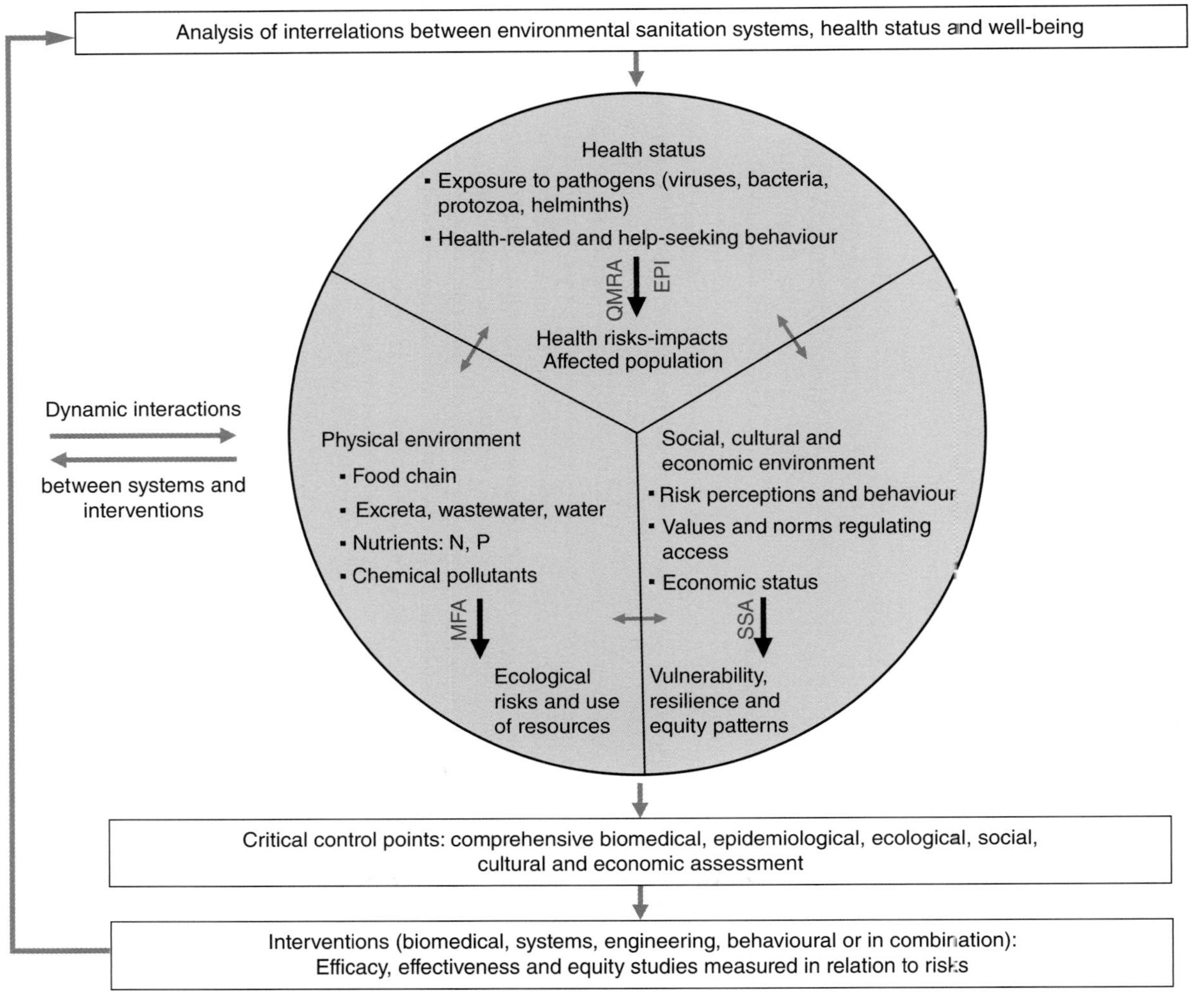


**Fig. 9.1.** Conceptual framework of integrated assessment for health, environmental sanitation and society (reproduced from Nguyen-Viet *et al.*, 2009).

assessments and is recommended in risk assessments for the safe use of wastewater, excreta and grey water and for drinking water quality (WHO, 2006b,c). The addition of QMRA to epidemiology is motivated by the quantitative aspect of this method, which calculates the estimated risk of having infection and disease burden related to pathogen exposure by combining available information on exposure and dose–response (Haas *et al.*, 1999; Vose, 2000; Pintar *et al.*, 2012). QMRA has been used in various risk assessments and shown to be effectively applied in developing countries, even with limited data (Howard *et al.*, 2006; Benke and Hamilton, 2008). The identification of pathogens (viruses, bacteria, protozoa and helminths) will effectively complement the epidemiological methods (Fig. 9.1).

#### Comprehensive critical control points

CCPs are conventionally defined, in food safety, as any step at which control can be applied and is essential to prevent or eliminate a food safety hazard or reduce it to an acceptable level (National Advisory Committee on Microbiological Criteria for Foods, 1997). CCPs in our framework resulted from the analyses of the three components described above. Therefore, integrated CCPs are taken into account and identified from different perspectives such as comprehensive biomedical, epidemiological (health), social, cultural and economic assessment (social sciences) and environmental assessment (physical environment) (Fig. 9.1). Our CCPs retain the traditional definition related to food chains, but are further complemented by other risks relating to pathogens in drinking water, wastewater, excreta and solid waste. They also include the social and cultural perspectives that consider the concept of vulnerability and resilience.

#### Interventions

Once CCPs are identified, interventions can be comparatively assessed for optimal contribution to improving health and minimizing impact on the environment and the use of resources in a given area. Interventions established based on these components will be integrated as they will take into account the needs and the demand of the populations concerned. Consequently, this will allow priority setting based on reconciled needs and demands. Figure 9.1 further shows the dynamics between the components of the framework and the interventions. The iterative process ensures that interventions are tailored to the needs and demands of any given setting and allows respective readjustments and strengthening of any intervention or component of an intervention.

### Integrated Human and Animal Waste Management in Vietnam: Application of the Framework for Combined Assessment

We applied this framework as a case study in Hanam Province, Vietnam. This section discusses how the framework is useful to comprehensively assess the impact of combined human and animal sanitation and address the One Health application for the sanitation issue. Hanam was selected as a peri-urban study site, because it offered a good setting to studying a system combining human and animal sanitation. In this area, human excreta and animal manure have been used together with wastewater in agriculture and aquaculture (Fig. 9.2). Most households (85%) have been engaged in agricultural activities; they are predominantly smallholders and often raise 2–20 pigs on land that is simultaneously residential, agricultural, aquacultural and horticultural. This use of waste raised issues for environmental sanitation, agriculture and health and well-being. Three components of the framework were implemented, namely environmental, health and socio-economic assessment leading to the identification of CCPs.

#### Physical environment

We used MFA for analysing environmental sanitation and agricultural systems with the

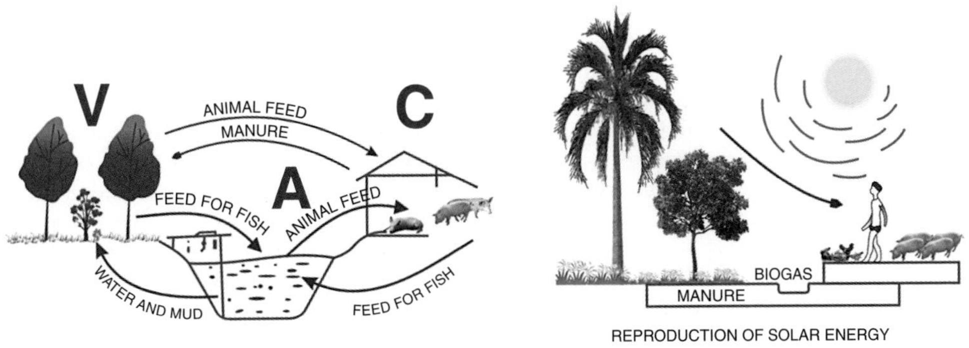


**Fig. 9.2.** Integrated crop (V) – fishery (A) – livestock (C) (V-A-C) in Vietnam (adapted from http://ccrd.com.vn/NewsDetail.asp?m=1&IDMain=l&ID=533&IDdetail=693).

emphasis on nutrient flows of nitrogen (N) and phosphorus (P). The results revealed that the agricultural system was a significant source of nutrients (N and P), which affect the surrounding environment and was mainly due to the overuse of chemical fertilizers (CCPs) (Nga *et al.*, 2011). In the study area and every year as of 2008, there were 103 ± 39 t of N released into the atmosphere, 25 ± 3 t of N leached to the surface water, and 14 ± 2 t of P accumulated in the soil, all originating from the applied chemical fertilizers. In addition, the sanitation system was also a critical source of nutrients that entered the surface water. A volume of 69 ± 6 t of N and 23 ± 4 t of P came from households through effluents of on-site sanitation systems (such as latrines and septic tanks) and were directly discharged to surface water every year. Moreover, the whole system annually generated a large nutrient source (214 ± 56 t of N (mean ± standard error); 58 ± 16 t of P) in the form of wastewater, faecal sludge, animal manure and organic solid waste. The validated MFA was used to model different scenarios for the study site. The first scenario demonstrated that if nutrient management was not improved, wastewater as well as faecal sludge and organic solid waste would be expected to double in the year 2020 as compared to that in 2008. The second and third scenarios revealed possible strategies to significantly reduce environmental pollution and reused nutrient sources predicted to be available in the year 2020 (Nga *et al.*, 2011).

## Health status

A set of epidemiological and QMRA studies have been carried out to look at the health effects of wastewater and excreta reuse. Two cross-sectional surveys were conducted during the rainy and dry season in Hanam to identify prevalence and risk factors for helminth and protozoal infections (Pham-Duc *et al.*, 2013). Results showed that 302 people (47.6%) were infected with at least one of the three helminth species in the rainy season and 336 people (46.3%) in the dry season. Furthermore, protozoal intestinal infections were also diagnosed. *Entamoeba histolytica* (6%) and *Giardia lamblia* (2.4%) were recorded in the rainy season and *E. histolytica* (6.7%), *Cryptosporidium parvum* (9.6%) and *Cyclospora cayetenensis* (2%) in the dry season (Pham-Duc *et al.*, 2013). A case control study for *E. histolytica* infection was also conducted to assess the risk factors associated with handling practices of wastewater and excreta use in agriculture and aquaculture in Hanam (Pham-Duc *et al.*, 2011). Analyses revealed that the risk factors included: direct contact with a domestic animal, not using or rarely using soap for hand washing, and lower socio-economic status. A nested case-control study assessed the incidence of and risk factors for diarrhoeal disease among people living and working in the same areas. The estimated annual risks of diarrhoea values were at least threefold greater than the upper threshold risk of $10^{-3}$ per person per year; and the annual burden of diarrhoeal disease was significantly higher than the health target of $10^{-6}$ disability-adjusted life years (DALYs) (≤1DALY/million persons) recommended by the World Health Organization (WHO). Further research may look at other microorganisms such as *Salmonella* or *Campylobacter*, which could reveal zoonotic transmission patterns.

## Social, economic and cultural environment

One of our studies investigated the perception of health risk and ability to prevent risk caused by wastewater and excreta reuse. The first survey focusing on threat appraisal found that people recognized the black colour and smell of wastewater, smell of excreta, inappropriate practices of excreta management and suspected diseases associated with contact with excreta and wastewater as threats (Tu *et al.*, 2011). We have also implemented a study in Kim Bang District, Hanam Province to assess the willingness-to-pay for construction of flush toilets at the household level. The contingent valuation method (CVM) was used in this study; it is a survey-based economic technique, which directly questions individuals as to how much they are willing to pay for a change in quantity or quality (or both) of a particular commodity. We found that 63% of the studied households were willing to pay for construction of flush toilets. The average willingness-to-pay level was VND16 million (US$800). There was no statistically significant difference in the willingness-to-pay level by socio-economic status.

The application of the framework for the specific case study in Vietnam identified the distinctions between the theoretical organization of the framework and the fluid interactions that occurred in the real-life case study. Ideally, all components of the framework should be prepared such that they begin at the same time. This would allow complementary components to be combined to identify CCPs, particularly for the QMRA and MFA. In practice, diverse information from the three components was combined as follows. The result of MFA identified the CCPs in the environment, providing a basis for health status research. The actual risks identified by the epidemiological studies supported and complemented the QMRA, which assessed the risk of infection, giving CCPs in terms of health risk. The socio-economic and cultural assessment looked at the behaviour and perception of participants with regards to these CCPs and the cost and willingness to pay for sanitation options. Our research revealed that participant perceptions of the health and environmental risks of intensive waste recycling and reuse within their agroecosystem was not consistent with the actual risks measured. However, they were willing to pay for better sanitation facilities. The combined assessment showed the importance of identifying CCPs in this system to be targeted for interventions. On-site sanitation systems and the combined management of human and animal waste (see next section) appear to be promising interventions. The CCPs also rely on the perceptions of the community that need to be addressed in the intervention so that it can be effectively implemented. Interventions identified by the concerned communities should be used to further validate the proposed integrated framework.

## Benefit of One Health for Sanitation: Combined Treatment of Human and Animal Waste

Vietnamese livestock production is increasing rapidly, particularly for ruminants and the development of a dairy industry, which is reflected in the increasing annual per capita milk consumption. In 1990, the ruminant (cattle and goat) population was 3.5 million – by 2008, it had grown to 8 million. The pig and chicken populations have increased steadily over these two decades, but slowed down with the steep increase of ruminants; in 2009, there were 27.6 million pigs and 200 million chickens. Subsequently, large amounts of manure are produced, which may be a hazard to the environment (e.g. pollution of surface and groundwater by excess nutrients and chemicals) and human health. Currently, there is national and international attention on environmental risk management (including cost-benefit assessments, for example, in biogas production from livestock waste) with regard to climate change and environmental hazards. However, there is no combined tool that balances human health and preserving ecosystem services.

In most rural and peri-urban settings of the country, mixed agricultural and residential land use causes humans and animals to live in close proximity, highlighting the importance of managing the health and environmental risks of human and animal waste (Fig. 9.2). Despite the national government's attempt to manage these through the new livestock centralization policy, it is unlikely that it will be implemented in the near future. As current practice, animal and human waste are separately treated or, in some places, they are mixed for treatment prior to use as fertilizer. While the risks of human waste are largely known, the risks associated with livestock waste are not so well known and tend to be perceived as causing lower risks than human waste. Human health hazards of livestock waste, which are often processed together with crop residues, may include zoonotic pathogens and residues of agrochemicals and drugs. Due to the proximity of animal and human waste disposal, storage and reuse, as well as the close proximity of human and animal living quarters, good practices in livestock and human waste management are needed for mitigating risks posed to human health and the environment. As such a task is multifaceted, participatory action research, involving a wide range of stakeholders, institutions and policy makers can promote better water management practices that integrate management of wastewater, human and animal waste and agricultural runoff.

We conducted a field intervention examining how the combination of human and animal excreta composting influences helminth egg die-off in excreta, while maintaining its nutrient value. The intervention aimed to improve the current storage practices of human excreta and identify the best option for the safe use of excreta in agriculture. Samples were taken from the experiments of ten combined composting prototypes in ten households in Hanam. This occurred biweekly and monthly, over a 6 month period. Our quantitative results and analyses included measurements of live and dead *Ascaris lumbricoides* egg counts, the nutrient parameter (N), pH, temperature and moisture content. The results showed that variation of the *A. lumbricoides* concentrations in the different sampling dates was influenced by composting options and time of composting. The average number of *A. lumbricoides* eggs was less than 1 egg/g in all of the composting options after 84 days (Plate 4). This parasite egg reduction meets the WHO standard (1 egg/l) for safe use of wastewater, excreta and grey water in agriculture and aquaculture (WHO, 2006a). This implies a significant reduction of estimated annual risk of infections. Therefore the combined human and animal waste management strategy shows the benefit of financial savings for the treatment option investment, which helps reduce environmental and health risk. The model is currently being promoted in Hanam (Plate 4).

## Challenges of Chemical Contamination in Vietnam

Our research has focused mainly on the effects of microbial contamination of human and animal waste on human health and the environment, as this is an important issue in developing countries. However, this is only a facet of the complex environmental sanitation picture. Among other types, large volumes of mixed domestic, hospital and industrial wastewater are discharged into water bodies, and in Vietnam, only about 20% are treated. This presents a threat as groundwater contamination, but more importantly for surface water in the peri-urban environment, where this wastewater is used to irrigate crops and feeds into aquaculture. The health and environmental impacts include, for example, the accumulation of heavy metals in vegetables and fish fed by wastewater, which will be consumed by humans (Fitamo *et al.*, 2007). Such high concentrations were observed in morning glory spinach, fish, and water from the To Lich and Nhue rivers and in the river basins within Hanoi and Hanam provinces (Marcussen *et al.*, 2008, 2012; Ingvertsen *et al.*, 2013).

The whole issue of chemical, soil and groundwater contamination is challenging for the country, as this is driven by economic growth and environmental degradation. Past experience from developed countries with environmental degradation related to the Industrial Revolution provides important lessons for developing countries, including Vietnam. However, these do not seem to be currently addressed, as countries like Vietnam and China are experiencing rapid economic growth, with huge impacts on health and the environment. Although balancing economic growth and environmental and health protection are difficult, strong political will and that from civil society organizations are needed. For this, a One Health approach might be useful to bring different people to work together.

## Conclusion and the Way Forward

The MDGs for water and sanitation provide specific targets for some very ambitious goals. Our field experience with the case study in Vietnam shows that sanitation is clearly a complex issue that requires more than behavioural change and large financial investments. The goal of meeting these targets to improve the health of people, while preserving sustainable environments, is a task that requires the perspectives of multiple sectors and stakeholders. The conceptual framework that informs our research provides the starting point for how to integrate aspects that have traditionally been done separately. It has been through asking different research questions of the problem of sanitation that has led us to address the different aspects found in the conceptual framework. In consideration of the local context, the boundaries of the problem of sanitation are not clear and research designed to address sanitation must draw its own boundaries for practical sake. Within these boundaries, what has been the progress thus far is the empirical data collected, which act as pieces of a puzzle and there remains the challenge of stitching these together to obtain a more complete picture. One broad area that remains to be integrated is an assessment of the benefits, in terms of ecological services and economic development, of different methods of recycling the excreta and other organic wastes (such as composting, biogas and other energy production, and fertilizer use). Excreta need to be evaluated both as a valuable source of energy and nutrients, enhancing environmental health and economic development, and in terms of the risks posed to human and animal health. This would enable policy makers to gain a clearer understanding of the financial gains, and not simply costs, of integrated approaches versus more simplistic treatments assessed only on the basis of improved public health or agricultural gains.

Integration can mean many different things. In our case, we are referring to the combination of knowledge and perspective of different sectors and stakeholders in such a way that brings about different ways of participating in the problem of interest and processes to uncover knowledge that addresses this (Charron, 2012). In this sense, a One Health approach offers an interesting conceptual and operational framework for jointly managing the human and animal waste in developing countries where the reuse and recycling of waste for agriculture is important, which is beneficial to the environment, health and the economy.

## References

An, Y.J., Yoon, C.G., Jung, K.W. and Ham, J.H. (2007) Estimating the microbial risk of *E-coli* in reclaimed wastewater irrigation on paddy field. *Environmental Monitoring and Assessment* 129, 53–60.

Anderson, L.M., Scrimshaw, S.C., Fullilove, M.T. and Fielding, J.E. (2003) The Community Guide's model for linking the social environment to health. *American Journal of Preventive Medicine* 24, 12–20.

Baccini, P. and Brunner, P.H. (1991) *Metabolism of the Anthroposphere*. Springer, New York.

Beaglehole, R., Bonita, R. and Kjellström, T. (2005) *Basic Epidemiology*. World Health Organization, Geneva.

Belevi, H. (2002) Material flow analysis as a strategic planning tool for regional waste water and solid waste management. Available at: http://www2.gtz.de/Dokumente/oe44/ecosan/en-material-flow-analysis-wastewater-and-waste-management-2002.pdf (accessed 26 October 2014).

Benke, K.K. and Hamilton, A.J. (2008) Quantitative microbial risk assessment: uncertainty and measures of central tendency for skewed distributions. *Stochastic Environmental Research and Risk Assessment* 22, 533–539.

Bonfoh, B., Roth, C., Traore, A.N., Fane, A., Simbe, C.F., Alfaroukh, I.O., Nicolet, J., Farah, Z. and Zinsstag, J. (2006) Effect of washing and disinfecting containers on the microbiological quality of fresh milk sold in Bamako (Mali). *Food Control* 17, 153–161.

Brunner, P.H. and Rechberger, H. (2004) *Pratical Handbook of Material Flow Analysis*. Lewis Publishers, Boca Raton, Florida.

Charron, D.F. (2012) *Ecohealth Research in Practice: Innovative Applications of an Ecosystem Approach to Health, Insight and Innovation in Development*. Springer and International Development Research Centre, New York and Ottawa.

Diallo, M.B.C., Anceno, A.J., Tawatsupa, B., Houpt, E.R., Wangsuphachart, V. and Shipin, O.V. (2008) Infection risk assessment of diarrhea-related pathogens in a tropical canal network. *Science of the Total Environment* 407, 223–232.

Eisenberg, J.N.S., Moore, K., Soller, J.A., Eisenberg, D. and Colford, J.M. (2008) Microbial risk assessment framework for exposure to amended sludge projects. *Environmental Health Perspectives* 116, 727–733.

Fitamo, D., Itana, F. and Olsson, M. (2007) Total contents and sequential extraction of heavy metals in soils irrigated with wastewater, Akaki, Ethiopia. *Journal of Environmental Management* 39, 178–193.

Gold, M.R., Siegel, J.E., Russell, L.B. and Weinstein, M.C. (1996) *Cost-effectiveness in Health and Medicine*. Oxford University Press, New York.

Haas, C.N., Rose, J.B. and Gerba, C.P. (1999) *Quantitative Microbial Risk Assessment*. John Wiley & Sons, New York.

Howard, G., Pedley, S. and Tibatemwa, S. (2006) Quantitative microbial risk assessment to estimate health risks attributable to water supply: can the technique be applied in developing countries with limited data? *Journal of Water and Health* 4, 49–65.

Huang, D.B., Bader, H.P., Scheidegger, R., Schertenleib, R. and Gujer, W. (2007) Confronting limitations: new solutions required for urban water management in Kunming City. *Journal of Environmental Management* 84, 49–61.

Hutton, G. (2000) *Considerations in Evaluating the Cost-effectiveness of Environmental Health Interventions: protection of the human environment*. World Health Organization, Geneva.

Ingvertsen, S.T., Marcussen, H. and Holm, P.E. (2013) Pollution and potential mobility of Cd, Ni and Pb in the sediments of a wastewater-receiving river in Hanoi, Vietnam. *Environmental Monitoring and Assessment* 185, 9531–9548.

Kleinman, A. (1981) *Patients and Healers in the Context of Culture, An Exploration of the Borderland between Anthropology, Medicine and Psychiatry*. University of California Press, Berkeley, California.

Mara, D.D., Sleigh, P.A., Blumenthal, U.J. and Carr, R.M. (2007) Health risks in wastewater irrigation: comparing estimates from quantitative microbial risk analyses and epidemiological studies. *Journal of Water and Health* 5, 39–50.

Marcussen, H., Joergensen, K., Holm, P.E., Brocca, D., Simmons, R.W. and Dalsgaard, A. (2008) Element contents and food safety of water spinach (*Ipomoea aquatica* Forssk.) cultivated with wastewater in Hanoi, Vietnam. *Environmental Monitoring and Assessment* 139, 77–91.

Marcussen, H., Hale, T., Polprasert, C. and Holm, P.E. (2012) Contents and mass balances of cadmium and arsenic in a wastewater-fed fish pond of Hoang Mai, Hanoi, Vietnam. *Journal of Environmental Science and Health. Part A, Toxic/hazardous Substances & Environmental Engineering* 47, 2246–2253.

Marmot, M. (2005) The social environment and health. *Clinical Medicine* 5, 244–248.

Marmot, M.G. (1998) Improvement of social environment to improve health. *The Lancet* 351, 57–60.

McMichael, A.J. (2000) The urban environment and health in a world of increasing globalization: issues for developing countries. *Bulletin of the World Health Organization* 78, 1117–1126.

Miller, G.W. (2006) Integrated concepts in water reuse: managing global water needs. *Desalination* 187, 65–75.

Montangero, A. (2007) Material Flow Analysis for Environmental Sanitation Planning in Developing Countries - An approach to assess material flows with limited data availability. PhD thesis, Leopold-Franzens-University, Innsbruck, Austria.

Montangero, A., Cau, L.N., Anh, N.V., Tuan, V.D., Nga, P.T. and Belevi, H. (2007) Optimising water and phosphorus management in the urban environmental sanitation system in Hanoi, Vietnam. *Science of the Total Environment* 384, 55–66.

Montgomery, M.A. and Elimelech, M. (2007) Water and sanitation in developing countries: including health in the equation. *Environmental Science & Technology* 41, 17–24.

Moore, M., Gould, P. and Keary, B.S. (2003) Global urbanization and impact on health. *International Journal of Hygiene and Environmental Health* 206, 269–278.

Morris, G.P., Beck, S.A., Hanlon, P. and Robertson, R. (2006) Getting strategic about the environment and health. *Public Health* 120, 889–903.

National Advisory Committee on Microbiological Criteria for Foods (1997) *HACCP guidelines*. US Food and Drug Administration, US Department of Agriculture, National Advisory Committee on Microbiological Criteria for Foods.

Nga, D.T., Morel, A., Hung, N.V., Phuc, P.D., Nishida, K. and Kootattep, T. (2011) Assessing nutrient fluxes in a Vietnamese rural area despite limited and highly uncertain data. *Resources Conservation and Recycling* 55, 849–856.

Nguyen-Viet, H., Zinsstag, J., Schertenleib, R., Zurbrugg, C., Obrist, B., Montangero, A., Surkinkul, N., Kone, D., Morel, A., Cisse, G., Koottatep, T., Bonfoh, B. and Tanner, M. (2009) Improving environmental sanitation, health, and well-being: a conceptual framework for integral interventions. *EcoHealth* 6, 180–191.

Nhapi, I., Gijzen, H.J. and Siebel, M.A. (2003) A conceptual framework for the sustainable management of wastewater in Harare, Zimbabwe. *Water Science and Technology* 47, 11–18.

Obrist, B. (2006) *Struggling for Health in the City. An Anthropological Inquiry of Health, Vulnerability And Resilience in Dar Es Salaam, Tanzania*. Peter Lang, Bern.

Obrist, B., Iteba, N., Lengeler, C., Makemba, A., Mshana, C., Nathan, R., Alba, S., Dillip, A., Hetzel, M.W., Mayumana, I., Schulze, A. and Mshinda, H. (2007) Access to health care in contexts of livelihood insecurity: a framework for analysis and action. *PLoS Medicine* 4, 1584–1588.

Pham-Duc, P., Nguyen-Viet, H., Hattendorf, J., Zinsstag, J., Cam, P.D. and Odermatt, P. (2011) Risk factors for *Entamoeba histolytica* infection in an agricultural community in Hanam province, Vietnam. *Parasites & Vectors* 4, 102.

Pham-Duc, P., Nguyen-Viet, H., Hattendorf, J., Zinsstag, J., Cam, P.D., Zurbrugg, C. and Odermatt, P. (2013) *Ascaris lumbricoides* and *Trichuris trichiura* infections associated with wastewater and human excreta use in agriculture in Vietnam. *Parasitology International* 62, 172–180.

Pintar, K.D., Fazil, A., Pollari, F., Waltner-Toews, D., Charron, D.F., McEwen, S.A. and Walton, T. (2012) Considering the risk of infection by *Cryptosporidium* via consumption of municipally treated drinking water from a surface source in a Southwestern Ontario Community. *Risk Analysis* 32, 1122–1138.

Seidu, R., Heistad, A., Amoah, P., Drechsel, P., Jenssen, P.D. and Stenstrom, T.A. (2008) Quantification of the health risk associated with wastewater reuse in Accra, Ghana: a contribution toward local guidelines. *Journal of Water and Health* 6, 461–471.

Tu, V.v., Huong, N., Phuc, P.D., Hung, N.V. and Zurbrugg, C. (2011) Developing a questionnaire to measure awareness and behaviours of people in relation to wastewater use in agriculture at Hoang Tay commune and Nhat Tan commune. *Vietnam Journal of Public Health* 22, 14–20.

United Nations (2006) The eight Millennium Development Goals (MDGs). Available at: http://www.un.org/millenniumgoals/index.html (accessed 18 December 2006).

van Lieverloo, J.H.M., Blokker, E.J.M. and Medema, G. (2007) Quantitative microbial risk assessment of distributed drinking water using faecal indicator incidence and concentrations. *Journal of Water and Health* 5, 131–149.

Vose, D. (2000) *Risk Analysis: A Quantitative Guide*. John Wiley & Sons, Chichester, UK.

Waltner-Toews, D. (2013) *The Origin of Feces: What Excrement Tells us about Evolution, Ecology, and Sustainable Development*. ECW, Toronto, Canada.

Weiss, M.G. (2001) Cultural epidemiology: an introduction and overview. *Anthropology & Medicine* 8, 1–29.

Westrell, T., Schonning, C., Stenstrom, T.A. and Ashbolt, N.J. (2004) QMRA (quantitative microbial risk assessment) and HACCP (hazard analysis and critical control points) for management of pathogens in wastewater and sewage sludge treatment and reuse. *Water Science and Technology* 50, 23–30.

WHO (2006a) *WHO Guidelines for the Safe Use of Wastewater, Excreta and Greywater – Vol. 4: Excreta and Greywater use in agriculture*. World Health Organization, Geneva, Switzerland.

WHO (2006b) *WHO Guidelines for Drinking-water Quality*, 3rd edn, incorporating first addendum. Vol. 1: *Recommendations*. World Health Organization, Geneva.

WHO (2006c) *WHO Guidelines for the Safe Use of Wastewater, Excreta and Greywater, Vol. 2: Wastewater use in agriculture*. World Health Organization, Geneva.

WHO/UNICEF (2013) *Progress on Sanitation and Drinking-water-2013 Update: Joint Monitoring Programme for Water Supply and Sanitation*. WHO/UNICEF Joint Monitoring Programme for Water Supply and Sanitation.

Yen, I.H. and Syme, S.L. (1999) The social environment and health: a discussion of the epidemiologic literature. *Annual Review of Public Health* 20, 287–308.

Zinsstag, J., Meisser, A., Schelling, E., Bonfoh, B. and Tanner, M. (2012) From 'two medicines' to 'One Health' and beyond. *Onderstepoort Journal of Veterinary Research* 79, E1–5.

1

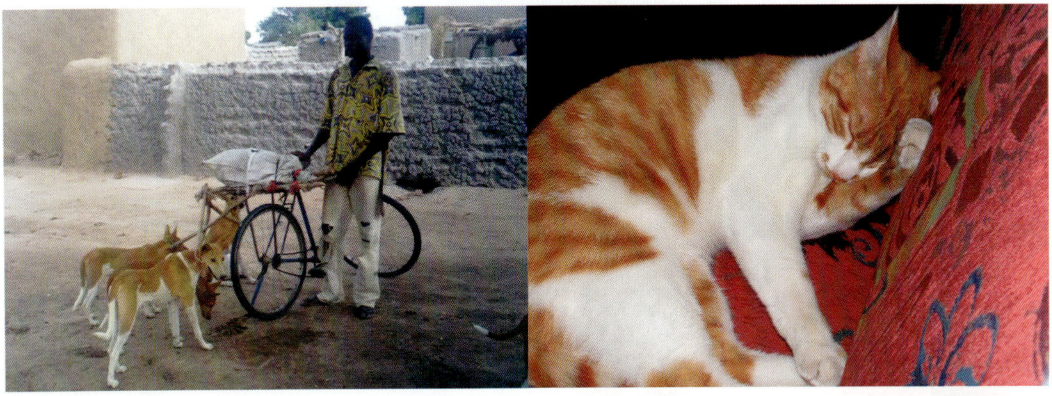

2

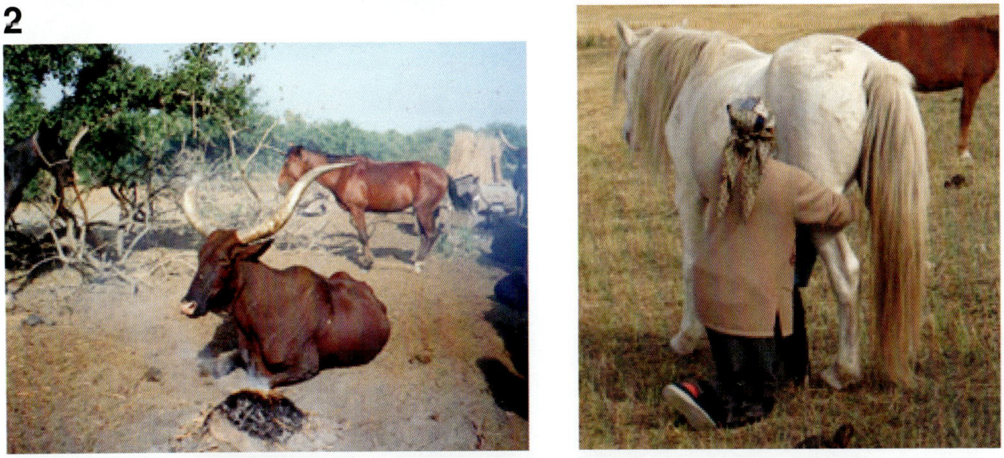

3

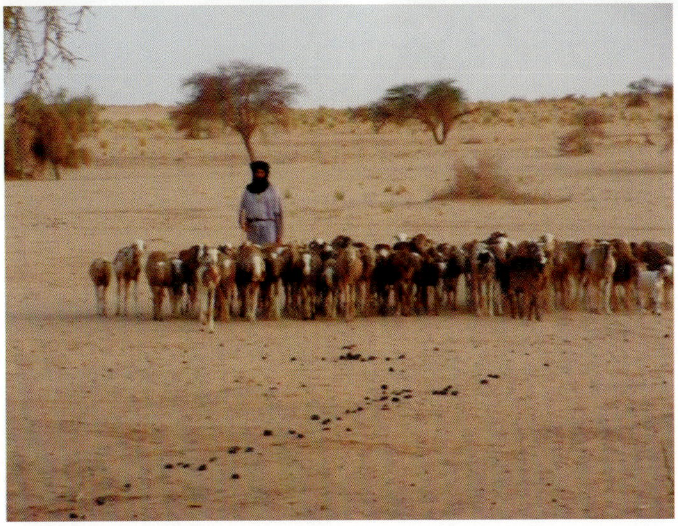

**Plate 1.** A dog trader on his way to the market in Eastern Mali, West Africa and a pet cat in a household in Switzerland (photos: J. Zinsstag).

**Plate 2.** Fulani cattle and horses in Chad (photo: J. Nicolet) and a woman milking a horse in Kyrgyzstan (photo: J. Zinsstag).

**Plate 3.** Livelihood and food security of mobile pastoralists depend highly on their livestock and climatic conditions (photo: J. Zinsstag, North Mali, 2005).

4

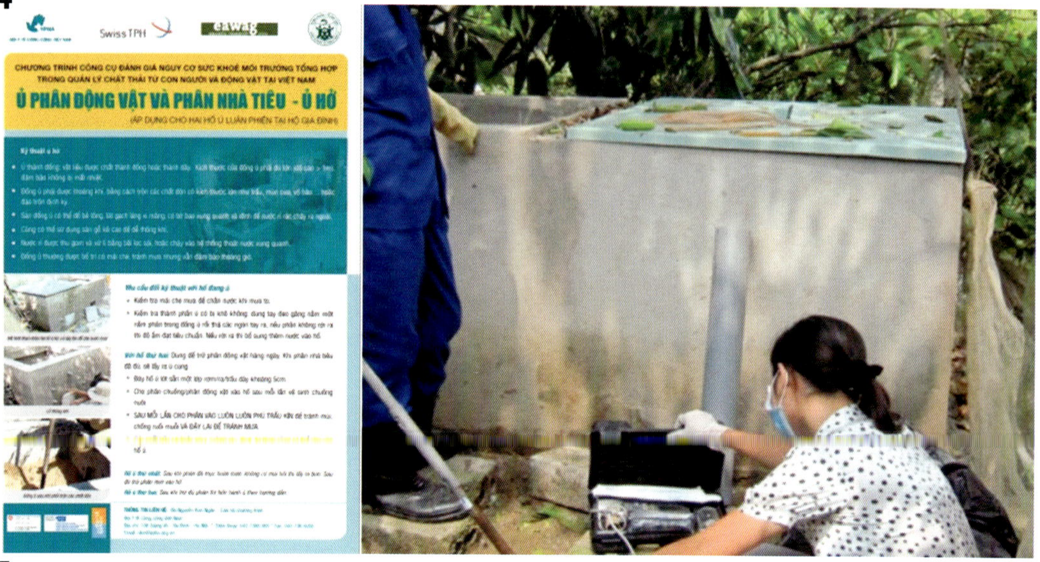


5

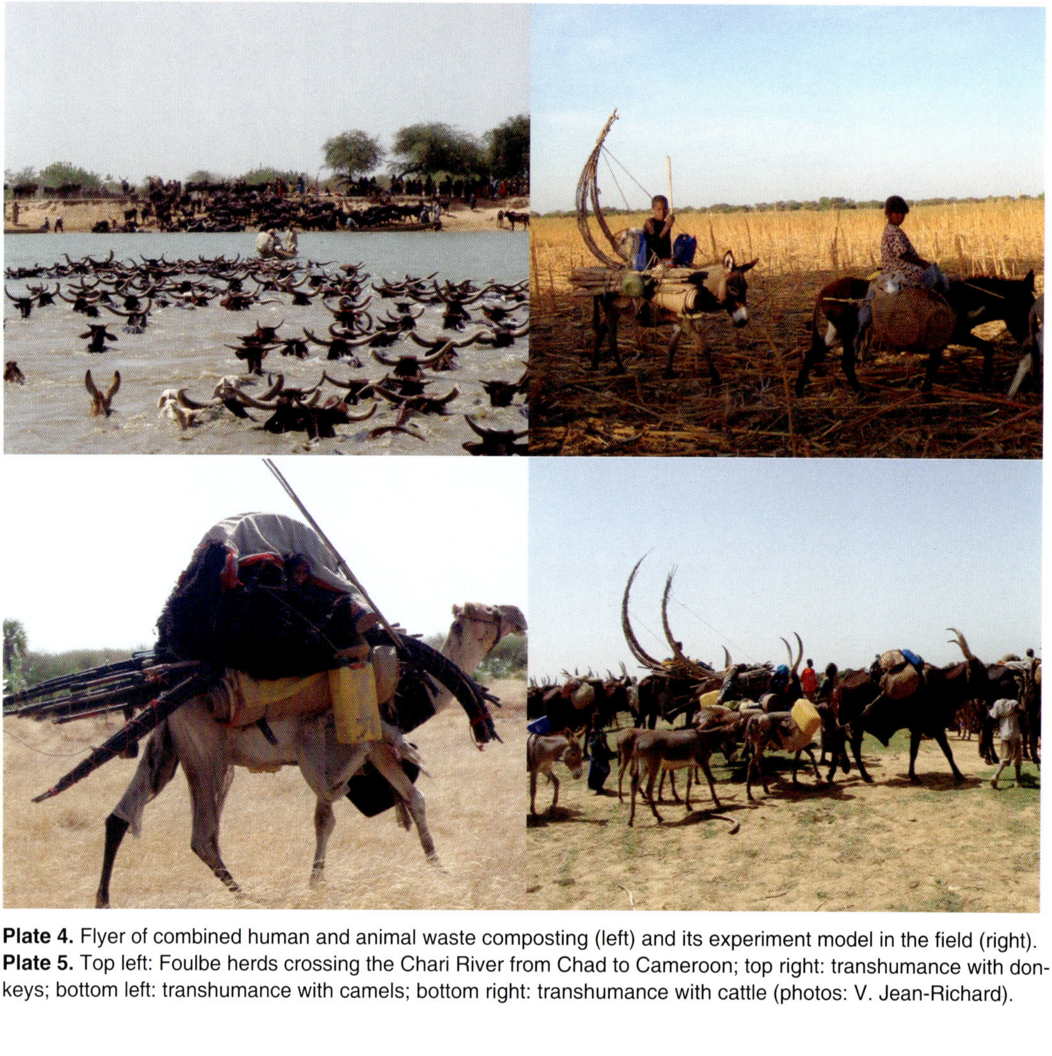

**Plate 4.** Flyer of combined human and animal waste composting (left) and its experiment model in the field (right).
**Plate 5.** Top left: Foulbe herds crossing the Chari River from Chad to Cameroon; top right: transhumance with donkeys; bottom left: transhumance with camels; bottom right: transhumance with cattle (photos: V. Jean-Richard).

6

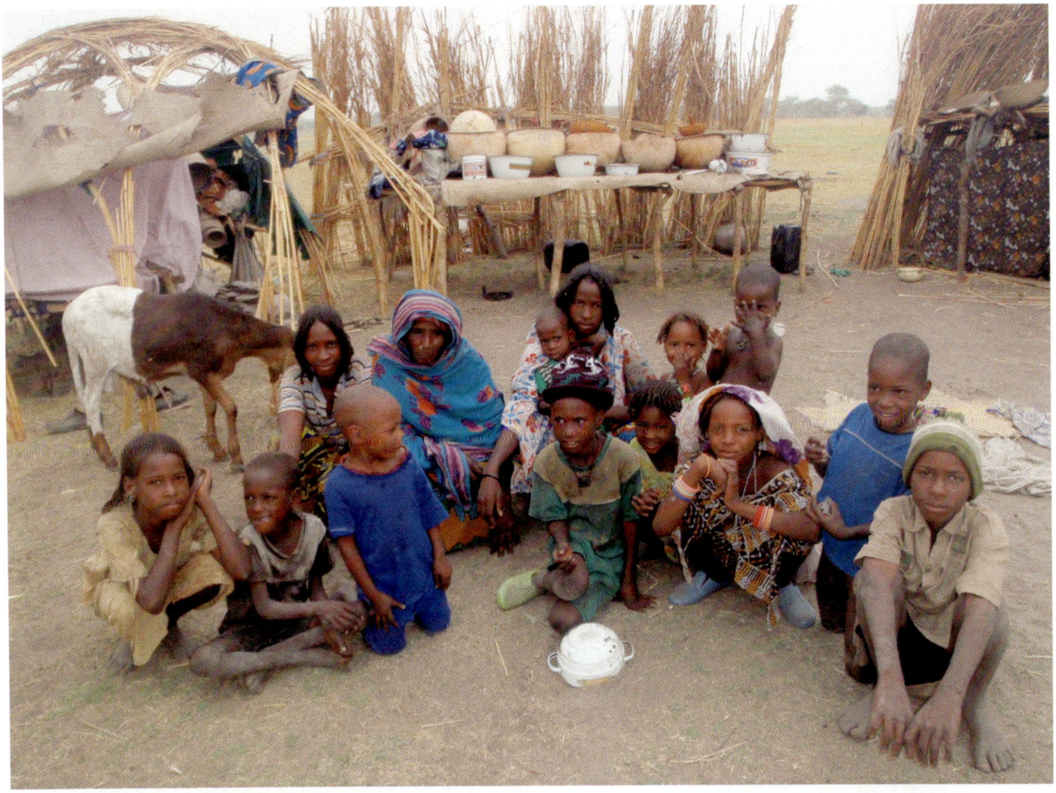

7

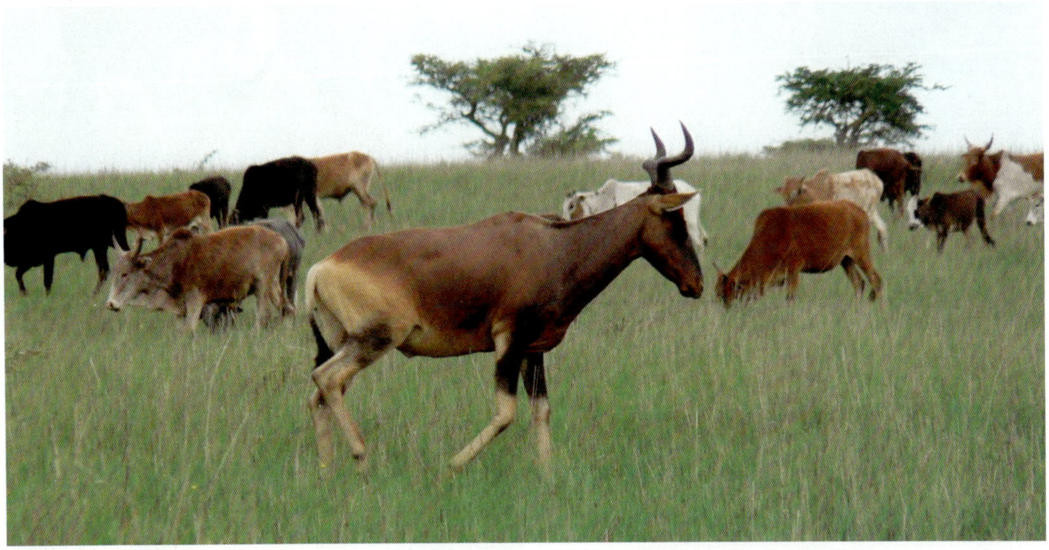

**Plate 6.** A participating Foulbe household from the small-scale human–animal demographic surveillance system (photo: V. Jean-Richard).
**Plate 7.** Swayne's hartebeest (*Alcelaphus buselaphus swaynei*) grazing with domestic cattle in Senkele Swayne's Hartebeest Sanctuary, Ethiopia (photo: L. Siege).

8

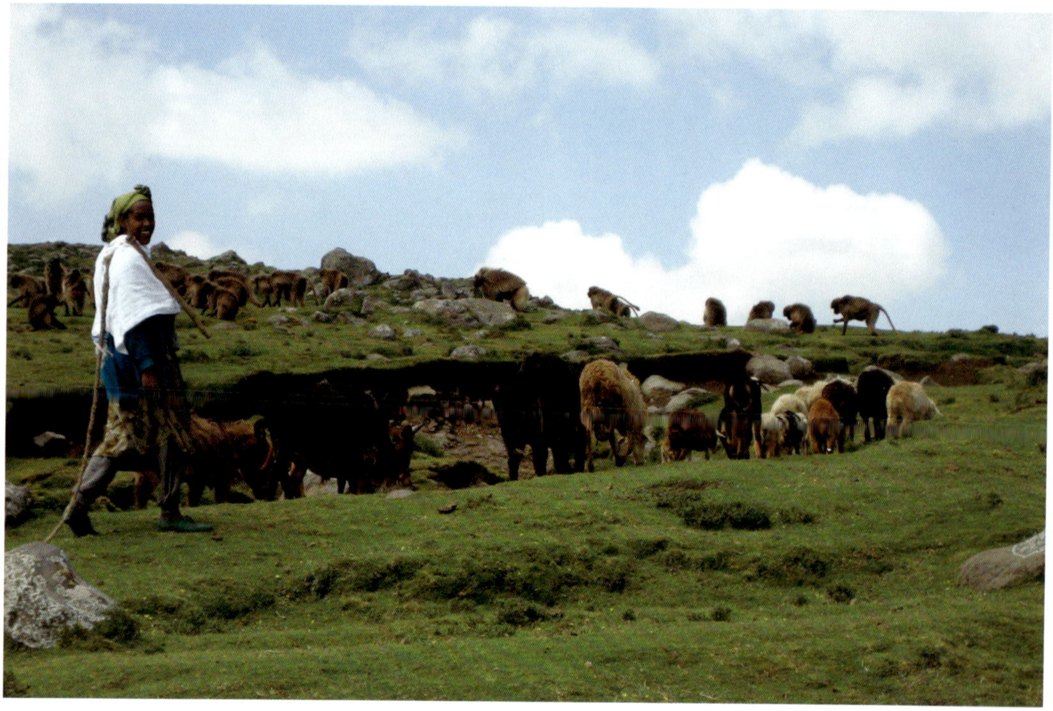

9

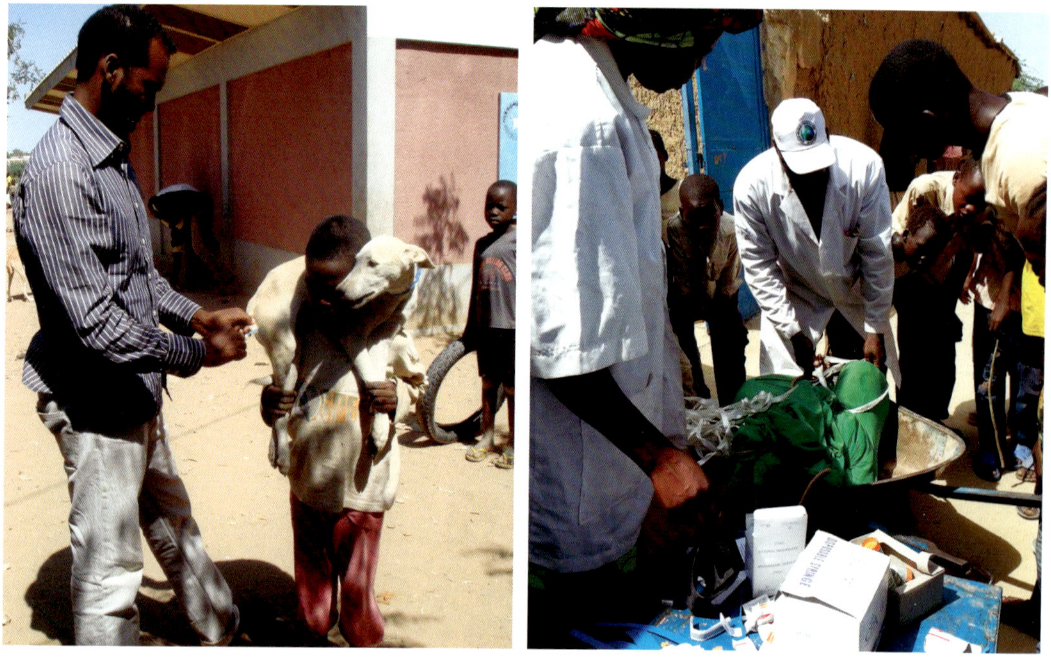

**Plate 8.** Human–livestock–wildlife interface in the Ethiopian Highlands (photo: R. Tschopp).
**Plate 9.** Differences in willingness of dogs to be handled illustrated by an easy-to-vaccinate dog on the left and a difficult dog that has been brought to the vaccination post on a wheelbarrow in a mosquito net on the right (photos: M. Léchenne).

**10**

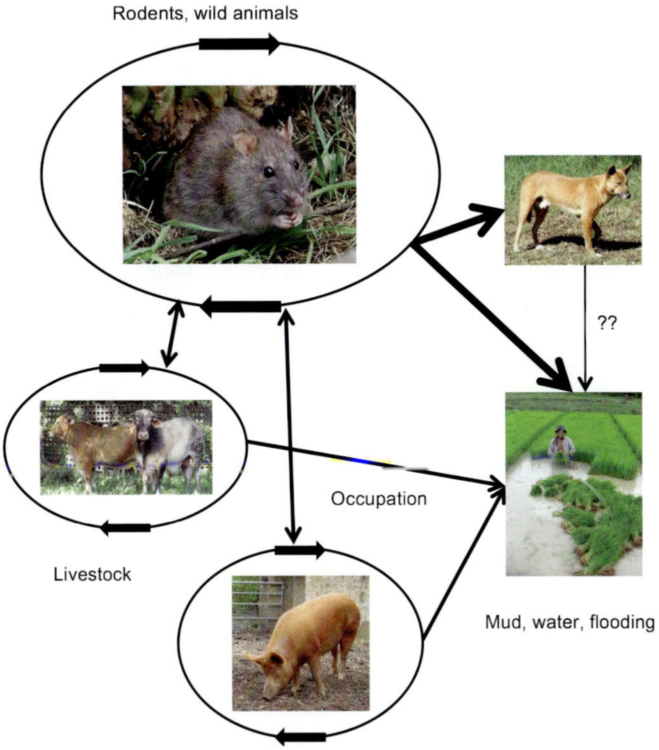


**11**

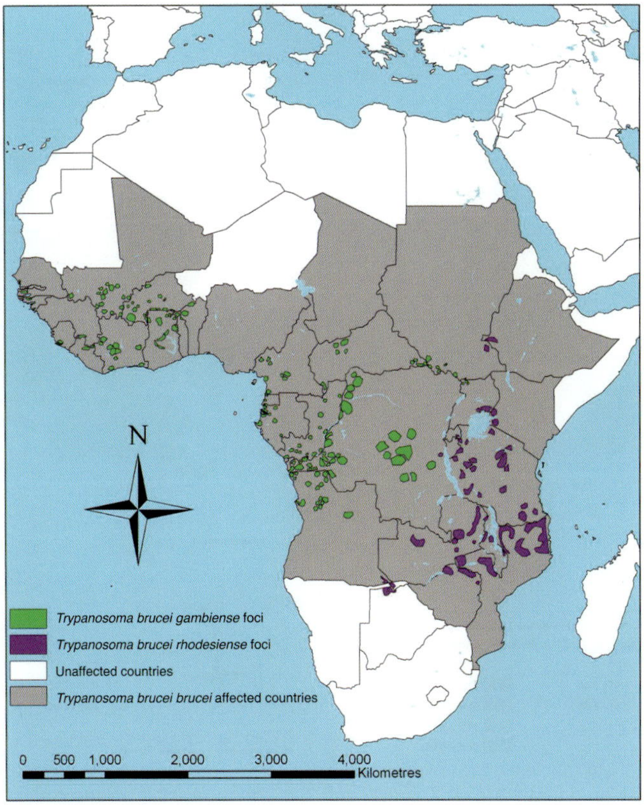


**Plate 10.** The epidemiology of leptospirosis.
**Plate 11.** HAT foci across sub-Saharan Africa (adapted from Welburn *et al.*, 2001).

# 12

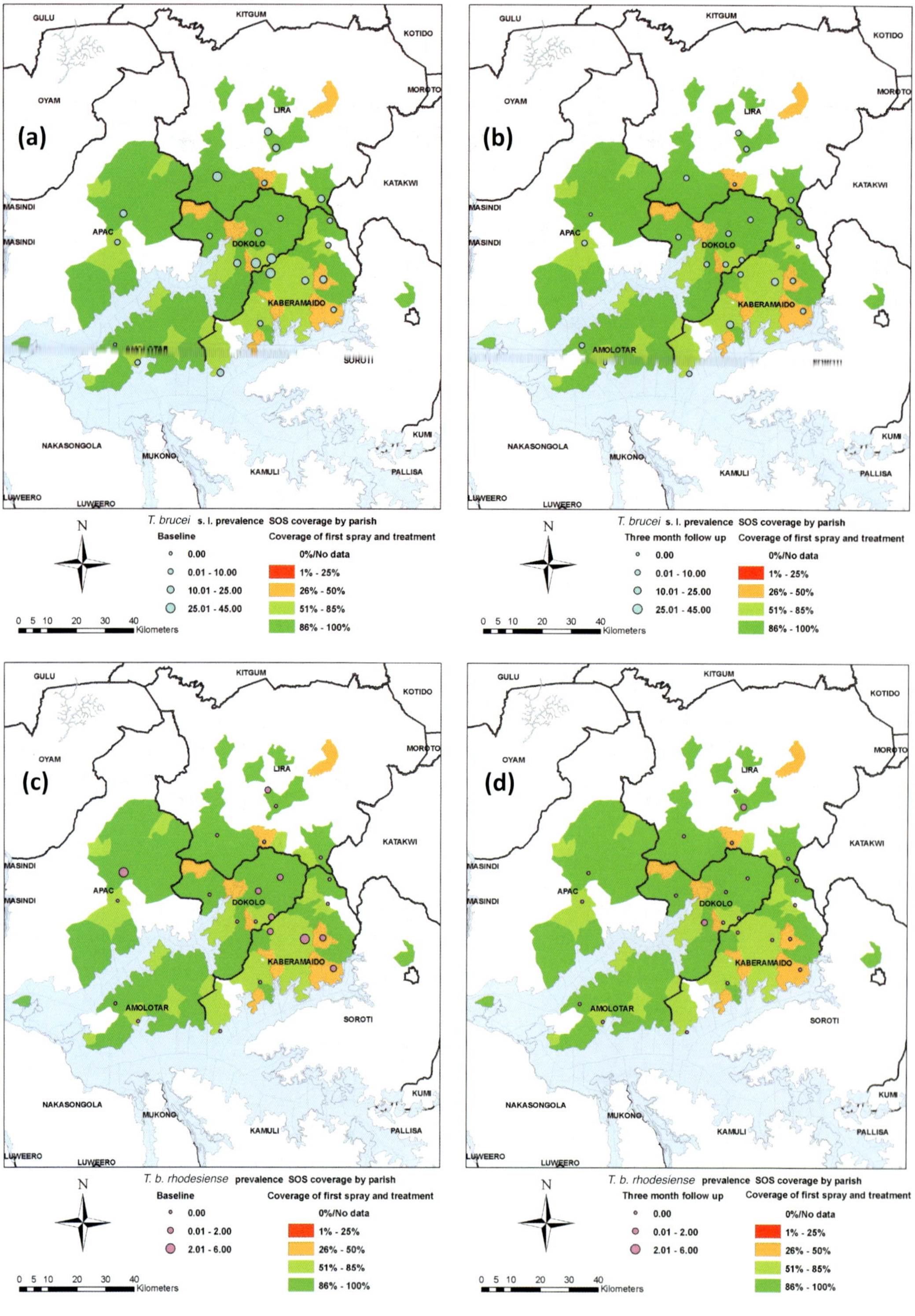


**Plate 12.** Impact of mass drug treatment on *T. brucei* and *T. b. rhodesiense* in village cattle. *T. b. brucei* before (a) and 3 months after (b) mass treatment with trypanocides and *T. b. rhodesiense* before (c) and 3 months after (d) mass treatment with trypanocides.

13

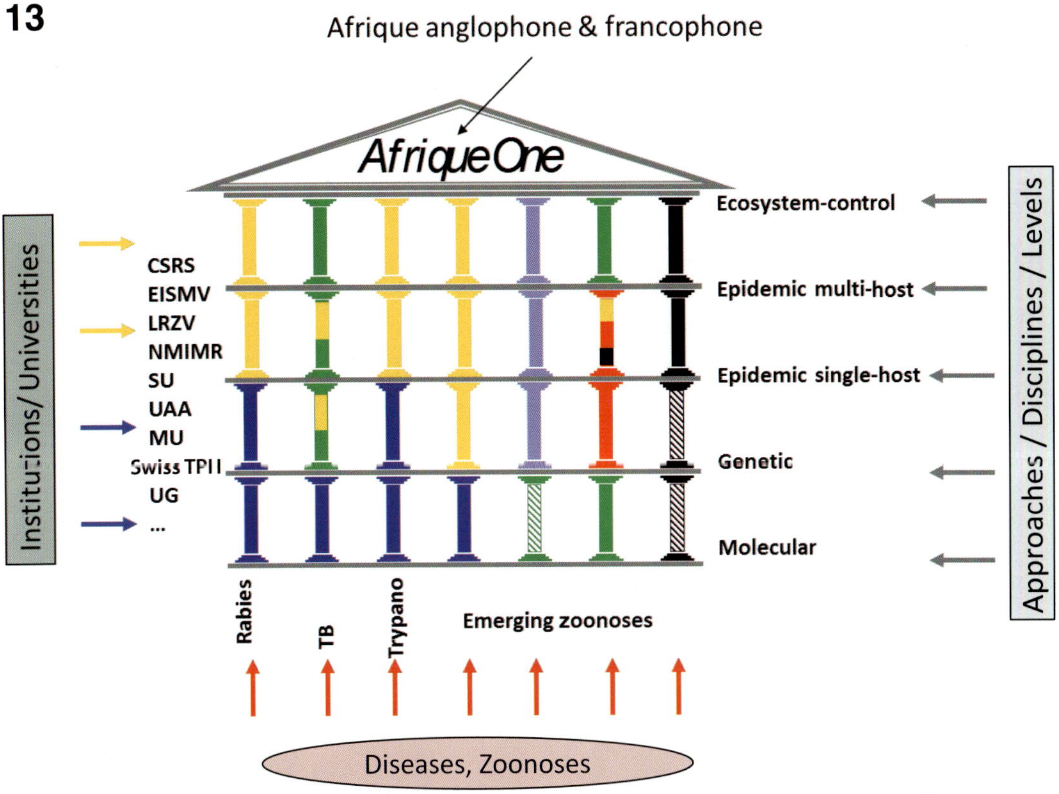


14

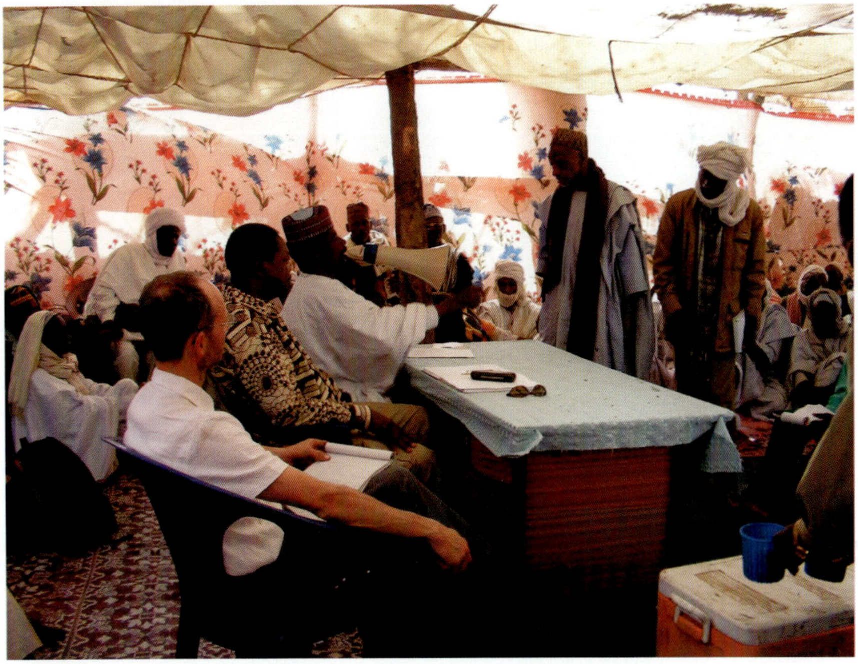

**Plate 13.** Conceptual framework of the Afrique One consortium. Note that the house with its floors and pillars is also the logo of the consortium.

**Plate 14.** Transdisciplinary stakeholder workshop on the shores of Lake Chad, bringing together national Chadian authorities, pastoralist communities and scientists (photo: J. Zinsstag).

**15**

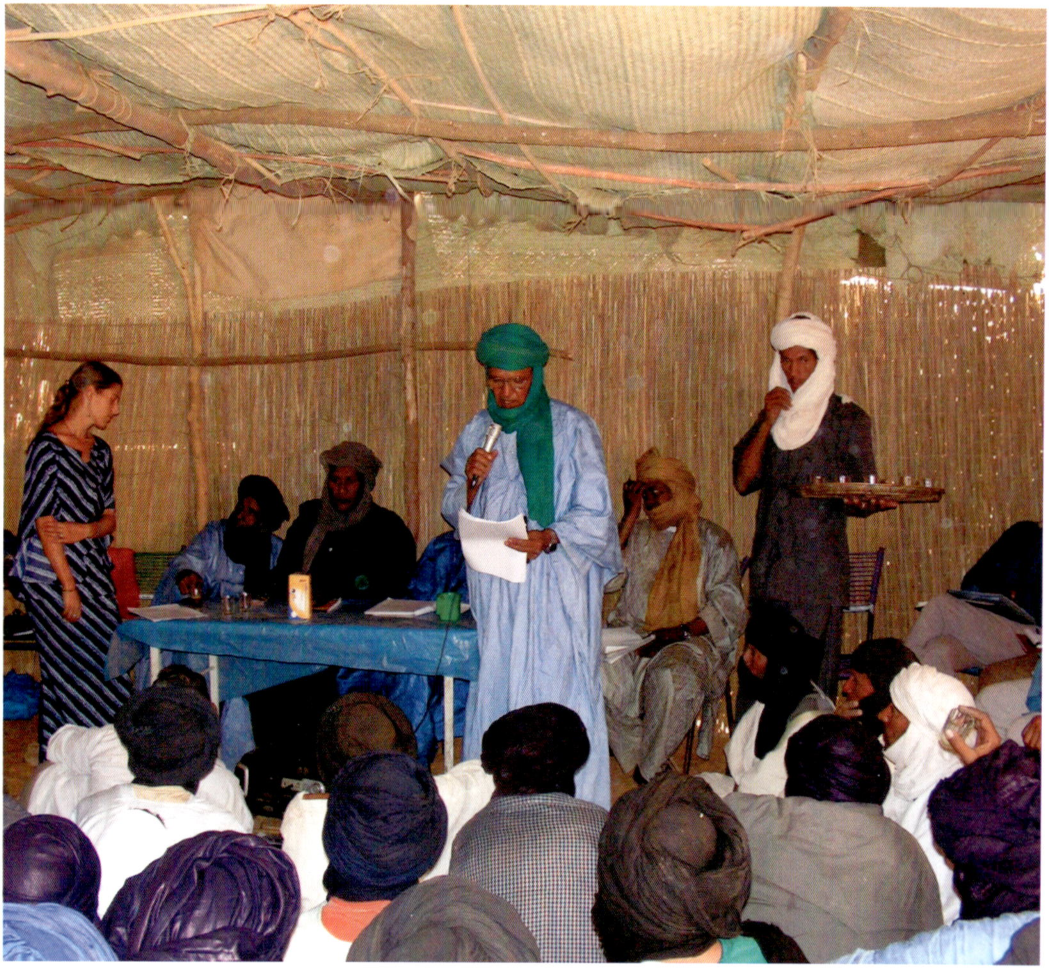

**Plate 15.** Stakeholder workshop north of Timbuktu, Mali. Political authorities and Kel Tamacheq communities discuss with scientists the provision of health care (photo: J. Zinsstag).

# 10 One Health Study Designs

**Esther Schelling*** **and Jan Hattendorf**
*Swiss Tropical and Public Health Institute, Basel, Switzerland and University of Basel, Basel, Switzerland*

## What is a One Health Study?

Human and animal health epidemiological studies use field surveys or secondary data analyses. Data collection and data interpretation are traditionally done within animal and human health sectors and during different periods, and also when an identical health topic is approached, which leads to unneeded duplication of field studies. Studies on zoonoses and foodborne pathogens are mainly led by veterinarians. A classical livestock sector approach to foodborne pathogens is risk assessment along the production and marketing chain. This allows the identification of the point of greatest leverage of control measures. However, human incidences are not assessed. Human health hazards are identified and impacts on human health are extrapolated from numbers. It is encouraging to see that risk assessors of foodborne diseases increasingly reach out to their colleagues in the public health sector and shortcuts to risk identification and quantification can be achieved. New integrated disease surveillance systems are under evaluation (Wendt *et al.*, 2014).

From separated studies it is difficult to draw coherent conclusions on linkages between human and animal health. Questions such as 'Which is the most important livestock species involved in brucellosis transmission to people in West Africa?' can hardly be answered. Results from other regions such as the Middle East, where people are mainly infected with *Brucella melitensis* from small ruminants, may not be valid. Epidemiological associations between positive human cases and positive livestock cases in different livestock species are best assessed in simultaneous studies of both people and animals with an emphasis on identifying those animal species acting as reservoir for *Brucella* spp. Knowing the main source of human infection is important to achieve the greatest leverage in reduction of human infections.

A One Health study implies that data on human and animal health, possibly also on ecological indicators, are analysed in an integrated way and are interpreted together. Sometimes these data are from different studies or data sources, but they should be comparable in terms of location, time, level of aggregation, details and quality, and a multidisciplinary team should publish their results together. A One Health study should lead to insights that would not be visible without intersectoral collaboration such as impacts of

*E-mail: esther.schelling@unibas.ch

multi-host infections on humans, animal and ecosystem health and economics (Zinsstag *et al.*, Chapter 5, this volume). Rabinowitz *et al.* (2013) have defined a One Health approach similarly: 'Integrated approaches that consider human, animal, and environmental health components that can improve prediction and control of certain diseases'. This is not only true for infectious diseases, but also for non-communicable diseases and health-system strengthening. The aim is not necessarily improved human health or averted human burden of disease. Messenger *et al.* (2014) showed that an increasing number of reports indicate that humans are transmitting pathogens to animals. Recent examples include methicillin-resistant *Staphylococcus aureus*, influenza A virus, *Cryptosporidium parvum* and *Ascaris lumbricoides*. A One Health study would show bi- and multidirectional relations between human and animal health and their health in relation to the health of their ecosystem (Zinsstag, 2012). Thus the aim is ideally improved human, animal and ecosystem health.

The most difficult step of a One Health study remains the initiation of a process that leads to change and health improvement. Solutions for successful control of neglected zoonoses may be outside the health sectors; for example policies may need to be mainstreamed into poverty reduction strategies and continuous training to build health service skills and competences. Networking and regional approaches have been successfully used for zoonoses control (Parkes *et al.*, 2012). Avian influenza led to the establishment of highly recognized networks for exchange of information and lessons such as from the Asian Partnership for Emerging Infectious Diseases Research and the Mekong Basin Disease Surveillance (Grace *et al.*, 2011). For most zoonoses, one country alone can hardly implement successful control measures without the neighbouring countries doing likewise. Disease-control programmes designed in developed countries for industry-wide application cannot be transferred without appropriate adaptation to other settings (Randolph *et al.*, 2007). Many factors critical to successful disease control cannot be assessed quantitatively. The way forward is to enhance interdisciplinary cooperation between the social and health-related sciences (Whittaker, Chapter 6, this volume). Note that the literature is richer on studies describing broader socio-cultural considerations for emerging than endemic zoonoses. These are, for example, human encroachment into forests with potential exposure to new pathogens, global travel and eating of bush meat. While One Health recognizes the importance of understanding the social and cultural factors in disease transmission dynamics and the planning of control interventions, anthropological studies on zoonoses are sparse and limited (Bardosh and Thys, 2012). Socio-cultural One Health surveys and the role of social sciences are described elsewhere in this book (Whittaker, Chapter 6, this volume).

In this chapter we focus on population-based quantitative One Health study designs with emphasis on planning of field surveys. Such studies are central to the understanding of disease dynamics and for evaluating evidence-based testing of control measures. In addition, data for cost–benefit and cost-effectiveness calculations (Zinsstag *et al.*, 2007; Zinsstag *et al.*, Chapter 12, this volume) are hardly available at central level alone and good quality field data is needed. Therefore, laboratory-based studies using competencies from different sectors are not presented, although these largely contribute to, for example, improved and new vaccines against zoonoses and comparative pathology. We do not focus on early detection of emerging diseases but rather on endemic zoonoses. The incidences of the latter are believed to be much higher, however are under-reported due to low capacity to recognize and diagnose the causative agents of zoonoses. Health of ecosystems is difficult to define. They are inherently dynamic and changing (Cumming and Cumming, Chapter 4, this volume). The simultaneous assessment of human and animal health outcomes should lead to a better understanding of the context and associated different disciplines (see Chapters 14 through 18, this volume).

A key discipline in One Health field studies is epidemiology, thus the study of health and disease in populations or, according to another broad description of the young discipline that only emerged in the 19th century, the study of the frequency, distribution and determinants of health and disease in populations. Epidemiology derives from Greek and literally means 'the study of what is upon the people'; 'demos' meaning 'people, district' (Omran, 1971). This may suggest that epidemiology applies only to human populations. Most veterinary epidemiologists believe, however, that it is pointless to use different terms such as epizootiology, epizootic, or enzootic when referring to a disease in an animal population. The words 'epidemiology', 'epidemic' and 'endemic' should be used to describe disease occurrence in all host species. Epidemiology has also been applied to studies of plant populations (Bartlett and Judge, 1997; Nutter, 1999). Common in epidemiology is that a health-related question leads to a hypothesis and defines an objective, which leads to the appropriate study design to use.

We first provide examples on joint surveys and surveillance, then on practical information on planning of a field study design and conclude on the advantages of One Health study designs. We also mention possible constraints for their implementation given that there are only a few One Health studies to date. For the examples, the main epidemiological considerations and the results that could not be achieved with single sector approaches are highlighted.

## Examples of One Health Surveys and Surveillance

Joint human and animal health surveys are either done during the same period or in the same geographical area and at different levels of aggregation. Levels of aggregation are from individual, for example an owner–pet relation, household and village levels, and also communities and their animals, districts, provinces or countries.

### Simultaneous human and animal health assessment

A simultaneous assessment of livestock milk and human sera vitamin levels, combined with a 24 h nutrition recall study, showed that milk was the most important source of vitamin A for pastoralists, but 17% of tested women were severely retinol-deficient. Therefore the consumption of more vegetables and fruits needs to be promoted (Zinsstag *et al.*, 2002). The latter survey could show the linkages between livestock and human nutrition, but was only done in one specific community. A comparison community of the same region in the survey would have better allowed to conclude on specificities and generalities of the findings.

A mixed team composed of medical and veterinary staff assessed during repeated cross-sectional surveys health and health-related issues of mobile pastoralists and their livestock using standardized clinical examination forms and questionnaires. The main diseases and conditions found among mobile pastoralists did not differ substantially from morbidity typical for the Sahelian zone such as respiratory diseases, malaria and diarrhoea. Despite frequent diarrhoea and fevers, respiratory infections including lower tract infections in children and tuberculosis in adults, and malaria, had more impact on individual and community health than food-poisoning and zoonotic diseases such as brucellosis. Therefore, a programme on control of zoonoses should not ignore other prevailing health problems of the communities. This simultaneous health assessment also showed that there was no fully immunized pastoralist child in the study population. In contrast, livestock had been vaccinated by veterinarians visiting the pastoralist camps during compulsory vaccination campaigns (Schelling *et al.*, 2005). Based on this finding and in agreement with the communities and the Chadian national and local authorities, joint human and animal vaccination services were conducted and evaluated (Schelling *et al.*, 2007; Schelling *et al.*, Chapter 20, this volume).

Health impact assessments of industrial development projects (Winkler *et al.*, 2012) could be extended to simultaneously assess livestock health, if veterinarians were associated. Projects such as construction of dams and mining can adversely affect the health of the livestock kept by the surveyed households and have implications on their livelihoods and income. Hence health impact assessment could be extended to One Health Impact Assessment (OHIA).

### Field surveys on zoonoses

Simultaneous assessment of zoonotic incidences and prevalences in animals and people at the same levels and same quality, for example regarding selection, helps to establish epidemiologic links. In Chad, human Q-fever seropositivity was associated with keeping of camels but not of cattle (Schelling *et al.*, 2003); in Kyrgyzstan and Egypt human brucellosis sero-prevalences were most closely related to keeping of sheep (El Sherbini *et al.*, 2007; Bonfoh *et al.*, 2012) and thus small ruminants cannot be excluded in a control programme. In Togo, human seropositivity was astonishingly low (below 1%), although cattle seropositivity was high (9% in village and 7% in transhumant cattle) (Dean *et al.*, 2013). The isolated *Brucella abortus* strains from cattle harboured a large deletion in a gene (*bruAb2_0168*) encoding for a putative autotransporter. This gene is of particular interest because it is used as a target for PCR in the identification of the species *B. abortus* and it encodes for a putative autotransporter, which might be involved in virulence and/or host predilection (Dean *et al.*, 2014). Further laboratory-based virulence studies will likely better explain the observations from the field (Zinsstag *et al.*, Chapter 14, this volume).

In Ethiopia, *Mycobacterium bovis* in human TB infection is very low (4 *M. bovis* isolates compared to 1000 *M. tuberculosis* isolates from clinical suspects of pulmonary and extra-pulmonary TB) (Firdessa *et al.*, 2013). Interestingly, *M. tuberculosis* was isolated from cattle and one camel (Gumi *et al.*, 2012). The latter study was a combined field, slaughterhouse and hospital study with data collection during the same period (Tschopp, Chapter 15, this volume). In 2006, the Health for Animals and Livelihood Improvement (HALI) project was initiated to test the feasibility of a One Health approach to find creative solutions to health problems in communities living in the water-limited Ruaha ecosystem of Tanzania. Simultaneous investigations of medical, ecological, socio-economic and policy issues driving the ecosystem were implemented. Based on input from local stakeholders, waterborne diarrhoeal diseases and cattle diseases were also assessed to identify geographic areas with varying water availability, where risk of transmission may be highest (Mazet *et al.*, 2009). The researchers could show with the example of bovine tuberculosis that there was livestock–wildlife pathogen transmission in the Ruaha ecosystem (Clifford *et al.*, 2013).

### Food- and waterborne zoonoses

Control of foodborne and waterborne infections requires input from public health, environmental health and veterinary public health practitioners as well as regulatory authorities responsible for safe food and water. They also require a deep understanding of how social, economic, environmental and cultural factors interact with dynamics of disease transmission and the acceptability of control measures (VWB/VSF Canada, 2010).

The Caribbean Eco-Health Program (CEHP) has supported interdisciplinary training, particularly of human and environmental health agents and assisted to identify regional knowledge gaps in environmental health threats such as pesticide residues, which were important to users and policy makers. The Atlantis Mobile Laboratory could move throughout the Caribbean and be able to respond to calls for specific research concerns and capacity-building opportunities (Forde *et al.*, 2011).

Total bacteria, *Streptococcus/Enterococcus*, yeast and mould, Enterobacteriaceae and *Staphylococcus* counts all increased along the chain from milk at milking to marketed milk in Kenya, indicating a human health hazard according to Kenyan quality standards. To test this, an unmatched nested case-control study – constructed from a cross-sectional survey – confirmed that gastrointestinal illness was significantly associated with consumption of certain vegetables and camel milk (Kaindi *et al.*, 2012). This study led to revitalizing the past efforts of seeing that milk collectors use containers that can be easily washed with water and soap (Bonfoh *et al.*, 2003). High levels of pathogens and other hazards in milk and milk products are reported from both the formal and informal dairy sectors. The role of food safety in dairy policy potentially constrains the shift of policy to more pro-poor policies because informal markets are a priori excluded.

### Survey and surveillance of antimicrobial resistance

Pets are often companions used for psychological support in the therapy of nursing home residents but have also been described as reservoirs for antibiotic-resistant bacteria. To investigate the role of healthy pets as reservoirs of multidrug-resistant staphylococci or Extended Spectrum Beta-Lactamase (ESBL) producing Enterbacteriaceae, several studies have assessed these with the same approach in both people and pets in nursing homes and the general population (reviewed in Messenger *et al.*, 2014). Although identical genomic patterns from people and from animals have been found, the direction of transmission often remains unclear. The same issues arose for example in tuberculosis. Cattle were infected with *M. tuberculosis* and could have acquired infection from people or from other cattle (Gumi *et al.*, 2012). Likely the question on 'who infects whom' is not necessarily the primary question since people and animals share the same ecosystem and evolve together, but rather which control measure has highest leverage in both people and animals (Tschopp, Chapter 15, this volume).

The Canadian Integrated Program for Antimicrobial Resistance Surveillance (CIPARS) unifies surveillance components, which can be linked to examine the relationship between antimicrobials used in food-animals and humans and the associated health impacts. Analysis of CIPARS data identified a link between ceftiofur (an antimicrobial of high importance to human medicine) usage in poultry and ceftiofur-resistant *Salmonella* Heidelberg isolates obtained from people and chicken meat in Quebec. Communication of this information led to a voluntary ban on the use of ceftiofur in 2005 (CIPARS, 2007). It would be interesting to have more information on costs of running this nationwide programme, which, in turn, can inform other countries on investing in a shared intersectoral system for evidence-based guidance to physicians and veterinarians in their selection of appropriate antimicrobials.

### Joint disease surveillance systems and use of routine data

In the Q-fever outbreak in the Netherlands (2007–2010), there were 4000 confirmed human Q-fever cases with 11 deaths and huge economic losses among dairy goat herds given the 40,000 slaughtered pregnant goats (Enserink, 2010). Could the outbreak have been controlled earlier if the health and veterinary sectors had exchanged data and communicated at an earlier stage? Most abnormal disease events are seen rather late in the human health and veterinary sectors, despite the fact that early detection is a core objective of surveillance systems. The cohort study set up in the Netherlands between 2007 and 2011 (van Loenhout *et al.*, 2012) included only people. A parallel cohort in goats may have led to additional links seen between events in people and goats.

Surveillance and monitoring efforts are major components and central to disease prevention and control programmes. Joint human and animal surveillance networks could be more effective in terms of earlier detection or lower fixed costs than active surveys. Currently such surveillance systems are being tested. Since they have been set up more recently, the results on possible added value are not yet available. Wendt *et al.* (2014) have reviewed these recent systems and found that the majority of the 27 identified human and animal surveillance systems world-wide were established for the purpose of early detection and tend to focus predominantly on emerging pandemic threats. Most systems use different data sources, and secondary data, methods and frameworks on the integration of disparate and secondary data are of great interest. Information integration is possible to achieve despite the fact that data have been collected in different surroundings and often for different purposes and thus differ in content, quality and terminology and are stored in different locations or formats. However, transforming and cleaning procedures have to be applied and this requires time and effort as long as the different data sources have not been standardized or prepared for an easy linkage. Above all, cross-sectoral structures, trust and good communication networks are required (Wendt *et al.*, 2014).

Regional and national intersectoral data exchange cannot be expected to work if there are no collaborations at all levels of data reporting, at least to briefly cross-check reports. There is a need for consistent, reliable data at a national level – over a longer term – but also – in the shorter term – the need for reliable data to demonstrate the neglected status of the diseases. The lack of diagnostic facilities and regional reference laboratories for diagnosis of zoonoses in many parts of the world is a constraint to this, since most current joint surveillance systems rely on routine data from diagnostic laboratories (WHO *et al.*, 2009; Wendt *et al.*, 2014). In future more alternative surveillance systems will be evaluated – such as syndromic surveillance, participatory epidemiology and risk-based joint surveillance systems. However, these systems still need to show that they can be effective in detection of abnormal events and are not too costly to be maintained. Also, to achieve added value of integrated surveillance systems requires shared objectives and strategies for institutional integration at the appropriate level (Mariner *et al.*, 2011).

Use of modern mobile technology for near real-time reporting will be used more frequently in future, for One Health and other surveillance systems (Karimuribo *et al.*, 2012; Jean-Richard and Crump, Chapter 13, this volume). But no near real-time reporting system should be established without giving possibilities of reacting to reported events. The lack of response capacity has stopped several surveillance systems in the past, because reporting ceased when the communities did not see any result to their reporting efforts (Karimuribo *et al.*, 2012). Also, monitoring can include other parameters than diseases or antimicrobial resistances. Stakeholders in zoonoses control and response capacity of the health and veterinary sectors can and should be monitored. For Rift Valley fever (RVF) in Kenya, a stakeholder analysis showed that the 28 relevant agencies in prevention/control of RVF go beyond the line of the livestock and public health sectors. A survey just after the RVF outbreak in 2006/2007 showed that the veterinary sector is understaffed to respond adequately to such an epidemic. The public health sector could deploy five times more staff than the veterinary sector, although the latter had more tasks during the outbreak situation (Schelling and Kimani, 2007).

Routine data is often compared with survey data to estimate under-reporting. For example, Cleaveland *et al.* (2002) found that active detection of human rabies deaths is difficult due to low incidence and the need to set up specific detection studies such as collection of verbal autopsy data from household surveys. Passive surveillance may be insufficient, leading to vast under-reporting of human rabies cases. However, animal bites can be surveyed given their rather high incidence and the likelihood of victims to seek professional care. Cleaveland *et al.* (2002) used a probability decision tree to estimate human mortality from information provided by animal bite victims. After validation with field studies, the authors estimated that in rural Tanzania the true incidence of human rabies was 10–100 times higher than the officially reported human rabies incidence.

Good routine data can be used for mathematical models (Zinsstag *et al.*, Chapter 11, this volume) – for example avian influenza. A mathematical model of avian influenza transmission between wild birds and domestic poultry was used to provide proof of concept for a proposed integrated intervention involving human, animal and environmental health to interrupt such transmission (Guan *et al.*, 2007). However, modelling of prediction is only possible where suitable primary (field-based) data are available. No model can improve data of doubtful quality.

## Practical Considerations for One Health Studies

### Study types in public health and veterinary epidemiology

Epidemiological research can be broadly classified into field-based and hospital-based studies. In veterinary epidemiology, studies at veterinary clinics are less common than in public health at health centres, and the main categories are field-based and abattoir/slaughterhouse-based studies. Obviously, field-based studies represent the general population much better than studies conducted in slaughterhouses, since the age distribution of the animals is different. Reviews found significantly higher prevalences in slaughterhouses compared to field-based surveys (Agrawal, 2012). In some settings, animal producers preferentially send their old, unproductive or infertile cattle for slaughter, which increases the chance of detecting more chronic infections than in the population. Conversely, farmers may prefer home slaughter if they fear condemnation of carcasses at abattoirs. Another constraint is the limited amount of additional information on the animals. Since intermediary traders are common in many parts of the world, information about origin, herd size or farming system is missing. On the other hand, field-based studies are much more resource intensive in terms of costs, time and administration. Besides more time and needed transportation, they also require higher logistical skills such as storage of samples until processing in laboratories.

Besides the study population, the study design is strongly linked to the associated level of evidence. For example, cross-sectional studies have a high risk of bias, which raises questions about the validity of the findings. One considers a systematic review of high quality studies as having a high level of evidence. In 1972, Archie Cochrane highlighted the lack of reliable reviews of available evidence and established the concept of evidence-based medicine. It was soon recognized that there was a need to develop also systematic approaches to assess the study quality in other health sectors. Consequently, evidence-based veterinary medicine and evidence-based public health evolved. Unfortunately, until today no attempt has been made to adapt the evidence base concept into the One Health context. However, numerous tools and checklists for assessing study quality are available and the main aspects apply also to One Health studies. The main constraints that prevent a causal interpretation are bias, confounding and chance. One of the seminal papers on this subject was by Sir Austin Bradford Hill (Hill, 1965). The highest level of evidence is provided by experiments, i.e. cluster randomized controlled clinical trials. However, such trials are often not feasible for ethical, operational or financial reasons. Properly designed large cohort studies are usually graded as high quality. It is noteworthy that not only the level of evidence defines the most suitable study design, but also disease and exposure characteristics. For example, cohort studies are inappropriate if the outcome of interest is rare.

### Sampling and sampling frame

In particular, young researchers commonly underestimate the complexity of planning and conducting sampling in resource-limited settings. However, an improperly drawn and not representative sample might introduce serious bias, which can easily double or halve the observed effective size. Unfortunately, only if controversial publications are published, will the importance of proper sampling attract more attention (for example, Burnham *et al.*, 2006, which led to numerous discussions on 'main street bias' and showed the difficulties associated with proper sampling in urban settings). Next to a careful sampling, a detailed description of the sampling approach used is mandatory. There are too many publications with an incomplete description of the sampling procedure. Likewise, research on sampling approaches and theory has been neglected by the scientific communities in both human health and veterinary epidemiology. There are only a few studies investigating appropriateness or bias associated with common but non-random sampling techniques such as 'spin the bottle' (i.e. spinning a bottle on the ground to select a direction). The potential of as unbiased as possible sampling using modern techniques using GIS and satellite images also remains underexploited.

Most statistical techniques require the theoretical assumption of a simple random sample, i.e. each individual from the population has the same probability to be selected and enrolled in the study. The sampling frame is a list of all members – or as complete as possible – from the population. Individuals are randomly drawn from the sampling frame and all individuals have the same chance to be enrolled in the study. Where no complete registries of humans or animals exist, as is the case in most studies a multi-stage cluster sampling is commonly used. In a first stage, clusters, i.e. administrative units such as villages or neighbourhoods, are randomly selected. If a nationwide study is done, selection may start at a higher level, such as provinces. Afterwards households or animal-keeping households are randomly selected within each cluster. In a final step, either all animals or a random subset of animals is selected. Cluster sampling is the natural sampling design in veterinary epidemiology, since livestock populations are typically clustered into herds or flocks. Surprisingly, cluster sampling is often confused with stratified sampling. Cluster sampling requires a higher sample size, which is not the case for stratified sampling compared to simple random sampling. The differences are explained in Box 10.1.

### Random selection of clusters

In contrast to lists with individuals, a sampling frame at cluster level, like a list of all villages in a certain district, is usually available or can be established. There are two main approaches to select the clusters, either by simple random sampling, or, if the number of individuals within each cluster is known, sampling with probability proportional to size (PPS). For the former approach, the probability of individuals to be selected is higher in smaller clusters. Almost all statistical software packages are able to perform a weighted sampling. If there is no software available, the method can also be applied without computer assistance as described in Box 10.2. The main advantage of sampling proportional to size is that each individual in the population has the same probability of being selected. Since the risk of infectious diseases is usually density dependent, this approach provides an unbiased prevalence estimate. A challenge in a One Health study is that humans and animals are investigated simultaneously. One needs to consider that selection probabilities can only be assigned to one population, thus either to the number of humans of interest or animals at the same time. One could argue to select the main presumptive reservoir host as sampling frame. During data analysis, sampling weights can be used to produce representative estimates.

If a list of villages or neighbourhoods cannot be established – for example slums are challenging in this context because they are very dynamic – alternative approaches have to be applied. But the approach needs to be selected carefully, given that virtually all are subject to selection bias. One methodology that is assumed to be tolerably unbiased is the random generation of geo-coordinates within the study area using GIS or alternative software and selection of the community closest to the generated point. However, bias may be introduced because villages in sparsely populated areas have a higher probability to be selected compared to villages from densely populated areas.

As for humans and animals, inclusion and exclusion criteria must be clearly stated in the study protocol, e.g. villages must be accessible by car during the rainy season or must have at least one cattle-keeping household. Likewise, the study area must be clearly defined. This is not the case with statements like 'villages within X hours driving time'. Sampling procedures like 'villages were selected on the basis of proximity to' is clearly a purposive selection approach and, therefore, unsuitable for quantitative data collection.

### Sampling of humans within villages or communities

The by far most common approach in selection of people in a rural community is via random selection of eligible households, but this approach requires a list of all households as the sampling frame. Such a list can usually be compiled together with the village head, who needs to be informed about the research activities anyway. To draw a map or to use a satellite image might be worth considering in longitudinal

**Box 10.1.** Stratified random sampling versus cluster sampling.

In a *stratified random sampling*, the individuals of the target population are first divided into subgroups called strata. Each individual belongs to one stratum. Then a random sample is drawn from each stratum, e.g. 10% of the population. This approach is advantageous if subpopulations vary greatly and the estimates in each subgroup or the differences between subgroups are of particular interest. *Cluster sampling* is an approach in which clusters of individuals rather than individuals are randomly selected. Like stratified random sampling, the population is divided into separate groups such that each individual belongs to exactly one cluster. Clusters are usually defined by geographic boundaries or administrative units (in contrast, strata can be defined as age groups, sex, etc., Fig. 10.1). Natural clusters are herds and households or villages. Depending on the research question, the cluster can be selected via simple random sampling or with a probability proportional to their size. Cluster sampling requires rather sophisticated analytical methods and a larger sample size.

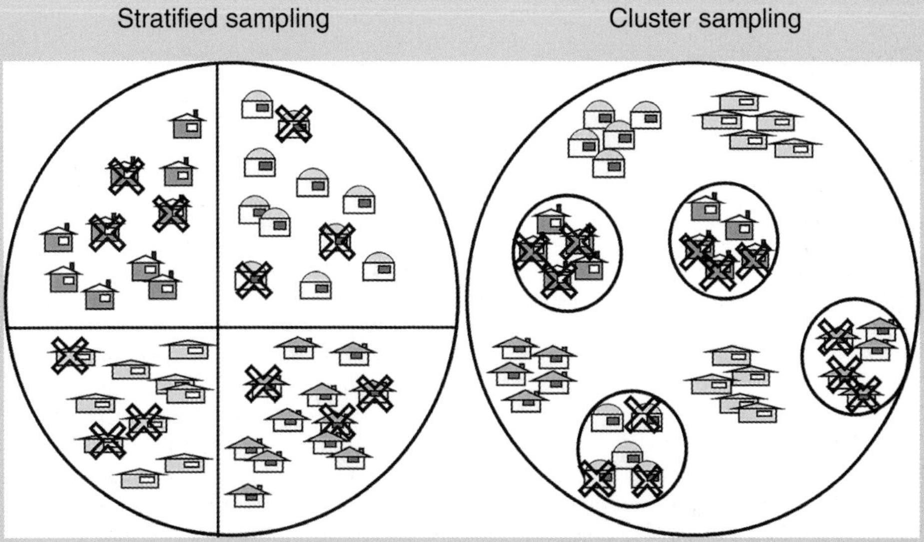


**Fig. 10.1.** Stratified random sampling versus cluster sampling.

studies. Which households are eligible, e.g. only animal-keeping households or all households, depends on the disease, the cultural setting and the research question. When the priority is to cover as many villages as possible, e.g. for estimation of vaccination coverage, alternative procedures such as segmentation techniques and random transects (spin the bottle) are commonly applied, but especially the latter approach is more prone to bias.

After random selection of households, the next step is to sample persons living within the households. For certain research questions only people with intense animal contacts may be of interest, but for a detailed understanding of the epidemiology and transmission pathways all family members are often considered eligible (whereby for ethical and practical reasons sometimes children or young children are excluded). In the ideal case, all family members are enrolled. But if the diagnostic procedures are time consuming or costly, it may be better to sample only some household members to ensure that the number of households will not be compromised. If only a single or few household members are selected, it is important to be aware of the 'household size bias'. Since all households have the same probability to be selected and a single person per household is randomly chosen, individuals in small households have obviously a higher selection probability compared to households with many family

**Box 10.2.** Sampling examples.

*Example A*: A simple method for sampling proportional to size as described by Bennett *et al.* (1991)

- Step 1 Randomly order the clusters in your study area with their populations;
- Step 2 Calculate the cumulative population numbers (say 6700);
- Step 3 Select a random starting point: a random number between 1 and the total population size. In our example 1814;
- Step 4 Calculate the sampling interval as number of clusters to be selected (say 3) divided by the total population. In our example 6700/3 = 2233;
- Step 5 Select the clusters with the cumulative population number higher than the starting point then add the next sampling interval.

*Example B*: It is sometimes ignored that the population size of the biggest cluster must be smaller than the sampling interval. If the A cluster is larger than the sampling interval – as is the case in Example B – there is no valid sampling plan for equal individual selection probability; unless the research question and the study design allow that clusters can be selected more than once, for example child vaccination coverage. Different statistical software packages will handle this problem in different ways. The software environment R (v3.0.1) will sample sequentially, which will not result in a sampling proportional to size. SAS (proc surveyselect) will return an error if a unit is too large. Stata does not have an inbuilt command to select proportional to size. The user written command 'gsample' will also stop with an error message.

| | Example A | | | | Example B | | | |
|---|---|---|---|---|---|---|---|---|
| Community | Population | Cumulative population | Selection probability of cluster | Start + X* interval | Population | Cumulative population | Selection probability of cluster | Start + X* interval |
| 1 | 1000 | 1000 | 0.45 | | 1000 | 1000 | ? | |
| 2 | 400 | 1400 | 0.18 | | 400 | 1400 | ? | |
| 3 | 200 | 1600 | 0.09 | | 200 | 1600 | ? | |
| **4** | **300** | **1900** | 0.13 | **1814** | **300** | **1900** | ? | **1814** |
| 5 | 1200 | 3100 | 0.54 | | 1200 | 3100 | ? | |
| **6** | **1000** | **4100** | 0.45 | **4047** | 300 | 3400 | ? | |
| 7 | 1600 | 5700 | 0.72 | | ***2300*** | ***5700*** | ***1*** | ***4047*** |
| 8 | 200 | 5900 | 0.09 | | 200 | 5900 | ? | |
| 9 | 350 | 6250 | 0.16 | | 350 | 6250 | ? | |
| 10 | **450** | **6700** | 0.20 | **6280** | **450** | **6700** | ? | **6280** |

members. Since household size is associated with the age structure – and many diseases have age-dependent distribution – the bias might be substantial.

### Random selection of animals

Informed consent is sought before the sampling from all animal owners (see ethical considerations below). The investigator must be in charge of the random selection of animals. Animal owners have the tendency to catch less healthy animals hoping that the present veterinarian would provide a treatment and thus one should make sure that owners influence the selection as little as possible. If the owner has a complete list of all eligible animals, a simple random selection can be drawn. However, the most common sampling method is that livestock owners are asked to drive the animals into an enclosure or pen. The total number of the herd (e.g. 100 sheep) is divided by the sample size (e.g. 10), which gives the sampling interval (in our case 10). Every tenth sheep coming out of the pen is then sampled, whereby the first sheep is selected with a random number from 1 to the sampling interval, for example by drawing a number from a bag or a dice if the sampling interval is smaller or equal to 6.

### Herd-level prevalence

For many diseases, not only the animal-level prevalence, but also the herd-prevalence is of interest. When all animals of the herd are sampled and a perfect diagnostic test is applied, no bias derives from the calculation of the herd-level prevalence. It becomes more complicated if the estimate needs to be corrected for imperfect test sensitivity and specificity and when only a small fraction of all animals is sampled. If animals were randomly chosen from each herd, the animal-level prevalence estimate will be unbiased, but this is not true for the herd-level prevalence. Formulae are available to calculate the corresponding herd-level prevalences (Faes *et al.*, 2011).

### Statistical analysis

Since cluster sampling is a study design feature and the outcome of interest is likely to be correlated within clusters, the data analysis has to take this into account. A comprehensive introduction goes beyond the scope of this chapter. We present some key aspects, which should be considered in the analysis. Theoretically, modern statistical software is in most cases able to handle several levels of clustering, i.e. animals within herds, herds within villages, villages within administrative units. However, in practice, only one level of clustering is considered in the analysis. The main question in this context is: which is the ecological unit? If all animals within a certain village are free roaming and mixing at water points and during grazing, all animals from this village should be considered as one herd. If animals are held in fenced and dispersed pastures, the ecological unit is more likely the individual herd. An increasingly popular statistical method that accounts for the cluster level sampling is the generalized linear mixed model (GLMM). This method also handles multi-stage cluster sampling. The disadvantage of this method is that it relies on strong assumptions, which are difficult to assess and rarely checked in practice. In particular, if there are many clusters with zero prevalence, the assumptions are likely to be violated. Alternatively, generalized estimating equation models (GEE) can be used. They are relatively easy to apply, but result in too narrow confidence intervals if the number of clusters is small (e.g. less than 30). In addition it is not possible to estimate the intra-cluster correlation coefficient (see below) and the interpretation is slightly different.

The combined analysis of human and animal data is challenging, since a certain person can only be linked to a certain animal under certain conditions. A joint analysis usually requires some level of aggregation or abstraction. However, for many research questions like evaluating the impact of an intervention simultaneously on humans and animals, the joint statistical analysis is less important than the joint presentation and interpretation of the results.

### Sample size considerations

The sample size determination in cluster sampling is more sophisticated, since individuals within the same cluster may be correlated. This seems obvious for infectious diseases, but can also be due to the fact that individuals within one cluster are more similar with respect to environmental exposure, nutrition, cultural behaviour or genetic factors. This similarity is expressed by the intra-cluster correlation coefficient rho ($\rho$). Rho is calculated from the within-cluster variance and the between-cluster variance. Rho and the average cluster size ($b$) can be used to calculate the design effect, which can be interpreted as a correction factor. The sample size calculated for simple random sampling has to be multiplied by the design effect (DE) to get the final sample size (Bennett *et al.*, 1991).

$$DE = 1 + (b - 1) \times \rho$$

Rho is most often unknown at the planning stage and difficult to predict. If no information from previous comparable studies in similar settings is available, rho is usually set to 0.2. This value is chosen because it has been shown that rho seldom exceeds 0.3 and is often below 0.2. Unless the number of individuals sampled is low, increasing the number of clusters will usually have a stronger effect on the sample size than increasing the number of individuals per cluster. With the exception of very rare outcomes, it rarely makes sense to sample more than 30 to 50 individuals per cluster. Still, practical considerations should be taken into account. Where the distance between clusters is high, the number of individuals per cluster should be chosen so that the data collection can be completed in 1 or 2 full days. Finally, non-consent and, in longitudinal studies, loss to follow-up should be considered when determining the final sample size.

### Ethical considerations in One Health studies

The common goal of veterinarians and physicians is to promote the health and well-being of their patients and to provide treatment where possible. There is overlap between the two sectors regarding individual versus community ethics such as cost containment, best use of resources (priority to most cost-beneficial and cost-effective approaches), herd immunity, sanitation and high risk groups. Public health ethics has a broad scope that includes ethical and social issues arising in health promotion and disease prevention, epidemiologic research and public health practice (Coughlin, 2006). Ethical concerns in public health often relate to the dual obligations of public health professionals to acquire and apply scientific knowledge aimed at restoring and protecting the public's health while respecting individual autonomy. In veterinary medicine, the client (normally the owner of the animal) making the choice for treatment is not the patient. Nevertheless, there is a duty to communicate and disclose risks as in human medicine (Johnston, 2013). Epidemics affect not only farmers, but also the entire agricultural sector and even the national economy. Van Vlissingen (2001) published a list summarizing factors that play a role in the ethical evaluation of policies and actions on suspected cases of animal diseases. The list includes aspects of animals' interests, owners' interests, veterinarians' interests, interests of an animal population, public health interests and economic interests (Zinsstag *et al.*, Chapter 2, this volume; Wettlaufer *et al.*, Chapter 3, this volume).

Any survey raises ethical considerations, which is also true for surveys on zoonoses without sampling or testing of people. Informed consent is needed from all interviewees. Participants have the right to know the results of the testing of their animals since a positive result can present a health risk for themselves, their families and the consumers of their livestock products. A study on zoonoses requires close collaboration with governmental bodies. It cannot be, for example, that the government would slaughter animals (without compensation) that have tested positive for brucellosis in the framework of a survey. Collaboration with authorities can also better ensure that the results are used to identify interventions that are fully carried by the communities. Appropriate protective measures must be promoted and their application facilitated by the project (Schelling and Zinsstag, Chapter 30, this volume).

## Advantages of and Possible Barriers to One Health Studies

Rabinowitz *et al.* (2013) concluded that all studies qualifying as 'proof of concept' of One Health did not use the term 'One Health' in their publications. Others, in turn, may refer to One Health, but do not necessarily comply with our criteria above. The pressure to publish in high impact journals – and the highest impact journals are disciplinary – forces researchers to split their findings and publish them according to the disciplinary strengths. Interdisciplinary/intersectoral efforts can get lost in this publication context. It is currently easier than in the past to publish interdisciplinary findings. But in one interdisciplinary manuscript, the disciplinary rigour of respective disciplines can only be sketchily presented, which, in turn, often does not satisfy reviewers of a given disciplinary background. Also, interdisciplinary journals may not reach the primary target audience. For example, a veterinarian more likely consults veterinary journals and not, for example, an ecohealth journal, despite the fact that these may have articles relevant to his/her work.

Most One Health studies are driven by veterinarians. Historically, the veterinary medical profession has held a focus on protecting and improving animal and human health. Unlike their contemporary human medicine counterparts, veterinarians must have multiple species knowledge (Kahn *et al.*, 2007). Doctors are rather strictly trained to do clinical work, and less to consider interactions with the closer and broader environment. Above we have presented only a few examples of projects considering ecosystem factors, although there should be a greater incorporation of environmental and ecosystem factors into disease assessments and interventions (Rabinowitz *et al.*, 2013). An evaluation of the social-ecological systemic impacts of agricultural developments on human, animal and ecosystem health and well-being may lead to more balanced assessments of the value of changes in one sector, and possible unintended consequences that need to be guarded against (Zinsstag *et al.*, 2011).

Joint surveillance systems should ensure that the data between the sectors are harmonized from local to national levels. Surveillance systems should also be in a position to react to reported abnormal disease events. Existing systems are currently under evaluation and new approaches such as syndromic surveillance and risk-based surveillance or use of alternative sources of information are being evaluated, but likewise need to show that they can generate useful information – and that they can use synergies between sectors and thus save costs. Using existing data, which have been previously collected for another purpose, makes data integration more time-consuming. Too often, people are still sentinels for zoonotic disease outbreaks, despite the fact that zoonoses could be picked up earlier in animals. To note, surveillance and monitoring is not carried out on diseases alone. There is and should also be monitoring of stakeholders, demographic health indicators and response capacity.

Since One Health studies most often feature concurrent sampling of humans and animals, proper planning and implementation needs more attention, and may require more funding. Data acquired from different sources are associated with more causes of variation and possibly bias and confounding. Data quality is always paramount and a particular challenge in a One Health study because every chain is only as strong as its weakest link and there are more links. Potential sources of errors range from selection bias to misclassification due to poor diagnostic test performance, all compromising the validity of the findings.

We see the following advantages of a One Health study design.

**1.** Simultaneous studies of human and animal health can better assess epidemiological linkages of zoonoses, including foodborne pathogens and antibiotic resistances that would otherwise not be seen.
**2.** Joint field research by mixed teams can serve as a nucleus for intersectoral collaboration and enhanced sharing of information in a country and a region.
**3.** A One Health perspective enhances intersectoral surveillance and communication, for example for rabies, and zoonotic disease outbreaks can be detected earlier if animals are used as sentinels.
**4.** Joint monitoring of an intervention, for example on brucellosis, can indicate if corrective actions are needed in the implementation of the livestock intervention and a decrease of human brucellosis incidence over time may be the most sensitive outcome of successful livestock vaccination.
**5.** Assessment of response and service provision capacity can lead to revived discussions on human and financial needs of sectors to manage zoonotic outbreaks.

## References

Agrawal, M. (2012) *Schistosomes and Schistosomiasis in South Asia*. Springer, New Delhi.

Bardosh, K. and Thys, S. (2012) Socio-cultural research on neglected zoonoses in Africa: a literature review analysis. Poster presented at the Ecohealth conference, Kunming, 2012.

Bartlett, P.C. and Judge, L.J. (1997) The role of epidemiology in public health. *Revue Scientifique et Technique OIE* 16, 331–336.

Bennett, S., Woods, T., Liyanage, W.M. and Smith, D.L. (1991) A simplified general method for cluster-sample surveys of health in developing countries. *World Health Statistics Quarterly* 44, 98–106.

Bonfoh, B., Wasem, A., Traoré, A.N., Fané, A., Spillmann, H., Simbé, C.F., Alfaroukh, I.O., Nicolet, J., Farah, Z. and Zinsstag, J. (2003) Microbiological quality of cows' milk taken at different intervals from the udder to the selling point in Bamako (Mali). *Food Control* 14, 495–500.

Bonfoh, B., Kasymbekov, J., Durr, S., Toktobaev, N., Doherr, M.G., Schueth, T., Zinsstag, J. and Schelling, E. (2012) Representative seroprevalences of brucellosis in humans and livestock in Kyrgyzstan. *EcoHealth* 9(2), 132–138.

Burnham, G., Lafta, R., Doocy, S. and Roberts, L. (2006) Mortality after the 2003 invasion of Iraq: a cross-sectional cluster sample survey. *Lancet* 368, 1421–1428.

Canadian Integrated Program for Antimicrobial Resistance Surveillance (CIPARS) (2007) *Salmonella* Heidelberg ceftiofur-related resistance in human and retail chicken isolates. Available at: http://www.phac-aspc.gc.ca/cipars-picra/heidelberg/heidelberg-eng.php (accessed 10 October 2014).

Cleaveland, S., Fevre, E.M., Kaare, M. and Coleman, P.G. (2002) Estimating human rabies mortality in the United Republic of Tanzania from dog bite injuries. *Bulletin of the World Health Organization* 80, 304–310.

Clifford, D.L., Kazwala, R.R., Sadiki, H., Roug, A., Muse, E.A., Coppolillo, P.C. and Mazet, J.A. (2013) Tuberculosis infection in wildlife from the Ruaha ecosystem Tanzania: implications for wildlife, domestic animals, and human health. *Epidemiology & Infection* 141, 1371–1381.

Coughlin, S.S. (2006) Ethical issues in epidemiologic research and public health practice. *Emerging Themes in Epidemiology* 3, 16.

Dean, A.S., Bonfoh, B., Kulo, A.E., Boukaya, G.A., Amidou, M., Hattendorf, J., Pilo, P. and Schelling, E. (2013) Epidemiology of brucellosis and Q Fever in linked human and animal populations in northern Togo. *PLoS One* 8, e71501.

Dean, A.S., Schelling, E., Bonfoh, B., Kulo, A.E., Boukaya, G.A. and Pilo, P. (2014) Deletion in the gene BruAb2_0168 of *Brucella abortus* strains: diagnostic challenges. *Clinical Microbiology and Infection* 20, 0550–0553.

El Sherbini, A., Kabbash, I., Schelling, E., El Shennawy, S., Shalapy, N., Elnaby, G.H., Helmy, A.A. and Eisa, A. (2007) Seroprevalences and local variation of human and livestock brucellosis in two villages in Gharbia Governorate, Egypt. *Transactions of the Royal Society of Tropical Medicine and Hygiene* 101, 923–928.

Enserink, M. (2010) Infectious diseases. Questions abound in Q-fever explosion in the Netherlands. *Science* 327, 266–267.

Faes, C., Aerts, M., Litiere, S., Meroc, E., Van der Stede, Y. and Mintiens, K. (2011) Estimating herd prevalence on the basis of aggregate testing of animals. *Journal of the Royal Statistical Society Series A – Statistics in Society* 174, 155–174.

Firdessa, R., Berg, S., Hailu, E., Schelling, E., Gumi, B., Erenso, G., Gadisa, E., Kiros, T., Habtamu, M., Hussein, J., Zinsstag, J., Robertson, B.D., Ameni, G., Lohan, A.J., Loftus, B., Comas, I., Gagneux, S., Tschopp, R., Yamuah, L., Hewinson, G., Gordon, S.V., Young, D.B. and Aseffa, A. (2013) Mycobacterial lineages causing pulmonary and extrapulmonary tuberculosis, Ethiopia. *Emerging Infectious Diseases* 19, 460–463.

Forde, M., Morrison, K., Dewailly, E., Badrie, N. and Robertson, L. (2011) Strengthening integrated research and capacity development within the Caribbean region. *BMC International Health and Human Rights* 11(Suppl. 2), S7.

Grace, D., Gilbert, J., Lapar, M.L., Unger, F., Fevre, S., Nguyen-Viet, H. and Schelling, E. (2011) Zoonotic emerging infectious disease in selected countries in southeast Asia: insights from ecohealth. *EcoHealth* 8, 55–62.

Guan, Y., Chen, H., Li, K., Riley, S., Leung, G., Webster, R., Peiris, J. and Yuen, K. (2007) A model to control the epidemic of H5N1 influenza at the source. *BMC Infectious Diseases* 7, 132.

Gumi, B., Schelling, E., Berg, S., Firdessa, R., Erenso, G., Mekonnen, W., Hailu, E., Melese, E., Hussein, J., Aseffa, A. and Zinsstag, J. (2012) Zoonotic transmission of tuberculosis between pastoralists and their livestock in South-East Ethiopia. *EcoHealth* 9, 139–149.

Hill, A.B. (1965) The environment and disease: association or causation? *Proceedings of the Royal Society of Medicine* 58, 295–300.

Johnston, C. (2013) Lessons from medical ethics. In: Wathes, C.M., Corr, S.A., May, S.A., McCulloch, S.P. and Whiting, M.C. (eds) *Veterinary & Animal Ethics*. Blackwell Publishing Ltd, Oxford, UK.

Kahn, L.H., Kaplan, B. and Steele, J.H. (2007) Confronting zoonoses through closer collaboration between medicine and veterinary medicine (as 'one medicine'). *Veterinaria Italiana* 43, 5–19.

Kaindi, D.W., Schelling, E., Wangoh, J.M., Imungi, J.K., Farah, Z. and Meile, L. (2012) Risk factors for symptoms of gastrointestinal illness in rural town Isiolo, Kenya. *Zoonoses and Public Health* 59, 118–125.

Karimuribo, E.D., Sayalel, K., Beda, E., Short, N., Wambura, P., Mboera, L.G., Kusiluka, L.J. and Rweyemamu, M.M. (2012) Towards one health disease surveillance: the Southern African Centre for Infectious Disease Surveillance approach. *The Onderstepoort Journal of Veterinary Research* 79, 454.
Mariner, J.C., Pfeiffer, D.U., Costard, S., Knopf, L., Zingeser, J., Chibeu, D., Parmley, J., Musenero, M., Pisang, C., Okuthe, S., Boland, P., Jost, C.C., Hendrickx, S. and Mehta, P. (2011) *Surveillance for the Present and the Future. Challenges of Animal Health Information Systems and Surveillance for Animal Diseases and Zoonoses*. FAO, Rome.
Mazet, J.A., Clifford, D.L., Coppolillo, P.B., Deolalikar, A.B., Erickson, J.D. and Kazwala, R.R. (2009) A 'one health' approach to address emerging zoonoses: the HALI project in Tanzania. *Plos Medicine* 6, e1000190.
Messenger, A.M., Barnes, A.N. and Gray, G.C. (2014) Reverse zoonotic disease transmission (zooanthroponosis): a systematic review of seldom-documented human biological threats to animals. *PLoS One* 9, e89055.
Nutter, F.W. (1999) Understanding the interrelationships between botanical, human, and veterinary epidemiology: the Ys and Rs of it all. *Ecosystem Health* 5, 131–140.
Omran, A.R. (1971) The epidemiologic transition. A theory of the epidemiology of population change. *The Milbank Quarterly* 49, 509–538.
Parkes, M.W., Charron, D.F. and Sanchez, A. (2012) Better together: field-building networks at the frontiers of ecohealth research. In: Charron, D.F. (ed.) *Ecohealth Research in Practice: Innovative Applications of an Ecosystem Approach to Health*. Springer and International Development Research Centre, Ottawa.
Rabinowitz, P.M., Kock, R., Kachani, M., Kunkel, R., Thomas, J., Gilbert, J., Wallace, R., Blackmore, C., Wong, D., Karesh, W., Natterson, B., Dugas, R. and Rubin, C. (2013) Toward proof of concept of a one health approach to disease prediction and control. *Emerging Infectious Diseases* 19(12).
Randolph, T.F., Schelling, E., Grace, D., Nicholson, C.F., Leroy, J.L., Cole, D.C., Demment, M.W., Omore, A., Zinsstag, J. and Ruel, M. (2007) Invited review: Role of livestock in human nutrition and health for poverty reduction in developing countries. *Journal of Animal Science* 85, 2788–2800.
Schelling, E. and Kimani, T. (2007) Human and animal health response capacity and costs: a rapid appraisal of the 2007 Rift Valley fever outbreak in Kenya. International Livestock Research Institute.
Schelling, E., Diguimbaye, C., Daoud, S., Nicolet, J., Boerlin, P., Tanner, M. and Zinsstag, J. (2003) Brucellosis and Q-fever seroprevalences of nomadic pastoralists and their livestock in Chad. *Preventive Veterinary Medicine* 61, 279–293.
Schelling, E., Daoud, S., Daugla, D.M., Diallo, P., Tanner, M. and Zinsstag, J. (2005) Morbidity and nutrition patterns of three nomadic pastoralist communities of Chad. *Acta Tropica* 95, 16–25.
Schelling, E., Bechir, M., Ahmed, M.A., Wyss, K., Randolph, T.F. and Zinsstag, J. (2007) Human and animal vaccination delivery to remote nomadic families, Chad. *Emerging Infectious Diseases* 13, 373–379.
van Loenhout, J.A., Paget, W.J., Vercoulen, J.H., Wijkmans, C.J., Hautvast, J.L.A. and van der Velden, K. (2012) Assessing the long-term health impact of Q-fever in the Netherlands: a prospective cohort study started in 2007 on the largest documented Q-fever outbreak to date. *BMC Infectious Diseases* 12, 280.
van Vlissingen, M. (2001) Professional ethics in veterinary science – considering the consequences as a tool for problem solving. *Veterinary Sciences for Tomorrow* 1, 1–8.
VWB/VSF Canada (2010) One Health for One World: A Compendium of Case Studies. Available at: https://www.vetswithoutborders.ca/images/pdfs/OHOW%20Compendium%20Case%20Studies.pdf (accessed 10 October 2014).
Wendt, A., Kreienbrock, L. and Campe, A. (2014) Zoonotic Disease Surveillance – Inventory of Systems Integrating Human and Animal Disease Information. *Zoonoses and Public Health* doi: 10.1111/zph.12120.
WHO, EU, ILRI, DBL, FAO, OIE and AU (2009) Integrated Control of Neglected Zoonotic Diseases in Africa / Applying the 'One Health' Concept, Nairobi, 13–15 November 2007. Available at: http://whqlibdoc.who.int/hq/2008/WHO_HTM_NTD_NZD_2008.1_eng.pdf (accessed 10 October 2014).
Winkler, M.S., Krieger, G.R., Divall, M.J., Singer, B.H. and Utzinger, J. (2012) Health impact assessment of industrial development projects: a spatio-temporal visualization. *Geospatial Health* 6, 299–301.
Zinsstag, J. (2012) Convergence of EcoHealth and One Health. *EcoHealth* 9, 371–373.
Zinsstag, J., Schelling, E., Daoud, S., Schierle, J., Hofmann, P., Diguimbaye, C., Daugla, D.M., Ndoutamia, G., Knopf, L., Vounatsou, P. and Tanner, M. (2002) Serum retinol of Chadian nomadic pastoralist women in relation to their livestocks' milk retinol and beta-carotene content. *International Journal for Vitamin and Nutrition Research* 72, 221–228.
Zinsstag, J., Schelling, E., Roth, F., Bonfoh, B., de Savigny, D. and Tanner, M. (2007) Human benefits of animal interventions for zoonosis control. *Emerging Infectious Diseases* 13, 527–531.
Zinsstag, J., Schelling, E., Waltner-Toews, D. and Tanner, M. (2011) From 'one medicine' to 'one health' and systemic approaches to health and well-being. *Preventive Veterinary Medicine* 101, 148–156.

# 11 Animal–Human Transmission Models

**Jakob Zinsstag,* Samuel Fuhrimann, Jan Hattendorf and Nakul Chitnis**
*Swiss Tropical and Public Health Institute, Basel, Switzerland and University of Basel, Basel, Switzerland*

## Introduction

More than 60% of human infectious diseases are caused by pathogens shared with animals (Karesh *et al.*, 2012). While there is a large body of knowledge of intra-species transmission of infectious disease, we know surprisingly little about the dynamics of between-species transmission of zoonotic pathogens (Lloyd-Smith *et al.*, 2009). Yet, to understand the animal–human interface, assess the best interventions and make cross-sector economic analyses of the cost of zoonoses, it is critical to understand the animal–human transmission dynamics. Understanding animal–human transmission of disease is difficult because it requires an understanding of animal and human ecological and demographic processes as well as the pathogens that circulate between them. This is a prime One Health topic as it not only involves human and veterinary medicine but also ecology, microbiology and the social sciences. Understanding One Health as the added value of closer cooperation between human and animal health, animal–human transmission models are at the heart of assessing the animal–human interface. They are a necessary requirement for the comparative analyses of the profitability and cost-effectiveness of interventions in humans, animals and the environment. The primary purpose of this chapter is to provide examples of animal–human transmission models of zoonotic diseases in view of cross-sector economic analyses (Zinsstag *et al.*, Chapter 12, this volume).

Understanding of the ecology of the transmission of zoonoses between animals and humans is a fundamental requirement on the way towards their efficient control and elimination. Often the human medical sector concentrates on clinical issues of rabies or brucellosis patients and does not address the diseases at their roots, which would lead towards primary prevention of transmission, avoiding future human cases (Madkour, 2001; Diop *et al.*, 2007). From the perspective of disease ecology, such an approach ignores at which level the transmission of a zoonosis could successfully be interrupted. Towards this end, we mention here the well-known concept of the basic reproductive number. The basic reproductive number ($R_0$) is defined as the average number of secondary infections produced when one infected individual is introduced into a host population in which every host is susceptible. The $R_0$ describes the potential of spread of an infectious disease

*E-mail: jakob.zinsstag@unibas.ch

and its regulation in a host population. If $R_0$ is above 1 the disease keeps spreading, if $R_0$ is below 1 the disease will go extinct. In the course of an epidemic, $R_0$ is called the effective reproductive number $R_e$ reflecting the number of secondary infections produced at a given moment after the onset of the epidemic. The use of $R_0$ can be applied to the transmission between animal and human hosts.

There are of course many animal infectious diseases that are not transmissible to humans. Of those transmissible to humans, we can distinguish three main levels, according to their transmissibility in humans: (i) diseases like brucellosis and rabies which are transmitted to humans without human-to-human transmission. In this category $R_0$ >1 in animals and <1 in humans; (ii) pathogens that spill over into populations with limited human-to-human transmission (e.g. monkeypox). $R_0$ in humans is close to 1 and may lead to 'stuttering transmission'; and (iii) diseases like influenza that persist in animal reservoirs but once transmitted to humans may cause persistent and even epidemic transmission in humans with $R_0$ >1 (Lloyd-Smith *et al.*, 2009). In this chapter we focus on diseases of the first category, i.e. without human-to-human transmission, which clearly require an intervention in the animal reservoir and in food safety, in order to interrupt transmission to humans.

Zoonotic diseases can also be characterized by their route of transmission: (i) direct animal–human transmission; (ii) vector-borne transmission; and (iii) environment (water, soil, food)-borne transmission. Although some diseases exhibit multiple modes of transmission and the relative importance of each is commonly unknown, there is often still a primary mode. We should not forget the role of animals as sources of blood meals for vectors but who are not competent host reservoirs (i.e. malaria vectors feed on cattle), or transmission of disease from humans, like measles or tuberculosis to wild and captive primates. This case illustrates $R_0$ >1 in humans and <1 in animals. We discuss briefly the mathematical concepts for addressing the three types of transmission and concentrate on examples of direct animal–human zoonoses transmission to improve our understanding of their transmission dynamics, and to assess the economic aspects of zoonoses control.

Mathematical transmission models are simplified and abstracted representations of transmission processes of infectious diseases, as described in detail in many textbooks (Anderson and May, 1991; Diekmann and Heesterbeek, 2000; Keeling, 2008). Mathematical models can generally be classified as deterministic (which assume that the system always follows a fixed rule with no randomness or chance) or stochastic (where randomness is present and one state may lead to multiple different states). Deterministic models are easier to analyse, and provide general statements that improve our understanding of disease dynamics. Stochastic models are difficult to analyse but provide more information away from the mean behaviour of the system, such as the effects or occurrence of low probability events.

Furthermore, models are either population-based (where populations or subsets of populations are treated homogeneously) or individual-based (where each individual human or animal is treated separately). Population-based models can either be deterministic or stochastic but are often deterministic. Individual-based models are almost always stochastic. Population-based models can be further classified as prevalence models (suitable for microparasites where the state variables are the proportions of hosts in different disease categories such as susceptible, infected, asymptomatic or immune) or burden models (suitable for macroparasites where the state variables are usually the mean number of different stages of the parasite per host).

Most deterministic population-based models are based on the seminal work of Kermack and McKendrick (1927) that divided the human population into susceptible, infected and recovered classes, and assumed mass action dynamics for their interaction and the transmission of disease. These models have formed the basis of much of mathematical epidemiology and led to many insights in the understanding and control of infectious diseases like the above mentioned $R_0$. Newer stochastic individual-based models have further improved our understanding and are better suited to simultaneously include different kinds of heterogeneity and to capture more detailed aspects of disease transmission. However, they are computationally more intensive and require more detailed data for their validation. Such data are often not available, and we must strike a balance between model detail and the scarcity of data.

The most appropriate model is the most economical one that answers the question posed, and not the most detailed. Models will always be representations which abstract a constructed reality with a certain level of imprecision and are most useful if they have a clear purpose. For this reason it is important to state the purpose of the model prior to its development. We began writing animal–human transmission models because we wanted to answer practical questions like: 'Is it cost-beneficial to mass vaccinate cattle, sheep and goats to prevent human brucellosis?' or 'Should we mass vaccinate dogs against rabies or rely on human post exposure prophylaxis in an African city'? Based on these practical questions, the purpose of the animal–human transmission models presented in this chapter is to relate human disease frequency to the animal reservoir, providing a mechanism for the comparison of the effectiveness of interventions in humans and animals.

## Directly Transmitted Zoonoses

In their textbook on modelling of infectious diseases, Keeling and Rohani (2008) emphasize the importance of animal–human transmission models of directly transmitted zoonoses for decisions on public health-related action. They criticize the scarcity of such models and present a generic framework for animal–human zoonoses transmission. Since cross-species transmission is the main characteristic of zoonoses, an ecological understanding involving all related hosts is of particular importance for understanding the occurrence in humans (Keeling, 2008). The force of human infection depends on the prevalence in the animal reservoir, the rate of human–animal contacts and the probability of infection per contact. The frequency, duration and quality of the contact are different in zoonoses transmitted by wildlife, domestic animals or pets (Lloyd-Smith *et al.*, 2009). Methods have been developed for the simultaneous assessment of human and animal zoonosis seroprevalence, allowing for the identification of the main source of transmission (Schelling *et al.*, 2003; Bonfoh *et al.*, 2011). Time series of such data are the most suitable for estimating animal–human transmission model parameters (Kayali *et al.*, 2003a). A detailed description of such One Health study designs is presented in Schelling and Hattendorf (Chapter 10, this volume).

### Brucellosis

Brucellosis re-emerged as a preventable public health problem in the post-socialist years in Mongolia after 1990 (Zinsstag *et al.*, Chapter 14, this volume). International experts recommended that Mongolia reinstate livestock mass vaccination to prevent human brucellosis. At this stage, we were asked by the World Health Organization (WHO) to answer if brucellosis mass vaccination was cost-beneficial for the prevention of human brucellosis in Mongolia. For the purpose of a cross-sector economic analysis of brucellosis control, we established a livestock–human transmission model for brucellosis (Fig. 11.1) (Roth *et al.*, 2003). We assumed that most of the transmission of brucellosis should originate from cattle, sheep and goats. For the estimation of parameters we used official data from the Mongolian statistical office, the ministry of health and the ministry of agriculture. The model takes Mongolian health policy into account, to adapt assessments to local health policy decision pathways (Habicht *et al.*, 1999). To keep the model as simple as possible we pooled sheep and goats as one group and did not consider age and sex structure of livestock and human populations.

A more detailed approach is currently being prepared based on new field data, using age and sex structured disease data and new livestock demographic models (Shabb *et al.*, 2013). With the current model, effects of brucellosis on livestock productivity were simulated separately; age- and sex-structured models would allow estimating them directly. Data on effects of zoonoses on livestock

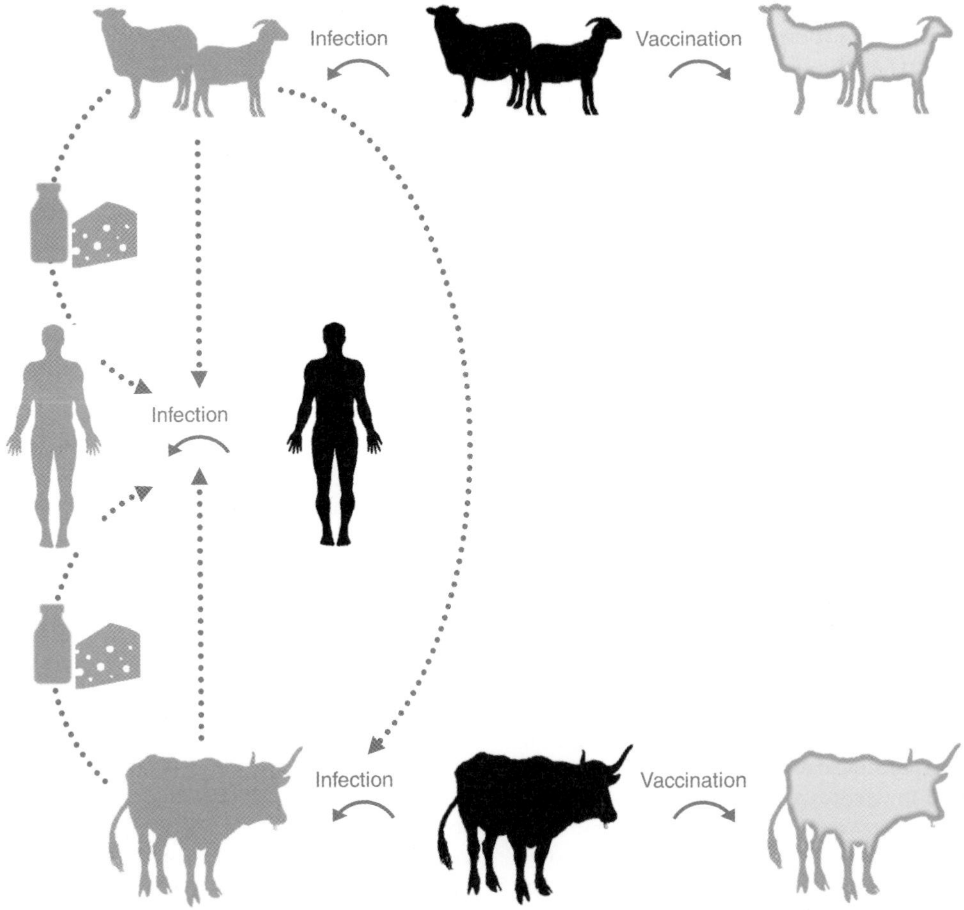


**Fig. 11.1.** Flow chart of brucellosis transmission.

production are very scarce and would be urgently required for economic assessments. For the transmission of brucellosis, only serological data was available from livestock. Hence we had to consider a proportion of infectious animals among the seropositive (Zinsstag *et al.*, 2005). The transmission to humans of cattle and small ruminant brucellosis was fitted simultaneously, and showed that the transmission from small ruminants dominated. This has recently been confirmed by bacteriological analyses in human brucellosis cases, finding dominantly *Brucella melitensis* and only a few *Brucella abortus* cases (Baljinnyam, 2014, Switzerland, personal communication). Average effective reproductive numbers $R_e$ for the year 1999 were 1.2 for sheep and 1.7 for cattle, indicating relatively low threshold vaccination coverage needed for the interruption of transmission. The livestock–human brucellosis model hence not only elucidated disease ecological aspects but served as the backbone for the cross-sector economic analysis (Zinsstag *et al.*, Chapter 12, this volume). While livestock brucellosis mass vaccination is not cost-beneficial for public health alone, it becomes highly profitable at a benefit–cost ratio of 3.1 from a societal perspective.

## Rabies

Motivated by the Chadian veterinary authorities, a project on dog rabies surveillance and control began in the year 2000. Dog rabies and human exposure data collection was initiated (Kayali *et al.*, 2003a) and complemented by dog demographic studies (Mindekem *et al.*, 2005). Small-scale dog mass-vaccination trials showed that a vaccination coverage of 70% could be achieved and that community participation was high (Kayali *et al.*, 2003b), provided the vaccination was free to the owner (Dürr *et al.*, 2008). However, neither the ministry of health nor the ministry of agriculture wanted to engage in dog mass vaccination. The ministry of health maintained a policy of exclusive provision of post-exposure prophylaxis to exposed humans, which is not always available. This motivated the question of whether, in an African city, dog rabies mass vaccination or human post-exposure prophylaxis was more costly to prevent human rabies. Based on the dog demographic data and 6 years of dog–human rabies surveillance data, a dog–human rabies transmission model was developed for the city of Ndjamena, Chad (Fig. 11.2) (Zinsstag *et al.*, 2009). The model included dog-bite localization and the respective probabilities of developing clinical rabies (Cleaveland *et al.*, 2002). The dog to dog transmission constant was 0.0807 $km^2/(dog \times week)$, whereas the dog–human transmission constant was 403 times lower with 0.0002 $km^2/(dog \times week)$. On average, every rabid dog exposed 2.3 humans, for a dog:human ratio of about 1 dog for 33 humans. Obviously no data were available for the number of exposed (incubating) dogs. Using data on the incubation period in dogs, this compartment could be estimated. Once the model parameters were fitted, mass vaccination and dog culling interventions were simulated; the most favourable scenario was dog mass vaccination coverage reaching at least 70%. The effective reproductive number $R_e$ was 1.01, indicating a high potential for fast elimination. Most importantly, the transmission data for humans and animals served as a basis for a cross-sector economic analysis, which is detailed in Chapter 12, this volume. Under the data conditions used, dog-rabies mass vaccination becomes more profitable after 6 years when compared to human post-exposure prophylaxis only. In parallel, we developed a stochastic model of rabies transmission which better represented the spiky nature of the rabies incidence pattern. However, the stochastic process led regularly to disease extinction without any intervention. We can argue that, despite the shortfalls of a deterministic model of dog rabies, its use for the simulation of interventions is more conservative, as the process is not interrupted by stochastic effects.

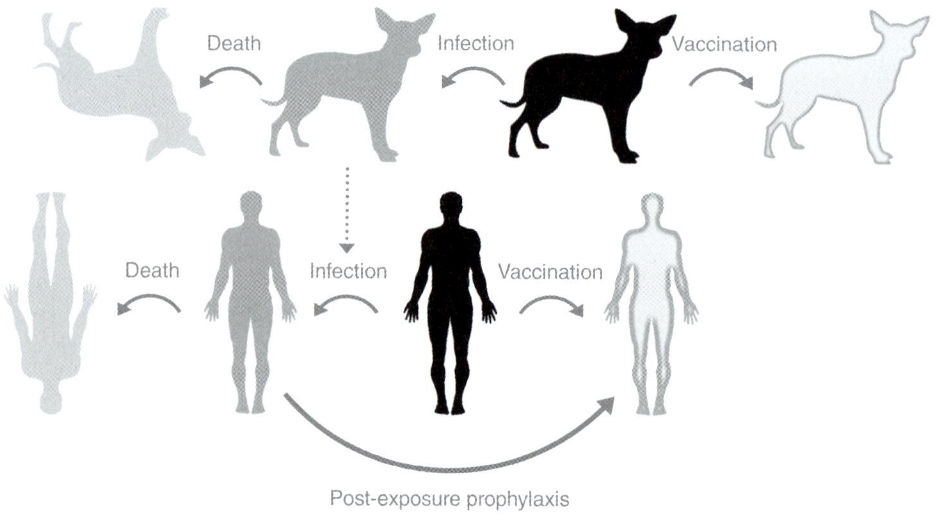


**Fig. 11.2.** Flow chart of dog–human rabies transmission.

## Vector-borne Transmission

Mathematical modelling of vector-borne diseases began with Ronald Ross' work in developing and analysing a model to determine a threshold condition for the density of mosquitoes required to transmit malaria (Ross, 1908, 1911; Macdonald, 1956; Smith *et al.*, 2012); George Macdonald fitted this to entomological and epidemiological data. David Rogers extended this Ross-Macdonald model to include both human and animal (cattle) hosts for analysing the dynamics of African trypanosomiases (Rogers, 1988; Welburn and Coleman, Chapter 18, this volume). Since then, models of vector-borne zoonoses have focused on either African trypanosomiases or arboviruses such as West Nile virus and Rift Valley fever virus (RVF), with some more recent models of *Plasmodium knowlesi* malaria in South-east Asia.

Most of these models have been deterministic compartmental models primarily used to investigate the relative effectiveness of control strategies in reducing transmission. However, they have also been analysed to answer such questions as: 'Are animals responsible for the sustained transmission of human African trypanosomiasis?'; 'What is the role of vertical transmission in mosquitoes in the persistence of RVF virus?'; and 'How does West Nile virus persist through the winter in North America?' Some detailed individual-based models have also been developed for RVF and human African trypanosomiasis (Muller *et al.*, 2004). As a further example, we describe a conceptual framework for an RFV model of mosquito–livestock–human transmission (Box 11.1).

## Rift Valley Fever

RVF is a viral zoonosis of increasing global importance (Clements *et al.*, 2007). This acute mosquito-borne disease is caused by a phlebovirus in the family Bunyaviridae (Xu *et al.*, 2007) and mainly affects livestock, but does affect humans and wildlife as well (Evans *et al.*, 2008). Primary transmission of Rift Valley fever virus (RVFV) to animals results from bites of infected mosquitoes, while most humans become infected by direct exposure to the blood, body fluids, or tissue of infected animals (Nguku *et al.*, 2010). RVF infection leads to high mortality and abortion in livestock, and significant morbidity and mortality in humans (Anyangu *et al.*, 2010). To trigger an RVF epidemic, it is assumed that three main factors need to appear together: (i) infected vectors; (ii) flooding of mosquito breeding sites; and (iii) susceptible host populations (Bird *et al.*, 2009). In the past years much research focused on vector and climate conditions. Results showed an association between the weather phenomenon El Niño, resulting in prolonged rains together with extended flooding in East Africa, and the subsequent occurrence of large RVF-infected mosquito populations (Anyamba *et al.*, 2010). Although many outbreaks from the past could be linked with such events, remote sensing appears to be insufficient to predict RVF outbreaks accurately and strategies to control the disease in livestock and humans are poorly understood and not yet sufficient to significantly reduce the impact of an epidemic (Geering *et al.*, 2002; Schelling and Kimani, 2007).

We conceptualized an individual base model (IBM) for pastoral livestock populations to assess the impact of interventions and determine which are the most cost-effective for RVF in East Africa, namely Kenya. In a simplified way, the model reflects the demographic dynamics of the most economically important animals (cattle, sheep, goats and camels) in normal and drought periods, with and without epidemics of RVF, as well as simulating livestock parameters with and without RFV control measures. The IBM gave the possibility to track each animal with its individual state (species, sex, age) over days and years, and observe what happens to animals during an RVF epidemic situation if a so-called SEIR-states approach (susceptible, exposed, infectious and recovered) is applied. RVF induced mortality and abortion on an individual livestock level. From the model, we can also determine how many infected animals are being sold or slaughtered and therefore pose risks for human infection. With such detailed information, we have the additional option to simulate the implementation of RVF control strategies and see the influence on livestock infection resulting in

**Box 11.1.** Flow chart of the individual-based RVF transmission model.

The simulation assigns each host to the state variables species, gender and age, to simulate the livestock herd structure. The model simulates dynamic processes on an individual level. Hosts can be removed from the model, given the turnover probabilities of mortality, selling and slaughtering. When a female host reaches the adult age, it is assigned to the state variable fertile and, further, will have a probability of becoming pregnant and going through a gestation period. If the pregnancy is not ended by abortion, it will give birth to an offspring. After such birth or abortion, the female enters a waiting stage in which it cannot get pregnant for a certain period. Rift Valley fever is simulated with the concept of an S-E-I-R model, therefore a host can be assigned to any one of the state variables: susceptible, exposed, infectious or recovered from RVF. During a specified time period, a susceptible host can become infected with RVF with a constant infection probability. After being infected it enters the incubation period (exposed state) before becoming infectious – also to people – and for the time of acute infection. During the latter stage, the host has an increased probability to die or to abort. Survivors recover with a lifelong immunity to the disease (Fuhrimann, 2011). The transmission to humans is considered proportional to infectiousness in animals.

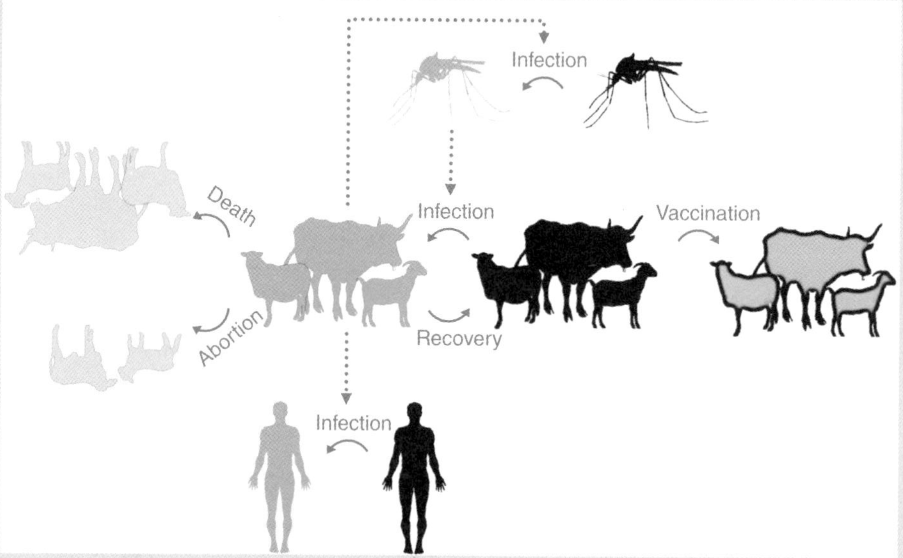


**Fig. 11.3.** Flow chart of the individual-based RVF transmission model.

human risk and livestock mortality. Furthermore, the model allows us to follow the immunization levels of animals after an RVF infection or a vaccination, to identify the time period when the animal host population is not at risk for a subsequent RVF epidemic (Box 11.1) (Fuhrimann, 2011).

The IBM approach improved our understanding of pastoralists' livestock management during normal and drought periods. Based on the outcomes of the different model scenarios, recommendations on control options can be formulated from the societal perspective for more appropriate allocation of limited resources and to facilitate inter-sector RVF planning by governmental and non-governmental agencies. Our model allows obtaining the proportion of affected animals, grouped by species, age classes and sex. Therefore, the baseline and RVF-attributable mortalities can be compared, to emphasize the huge impact of RVF. We have determined that infected sheep and goats are most likely to spread the disease through livestock trade. Also, we discovered that slaughtered infected sheep are an important risk factor to human RVF infection. Our results assist the development of future studies to assess the effect of control measures against RVF before an outbreak occurs. The ratio of susceptible:immune hosts can also support the existing prediction system by further consideration of the susceptibility of a host population. The model can be extended to include transmission to humans, which provides the interface to public health. Such a model would allow assessing the effects of interventions in animals on human health, similar to the brucellosis and rabies models above. To validate such an extended livestock–human RVF model, a time series of RVF incidence in livestock and humans will be needed. A validated model could then provide insight into future joint livestock and public health contingency plans (Fuhrimann, 2011). Due to lack of available data, the model does not explicitly model cross-species transmission to humans, which would be a valuable extension. This example sheds light on various ways that models can be parameterized. As applied here, a 'bottom-up' approach estimates parameter values (ideally with distributions) from the literature. Alternatively, models can be fitted to observations (of prevalence or incidence) as in the above examples on brucellosis and rabies. The latter is much less common but potentially more robust, and provides greater confidence in predicting outside the observed situations.

## Environmental and Foodborne Transmission

Animal-borne infectious diseases can be transmitted to humans by the environment. Cattle may die from anthrax and be consumed by humans. Rodents excrete *Leptospira* spp. in their urine and contaminate stagnant water from which humans become infected. Food contaminated with *Salmonella*, *Campylobacter* or *Escherichia coli* originating from animals is the source of a huge burden of foodborne illnesses. The mathematical treatment of infection of humans is straightforward, but the simulation of contamination is not. Figure 11.4 shows a simplified schematic of how animals may contaminate the environment (soil, water) and food, which are then a source of infection for humans. The transmission is proportional to the incidence ($i$) and the number of susceptible ($S$) at risk. At time 0, the number susceptible $S(0)=S_0$. Under the special condition of a constant incidence $i$,

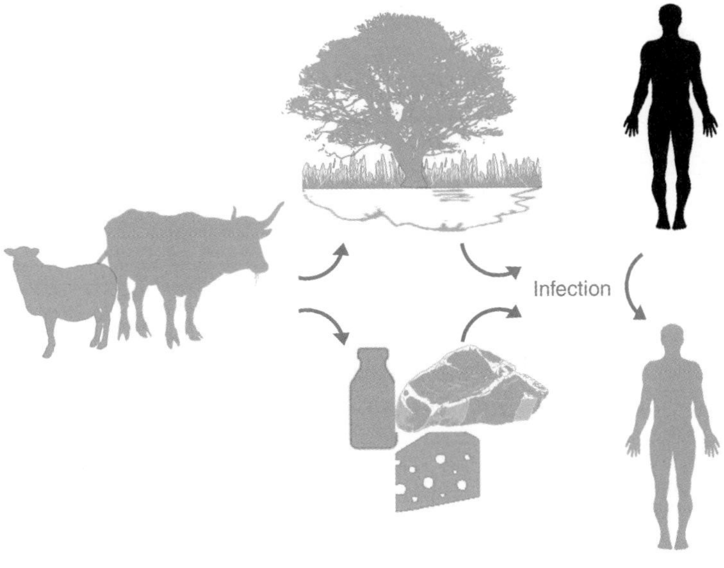


**Fig. 11.4.** Simplified schematic of environmental and foodborne transmission of zoonoses.

we obtain a simple exponential form which has an analytical solution.

$$\frac{dS}{dt} = -iS \Rightarrow S = S_0 e^{-it} \qquad (11.1)$$

The average time to infection in this simple exponential decay model is $1/i$ (Scott and Smith, 1994).

This type of transmission model does not include the animal component explicitly.

More detailed ecological studies are needed to estimate the contamination of the environment and food. Moreover, pathogens may decay in the environment or grow in food. As an example we can consider the contamination of milk with enterobacteria. Figure 11.5 presents the contamination level of milk in the peri-urban dairy production system of Bamako (Bonfoh *et al.*, 2006), where the bacterial contamination of the milk is measured at different control points in the food chain. This type of statistical modelling of contamination is called quantitative microbial risk assessment (QMRA), which has recently been combined with material flow analysis (MFA) for waste water-related disease risks (Nguyen-Viet *et al.*, 2008; Nguyen-Viet *et al.*, Chapter 9, this volume).

Adding the human interface to animal-source foodborne illnesses requires a detailed understanding of food processing and consumption patterns and frequencies. In the case example of milk consumption in Mali, we have attempted to add this aspect through a case-control study but have not established a direct interface with the food source (Hetzel *et al.*, 2004). More sophisticated models have been developed for *Campylobacter* transmission, where detailed data are available. For example, Nauta and colleagues (Nauta *et al.*, 2007) modelled the dynamics of the pathogen population from 'farm to fork'. The *Campylobacter* model incorporates all steps through the chicken meat production chain to the food storage and processing at home, including potential cross-contamination of salad. Integrated risk assessment for food safety is further detailed by Racloz *et al.* (Chapter 8, this volume).

More challenging are transmission models where the main route of infection is via the environment. Pathogen survival in the environment is determined by numerous factors simultaneously. A good example to demonstrate the complex interactions is *Leptospirosis*. Virtually all mammalian species can carry leptospires and may act as a source of infection to humans or other animals. However, livestock and rodents are of primary public

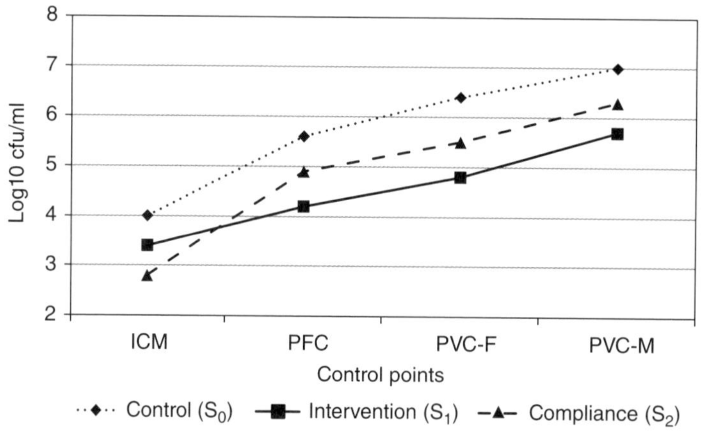


**Fig. 11.5.** Level of contamination of cow milk at different control points: from the individual cow's milk (ICM), to the pooled milk from the farmer's container (PFC), to the vendor's container at the farm gate (PVC-F) and to the vendor's container at the market (PVC-M). Control ($S_0$) was prior to an intervention, intervention ($S_1$) was after introducing better containers (wide opening for better cleaning) and hygienic milking procedures, and compliance ($S_2$) is the measurement some weeks after the introduction of the intervention (adapted from Bonfoh *et al.*, 2006).

health interest. There are about 250 pathogenic serovars, which have varying degrees of host specificity and differ in terms of pathogenicity and virulence. Leptospirosis in humans presents with a wide variety of clinical manifestations and mostly non-specific symptoms which resemble those of other febrile diseases. Hence it is frequently misdiagnosed as dengue fever, RVF, brucellosis or influenza, and under-reporting appears to be common in many countries. Transmission to humans can either be by direct contact with the urine of infected animals or by contact with a urine-contaminated environment. The disease exhibits a strong seasonal pattern, which is linked to rainfall, animal, agricultural or occupational cycles. However, the relationship between climatic, soil and anthropogenic variables is complex and poorly understood. Outbreaks of leptospirosis are common, and in countries with a high burden it is particularly difficult to differentiate between the seasonal endemic situation and local outbreaks, if only aggregated data are available. Outbreaks are often reported after heavy rainfall, floods and other natural disasters. The reasons range from more frequent human water contacts to less predatory pressure on rodent populations. Finally, there are two distinct epidemiological patterns of leptospirosis. In rural areas, the disease is strongly linked to agricultural activities; in urban slums sanitation infrastructure and sewage facilities are important determinants. How this system can be simplified depends on the setting but even more on the question that should be addressed. It is relatively easy to captures the dynamics of the seasonal variation with time series analysis (ARIMAX) models. However, those are not able to simulate the impact of potential intervention and are limited in the ability to forecast the future. Several deterministic models have been developed, but due to lack of detailed knowledge and data, a thorough model validation was not possible. Since an important objective is the prediction of future outbreaks, spatio-temporal Markov models, as recently developed for meningitis in Africa, might be a promising approach (Agier *et al.*, 2013).

## Conclusion

Animal–human transmission models require an ecological perspective, an understanding of the biology of the animal–human interface and specific methods to collect relevant spatio-temporal data. They further require an in-depth understanding of animal and human demographic processes and their interaction. Clearly, contact network heterogeneity and stochastic random processes cannot be captured by simple deterministic models. However, we must always point out the purpose of models, aiming for example at a deep understanding of the transmission dynamics or at the economics of interventions. Here we presented two examples of directly transmitted zoonoses, which provided the basis for cross-sector economic assessments of interventions in animals and humans. They provide new insight into the animal–human interface by estimating animal–human transmission constants that could not be estimated otherwise. Future research should: (i) address the heterogeneity and network nature of the animal–human interface, moving towards a more realistic representation of zoonoses transmission; (ii) include the ecological boundaries, such as competition over resources, which further determine animal demographic processes and indirectly the transmission of zoonoses; and (iii) complement animal–human models with a cross-sector economic framework to identify the most cost-effective interventions (Narrod *et al.*, 2012; Zinsstag *et al.*, Chapter 12, this volume).

## References

Agier, L., Stanton, M., Soga, G. and Diggle, P.J. (2013) A multi-state spatio-temporal Markov model for categorized incidence of meningitis in sub-Saharan Africa. *Epidemiology and Infection* 141(8), 1764–1771.

Anderson, R. and May, R. (1991) *Infectious Diseases of Humans*. Oxford University Press, Oxford, UK.

Anyamba, A., Linthicum, K.J., Small, J., Britch, S.C., Pak, E., de La Rocque, S., Formenty, P., Hightower, A.W., Breiman, R.F., Chretien, J.P., Tucker, C.J., Schnabel, D., Sang, R., Haagsma, K., Latham, M., Lewandowski, H.B., Magdi, S.O., Mohamed, M.A., Nguku, P.M., Reynes, J.M. and Swanepoel, R. (2010) Prediction, assessment of the Rift Valley fever activity in East and Southern Africa 2006–2008 and possible vector control strategies. *Am J Trop Med Hyg* 83(Suppl. 2), 43–51.

Anyangu, A.S., Gould, L.H., Sharif, S.K., Nguku, P.M., Omolo, J.O., Mutonga, D., Rao, C.Y., Lederman, E.R., Schnabel, D., Paweska, J.T., Katz, M., Hightower, A., Njenga, M.K., Feikin, D.R. and Breiman, R.F. (2010) Risk factors for severe Rift Valley fever infection in Kenya, 2007. *Am J Trop Med Hyg* 83(Suppl. 2), 14–21.

Bird, B.H., Ksiazek, T.G., Nichol, S.T. and Maclachlan, N.J. (2009) Rift Valley fever virus. *J Am Vet Med Assoc* 234(7), 883–893.

Bonfoh, B., Roth, C., Traore, A.N., Fane, A., Simbe, C.F., Alfaroukh, I.O., Nicolet, J., Farah, Z. and Zinsstag, J. (2006) Effect of washing and disinfecting containers on the microbiological quality of fresh milk sold in Bamako (Mali). *Food Control* 17(2), 153–161.

Bonfoh, B., Kasymbekov, J., Durr, S., Toktobaev, N., Doherr, M.G., Schueth, T., Zinsstag, J. and Schelling, E. (2011) Representative seroprevalences of Brucellosis in humans and livestock in Kyrgyzstan. *EcoHealth* 9(2), 132–138.

Cleaveland, S., Fevre, E.M., Kaare, M. and Coleman, P.G. (2002) Estimating human rabies mortality in the United Republic of Tanzania from dog bite injuries. *Bulletin of the World Health Organization* 80(4), 304–310.

Clements, A.C., Pfeiffer, D.U., Martin, V. and Otte, M.J. (2007) A Rift Valley fever atlas for Africa. *Prev Vet Med* 82(1–2), 72–82.

Diekmann, O. and Heesterbeek, J.A.P. (2000) *Mathematical Epidemiology of Infectious Diseases: model building, analysis and interpretation*. Wiley, New York.

Diop, S.A., Manga, N.M., Dia, N.M., Ndour, C.T., Seydi, M., Soumare, M., Diop, B.M. and Sow, P.S. (2007) [The point on human rabies in Senegal from 1986 to 2005]. *Médecine et maladies infectieuses* 37(12), 787–791.

Dürr, S., Meltzer, M., Mindekem, R. and Zinsstag, J. (2008) Owner valuation of rabies vaccination in dogs, Chad. *Emerging Infectious Diseases* 14(10), 1650–1652.

Evans, A., Gakuya, F., Paweska, J.T., Rostal, M., Akoolo, L., Van Vuren, P.J., Manyibe, T., Macharia, J.M., Ksiazek, T.G., Feikin, D.R., Breiman, R.F. and Kariuki Njenga, M. (2008) Prevalence of antibodies against Rift Valley fever virus in Kenyan wildlife. *Epidemiol Infect* 136(9), 1261–1269.

Fuhrimann, S. (2011) Rift Valley Fever in Kenyan pastoral livestock. MSc thesis, University of Basel.

Geering, W.A., Davies, F.G. and Martín, V. (2002) *Preparation of Rift Valley fever contingency plans*. Food and Agriculture Organization of the United Nations, Rome, p. 80.

Habicht, J.P., Victora, C.G. and Vaughan, J.P. (1999) Evaluation designs for adequacy, plausibility and probability of public health programme performance and impact. *International Journal of Epidemiology* 28(1), 10–18.

Hetzel, M., Bonfoh, B., Farah, Z., Traore, M., Simbe, C.F., Alfaroukh, I.O., Schelling, E., Tanner, M. and Zinsstag, J. (2004) Diarrhoea, vomiting and the role of milk consumption: perceived and identified risk in Bamako (Mali). *Tropical Medicine & International Health* 9(10), 1132–1138.

Karesh, W.B., Dobson, A., Lloyd-Smith, J.O., Lubroth, J., Dixon, M.A., Bennett, M., Aldrich, S., Harrington, T., Formenty, P., Loh, E.H., Machalaba, C.C., Thomas, M.J. and Heymann, D.L. (2012) Ecology of zoonoses: natural and unnatural histories. *Lancet* 380(9857), 1936–1945.

Kayali, U., Mindekem, R., Yemadji, N., Oussiguere, A., Naissengar, S., Ndoutamia, A.G. and Zinsstag, J. (2003a) Incidence of canine rabies in N'Djamena, Chad. *Preventive Veterinary Medicine* 61(3), 227–233.

Kayali, U., Mindekem, R., Yemadji, N., Vounatsou, P., Kaninga, Y., Ndoutamia, A.G. and Zinsstag, J. (2003b) Coverage of pilot parenteral vaccination campaign against canine rabies in N'Djamena, Chad. *Bulletin of the World Health Organization* 81(10), 739–744.

Keeling, M.J. and Rohani, P. (2008) *Modeling Infectious Disease*. Princeton University Press, Princeton, New Jersey.

Kermack, W.K. and McKendrick, A.G. (1927) A contribution to the mathematical theory of epidemics. *Proceedings of the Royal Society Series A* 115, 700–721.

Lloyd-Smith, J.O., George, D., Pepin, K.M., Pitzer, V.E., Pulliam, J.R., Dobson, A.P., Hudson, P.J. and Grenfell, B.T. (2009) Epidemic dynamics at the human-animal interface. *Science* 326(5958), 1362–1367.

Macdonald, G. (1956) Epidemiological basis of malaria control. *Bulletin of the World Health Organization* 15(3–5), 613–626.

Madkour, A.A. (2001) *Madkour's Brucellosis*. Heidelberg, Berlin.

Mindekem, R., Kayali, U., Yemadji, N., Ndoutamia, A.G. and Zinsstag, J. (2005) [Impact of canine demography on rabies transmission in N'djamena, Chad]. *Médecine tropicale: revue du Corps de santé colonial* 65(1), 53–58.

Muller, G., Grebaut, P. and Gouteux, J.P. (2004) An agent-based model of sleeping sickness: simulation trials of a forest focus in southern Cameroon. *Comptes Rendus Biologies* 327(1), 1–11.

Narrod, C., Zinsstag, J. and Tiongco, M. (2012) A One Health framework for estimating the economic costs of zoonotic diseases on society. *EcoHealth* 9(2) 150–162.

Nauta, M.J., Jacobs-Reitsma, W.F. and Havelaar, A.H. (2007) A risk assessment model for *Campylobacter* in broiler meat. *Risk Analysis* 27(4), 845–861.

Nguku, P.M., Sharif, S.K., Mutonga, D., Amwayi, S., Omolo, J., Mohammed, O., Farnon, E.C., Gould, L.H., Lederman, E., Rao, C., Sang, R., Schnabel, D., Feikin, D.R., Hightower, A., Njenga, M.K. and Breiman, R.F. (2010) An investigation of a major outbreak of Rift Valley fever in Kenya: 2006-2007. *Am J Trop Med Hyg, 83*(Suppl. 2), 5–13.

Nguyen-Viet, H., Zinsstag, J., Schertenleib, R., Zurbrügg, C., Obrist, B., Montangero, A., Surkinkul, N., Doulaye, K., Morel, A., Cisse, G., Koottatep, T., Wangsuphachart, V., Bonfoh, B. and Tanner, M. (2008) Improving environmental sanitation, health and well-being – a conceptual framework for integral interventions. *EcoHealth* 6(2), 180–191.

Rogers, D.J. (1988) A general model for the African trypanosomiases. *Parasitology* 97(1), 193–212.

Ross, R. (1908) *Report on the Prevention of Malaria in Mauritius*. Waterlow and Sons Ltd, London.

Ross, R. (1911) *The Prevention of Malaria*, 2nd edn. John Murray, London.

Roth, F., Zinsstag, J., Orkhon, D., Chimed-Ochir, G., Hutton, G., Cosivi, O., Carrin, G. and Otte, J. (2003) Human health benefits from livestock vaccination for brucellosis: case study. *Bulletin of the World Health Organization* 81(12), 867–876.

Schelling, E. and Kimani, T. (2007) *Human and animal health response capacity and costs: a rapid appraisal of the 2007 Rift Valley fever outbreak in Kenya*. International Livestock Research Institute, Kenya and Swiss Tropical and Public Health Institute.

Schelling, E., Diguimbaye, C., Daoud, S., Nicolet, J., Boerlin, P., Tanner, M. and Zinsstag, J. (2003) Brucellosis and Q-fever seroprevalences of nomadic pastoralists and their livestock in Chad. *Preventive Veterinary Medicine* 61(4), 279–293.

Scott, M.E. and Smith, G. (1994) *Parasitic and Infectious Diseases: epidemiology and ecology*, Academic Press, New York.

Shabb, D., Chitnis, N., Baljinnyam, Z., Saagii, S. and Zinsstag, J. (2013) A mathematical model of the dynamics of Mongolian livestock populations. *Livestock Science* 157, 280–288.

Smith, D.L., Battle, K.E., Hay, S.I., Barker, C.M., Scott, T.W. and McKenzie, F.E. (2012) Ross, Macdonald, and a theory for the dynamics and control of mosquito-transmitted pathogens. *PLoS Pathogens* 8(4), e1002588.

Xu, F., Liu, D., Nunes, M.R., da Rosa, A.P., Tesh, R.B. and Xiao, S.Y. (2007) Antigenic and genetic relationships among Rift Valley fever virus and other selected members of the genus *Phlebovirus* (Bunyaviridae). *Am J Trop Med Hyg* 76(6), 1194–200.

Zinsstag, J., Roth, F., Orkhon, D., Chimed-Ochir, G., Nansalmaa, M., Kolar, J. and Vounatsou, P. (2005) A model of animal-human brucellosis transmission in Mongolia. *Preventive Veterinary Medicine* 69(1–2), 77–95.

Zinsstag, J., Durr, S., Penny, M.A., Mindekem, R., Roth, F., Menendez Gonzalez, S., Naissengar, S. and Hattendorf, J. (2009) Transmission dynamics and economics of rabies control in dogs and humans in an African city. *Proceedings of the National Academy of Sciences* 106(35), 14996–15001.

# 12 One Health Economics

**Jakob Zinsstag,[1]* Adnan Choudhury,[2] Felix Roth[1] and Alexandra Shaw[3]**
[1]*Swiss Tropical and Public Health Institute, Basel and University of Basel, Switzerland;* [2]*University of Queensland, Brisbane, Australia;* [3]*The University of Edinburgh, UK*

## Introduction

One Health can be best explained by an economic metaphor as being the 'added value' of closer cooperation between human and animal health. Therefore understanding the nature of the cost-benefit and cost-effectiveness of greater integration of human and animal health interventions is central to effective advocacy for this approach. In this chapter, we present examples of how both costs and benefits of diseases and disease control can cross from animals to humans, and vice versa. These examples span from health services for mobile pastoralists in Chad and brucellosis control in Mongolia, to rabies control in an African city and the cost of bovine tuberculosis in Ethiopia. Each illustrates a particular aspect of One Health economics. Based on these four examples, we will infer some general principles of One Health economics. Finally, we will discuss the economics of the human–animal interface and provide an outlook on One Health financing options.

## Joint Human and Animal Vaccination Services for Mobile Pastoralists in Chad

Mobile pastoralists in Chad live closely together with the animals that form the basis of their livelihood. They live a mobile lifestyle in perpetual search of fodder and water for their livestock. As a result, they are almost completely excluded from currently available health services. Aiming towards a better understanding of the health status of pastoralists and their animals, we chose an integrated approach with a mixed team of veterinarians and public health personnel (Montavon *et al.*, 2013; Schelling and Hattendorf, Chapter 10, this volume). During these initial studies, pastoralists were also interviewed about their perceptions of human and animal vaccinations. To our surprise, the pastoralists reported a relatively high proportion of vaccinated cattle, whereas the vaccination coverage of children and women seemed very low. During the study, we did not find a single child who had been fully vaccinated by the standards of the Expanded Programme on Immunization (EPI). Based on these observations, joint health services were developed together with the Chadian public health and veterinary authorities (Schelling *et al.*, Chapter 20, this volume). When veterinarians, who were mobile, planned a vaccination campaign for cattle, they took along public health personnel who would then vaccinate children and women. Joint vaccination campaigns were operated strictly separately by veterinary and medical personnel,

*E-mail: jakob.zinsstag@unibas.ch

but both transport and the cold chain for vaccines were shared. The cost of running animal and public health services separately was compared to the cost of operating them jointly; the respective costs are presented in Table 12.1. The cost savings from joint human and animal health vaccine delivery was 15% in Gredaya when compared to providing separate human and veterinary services. This saving may seem modest but it is important to note that this approach was also the first time that childhood vaccination had ever been provided to these communities, who otherwise had no access to such services.

Combined human–animal vaccination campaigns may be not only cheaper, but they may also notably increase the percentage of humans, and perhaps even animals, vaccinated. The challenge, however, is to measure the number of vaccinated children among a nomadic population. This is particularly difficult, as pastoralists are mobile and cannot be found repeatedly in the same homestead at the same location. Initial attempts to measure vaccination coverage used a mark–release–recapture approach with electronic fingerprints for approximating the proportion of vaccinated individuals and the human demographic composition (Weibel, 2009; Weibel *et al.* 2011). Initially, vaccinated children and women were considered 'marked' after providing their fingerprints for an electronic database and receiving a vaccine card. The intervention areas were then revisited using random directions to find vaccinated women and children among unvaccinated ones, in order to estimate the level of vaccination coverage (Jean-Richard and Crump, Chapter 13, this volume). Recapture proportions, however, were too low to obtain reliable information.

In the first decade of the 21st century, the revolution of mobile communication radically changed the conditions of accessing mobile populations. Most pastoralist households today have a cellphone, and the network of communication is growing every day. Hence, we started testing the use of regular cellphone-based communication for health and demographic surveillance in mobile pastoralist communities. This was shown to be feasible for the recording of human and livestock population data

**Table 12.1.** Comparative cost summary of veterinary and public health services (adapted from Schelling *et al.*, 2007). Variable and fixed costs of vaccinations in the veterinary and public health sectors in Gredaya and AmDobak/Chaddra, Chad.[a]

| | Veterinary sector | | Public health sector | | | |
|---|---|---|---|---|---|---|
| | Gredaya | Chaddra/ AmDobak | Gredaya | | Chaddra/ AmDobak | |
| Cost | Euros (% fixed) | Euros (% fixed) | Euros (% fixed) | % Euros shared | Euros (% fixed) | % Euros shared |
| Personnel/ administration | 2,559 (0) | 475 (0) | 3,627 (0) | 10.6 | 3,376 (0) | 2.7 |
| Transportation | 2,835 (80) | 345 (75) | 4,004 (82) | 19.3 | 3,797 (79) | 3.3 |
| Cold chain | 62 (36) | 45 (56) | 1,185 (37) | 6.2 | 531 (36) | 10.1 |
| Vaccines and vaccine-related | 7,541 (29) | 214 (21) | 12,146 (12) | 0 | 4,072 (12) | 0 |
| Other (buildings, supplies) | 480 (95) | 152 (100) | 938 (98) | 25.4 | 938 (98) | 9.1 |
| Total costs | 13,476 | 1,231 | 21,900 | 6.7 | 12,712 | 2.8 |
| Total costs excl. vaccines | 5,935 | 1,025 | 9,754 | 15.1 | 8,641 | 4.1 |

[a]In Gredaya, three vaccination rounds were conducted jointly between veterinarians and public health professionals and another three rounds were conducted by the public health sector alone to fully immunize children, whereas in Chaddra/ AmDobak, only one of six rounds was conducted jointly with the veterinarians.
The cost-sharing scheme and the proportion of reduced costs due to the joint approach are described in the text.

(Jean-Richard *et al.*, 2014). In the future, vaccination coverage and population data could be collected this way, enabling more reliable estimations of the cost-effectiveness of joint human and animal interventions. Plans are already under way for a full scale mobile health and demographic surveillance system for mobile pastoralists (Jean-Richard and Crump, Chapter 13, this volume).

## Cross-Sector Analysis of Brucellosis Control in Mongolia

Brucellosis is a zoonotic disease that causes late-stage abortion in animals. It is one of the most important zoonoses worldwide, occurring mostly in areas with extensive production of small ruminants and cattle. Humans become infected by direct exposure while working as farmers, veterinarians or butchers, or through the consumption of unpasteurized milk and milk products. Human brucellosis is a severe chronic disease, characterized by recurrent fever and pain that can put people out of work for long periods (Dean *et al.*, 2012a,b). Brucellosis re-emerged as a major preventable disease in Mongolia after 1990, when the political and economic system changed from a socialist to a liberal market rule. Health and veterinary service provision collapsed, leading to a rapid increase in human cases. International experts recommended to the World Health Organization (WHO) that Mongolia should reinstate livestock mass vaccination to prevent brucellosis in humans. We were subsequently approached with the question: 'Is it cost-effective to mass vaccinate 25 million cattle, sheep and goats, in order to prevent human brucellosis?' We sought to answer the question: 'What is the effect of mass vaccination of livestock on human health?' For this purpose we developed the first livestock–human brucellosis transmission model, as a backbone for the economic assessment (Zinsstag *et al.*, Chapter 11, this volume). Costs and benefits are incurred in the private and public sectors for both human health and livestock production. Therefore, we needed an analysis that included human health and livestock production from a societal perspective.

Identifying all the sectors involved is an important aspect of a One Health economic assessment. This is most easily done by considering a flow chart of disease transmission between all involved species. It is important to start from the biological and ecological roots of disease transmission to identify the relevant sectors involved. In the case of brucellosis, this meant we considered sheep, goats, cattle and humans, but ignored yaks and camels. Once the transmission dynamics of the disease are understood, we can simulate the effect of interventions in humans and animals (Zinsstag *et al.*, Chapter 11, this volume) and the related costs. The first step is to develop cost menus for the public and private domains in human health and livestock production. For example, the cost of hospitalization has both public and private costs. Patients spend considerable sums of money privately on doctors' fees, transportation, laboratory and drug cost, in addition to lost income. If they must also employ other people to do their job, these are extra coping costs.

Data for the economic analysis were collected from government statistics and health information systems. Patient interviews revealed very important information on private costs. They showed the importance of private out-of-pocket expenses for transportation, drugs and informal treatments, i.e. by traditional healers. For information where data were missing, especially for livestock production, we used Delphi panels. Delphi panels are groups of experts who are interviewed for their opinion regarding information that is not readily available. For example, ten experts were asked to estimate the proportion of abortions among brucellosis seropositive animals. After calculation of the median value, in a second round, the experts are asked to revise their estimate in view of the median value of the first round. Costs are then summarized and presented by the respective sector (Fig. 12.1).

The savings to human public health totalled roughly US$3 million, which is notably lower than the US$8 million cost of intervention. From a public health perspective, it would therefore not be financially cost-effective to mass vaccinate the livestock in order to avert the public health cost. Combined savings, however, from the reduced burden of disease in human health, households and animal

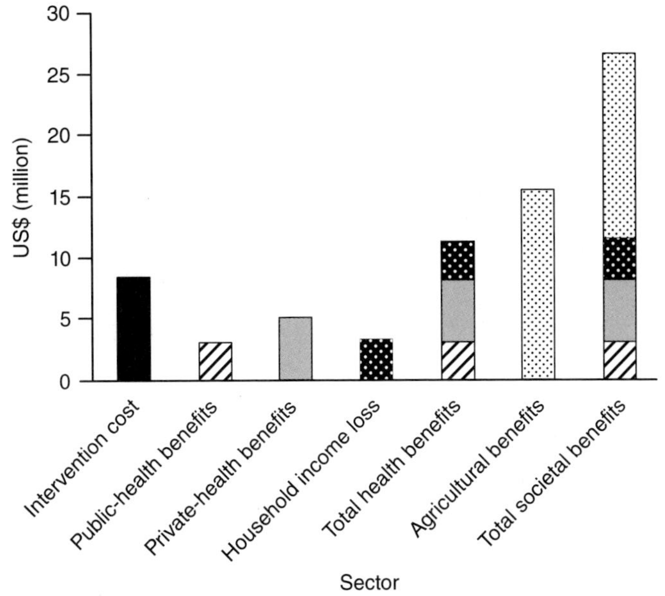


**Fig. 12.1.** Distribution of benefits in relation to the cost of intervention from brucellosis mass vaccination of livestock for the Mongolian society (adapted from Roth *et al.*, 2003).

production, totalled US$26 million, which is three times the US$8 million cost of the intervention (Fig. 12.1). This is a prime example of a One Health approach, showing that interventions become cost-beneficial when viewed from a broader societal perspective that is contrary to the single-sector point of view. Furthermore, if intervention costs are allocated proportionally to the monetary benefits, only 11% of the intervention costs would be debited against the public health sector. Including non-monetary benefits to human health, measured in DALYs, the cost per DALY averted amounts to US$19.1 (95% confidence interval 5.3–486.8). This is considered to be highly cost effective. Such cost-sharing models between the public health and livestock sectors illustrate another added value of a One Health approach (Roth *et al.*, 2003).

## Dog Rabies Elimination in an African City

Rabies is a viral disease transmitted most often in urban areas of Africa and Asia through dog bites (Knobel *et al.*, 2005; Léchenne *et al.*, Chapter 16, this volume). Human cases, which are invariably fatal, can be prevented by post-exposure prophylaxis (PEP), which is an active and passive immunization following a bite from a dog suspected to be rabid. Alternatively, dog rabies, and indirectly human rabies, can be eliminated by mass dog vaccination campaigns. Similar to the previously described example of brucellosis, one might ask: 'Is it cost-effective to prevent human rabies by mass vaccination of dogs in an African city?' This question arises through consideration of different intervention options. Indeed, WHO recommends both human PEP and dog mass vaccination, but the latter is rarely implemented in a systematic way. Based on 6 years of weekly observations of dog rabies cases and the number of exposed humans in N'Djamena, Chad, we estimated the transmission parameters of a dog–human rabies transmission model and then simulated the effects of different interventions (Zinsstag *et al.*, Chapter 11, this volume). Based on our experiences from small vaccination trials, we recorded the cost of dog mass vaccination (Kayali *et al.*, 2006). The actual cost of human PEP was collected from pharmacies and health centres. In this way, we could estimate the comparative cost of human PEP alone versus human PEP with dog mass vaccination (Fig. 12.2).

The cumulative cost of human PEP alone increases continuously because of ongoing transmission of dog rabies. In N'Djamena, every year more than 100 people are bitten by a rabid dog and, on average, seven of them die from rabies (Frey *et al.*, 2013). The cumulative cost of a single dog mass vaccination campaign with human PEP starts at a higher level, at approximately US$43,000, but does not increase much further because the transmission of dog rabies is interrupted, resulting in fewer human cases and thus less human PEP cost. The cumulated cost of human PEP with a single dog mass vaccination and human PEP alone reach the point of break-even at 6 years after the start of the interventions. After this period, the intervention of human PEP with a single dog mass vaccination is less costly than the cost of human PEP alone. Similar to the above example on brucellosis, the cost-effectiveness of the two compared interventions is expressed in cost per averted DALY (see Fig. 12.3).

For the first 5 years after the single vaccination intervention, cost-effectiveness of human PEP with dog mass vaccination is lower than human PEP alone, resulting in a higher cost per DALY averted. However in year 6 and beyond, human PEP with dog mass vaccination is more cost-effective. This example again shows the advantage of a One Health approach, taking an ecological perspective of the dog–human rabies transmission for the economic analysis of an intervention. It illustrates under which conditions and time frames an intervention in the dog reservoir can become more cost-effective compared to interventions in humans alone.

The above example is, however, highly context dependent. This means that the break-even points between the two interventions depend highly on the dog:human ratio and dog–human behaviour in a given location. Therefore, the analytical framework has been generalized in Fig. 12.4, showing different slope possibilities for the cumulative cost of dog mass vaccination and human PEP depending on a given context, for instance, cities in Asia and Africa. Finally, the comparative cost scenarios are also highly dependent on the rate of reintroduction of rabies. A country-wide approach, or even a regional approach similar to that used in Latin America (Hampson *et al.*, 2007), are most promising to reduce the risk of reintroduction of dog rabies.

## Cost of Bovine Tuberculosis in Ethiopia

Bovine tuberculosis belongs to the tuberculosis complex, which comprises a group of

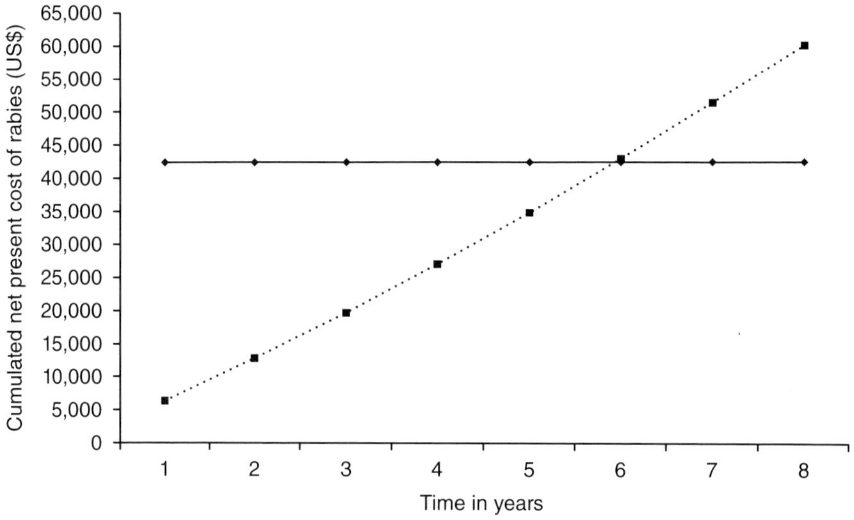


**Fig. 12.2.** Accumulated and discounted costs of human PEP alone (dotted line) and human PEP with dog vaccination (solid line) (adapted from Zinsstag *et al.*, 2009).

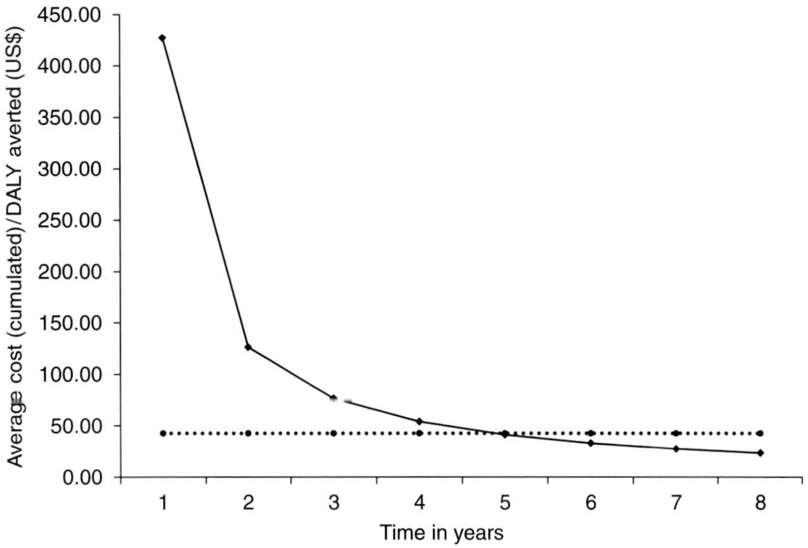


**Fig. 12.3.** Average and discounted cost-effectiveness of human PEP alone (dotted line) and human PEP with dog vaccination (solid line) (adapted from Zinsstag *et al.*, 2009).

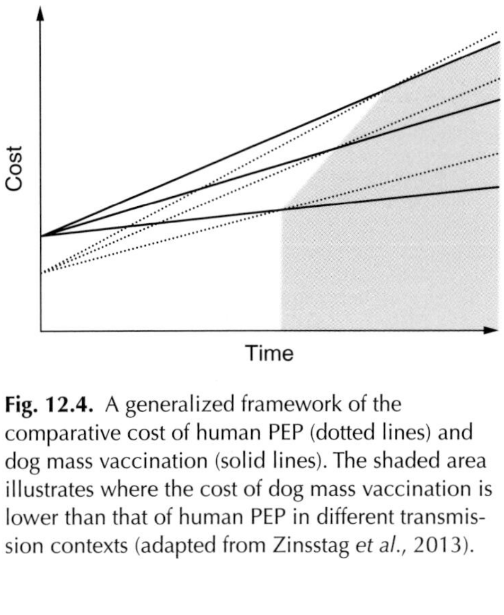


**Fig. 12.4.** A generalized framework of the comparative cost of human PEP (dotted lines) and dog mass vaccination (solid lines). The shaded area illustrates where the cost of dog mass vaccination is lower than that of human PEP in different transmission contexts (adapted from Zinsstag *et al.*, 2013).

bacteria causing tuberculosis in humans and animals. The causative pathogen is *Mycobacterium bovis*, which mainly infects cattle but can also be transmitted to humans, by the consumption of unpasteurized milk and by direct contact. The examples of brucellosis and rabies presented previously in this chapter can be extended to include a wildlife component (Tschopp, Chapter 15, this volume).

For bovine tuberculosis, the typical wildlife reservoirs are badgers in the UK and white-tailed deer in Michigan in the USA. In Africa, the spill-over of bovine tuberculosis from cattle to wildlife and the subsequent mortality of lions in the Kruger National Park demonstrate the additional costs that the disease imposes on the wildlife sector and the potential cost to the tourism industry (Renwick *et al.*, 2007). We have conceptualized this for future economic analysis in Fig. 12.5. Recent work on bovine tuberculosis in Ethiopia showed that the prevalence, as measured by the tuberculin test, was high in the peri-urban dairy production sector, and endemic at a low level in rural cattle (Tschopp *et al.*, 2010a,b). To date, very few human *M. bovis* cases have been detected, and no wildlife cases have been confirmed. Therefore, for a contemporary cost analysis of bovine tuberculosis in Ethiopia, we restricted the analysis to the cattle sector (Tschopp *et al.*, 2012).

In this analysis, we extended demographic models of cattle populations to incorporate stochastic parameter specifications using an existing bio-economic model called Livestock Development Planning System (http://www.fao.org/agriculture/lead/tools/livestock0/en). The uncertainty of parameter

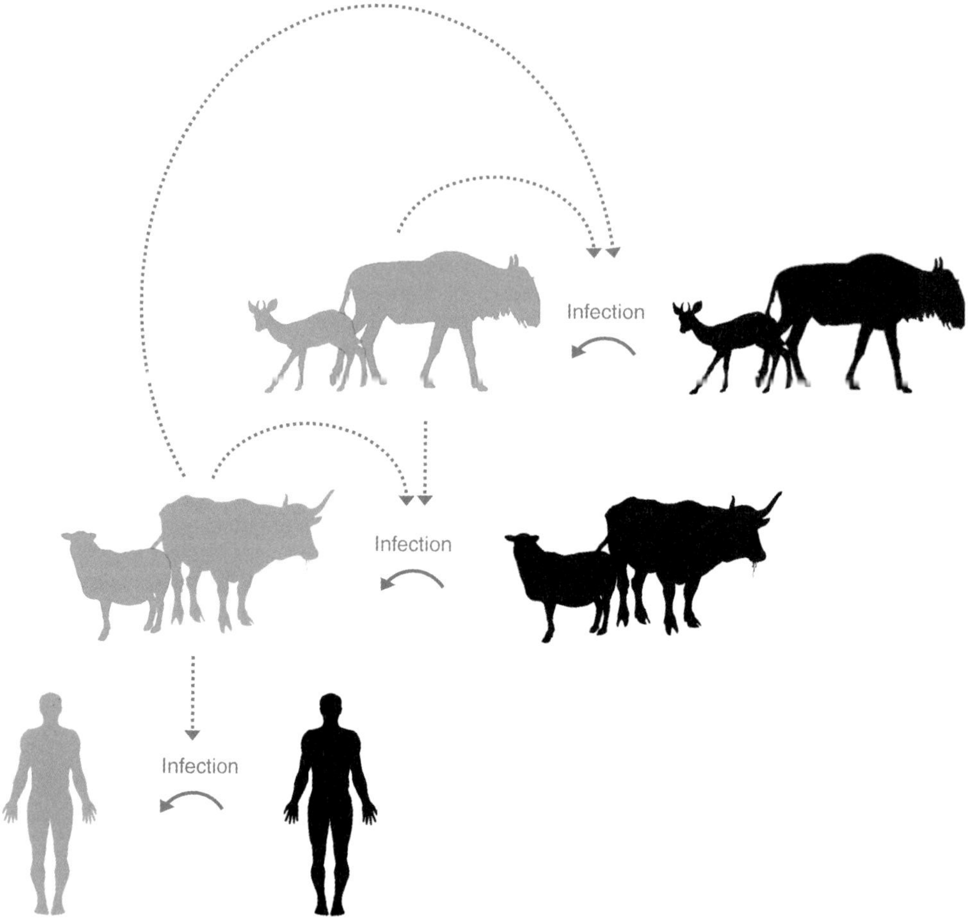


**Fig. 12.5.** Flow chart of the transmission of bovine tuberculosis used to underpin a dynamic cross-sector economic assessment (adapted from Zinsstag *et al.*, 2006).

values can be formally addressed by using Monte Carlo simulation; a low cost Monte Carlo application for Excel called Ersatz is currently available from http://www.epigear.com. Livestock numbers, offtake for meat, milk production and animal traction for ploughing were simulated with and without prevalence-dependent decreases of production parameters, such as milk yield and fertility. For example, the fertility rate in terms of number of calves born per cow per year for diseased animals is related to the base-line fertility rate, as shown in Eqn 12.1. We assumed that the disease effect is a 15% fertility reduction in tuberculin-positive animals (Bernues *et al.*, 1997).

$$\text{Fertility with bTB} = \text{Baseline Fertility} \times (1 - (0.15 \times \text{tuberculin prevalence})) \quad (12.1)$$

This formula is then used to estimate parameter values both 'with' and 'without' disease, for fertility, mortality and milk yields for the herd model.

In Fig. 12.6, the cumulative cost of bovine tuberculosis in urban dairy production is shown in terms of present value (PV) from 2005 to 2011. The yearly productivity from cattle with bovine tuberculosis would be reduced by approximately US$29 per animal, which is more than the cost of annual tuberculin testing per animal. However, if the aim of testing were to

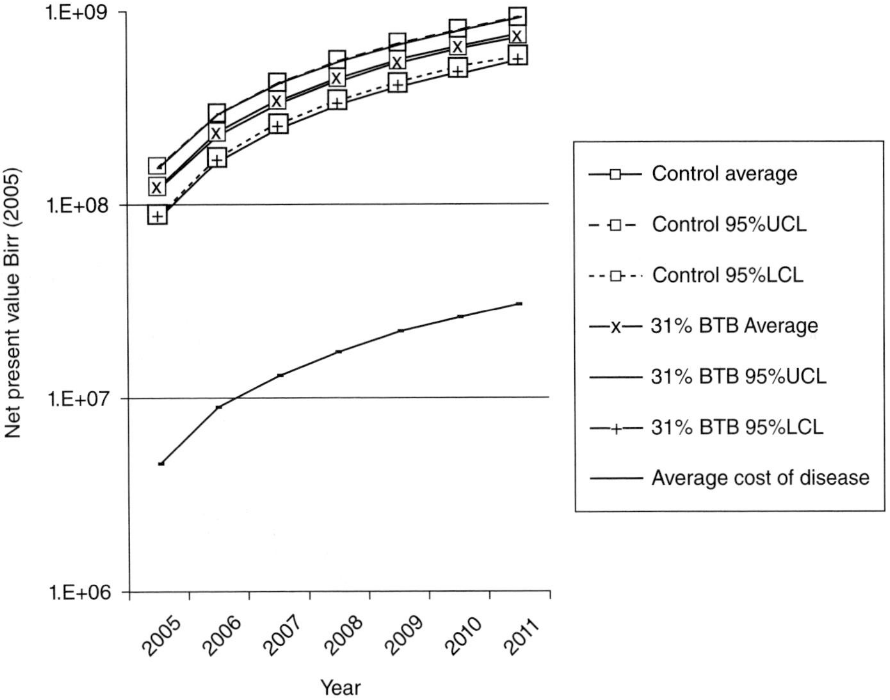


**Fig. 12.6.** Present value of urban cattle production (Addis Ababa), with and without 31% prevalence of bovine tuberculosis, and average present value of cost of disease (UCL, upper 95% confidence limit; LCL, lower 95% confidence limit; BTB, bovine tuberculosis, synonymous to bTB (adapted from Tschopp *et al.*, 2012).

remove test-positive animals, then the cost of removal, in terms of compensation to farmers for culled stock, would additionally need to be included. Such a test-and-slaughter intervention would almost certainly not be cost-beneficial given the current situation.

The fact that high numbers of human *M. bovis*-infected cases were not found (Gumi *et al.*, 2012) does not mean that there is no risk to people. Expanding and increasingly intensive dairy production in peri-urban areas, coupled with uncontrolled transmission of *M. bovis* in cattle, clearly represents a public health risk which should be addressed in a locally adapted way. In this example, there is no cross-sector One Health component; however, this illustration emphasizes the importance of a prior understanding of effective transmission pathways when structuring an economic analysis.

## Case Study Conclusions

Each of the four case studies described in this chapter presents one aspect of One Health economics. The Chadian pastoralist example provides clear evidence of the cost savings that can be made when health interventions target both people and livestock. The example of brucellosis in Mongolia shows that by pooling the human and animal benefits the intervention becomes highly cost-effective. The intervention is cost effective to the public health sector (measured as cost per DALY averted) when the intervention costs are allocated to sectors proportionally to their benefits. The rabies case study highlights how intervening in animals, here by mass dog vaccination, yields a net benefit in terms of cost saving on human treatments, in this case through reduced need for PEP. The bovine tuberculosis study in Ethiopia shows how a stochastic herd model can estimate overall benefit levels and can highlight the differences between cattle production systems. The method used in Ethiopia is currently extended to China and will also include costs to humans, a component that is difficult to produce in countries with insufficient data collection.

The case studies of this chapter have common features, which can be generalized in an overall framework (Narrod *et al.*, 2012). Most importantly, we do not attempt to introduce a joint metric for diseased humans and animals. For humans, there is a moral consensus that human life has a unique value, no matter who it is or where that person lives. This has been translated into a number of health- adjusted life-year measures, with DALY currently the most commonly used in a worldwide context. For animals, such a consensus is lacking. Developing a disability metric for animals would be highly controversial, as animals are valued differently, both in different cultures and even among individuals within a single economy. This may range from a high emotional value for a pet to a strictly commercial value that is based on the body weight of livestock. Furthermore, the lifespan for livestock is a function of the production system in which they are kept, in which humans determine when they should be culled or sold for slaughter. Thus, African cows often have longer lives than European dairy cows. In humans, a disability such as incurable lameness would receive a moderate disability weight; in many production animals, lameness would lead to culling. Thus for animals, monetary values are the most appropriate measure. For humans, attempts to put monetary values on human life do exist, for example, based on average national income or risk-based assessments, such as life insurances and the value of a statistical life (VSL), which is estimated on the basis of people's recorded expenditures to avoid risky situations which might lead to death. Unsurprisingly, these attempts yield widely different values within different economic contexts. These monetary values may be helpful in guiding expenditure levels on health interventions. In our view, however, DALY or other similar non-monetary measures are the most appropriate for quantifying human health outcomes. Therefore, we present composite outcomes in terms of cost-effectiveness of interventions, expressed as cost per DALY averted for the human component, and financial cost–benefit for the animal component. To address cultural differences, we recommend clear specification of the perspective of the analysis, in terms of cultural background. We have not addressed macroeconomic consequences of transboundary transmission of diseases like avian influenza, but such components could be added when needed.

## One Health Economics and the Human–Animal Interface

The application of One Health economics extends in both directions. Although thorough investigation of the impact of human diseases on animals is not common, there is literature available about these types of impacts (Lowder *et al.*, 2009; Thompson, 2013). Even in situations where humans have been strongly implicated as being a potential risk factor in the spread of diseases to animals (Ferguson *et al.*, 2001; McGarry and Shackleton, 2009), follow-up economic evaluation has been mostly non-existent in scientific literature. It is unlikely that research into the impact of human-to-animal diseases will receive funding priority in the near future. However, it is quite likely that further exploration of the impacts of human–animal diseases on human industries will receive increased attention, due to the potential for significant economic burden to society from the spread of zoonosis led by humans, e.g. pandemic spread of *Stapylococcus aureus* in the poultry industry (Lowder *et al.*, 2009). The One Health concept extends beyond zoonosis, however, as illness in one sector can spill over to another in indirect ways. The impact of HIV/AIDS on the livestock industry of sub-Saharan Africa has been the subject of some attention already. The livestock industry forms the backbone of income in many communities, and the impacts of the disease have profound effects for the industry, including loss of agricultural labour force (Lagu *et al.*, 2011), loss of key regional agricultural knowledge and the defaulting on group savings and credit schemes due to inability to pay for loans (Lengkeek *et al.*, 2008). At the same time, livestock is also seen as the primary buffer against financial shocks created by HIV/AIDS-related medical expenses for the most disadvantaged (Mutenje *et al.*, 2008), demonstrating that the relationship does go in both directions. Observations go as far as reporting that the impact of HIV leads some communities to hunt significantly more wildlife, including reptiles and insects, compared to non-HIV-affected communities, as a response to the financial burden of the disease (McGarry and Shackleton, 2009). Although One Health is growing as a concept, the current focus on research is primarily focused on proving the efficiency of the concept through the animal-to-human side of the relationship. This chapter shows demonstrable economic evidence of the advantages to bi-directional economic analysis across human and animal health-related sectors. Once the One Health concept is ready to evolve into a closer iteration of the holistic design, as initially envisioned, the human-to-animal interface will require further attention for the benefit of both animal and human health, respectively.

## Outlook on One Health Financing

One Health economics is not necessarily restricted to infectious diseases. The funding of zoonosis control is often difficult because public health sector awareness is low, and effective interventions are mostly outside the human health sector, targeting instead animal reservoirs or the environment. Globally, zoonoses will remain a problem in low income countries and will continue to threaten the rest of the world. The global cost of an emerging disease can be far higher than the cost of prevention at its source. Hence a global subsidiary principle, similar to the Global Fund to Fight AIDS, Tuberculosis and Malaria (GFATM), is recommended for emerging and possibly also for endemic zoonoses (Zinsstag *et al.*, 2007). More recent funding instruments, called Development Impact Bonds, share risk between donors and private investors in clearly defined projects that could include zoonosis elimination (Welburn and Coleman, Chapter 18, this volume). Economic analyses will play a key role in demonstrating an added value for closer cooperation of human and animal health. While interventions may not be cost-effective for one sector alone, they may become cost-effective by taking an overall societal perspective with the benefits aggregated for all sectors. Thus, economic analysis involving all related sectors has become a central element for providing evidence of the added value of a One Health approach.

## References


Bernues, A., Manrique, E. and Maza, M.T. (1997) Economic evaluation of bovine brucellosis and tuberculosis eradication programmes in a mountain area of Spain. *Preventive Veterinary Medicine* 30(2), 137–149.

Dean, A.S., Crump, L., Greter, H., Hattendorf, J., Schelling, E. and Zinsstag, J. (2012a) Clinical manifestations of human brucellosis: a systematic review and meta-analysis. *PLoS Neglected Tropical Diseases* 6(12), e1929.

Dean, A.S., Crump, L., Greter, H., Schelling, E. and Zinsstag, J. (2012b) Global burden of human brucellosis: a systematic review of disease frequency. *PLoS Neglected Tropical Diseases* 6(10), e1865.

Drummond, M.F., Sculpher, M.J., Torrance, G.W., O'Brien, B.J. and Stoddart, G.L. (2005) *Methods for the Economic Evaluation of Health Care Programmes*, 3rd edn. Oxford University Press, Oxford, UK.

Ferguson, N.M., Donnelly, C.A. and Anderson, R.M. (2001) The foot-and-mouth epidemic in Great Britain: pattern of spread and impact of interventions. *Science* 292(5519), 1155–1160.

Frey, J., Mindekem, R., Kessely, H., Doumagoum Moto, D., Naissengar, S., Zinsstag, J. and Schelling, E. (2013) Survey of animal bite injuries and their management for an estimate of human rabies deaths in N'Djamena, Chad. *Tropical Medicine & International Health* 18(12), 1555–1562.

Gumi, B., Schelling, E., Berg, S., Firdessa, R., Erenso, G., Mekonnen, W., Hailu, E., Melese, E., Aseffa, A., Young, D. and Zinsstag, J. (2012) Zoonotic transmission of tuberculosis in southeast Ethiopian pastoralists and their livestock. *EcoHealth* 9(2), 139–149.

Hampson, K., Dushoff, J., Bingham, J., Bruckner, G., Ali, Y.H. and Dobson, A. (2007) Synchronous cycles of domestic dog rabies in sub-Saharan Africa and the impact of control efforts. *Proceedings of the National Academy of Sciences* 104(18), 7717–7722.

Jean-Richard, V., Crump, L., Moto Daugla, D., Hattendorf, J., Schelling, E. and Zinsstag, J. (2014) The use of mobile phones for demographic surveillance of mobile pastoralists and their animals in Chad: proof of principle. *Global Health Action* 7, 23209.

Kayali, U., Mindekem, R., Hutton, G., Ndoutamia, A.G. and Zinsstag, J. (2006) Cost-description of a pilot parenteral vaccination campaign against rabies in dogs in N'Djamena, Chad. *Tropical Medicine & International Health* 11(7), 1058–1065.

Knobel, D.L., Cleaveland, S., Coleman, P.G., Fevre, E.M., Meltzer, M.I., Miranda, M.E., Shaw, A., Zinsstag, J. and Meslin, F.X. (2005) Re-evaluating the burden of rabies in Africa and Asia. *Bulletin of the World Health Organization* 83(5), 360–368.

Lagu, C., Mugisha, A. and Koma, L.M.P.K. (2011) Impact of HIV/AIDS on the livestock-producing communities of Uganda: case studies of Moyo and Kashumba sub counties. *Livestock Research for Rural Development* 23.

Lengkeek, A., Koster, M. and Salm, M. (2008) *Mitigating the effects of HIV/AIDS in small-scale farming, Agrodoks*. Agromisa CTA, Wageningen, the Netherlands.

Lowder, B.V., Guinane, C.M., Ben Zakour, N.L., Weinert, L.A., Conway-Morris, A., Cartwright, R.A., Simpson, A.J., Rambaut, A., Nübel, U. and Fitzgerald, J.R. (2009) Recent human-to-poultry host jump, adaptation, and pandemic spread of *Staphylococcus aureus*. *Proceedings of the National Academy of Sciences* 106(46), 19545–19550.

McGarry, D.K. and Shackleton, C.M. (2009) Is HIV/AIDS jeopardizing biodiversity? *Environmental Conservation* 36(01), 5–7.

Montavon, A., Jean-Richard, V., Bechir, M., Daugla, D.M., Abdoulaye, M., Bongo Nare, R.N., Diguimbaye-Djaibe, C., Alfarouk, I.O., Schelling, E., Wyss, K., Tanner, M. and Zinsstag, J. (2013) Health of mobile pastoralists in the Sahel - assessment of 15 years of research and development. *Tropical Medicine & International Health* 18(9), 1044–1052.

Mutenje, M.J., Mapiye, C., Mavunganidze, Z., Mwale, M., Muringai, V., Katsinde, C. and Gavumende, I. (2008) Livestock as a buffer against HIV and AIDS income shocks in the rural households of Zimbabwe. *Development Southern Africa 25*(1), 75–82.

Narrod, C., Zinsstag, J. and Tiongco, M. (2012) A one health framework for estimating the economic costs of zoonotic diseases on society. *EcoHealth* 9(2), 150–162.

Renwick, A.R., White, P.C. and Bengis, R.G. (2007) Bovine tuberculosis in southern African wildlife: a multi-species host-pathogen system. *Epidemiology and Infection* 135(4), 529–540.

Roth, F., Zinsstag, J., Orkhon, D., Chimed-Ochir, G., Hutton, G., Cosivi, O., Carrin, G. and Otte, J. (2003) Human health benefits from livestock vaccination for brucellosis: case study. *Bulletin of the World Health Organization* 81(12), 867–876.

Schelling, E., Bechir, M., Ahmed, M.A., Wyss, K., Randolph, T.F. and Zinsstag, J. (2007) Human and animal vaccination delivery to remote nomadic families, Chad. *Emerging Infectious Diseases* 13(3), 373–379.

Thompson, R.C.A. (2013) Parasite zoonoses and wildlife: One Health, spillover and human activity. *International Journal for Parasitology* 43(12–13), 1079–1088.

Tschopp, R., Berg, S., Argaw, K., Gadisa, E., Habtamu, M., Schelling, E., Young, D., Aseffa, A. and Zinsstag, J. (2010a) Bovine tuberculosis in Ethiopian wildlife. *Journal of Wildlife Diseases* 46(3), 753–762.

Tschopp, R., Schelling, E., Hattendorf, J., Young, D., Aseffa, A. and Zinsstag, J. (2010b) Repeated cross-sectional skin testing for bovine tuberculosis in cattle kept in a traditional husbandry system in Ethiopia. *Veterinary Record* 167(7), 250–256.

Tschopp, R., Hattendorf, J., Roth, F., Choudhoury, A., Shaw, A., Aseffa, A. and Zinsstag, J. (2012) Cost estimate of bovine tuberculosis to Ethiopia. *Current Topics in Microbiology and Immunology* 365, 249–268.

Weibel, D. (2009) Demographic surveillance of mobile pastoralists in Chad. Unpublished PhD, University of Basel, Switzerland.

Weibel, D., Bechir, M., Hattendorf, J., Bonfoh, B., Zinsstag, J. and Schelling, E. (2011) Random demographic household surveys in highly mobile pastoral communities in Chad. *Bulletin of the World Health Organization* 89(5), 385–389.

Zinsstag, J., Schelling, E., Roth, F. and Kazwala, R.R. (2006) Economics of bovine tuberculosis. In: Thoen, C.O., Steele, J.H. and Gilsdorf, M.J. (eds) *Mycobacterium Bovis Infection in Animals and Humans*. Blackwell Science, London, pp. 68–84.

Zinsstag, J., Schelling, E., Roth, F., Bonfoh, B., de Savigny, D. and Tanner, M. (2007) Human benefits of animal interventions for zoonosis control. *Emerging Infectious Diseases* 13(4), 527–531.

Zinsstag, J., Durr, S., Penny, M.A., Mindekem, R., Roth, F., Menendez Gonzalez, S., Naissengar, S. and Hattendorf, J. (2009) Transmission dynamics and economics of rabies control in dogs and humans in an African city. *Proceedings of the National Academy of Sciences* 106(35), 14996–15001.

Zinsstag, J., Lechenne, M., Mindekem, R., Naissengar, S. and Schelling, E. (2013) The economics of dog rabies control and the potential for combining it with other interventions. In: Office International des Epizooties (ed.) *OIE Global Conference on Rabies Control*. OIE, Seoul, South Korea, pp. 163–168.

# 13 Integrated Human and Animal Demographic Surveillance

**Vreni Jean-Richard* and Lisa Crump**
*Swiss Tropical and Public Health Institute, Basel, Switzerland and University of Basel, Basel, Switzerland*

## Introduction

This chapter describes integrated approaches for human and animal demographic surveillance. A case study illustrates how an innovative combined method increased both success, in terms of acceptability and accuracy, and cost-effectiveness. Demographic information is essential for expansion of social development concepts and planning of land management policies and social services, in particular health services. Without this information, it is impossible to assess accurately the effectiveness of interventions (Weibel *et al.*, 2008). Developing countries often lack a functioning demographic registration system, and the Routine Health Information Systems (RHIS) are often inadequately organized and unable to meet scientific demands for data. In most cases, only sedentary people are considered, with mobile pastoralists and the regions where they comprise a majority not included in demographic assessments (Homewood and Randall, 2009). There are very few studies investigating demographic indices in African mobile pastoralists (Hill and Randall, 1984; Brainard, 1986; Roth, 1994; Leslie and Little, 1999; Schelling *et al.*, 2005; Münch, 2012).

The International Network for the Demographic Evaluation of Populations and Their Health (INDEPTH), a global network of longitudinal health and demographic surveillance sites in low- and middle-income countries, has established 43 sites in 20 countries for demographic and health surveillance for research. The findings from these Demographic Surveillance Systems (DSS) sites are extrapolated for larger populations. However, tracking the details of migration remains one of the most complex aspects for INDEPTH network surveillance sites, and the site populations are unlikely to represent closely the surrounding population in logistically challenged areas (Sankoh and Byass, 2012). However, demographic surveillance, as conceived and developed for sedentary communities, is not feasible for mobile populations, because the regular visits need to occur in different locations depending on the migration routes. This chapter presents a case study from Chad to illustrate some lessons on the role of and the process for integrating the One Health approach into ongoing Demographic and Health Surveillance Systems (DHSS) globally.

## Background

In the mid-1990s, staff from a rural health centre in the Lake Chad area observed that

*E-mail: vreni@jean-richard.ch

many mobile pastoralists were passing close to the health centre without utilizing any of the offered services. The local primary health-care programme, implemented by the Centre de Support en Santé Internationale (CSSI), sought to develop more accessible services for mobile populations. A pre-study was conducted in 1996 to assess the access of mobile pastoralists to health services in Chad. Subsequently, a research partnership was established between the Laboratoire de Recherches Vétérinaires et Zootechniques de Farcha (LRVZ), the CSSI and the Chadian Ministry of Health. Stakeholders on the national and local level were involved in the research process from the outset.

The early research indicated that most of the livestock was adequately vaccinated, in contrast to the children, none of whom had received the complete recommended childhood vaccination programme (Bechir *et al.*, 2004). On the basis of workshops and discussions between the involved population, authorities and researchers, a joint human and animal vaccination programme was developed (Zinsstag *et al.*, 2005; Schelling *et al.*, 2007; Schelling *et al.*, Chapter 20, this volume).

Although 4022 nomadic children were fully immunized, 6284 women received at least two injections against tetanus and a total of 103,500 livestock were vaccinated, no vaccination coverage could be estimated due to a lack of baseline data for the mobile population (Schelling *et al.*, 2008). An evaluation of the programme on a population scale was not possible because the communities could rarely be located for a second time due to their mobility. In an effort to overcome these knowledge gaps, a new research area for population estimates and demography of mobile human and animal populations was undertaken.

## Rationale

In Chad, there is a sizeable mobile pastoralist population, with estimates ranging from less than 400,000, or 3.5% of the total population in the most recent national census (2009), up to 2 million (Thornton *et al.*, 2002; Rass, 2006). These mobile populations utilize a transhumant lifestyle, moving with their livestock from one grazing area to another, as shown in Plate 5. Although several authors have described the mobile pastoralist populations in the Lake Chad area (Wiese, 2006; Weibel *et al.*, 2008), longitudinal data describing the demographic development of the human and animal populations were lacking (Schelling *et al.*, 2003; Weibel *et al.*, 2011).

Demographic surveys in mobile communities in Africa have generally been focused on documenting fertility and mortality rates (Hampshire and Randall, 2000), although direct observation methods (Münch, 2012) are costly and not feasible for large populations. A few alternative approaches have been described for estimating population numbers and densities of mobile pastoralists. One example is the 'water point approach', where data are collected at wells or water bodies used by mobile pastoralists' livestock. The main drawback is uncertainty on completeness of numbers due to multiple water points usage, variable migration routes and the difficulty for personnel to cover all water points (Kalsbeek, 1986). This approach has also been proposed for a livestock census yet to be conducted in Chad in collaboration with FAO.

Aerial censuring is another method, but information must be validated in the field (e.g. for people and household structures) and it has a significant limitation in areas with many trees, where people and animals tend to rest during the main part of the day for protection from the sun (Anonymous, 1993).

Following the previously described joint vaccination campaign, an innovative approach to estimate the size of the mobile population in the south-eastern Lake Chad area was tested (Weibel *et al.*, 2008). The method of capture–mark–recapture, as developed for research in the ecology and wildlife sectors, was adapted for use in human populations. Biometric fingerprints were used to register and identify mobile pastoralist women, and random transects were conducted for the sampling method and also for re-encounter. The approach proved to be applicable, but the number of re-encounters was too low to estimate the population size for such a highly mobile population.

Up until this point in 2007, livestock assessment had not been included in the demographic surveillance, although mobile pastoralists are heavily dependent both economically and socially on the productivity of their livestock. Mobile populations are reported to own about half of all livestock and generate about half of the national meat production in Chad (Rass, 2006) and, therefore, represent great economic potential. Additionally, there is the issue of increasing resource scarcity in the Sahel zone, which is noticeable, for instance, through the spread of non-palatable plant species like *Calotropis procera*, and which has contributed to numerous small and larger scale conflicts. These conflicts develop between pastoralists and farmers over access to water and pasture areas or over damage from animals straying into crop fields to graze (Schelling *et al.*, 2008; Zinsstag *et al.*, 2010). Increasingly violent outcomes indicate the high stakes for all involved, who depend on availability of water and pastures for survival. The increasing demand for natural resources threatens the livelihoods of farmers and herders and is a community concern. Clearly, demographic information, about people as well as livestock, is urgently needed to plan and prioritize health interventions and to negotiate equitable, sustainable regulations governing land use.

## A Chadian Case Study

Many pastoralist communities stay seasonally in the south-eastern Lake Chad area, before migrating into other countries during the rainy season. This dynamic situation, along with a relative lack of infrastructure, complicated the task of defining and estimating the population size. Therefore, a unique approach was elaborated to estimate the seasonal density of people and livestock, rather than the total population. The method utilized randomly generated GPS coordinates, which were subsequently visited at regular intervals during 2 consecutive years. The sampling periods were at the beginning and at the end of the dry season, when the mobile population is most dense in close proximity to the lake. Two consecutive years were included to document the between-year as well as the between-season dynamics.

The areas around the randomly selected GPS coordinate points were visually scanned and then circles of 1 and then 2 km radius were driven in order to identify all camps or settlements. The assumed visibility was 500 m. With this approach, a circular area of 2.5 km radius (5 km diameter) was covered around each random coordinate point (Fig. 13.1). After registration of each camp, permission for an interview was requested, followed by an interview conducted with the camp or village leader to gather information about the human and animal population of the community. The inclusion criterion was that the house/tent of the village/camp leader (*'Boulama'*) was inside the 2.5 km radius around the random coordinate point. Human and animal densities were calculated and then extrapolated to estimate seasonal human and animal population densities. For livestock, Tropical Livestock Units[1] (TLU; Jahnke, 1982), as described by the Food and Agriculture Organization of the United Nations (FAO, 2014) were used. The results indicated a very high pressure of animals on the pastures, up to five times as high as carrying capacities estimated in earlier studies in comparable areas (Jean-Richard *et al.*, 2014a).

Although this kind of information represents a valid base for political negotiations and the development of regulations, it only provides a 'snapshot' of the situation at a point in time without revealing the dynamics within the communities. This aspect was addressed through another type of survey, which capitalized on the recent developments in the field of mobile phone technology. In the last decade, mobile phone communication increased rapidly in Africa with 45% penetration across the continent (Yonazi *et al.*, 2012). While one

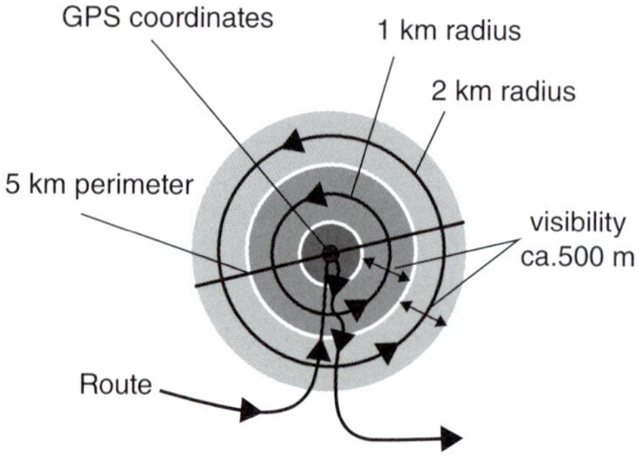


**Fig. 13.1.** Schematic illustration of the sampling method.

in three Chadians owned a mobile phone by the end of 2011 (Anonymous, 2013b), penetration rates in Chad are still reported to be far lower than the African average, with sporadic network coverage most notably in the remote areas (Anonymous, 2013a). Despite these limitations, mobile pastoralists profit from the use of mobile phones for exchanging information about family and herd positions, pasture availability and other relevant developments. The flat topography of the Sahel zone facilitates network coverage even with a low density of antennas.

A small-scale trial of a mobile human and animal demographic surveillance was established for 18 months (Jean-Richard *et al.*, 2014b). Twenty mobile pastoralist camps from three ethnic groups (Foulbe, Gorane and Arab) were selected by convenience from among those willing to participate. In each camp, one mixed livestock herd (defined as the animals regularly kept together) was chosen by the camp leader, according to cultural norms, as the sample livestock population. For the human population, all the households connected to this herd were included (three to seven households per herd). A household was defined, according to the local specification, as the members who eat and live together, as shown in Plate 6. Usually each wife had her own household, so in polygamous households the husband was counted only in the household of his first wife. Generally, several closely related households would keep their animals together. The herds consisted of cattle, small ruminants, donkeys, horses and camels, which were recorded stratified by sex and age groups for each species. Chickens were also included in the study. At the mid-point of the study, the cohort consisted of 579 people, 2869 cattle, 1183 goats, 1198 sheep, 338 donkeys, 99 horses, 35 camels and 315 chickens.

Every 2 to 4 weeks, a telephone interview was conducted with each participating community. The interviews were conducted first with the leader of the camp (or the included herd), who provided information about the herd and the current position of the camp. A further conversation was had with the leader's wife, who provided information about family members of all included households. This approach was chosen because more detailed information about pregnant women and the presence or absence of children could be collected from the women, while the men were able to provide the most accurate information about the livestock and migratory routes. When the wife was unavailable, the entire interview was conducted with the male participant. After each phone interview, a small amount of money (equivalent to about US$2) was transferred to the participant's phone account as compensation for participation. The transfer amount was doubled if the wife was also available for the interview, which was an incentive to allow women to participate in the pilot and seemed to contribute to a high degree of female participation. As an additional measure, an emergency service for medical and veterinary problems, using a shared cost system, was established and maintained to date. This regular personal contact built trust between the survey staff and study participants and improved the physical validation of interview data.

The calls were made from a central village in the area by a village health worker who was well known and trusted by the pastoralists. The participants made great efforts to be available for the interviews, sometimes climbing trees or travelling to an area with more consistent network coverage. This strong commitment resulted in no drop-outs during the course of the study with all the interviews conducted as planned. It also underlined the expressed desire of these marginalized communities to participate in political and social life outside the confines of their own communities.

Several interesting observations were registered during the study period in addition to the routine demographic information:

- Some communities separated into two groups and two herds towards the end of the dry season, when pastures were most scarce, and then joined together again when the rainy season started.
- The herd model that was calculated to show the consistency and validity of the livestock data showed growing herds, which was consistent with reports from the pastoralists who were attempting to recover their herd sizes after losses due to disease in recent years.

- The interviews with the women provided data about current human pregnancies, and it was possible to record the outcome of the pregnancies. A high number of pregnancies not resulting in a live birth (9 out of 24 pregnancies) was observed. As miscarriages are often considered a taboo topic, this method could provide novel opportunities to collect data and conduct and monitor interventions.
- The migratory routes of the communities clearly showed a pattern according to the ethnic groups. This pattern was consistent with the different husbandry practices.
- There was little in- and out-migration in the communities and only three human deaths, all due to disease, were registered during the sampling period.
- None of the children from the participating families attended school (although some boys attended Qur'an schools). In Chad, an average of 29% of boys and 47% of girls complete primary school (World Bank, 2011). This obvious inequitable access of mobile pastoralists should be urgently addressed by the authorities.

## Future Steps

Based on our experience with this small-scale study, adapted interventions for health and other social services can be developed. Technological advancements should enable GPS tracking of mobile communities. Information on migratory movements on a real-time basis would provide opportunities for specific measures, thus enabling monitoring and evaluation, and also maximize the spatio-temporal accessibility of camps for social service providers to increase coverage of interventions.

Our experiences underline the feasibility of a larger scale project. The costs for the small-scale study were low because we worked with local staff using locally available resources. The estimated costs of a scale-up to a full mobile DSS with 20,000 participants are about US$10 per participant per year (Jean-Richard, 2013).

This type of surveillance system would not only be low-cost, but also well accepted by the target population, while providing reliable real-time data. A longer term mobile demographic health and surveillance system could have benefits in many areas. Health and demographic data could be collected, as well as environmental and economic information, for instance, about rainfall, droughts, locusts and prices of cereals, milk and livestock. The real-time knowledge of camp locations and populations could facilitate health interventions such as vaccination delivery or sensitization and information campaigns. Through expansion of this small-scale surveillance system into a full-scale mobile DSS, for example, an ante-natal care visit, including a pregnancy test, could be conducted by health personnel soon after a participating woman is reported as being pregnant. Such an approach would provide the opportunity to collect specific detailed information and also improve healthcare for pregnant women. Additionally, it would enhance the motivation to report pregnancies as soon as possible, which would also lead to more accurate data about spontaneous abortion and to provision of adequate care. An emergency system using shared costs, similar to the one developed during the above described small-scale survey, would be greatly valued by the local population. Also, outbreaks of human and animal diseases such as cholera or anthrax could be monitored closely, enabling control measures to be taken within a short response-time. The combined health, ecological and economic information could be processed into an early warning system for humanitarian crisis situations, which regularly occur in the area (UN, 2012; Ford, 2013), and thereby facilitate a timely response.

## Conclusion

It is advantageous to maintain a combined human–animal approach due to the close interactions and interdependence between human and animal populations, which benefit from the added value of integrated approaches. Combined health interventions can be conducted with lower costs, through resource sharing. Information on diseases, including zoonotic diseases, becomes available to multiple sectors quickly and effectively. A systematic approach to animal health also opens the possibility to accurately document animal numbers, after a certain level of trust is established. Such information would be extremely valuable in regional and national land-use policy development.

The combined human–animal approach adapts demographic surveillance to the reality of these communities, where people rely on animals and reciprocally animals depend on people. It is crucial not to restrict the view to health, but to include related issues such as equitable resource use and access to social services, land rights and local cultural practices.

## Note

[1] Cattle = 0.7 TLU; camels = 1 TLU; small ruminants = 0.1 TLU; donkeys = 0.5 TLU; horses = 0.8 TLU.

## References


Anonymous (1993) *Survols aériens à basse altitude du cheptel, des habitations humaines et des ressources partorales dans la 'zone d'organisation pastorale', Tchad.* Resource Inventory and Management, Ltd, Jersey, Channel Islands, UK.

Anonymous (2013a) Chad - Telecoms, Mobile and Internet. Available at: http://www.budde.com.au/Research/Chad-Telecoms-Mobile-and-Internet.html (accessed 4 January 2014).

Anonymous (2013b) Telecoms overview for Chad, Ethiopia, Guinea, Cote d'Ivoire, Mozambique, Niger, DR Congo. Available at: http://www.oafrica.com/city-profile/telecoms-overview-for-chad-ethiopia-guinea-cote-divoire-mozambique-niger-dr-congo-as-of-2012 (accessed 4 January 2014).

Béchir, M., Schelling, E., Wyss, K., Daugla, D., Daoud, S., Tanner, M. and Zinsstag, J. (2004) [An innovative approach combining human and animal vaccination campaigns in nomadic settings of Chad: experiences and costs]. *Médecine tropicale: revue du Corps de santé colonial* 64(5), 497–502.

Brainard, J. (1986) Differential mortality in Turkana agriculturalists and pastoralists. *American Journal of Physical Anthropology* 70(4), 525–536.

FAO (2014) FAO Livestock and Environment Toolbox. Available at: http://www.fao.org/ag/againfo/programmes/en/lead/toolbox/Mixed1/TLU.htm (accessed 6 October 2014).

Ford, E. (2013) *Learning the Lessons in the Sahel.* Oxfam International.

Hampshire, K. and Randall, S. (2000) Pastoralists, agropastoralists and migrants: interactions between fertility and mobility in northern Burkina Faso. *Population Studies* 54(3), 247–261.

Hill, A. and Randall, S. (1984) Différences géographiques et sociales dans la mortalité infantile et juvénile au Mali. *Population* 6, 921–946.

Homewood, K. and Randall, S. (2009) African pastoralist demography. In: *Ecology of African Pastoralist Societies.* Ohio University Press, Athens, pp. 199–226.

Jahnke, H.E. (1982) *Livestock Production Systems and Livestock Development in Tropical Africa.* Kieler Wissenschaftsverlag Vauk, Kiel, Germany.

Jean-Richard, V. (2013) *Crowding at Lake Chad: An Integrated Approach to Demographic and Health Surveillance of Mobile Pastoralists and Their Animals.* University of Basel, Basel.

Jean-Richard, V., Crump, L., Abicho, A., Abakar, A., Il, A., Bechir, M., Eckert, S., Engesser, M., Hattendorf, J., Schelling, E. and Zinsstag, J. (2014a) Estimating population and livestock density of mobile pastoralists and sedentary settlements in the southeastern Lake Chad area, Chad. *Geospatial Health* (in press).

Jean-Richard, V., Crump, L., Daugla, D., Hattendorf, J., Schelling, E. and Zinsstag, J. (2014b) The use of mobile phones for demographic surveillance of mobile pastoralists and their animals in Chad: proof of principle. *Global Health Action* 7, 23209.

Kalsbeek, W. (1986) Nomad sampling: an analytic study of alternative design strategies. In: *Proceedings of the Section on Survey Research Methods.* American Statistical Association. Alexandria, Virginia.

Leslie, P. and Little, M. (1999) *Turkana Herders of the Dry Savanna: Ecology and Biobehavioral Response of Nomads to an Uncertain Environment.* Oxford University Press, Oxford, UK.

Münch, A. (2012) *Nomadic Women's Health Practice: Islamic Belief and Medical Care among Kel Alhafra Tuareg in Mali*. Schwabe Verlag, Basel.

Rass, N. (2006) *Policies and Strategies to Address the Vulnerability of Pastoralists in Sub-Saharan Africa*. FAO, Rome.

Roth, E. (1994) Demographic systems: two east African examples. In: *African Pastoral Systems: An Integrated Approach*. L. Rienner, Boulder, Colorado, pp. 133–146.

Sankoh, O. and Byass, P. (2012) The INDEPTH Network: filling vital gaps in global epidemiology. *International Journal of Epidemiology* 41(3), 579–588.

Schelling, E., Diguimbaye, C., Daoud, S., Nicolet, J., Boerlin, P., Tanner, M. and Zinsstag, J. (2003) Brucellosis and Q-fever seroprevalences of nomadic pastoralists and their livestock in Chad. *Preventive Veterinary Medicine* 61(4), 279–293.

Schelling, E., Wyss, K., Bechir, M., Daugla, D. and Zinsstag, J. (2005) Synergy between public health and veterinary services to deliver human and animal health interventions in rural low income settings. *BMJ (Clinical research edn)* 331(7527), 1264–1267.

Schelling, E., Bechir, M., Ahmed, M., Wyss, K., Randolph, T. and Zinsstag, J. (2007) Human and animal vaccination delivery to remote nomadic families, Chad. *Emerging Infectious Diseases* 13(3), 373–379.

Schelling, E., Wyss, K., Diguimbaye, C., Bechir, M., Taleb, M., Bonfoh, B., Tanner, M. and Zinsstag, J. (2008) Towards integrated and adapted health services for nomadic pastoralists and their animals: a North–South partnership. In: *Handbook of Transdisciplinary Research*. Springer, Heidelberg, pp. 277–291.

Thornton, P., Kruska., R., Henningerl, N., Kristjanson, P., Reid, R. and Atieno, F. (2002) ILRI - Mapping Poverty and Livestock in the Developing World. Available at: http://www.ilri.cgiar.org/InfoServ/Webpub/fulldocs/Mappoverty/media (accessed 24 October 2013).

UN (2012) *Sahel Regional Strategy 2013*. United Nations, New York.

Weibel, D., Schelling, E., Bonfoh, B., Utzinger, J., Hattendorf, J., Abdoulaye, M., Madjiade, T. and Zinsstag, J. (2008) Demographic and health surveillance of mobile pastoralists in Chad: integration of biometric fingerprint identification into a geographical information system. *Geospatial Health* 3(1), 113–124.

Weibel, D., Bechir, M., Hattendorf, J., Bonfoh, B., Zinsstag, J. and Schelling, E. (2011) Random demographic household surveys in highly mobile pastoral communities in Chad. *Bulletin of the World Health Organization* 89(5), 385–389.

Wiese, M. (2006) *Health-Vulnerability in a Complex Crisis Situation. Implications for providing health care to a nomadic people in Chad*. Verlag für Entwicklungspolitik, Saarbrucken.

World Bank (2011) Primary completion rate, (% of relevant age group) | Data | Table. Available at: http://data.worldbank.org/indicator/SE.PRM.CMPT.FE.ZS?order=wbapi_data_value_2012+wbapi_data_value+wbapi_data_value-last&sort=asc (accessed 30 October 2013).

Yonazi, E., Kelly, T., Halewood, N. and Blackman, C. (2012) The transformational use of information and communication technologies in Africa. Available at: http://siteresources.worldbank.org/extinformationandcommunicationandtechnologies/resources/282822-1346223280837/MainReport.pdf (accessed 4 January 2014).

Zinsstag, J., Schelling, E., Wyss, K. and Bechir, M. (2005) Potential of cooperation between human and animal health to strengthen health systems. *Lancet* 366(9503), 2142–2145.

Zinsstag, J., Bonfoh, B. and Schelling, E. (2010) Cohérence des systèmes de santé humaine et animale en Afrique: en route pour une santé unique. In: Gauthier-Clerc, M. and Thomas, F. (eds) *Écologie de la santé et biodiversité*. De Boeck, Brussels, pp. 400–406.

# 14 Brucellosis Surveillance and Control: a Case for One Health

**Jakob Zinsstag,[1,2]* Anna Dean,[1,2] Zolzaya Baljinnyam,[1,2,3] Felix Roth,[1,2] Joldoshbek Kasymbekov[1,2,3] and Esther Schelling[1,2]**

*[1]Swiss Tropical and Public Health Institute, Basel, Switzerland; [2]University of Basel, Basel, Switzerland; [3]Animal Health Project, Swiss Agency for Development and Cooperation, Ulaanbaatar, Mongolia; [4]Institute of Biotechnology of the National Academy of Sciences of the Kyrgyz Republic, Bishkek, Kyrgyzstan*

## Introduction

Brucellosis, a bacterial disease causing abortion in livestock and an often chronic illness in humans is endemic in both extensive pastoral settings as well as more intensive livestock systems throughout Asia, Latin America and Africa and some European countries (Pappas *et al.*, 2006; Dean *et al.*, 2012b). The most important preferential reservoir host for *Brucella abortus* is cattle and for *B. melitensis*, sheep and goats, among which *Brucella* spp. cause important productivity losses (Bernues *et al.*, 1997). *Brucella abortus* and *B. melitensis* can spill over into other livestock populations such as yak and camels. Wildlife reservoirs of *B. abortus* have been identified in North America and Africa (Godfroid *et al.*, 2013b). Humans are exposed through direct contact with infected animals or the consumption of unpasteurized milk or dairy products. As one of the most widespread zoonoses in the world, brucellosis provides a prime example of the importance of a One Health approach to disease prevention and control, demonstrating the added value achieved by closer cooperation of the human health and animal health sectors.

Most of the published research focuses solely on either human or livestock brucellosis (Li *et al.*, 2013), although some studies do recommend a One Health approach for more effective control (Boukary *et al.*, 2013), including the involvement of the social sciences (Marcotty *et al.*, 2009). Given the re-emergence of the disease in some areas, particularly in the countries of the former Soviet Union, and the prevailing endemic situation in many resource-poor countries, the planning of control measures must go beyond classical textbook approaches. Plumb and colleagues recognized that the challenges and opportunities for brucellosis management were fundamentally multivariate, multifaceted and integrative and called for a brucellosis One Health paradigm (Plumb *et al.*, 2013). The aim of this chapter is not to reiterate the biological characteristics and clinical understanding of brucellosis (Godfroid *et al.*, 2011; Zinsstag *et al.*, 2011). We summarize briefly key features of zoonotic brucellosis in Box 14.1. In this chapter, we instead concentrate on the way in which a One Health approach to brucellosis surveillance and control provides significant additional value when compared to human health or veterinary

*E-mail: jakob.zinsstag@unibas.ch

**Box 14.1.** Zoonotic brucellosis.

Brucellosis is one of the world's major zoonoses (Dean *et al.*, 2012b). Human infection results mainly from direct contact with infected animals (often occupational exposure) or by the consumption of contaminated raw milk or dairy products (consumer exposure). The most important causative agents are *B. melitensis* (sheep and goats), *B. abortus* (cattle), *B. suis* (pigs) and *B. canis* (dogs). *Brucella* are gram-negative coccobacillary bacteria with an intracellular predilection in the host. The main clinical feature in livestock is late-stage abortion, at which time bacteria are excreted in high numbers. *Brucella* may be shed during prolonged periods in milk after the cessation of clinical signs. Brucellosis causes mainly a loss of fertility and a reduction of milk production in sheep, goats and cattle.

Symptoms of the disease in people are highly variable. In general, *B. melitensis* causes a more severe illness, with less severe forms caused by *B. suis* and *B. abortus*. The main symptoms are fever, sweats, malaise, anorexia, headache, arthralgia, myalgia, backache and weight loss (Dean *et al.*, 2012a). The bacteria can localize anywhere in the body. Two-thirds of the cases become chronic and the illness can continue for years if patients do not receive appropriate treatment (Roth *et al.*, 2003). There is no or very rare human-to-human transmission of brucellosis. Acute human brucellosis without complications should be treated with combination therapy of doxycycline-streptomycin or doxycycline-gentamicin. Focal forms often require prolonged treatment.

Human brucellosis can only be prevented by its elimination in animals. Control and elimination in the animal host is most effectively achieved by mass vaccination and, if possible, subsequent test-and-slaughter programmes (see Control of Brucellosis) (Zinsstag *et al.*, 2011).

studies alone. Most of the examples are from Central Asia and Africa. We focus on the added value of One Health joint surveillance, livestock–human epidemiological assessments, cross-sector economics and practical control options in developing countries.

## Joint Surveillance of Brucellosis in Humans and Livestock

To understand the transmission of brucellosis from livestock to people, simultaneous investigation in humans and animals may reveal an epidemiological linkage to the source of infection, the level of under-reporting of cases or serve as the basis for animal–human transmission models (Godfroid *et al.*, 2011). Such results cannot be obtained from studies in animals or humans alone and thus represent a clear added value of joint animal–human investigation (Schelling and Hattendorf, Chapter 10, this volume). Godfroid and colleagues rightly point out the weaknesses of brucellosis serological studies with regard to *Brucella* species identification and the importance of *Brucella* strain isolation and characterization (Godfroid *et al.*, 2013a). In a livestock–human seroprevalence study in mobile pastoralists in Chad, no association between human seroprevalence and herd level seroprevalence in cattle, sheep or goats could be established. A single strain isolated from cattle was identified as *B. abortus* (Schelling *et al.*, 2003). However, in a larger representative cross-sectional study in cattle, sheep, goats and humans in Kyrgyzstan, human seroprevalence was associated with seroprevalence in sheep at the district level (Zinsstag *et al.*, 2009; Bonfoh *et al.*, 2012; Kasymbekov *et al.*, 2013) (Box 14.2).

The important role of sheep in the transmission dynamics of brucellosis in Kyrgyzstan could be further substantiated by the isolation and characterization of *B. melitensis* from both sheep and cattle. However, no human brucellosis strains from Kyrgyzstan have been characterized as yet to ascertain the animal source (Kasymbekov *et al.*, 2013). Multilocus variable number of tandem repeat analysis (MLVA) of *B. melitensis* in China showed homologous patterns in humans and goats from the Zheijiang region (Jiang *et al.*, 2013), indicating that goats are likely a source of transmission. But there were also homologous strains from geographically unrelated areas. In the first joint epidemiological study of human and animal brucellosis in Togo, livestock seropositivity was restricted to cattle only, with no seropositive small ruminants. *Brucella abortus* was

**Box 14.2.** Estimating incidence of clinical brucellosis from seroprevalence data.

A catalytic model was used to estimate human clinical brucellosis incidence from seroprevalence data, assuming that brucellosis antibodies would be detectable for 10.9 years after exposure (Eqns 14.1–14.3). In endemic stable transmission, Eqns 14.1 and 14.2 (the change in the number of susceptible and infected individuals over time, respectively) can be set to zero. The seroprevalence $P = I/(S+I)$ (where $I$ and $S$ are the numbers of infected and susceptible people, respectively) is then equal to $a/(a+b)$, where $a$ is the incidence of exposure and $b$ is the immunity loss rate. Solving for $a$ returns the incidence of exposure, of which 10–50% of new human cases may have clinical symptoms (Tsend *et al.*, 2014). However, the model cannot distinguish between acute and chronic cases or relapses. Given an apparent human seroprevalence of 8.8%, as determined by a serological survey conducted in Kyrgyzstan, the incidence of brucellosis exposure is estimated to be 880 per 100,000 per year (Bonfoh *et al.*, 2012).

$$\frac{\partial S}{\partial t} = -aS + bI \tag{14.1}$$

$$\frac{\partial I}{\partial t} = aS - bI \tag{14.2}$$

$$P = \frac{a}{(a+b)} \tag{14.3}$$

isolated from cattle joint hygromas. Brucellosis did not appear to be a human health problem in the study zone despite the evidence of exposure in the cattle population. It may be possible that the Togolese *B. abortus* has only a low potential for transmission or a lower pathogenic potential to humans (Dean *et al.*, 2013). The isolated *B. abortus* strains from cattle harboured a large deletion in a gene *bruAb2_0168*. This gene is of particular interest because it is used as a PCR target for the identification of the species *B. abortus* and it encodes a putative autotransporter which might be involved in virulence and/or host predilection (Dean *et al.*, 2014). Further laboratory-based virulence and epidemiological studies will likely better explain the observations from the field.

A recent study of human and animal brucellosis seroprevalence in Mongolia found a high human seroprevalence of 17% among rural populations which were likely to be exposed to brucellosis, suggesting significant under-reporting (Tsend *et al.*, 2014). Human seroprevalence was not associated with small ruminant and cattle seroprevalence. Among seropositive people, 58.5% had at least two symptoms and 31.5% at least three symptoms indicating active clinical brucellosis (Tsend *et al.*, 2014). Stratification of livestock seroprevalence by the age of the animal allows the estimation of the basic reproductive ratio, which is the number of secondary infections that one infectious individual may induce in a naive population (Zinsstag *et al.*, Chapter 11, this volume) (Box 14.3).

In light of the animal–human brucellosis studies mentioned above, it can be assumed that the assessment of brucellosis at the animal–human interface is influenced by the diagnostic testing methods used, the predominant circulating *Brucella* species, as well as contact networks and spatial heterogeneities (i.e. non-uniform distribution of disease frequency). A significant human–animal linkage is more likely to be detected at a higher spatial resolution (e.g. national level) than in a smaller geographical area (e.g. household, district or village level). A combination of serological and bacteriological studies in animals and humans proves to be a powerful tool to characterize the transmission of brucellosis from various livestock reservoirs to people and within livestock.

The consequences of a more comprehensive approach for surveillance are far reaching. The cross-sectional studies presented here, which can be considered to be active surveillance, show epidemiological linkages. Such joint human and animal surveillance can also be passive, with recording of cases in humans and animals within each respective sector whilst ensuring timely communication and joint action plans. In Mongolia, based on 10 years of

**Box 14.3.** Calculating $R_0$ from age prevalence data of livestock.

The basic reproductive ratio ($R_0$) of a disease is the number of secondary cases generated from one infectious case in a susceptible population at the onset of transmission, thereby giving an indication of the ability of the disease to spread within a population. Age prevalence data was used to estimate the basic reproductive ratio in sheep ($R_0$=1.03), goats (1.02) (*B. melitensis*) and cattle (1.09) (*B.abortus*), using the likelihood function for $R_0$ related to the age distribution of seropositive and seronegative animals (Eqn 14.4) (Baljinnyam, 2014), whereby μ is the average age and *a* and *b* are the respective ages of seropositive and seronegative animals at the time of sampling. Given that the estimated $R_0$ values for each species are close to 1, this indicates low-level endemic stable transmission of brucellosis in extensive pastoralist settings of Mongolia (Keeling, 2008).

$$\text{Likelihood} R_0 = \prod_{a=1}^{n} e^{(-a\mu(R_0-1))} \prod_{b=1}^{m} (1 - e^{(-b\mu(R_0-1))} \quad (14.4)$$

The values of $R_0$ calculated based on age prevalence data are lower than the effective $R_e$ estimated from a transmission model where $R_e$ = 1.2 and 1.7 for sheep and cattle, respectively (see below). The effective reproductive number $R_e$ represents the number of secondary infections during ongoing transmission, i.e. a non-naive population (Box 14.4). With regard to use of $R_0$ to calculate the minimum needed immunization coverage to interrupt transmission, it is appropriate to use the higher estimates of $R_e$ = 1.2 and 1.7. Assuming more conservatively $R_0$ = 2, a minimum threshold vaccination coverage $p_c$ of 80% is proposed for the Mongolian livestock population (Zinsstag *et al.*, 2005). The threshold vaccination coverage $p_c$ indicates the proportion of animals (sheep, goats and cattle) that should be immunized to interrupt transmission. It is calculated using Eqn 14.5. The term *v* is the efficacy of the vaccines (Rev1 and S19) in reducing transmission, which is assumed conservatively to be 65% including an assumed loss of efficacy from disruptions in the cold chain. More epidemiological research is needed to estimate the $R_0$ and $p_c$ of brucellosis in other contexts.

$$p_c = \frac{\left(1 - \frac{1}{R_0}\right)}{v} \quad (14.5)$$

official livestock serological data and routine reporting of human brucellosis cases, the first livestock–human brucellosis transmission model was developed (Zinsstag *et al.*, Chapter 11, this volume). Joint surveillance is also a critical element in the follow-up of interventions such as mass vaccination of livestock. Surveys of vaccination coverage can be done in the very same way by the concurrent assessment of livestock vaccination antibodies and the prevailing number of reported human cases. Such assessments will provide a sound evidence base for the success of the implementation of mass vaccination at high coverage.

## Animal–Human Brucellosis Transmission Models

Livestock–human transmission dynamics and the effects of mass vaccination of livestock on animal and human disease cannot be captured by linear statistical models. They are governed by non-linear processes, which require a mathematical approach. Time-series brucellosis data from animals and humans can be used for the development of animal–human mathematical transmission models. A simple compartmental deterministic model of livestock brucellosis transmission was developed, based on Mongolian government data on reported human cases and livestock serological data from 1990 to 1999 (Zinsstag *et al.*, 2005; Zinsstag *et al.*, Chapter 11, this volume). The model provided the mechanism for the simulation of animal–animal and animal–human transmission and the measurement of the estimated effect of animal vaccination on human brucellosis incidence (Fig. 14.1). It can be observed that the number of human cases decreases at varying rates depending on the proportion of livestock immunized. An intervention in livestock thus

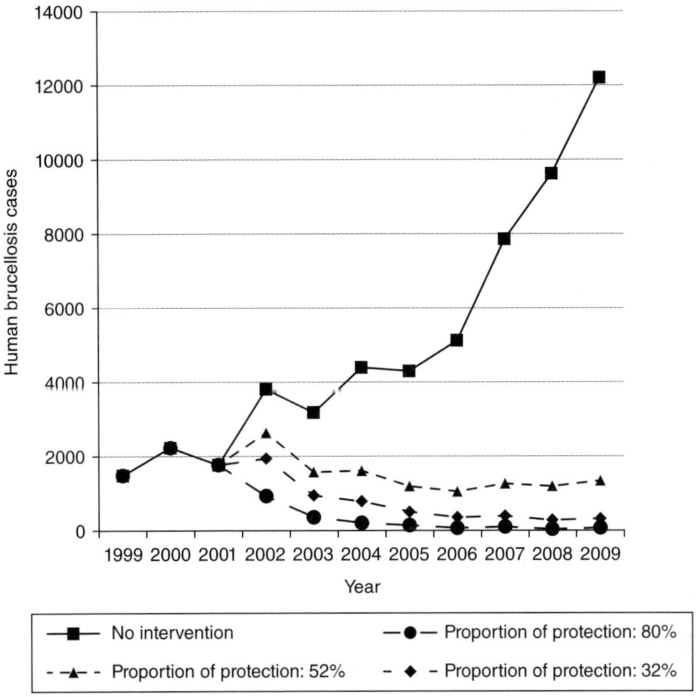


**Fig. 14.1.** Effect of livestock brucellosis vaccination of small ruminants and cattle populations on human annual cumulative incidence (adapted from Zinsstag *et al.*, 2005).

indirectly reduces the number of human brucellosis cases.

The small ruminant–small ruminant transmission constant (contact rate between infectious and susceptible individuals) (1.56 $e^{-7}$ (sheep × year)$^{-1}$) is 13 times higher than the small ruminant–human transmission constant (1.13 $e^{-8}$ (sheep × year)$^{-1}$). The cattle–cattle transmission constant (3.49 $e^{-7}$ (cattle × year)$^{-1}$) is 165 times higher than the cattle–human transmission constant of 2.11 $e^{-9}$ (cattle × year)$^{-1}$. The cattle–human transmission constant is five times lower than the small ruminant–human transmission constant. If the transmission constants are corrected for between-animal transmission, the cattle–human transmission efficiency is less than 10% of the efficiency of small ruminant–human transmission These findings indicate that in the given Mongolian livestock production system and husbandry practices, *B. abortus* is less easily transmitted to humans than *B. melitensis* and that the principal source of infection for people is small ruminants.

This should be interpreted with some caution, considering the risk of bias and under-reporting in routinely reported data and the difficulty in interpreting brucellosis serological data (Godfroid *et al.*, 2013a). Out of 11 Mongolian human brucellosis strains from a recent study, ten were *B. melitensis* and one was *B. abortus* (Baljinnyam, 2014), which would support the above observations. In the above model, the spill-over of *B. melitensis* to cattle was omitted. This could be introduced when more data are available on the proportion of *B. melitensis* and *B. abortus* isolated from Mongolian cattle.

Livestock–human brucellosis transmission models combined with molecular epidemiological studies provide insight into the interface between humans and animals and allow the quantification of the disease transmission dynamics between livestock, humans and reservoir hosts (Box 14.4). At the same time, such models serve as a backbone to a cross-sector economic analysis.

**Box 14.4.** Using transmission models to assess the persistence of brucellosis transmission in pastoral areas.

The change in the number of newly infected animals *I* can be considered to be at equilibrium if Eqn 14.6 can be set equal to zero. The effective reproductive ratio $R_e$ is determined by the geo-spatial density of susceptible animals *S*. If $R_e$ is greater than 1, transmission is ongoing; if it is less than 1, transmission is interrupted. Using estimated values for the parameters β (transmission constant, which is a multiplicative relationship of the capacity of transmission of the bacterium and the contact pattern between susceptible *S* and infectious animals *I*), γ (the proportion of infectious animals among the seropositive) and μ (mortality of infected animals), the threshold density of susceptible animals resulting in $R_e$ falling below 1 can be estimated, meaning that transmission is no longer maintained. In the Mongolian context, $R_e$ drops below 1 if the density of cattle is lower than 1.2 (min. 0.6, max. 8) cattle per km² and if the density of small ruminants is lower than 6.8 (min. 4.5, max. 21) small ruminants per km² (Racloz *et al.*, 2013).

$$\frac{\partial I}{\partial t} = -\gamma \beta S I - \mu I \tag{14.6}$$

$$R_e = \frac{\gamma \beta s}{\mu} \tag{14.7}$$

## Cross-sector Economics of Brucellosis

Brucellosis results in public and private health costs as well as major losses to livestock production. These costs vary in a non-linear way depending on the intensity of transmission or the effectiveness of an intervention as captured by animal–human transmission models (see above). A detailed description of such a cross-sector economic analysis is provided in Zinsstag *et al.* (Chapter 12, this volume), based on the work of Roth and colleagues (Roth *et al.*, 2003). There is very little information available on the impact of brucellosis on livestock production (Bernues *et al.*, 1997). The effect of brucellosis on African and Asian cattle and small-ruminant productivity is not known. Brucellosis mainly affects herd fertility and reduces milk production. In susceptible pregnant animals, most may abort in what is referred to as an 'abortion storm'. Subsequently, the frequency of abortions will be low under endemic circumstances. For the purpose of demographic simulation, we relate an overall reduction of fertility to brucellosis seroprevalence. The reduction of fertility, i.e. the annual calving rate per fertile female in a herd with brucellosis, can be calculated as baseline fertility *f* multiplied by a prevalence-dependent decrease (Eqn 14.8). For example, if the baseline fertility is 75% calving per fertile female per year, the overall fertility of a herd with a 10% seroprevalence and a 15% decrease of fertility because of abortions would be 73.9% (Bernues *et al.*, 1997).

$$f_{\text{disease}} = f_{\text{baseline}} \,(1 - (\text{proportion of decrease} \times \text{seroprevalence})) \tag{14.8}$$

Such a decrease in fertility may appear small but it has a significant effect on total animal numbers and livestock product availability such as meat and milk. For the estimation of losses to livestock production, comprehensive livestock demographic models are needed. One such example is the livestock development planning system (LDPS) of the Food and Agriculture Organization of the United Nations (FAO; Roth *et al.*, 2003).

Costs to human health and livestock production can be combined in a broader framework for assessing the economic impact of brucellosis. The top portion of Fig. 14.2 shows the importance of the first two sections of this chapter (joint surveillance and joint disease transmission models). The disease impact is assessed as costs to human health and livestock production both at the household and at national levels (Narrod *et al.*, 2012; McDermott *et al.*, 2013). For the assessment of interventions, reduced health costs and improved livestock production are valued against the cost of the intervention in terms of profitability. The cost-effectiveness of an intervention or, in other words, the cost to achieve a reduced burden of illness

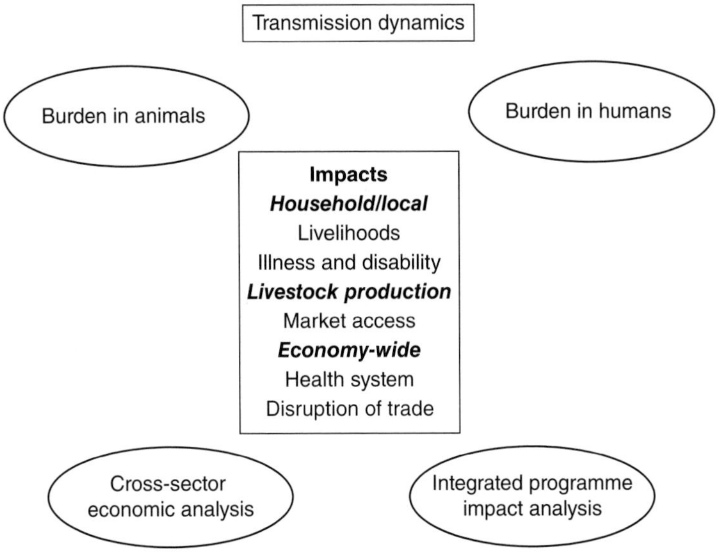


**Fig. 14.2.** Framework for assessing economic impacts of brucellosis linked to burden of disease, diagnostics, epidemiology and control programme considerations (adapted from Narrod *et al.*, 2012 and McDermott *et al.*, 2013).

in people, is expressed as the cost per number of disability adjusted live years (DALYs) averted. The advantage of such a One Health economic assessment is that it reveals broader societal benefits and options for cost-sharing scenarios between different sectors. While mass vaccination of livestock against brucellosis is not profitable to the public health sector alone, it becomes profitable if the benefits to all sectors are cumulated (Zinsstag *et al.*, Chapter 12, this volume). Such an overall benefit would not be apparent without a cross-sectoral human and animal economic analysis. Economic analyses are important steps in the process of disease control and elimination, especially in low income and transition countries. Ultimately, effective control programmes require close cross-sectoral coordination within an environment that fosters and enables such activities (Zinsstag *et al.*, 2012). The development of a health-related government policy often first requires the demonstration of benefits and the efficacy of interventions (e.g. the use of conjunctival versus subcutaneous livestock vaccination) within a country or a livestock production system.

## Control of Brucellosis

Effective interventions against brucellosis must be supported by certain enabling conditions: (i) public or private veterinary services that fully cover the geographical area of the intervention and have sufficient equipment and staff; (ii) there must be sufficient capacity of human health and veterinary laboratories at district and provincial levels to handle the testing of blood samples, as well as a laboratory at the central level that can cultivate and identify the pathogen – the vaccination of livestock requires an operational cold chain and trained veterinarians; and (iii) a reliable electricity supply is needed to produce vaccines (which should only be done where adequate technical capacity, high level biosafety and stringent quality control are available) and to keep vaccines cooled until they reach the animals to be vaccinated.

If test-and-slaughter systems are implemented, sufficient public funds to compensate farmers for culled stock and a relatively corruption-free environment is a condition *sine qua non*. If farmers are not compensated, they may sell infected animals illegally, thereby contributing to continued transmission of brucellosis. Further enabling requirements are an animal registration system with movement traceability and appropriate management and monitoring of the control programme, e.g. sufficient human resources, well-designed protocols and guidelines, ongoing assessment of incoming data and the ability to respond in a timely manner. Mobile livestock production systems, including nomadic or transhumant practices, allow the intermixing of tested and untested herds, thus rendering a test-and-slaughter approach impossible.

If brucellosis is detected in livestock, mass vaccination of livestock should be the first option, regardless of the number of animals infected. It is safer and the best practice for female animals to be vaccinated using eye drops (conjunctival vaccination) rather than a subcutaneous administration using a syringe. Different reservoir species require different types of vaccine: sheep and goats should be vaccinated with *B. melitensis* Rev-1 and cattle and yaks with an attenuated *B. abortus* S19 strain, depending on the knowledge of the principal reservoir species. Overall, more than 80% of the animals in an area should be vaccinated every year to reduce the risk of disease transmission (Box 14.3). Sheep and goats of any age and sex can be vaccinated using eye drops, including lactating animals. However, it is essential that vaccination takes place before the mating season, as vaccinating pregnant sheep can induce abortion. Vaccine-related abortions are more severe following subcutaneous vaccination in sheep and goats. In cattle, female animals of all ages can be vaccinated, but never males (Zinsstag *et al.*, 2012). The vaccine quality must be tested prior to annual campaigns. Vaccines should be procured from reliable sources (Zinsstag *et al.*, 2012).

A mass vaccination campaign should be followed after 3 weeks by a monitoring programme to assess the proportion of vaccinated animals. The recording of new human cases provides additional information on how effective the campaign has been. The number of new human cases should drop, although this will not be immediate, as infected animals are not culled during such a campaign and will remain in herds for several years. We lack sufficient knowledge on the outcome of vaccinating brucellosis-infected animals. Livestock vaccination campaigns raise awareness of the disease and subsequently more human patients may present themselves to health centres. It may therefore be most appropriate to monitor the incidence of human brucellosis for a period of several years after the implementation of the vaccination campaign.

A comprehensive follow-up of mass vaccination campaigns by coverage surveys and the monitoring of human cases provides the necessary information on the overall effectiveness of livestock mass vaccination and, if done well, is the One Health key to the success of brucellosis control. For this purpose, a workforce of district and provincial veterinarians and physicians should be trained in basic epidemiology and statistics, enabling them to plan, run and analyse vaccination coverage surveys and cross-sectoral prevalence surveys independently. The doctors need to evaluate the capacities of the primary health centres for human patients in light of the necessary human resources, diagnostic tools and drugs for treatment. The training of veterinarians and physicians should focus on identification of where corrective actions of implementation of national policies are most effective. Training together for brucellosis monitoring has a strong team-building effect and provides additional strength to control efforts. Monitoring teams should be independent from vaccination teams to ensure an independent, non-biased assessment. Involving communities and local authorities in the development of acceptable vaccination schemes creates ownership and encourages adherence to jointly decided activities (Schelling *et al.*, 2007). Microbiologists and molecular biologists should be trained in brucellosis isolation and characterization in order to monitor circulating and possible vaccine strains during ongoing brucellosis control. Brucellosis mass vaccination schemes could be further combined with other interventions, for example, foot and mouth disease (FMD), contagious bovine pleuropneumonia (CBPP) or rabies vaccinations. However, we have hardly any knowledge on the safety and efficacy of combined vaccination schemes, despite the fact that this has been recently identified as a priority by the FAO. Asian countries should share their experiences with African countries having no or very little experience with the implementation of brucellosis control strategies, including brucellosis vaccination in livestock. Conversely, African countries could inform Asian countries on the vaccination of livestock against anthrax. In Central Asia and Africa, with frequent cross-border mobility of pastoralist herds, regional control programmes should be envisaged.

Behaviour change communication strategies should be carried out in parallel to epidemiological interventions within the context of the control programme. Such activities require the expertise of social scientists to address effectively risk behaviours such as the consumption of unpasteurized dairy products, the handling of abortion materials and lack of hand-washing practices after contact with livestock, but particularly to identify locally adapted practices to lower exposure not only to brucellosis but also to other harmful zoonotic diseases. After such information campaigns, one would expect an increase of brucellosis patients seeking diagnosis and treatment at health centres. The additional need for diagnostic/treatment capacity should be anticipated and accounted for when monitoring the impact.

## Conclusion

A One Health approach contributes to brucellosis control at various levels, creating an added value that can only be achieved by human and animal health working closely together:

**1.** Joint human and animal surveillance reduces the time to the detection of the main source of human infection and thereby allows more targeted control interventions and allows an assessment of the level of under-reporting.
**2.** Molecular epidemiological studies, including *Brucella* strains isolated from humans and animals in the same setting, allow the ascertainment of the source of human infection.
**3.** Livestock–human transmission models demonstrate and quantify the effect of interventions in animals on public health, which cannot be shown by studying transmission in humans and livestock in isolation.
**4.** Cross-sectoral economic assessment of brucellosis control by mass vaccination of livestock demonstrates that, from a societal point of view, brucellosis control is cost-beneficial whereas from a public health perspective alone, it is not.
**5.** One Health brucellosis studies inform policy and control programmes as well as behaviour change strategies, advocating for much stronger collaboration between human and animal health sectors and other related disciplines, including a possible sharing of disease intervention costs.

A One Health approach thus clearly provides additional scientific insight, which is of eminent practical relevance for the control and elimination of brucellosis.

## References


Baljinnyam, Z. (2014) Molecular epidemiologiy of animal and human brucellosis in Mongolia. Unpublished PhD thesis, University of Basel, Basel, Switzerland.

Bernues, A., Manrique, E. and Maza, M.T. (1997) Economic evaluation of bovine brucellosis and tuberculosis eradication programmes in a mountain area of Spain. *Preventive Veterinary Medicine* 30(2), 137–149.

Bonfoh, B., Kasymbekov, J., Durr, S., Toktobaev, N., Doherr, M.G., Schueth, T., Zinsstag, J. and Schelling, E. (2012) Representative seroprevalences of brucellosis in humans and livestock in Kyrgyzstan. *EcoHealth* 9(2), 132–138.

Boukary, A.R., Saegerman, C., Abatih, E., Fretin, D., Alambedji Bada, R., De Deken, R., Harouna, H.A., Yenikoye, A. and Thys, E. (2013) Seroprevalence and potential risk factors for *Brucella* spp. infection in traditional cattle, sheep and goats reared in urban, periurban and rural areas of Niger. *PLoS One* 8(12), e83175.

Dean, A.S., Crump, L., Greter, H., Hattendorf, J., Schelling, E. and Zinsstag, J. (2012a) Clinical manifestations of human brucellosis: a systematic review and meta-analysis. *PLoS Neglected Tropical Diseases* 6(12), e1929.

Dean, A.S., Crump, L., Greter, H., Schelling, E. and Zinsstag, J. (2012b) Global burden of human brucellosis: a systematic review of disease frequency. *PLoS Neglected Tropical Diseases* 6(10), e1865.

Dean, A.S., Bonfoh, B., Kulo, A.E., Boukaya, G.A., Amidou, M., Hattendorf, J., Pilo, P. and Schelling, E. (2013) Epidemiology of brucellosis and Q-fever in linked human and animal populations in northern Togo. *PLoS One* 8(8), e71501.

Dean, A.S., Schelling, E.,Bonfoh, B., Kulo, A.E., Boukaya, G.A. and Pilo, P. (2014) Deletion in the gene BruAb2_0168 of *Brucella abortus* strains: diagnostic challenges. *Clinical Microbiology and Infection* (in press).

Godfroid, J., Scholz, H.C., Barbier, T., Nicolas, C., Wattiau, P., Fretin, D., Whatmore, A.M., Cloeckaert, A., Blasco, J.M., Moriyon, I., Saegerman, C., Muma, J.B., Al Dahouk, S., Neubauer, H. and Letesson, J.J. (2011) Brucellosis at the animal/ecosystem/human interface at the beginning of the 21st century. *Preventive Veterinary Medicine* 102(2), 118–131.

Godfroid, J., Al Dahouk, S., Pappas, G., Roth, F., Matope, G., Muma, J., Marcotty, T., Pfeiffer, D. and Skjerve, E. (2013a) A 'One Health' surveillance and control of brucellosis in developing countries: moving away from improvisation. *Comparative Immunology, Microbiology and Infectious Diseases* 36(3), 241–248.

Godfroid, J., Garin-Bastuji, B., Saegerman, C. and Blasco, J.M. (2013b) Brucellosis in terrestrial wildlife. *Revue Scientifique et Technique* 32(1), 27–42.

Jiang, H., Wang, H., Xu, L., Hu, G., Ma, J., Xiao, P., Fan, W., Di, D., Tian, G., Fan, M., Mi, J., Yu, R., Song, L., Zhao, H., Piao, D. and Cui, B. (2013) MLVA genotyping of *Brucella melitensis* and *Brucella abortus* isolates from different animal species and humans and identification of *Brucella suis* vaccine strain S2 from cattle in China. *PLoS One* 8(10), e76332.

Kasymbekov, J., Imanseitov, J., Ballif, M., Schurch, N., Paniga, S., Pilo, P., Tonolla, M., Benagli, C., Akylbekova, K., Jumakanova, Z., Schelling, E. and Zinsstag, J. (2013) Molecular epidemiology and antibiotic susceptibility of livestock *Brucella melitensis* isolates from Naryn Oblast, Kyrgyzstan. *PLoS Neglected Tropical Diseases* 7(2), e2047.

Keeling, M.J.R.P. (2008) *Modeling Infectious Disease*. Princeton University Press, Princeton, New Jersey.

Li, Y.J., Li, X.L., Liang, S., Fang, L.Q. and Cao, W.C. (2013) Epidemiological features and risk factors associated with the spatial and temporal distribution of human brucellosis in China. *BMC Infectious Diseases* 13(1), 547.

Marcotty, T., Matthys, F., Godfroid, J., Rigouts, L., Ameni, G., Gey van, P.N., Kazwala, R., Muma, J., van, H.P., Walravens, K., de Klerk, L.M., Geoghegan, C., Mbotha, D., Otte, M., Amenu, K., Abu, S.N., Botha, C., Ekron, M., Jenkins, A., Jori, F., Kriek, N., McCrindle, C., Michel, A., Morar, D., Roger, F., Thys, E. and Van Den, B.P. (2009) Zoonotic tuberculosis and brucellosis in Africa: neglected zoonoses or minor public-health issues? The outcomes of a multi-disciplinary workshop. *Annals of Tropical Medicine and Parasitology* 103(5), 401–411.

McDermott, J., Grace, D. and Zinsstag, J. (2013) Economics of brucellosis impact and control in low-income countries. *Revue Scientifique et Technique* 32(1), 249–261.

Narrod, C., Zinsstag, J. and Tiongco, M. (2012) A one health framework for estimating the economic costs of zoonotic diseases on society. *EcoHealth* 9(2), 150–162.

Pappas, G., Papadimitriou, P., Akritidis, N., Christou, L. and Tsianos, E.V. (2006) The new global map of human brucellosis. *Lancet Infectious Diseases* 6(2), 91–99.

Plumb, G.E., Olsen, S.C. and Buttke, D. (2013) Brucellosis: 'One Health' challenges and opportunities. *Revue Scientifique et Technique* 32(1), 271–278.

Racloz, V., Schelling, E., Chitnis, N., Roth, F. and Zinsstag, J. (2013) Persistence of brucellosis in pastoral systems. *Revue Scientifique et Technique* 32(1), 61–70.

Roth, F., Zinsstag, J., Orkhon, D., Chimed-Ochir, G., Hutton, G., Cosivi, O., Carrin, G. and Otte, J. (2003) Human health benefits from livestock vaccination for brucellosis: case study. *Bulletin of the World Health Organization* 81(12), 867–876.

Schelling, E., Diguimbaye, C., Daoud, S., Nicolet, J., Boerlin, P., Tanner, M. and Zinsstag, J. (2003) Brucellosis and Q-fever seroprevalences of nomadic pastoralists and their livestock in Chad. *Preventive Veterinary Medicine* 61(4), 279–293.

Schelling, E., Wyss, K., Diguimbaye, C., Bechir, M., Taleb, M.O., Bonfoh, B., Tanner, M. and Zinnstag, J. (2007) Towards integrated and adapted health services for nomadic pastoralists. In: Hirsch Hadorn, G., Hoffmann-Reim, H., Biber-Klemm, S., Grossenbacher, W., Joye, D., Pohl, C., Wiesmann, U. and Zemp, E. (eds) *Handbook of Transdisciplinary Research*. Springer, Heidelberg, pp. 277–291.

Tsend, S., Baljinnyam, Z., Suuri, B., Dahbal, E., Zinsstag, J., Roth, F., Oidov, B., Schelling, E. and Dambadarjaa, D. (2014) Representative survey on human brucellosis among rural people in Mongolia. *Western Pacific Surveillance and Response Journal* (in press).

Zinsstag, J., Roth, F., Orkhon, D., Chimed-Ochir, G., Nansalmaa, M., Kolar, J. and Vounatsou, P. (2005) A model of animal-human brucellosis transmission in Mongolia. *Preventive Veterinary Medicine* 69(1–2), 77–95.

Zinsstag, J., Schelling, E., Bonfoh, B., Fooks, A.R., Kasymbekov, J., Waltner-Toews, D. and Tanner, M. (2009) Towards a 'one health' research and application tool box. *Veterinaria Italiana* 45(1), 121–133.

Zinsstag, J., Schelling, E., Solera, J., Blasco, J. and Moriyon, I. (2011) Brucellosis. In: Palmer, S., Soulsby, L., Torgerson, P. and Brown, D. (eds) *Oxford Textbook of Zoonoses*. Oxford University Press, Oxford, UK, pp. 54–62.

Zinsstag, J., Kasymbekov, J., Schelling, E. and Bonfoh, B. (2012) It's time to control brucellosis in Central Asia. In: Aryonova, M. and Bonfoh, B. (eds) *Evidence for Policy Series, Regional Edition Central Asia*, No 2. Bishkek, Kyrgyzstan and Abidjan, Côte d'Ivoire. pp. 1–4.

# 15 Bovine Tuberculosis at the Human–Livestock–Wildlife Interface in Sub-Saharan Africa

**Rea Tschopp***
*Swiss Tropical and Public Health Institute, Basel, Switzerland; University of Basel, Basel, Switzerland; and Armauer Hansen Research Institute, Addis Ababa, Ethiopia*

## Introduction

The majority (60%) of all infectious diseases are of zoonotic nature and of these over two-thirds have a wildlife reservoir (Jones *et al.*, 2008). Livestock diseases cause the loss of more than 40% of the global food supply. While threatening the economy of developing nations and food security, livestock diseases cost globally US$200 billion in the last 10 years in loss of trade, tourism and tax revenue (Cartin-Rojas, 2012).

The outbreaks of SARS in 2002 in China, Nipah in Malaysia and recently Mers virus in the Middle East are some of the zoonoses highlighting the importance of wildlife reservoirs for human health. However, the main drivers for infectious disease outbreaks and emerging infectious diseases (EID) remain human population density and growth and their associated anthropogenic land-use change (Daszak *et al.*, 2001; Patz *et al.*, 2004; Jones *et al.*, 2008).

This chapter focuses on bovine tuberculosis (BTB) in sub-Saharan Africa, which is an example of a pathogen shared at the human–livestock–wildlife interface. It will describe how interfaces are multiple, fluid and dynamic in nature, and very poorly studied in the African context. The importance of wildlife in sub-Saharan Africa will be highlighted and the chapter will conclude with the One Health approach to control the disease and illustrate its societal benefit from the wildlife side.

## Bovine Tuberculosis

Bovine tuberculosis is a bacterial disease found in humans, livestock and wildlife. It is caused by *Mycobacterium bovis*, a bacterium belonging to the mycobacterium tuberculosis complex (MTC), a group of seven genetically and clinically closely related *Mycobacteria* species that show host preferences. Some MTC, such as the human-associated *M. tuberculosis*, *M. africanum* and *M. canetti*, and the predominantly rodent pathogen *M. microti*, are host specific while others (*M. bovis*, *M. caprae*) have a broader host range (Brosch *et al.*, 2002; Mostowy *et al.*, 2005; Smith *et al.*, 2006; de Jong *et al.*, 2010). Domestic cattle are the main host for *M. bovis* (Cosivi *et al.*, 1998). However, a wide range of domestic and wildlife mammals can acquire the disease and act either as reservoir or spill-over hosts (de Lisle *et al.*, 2002). A reservoir host is defined as having a persistent BTB infection within the population even in

*E-mail: rea.tschopp@unibas.ch

the absence of a constant infection source and can thus transmit the agent to other species. Spill-over hosts, on the other hand, have only limited capacity of maintaining the disease in their populations if a persistent source of infection is absent (Renwick *et al.*, 2007). Some classical examples of known wildlife reservoir hosts are the brushtail possum (*Trichosurus vulpecula*) in New Zealand, the Eurasian badger (*Meles meles*) in the UK and the African buffalo (*Syncerus caffer*) in Southern Africa (Coleman and Cooke, 2001; Rodwell *et al.*, 2001; Griffin *et al.*, 2005).

The main routes of disease transmission are by inhalation or ingestion of infected raw animal products (Cosivi *et al.*, 1998). In most industrialized countries, BTB has been eliminated or controlled through costly national test and slaughter programmes as well as decades of milk pasteurization. However, there is a resurgence of BTB for instance in Spain and the UK, linked to existing wildlife reservoirs (Phillips *et al.*, 2003; Naranjo *et al.*, 2008). The disease remains largely prevalent in sub-Saharan Africa, where the control programmes are often logistically and financially not feasible (Ayele *et al.*, 2004).

## Bovine tuberculosis in African livestock

BTB is endemic in sub-Saharan African cattle and has been reported in 42 of the 54 African nations (de Garine-Wichatitsky *et al.*, 2013). Prevalence varies across the regions, the breeds involved and the husbandry type. Higher prevalence is generally found in exotic and cross-breeds, which were found to be more susceptible to *M. bovis* than local breeds (Vordermeier *et al.*, 2012). Prevalence tends to be higher in intensive husbandry dairy systems (found usually in urban and peri-urban areas) than in traditional rural extensive husbandry systems (Fofana, 2003; Diguimbaye-Djaibé *et al.*, 2006; Müller *et al.*, 2008; Tschopp *et al.*, 2010c; Boukary *et al.*, 2011; Firdessa *et al.*, 2012; Swai and Schoonman, 2012). Three clonal complexes of *M. bovis* (European 1, African 1 and 2) have been characterized in cattle in Africa to date suggesting geographical clustering of the pathogen and possibly shedding some light on the evolutionary history of BTB in Africa (Müller *et al.*, 2009; Berg *et al.*, 2011; Smith *et al.*, 2011). For instance, European 1 clonal complex was isolated in cattle from Zambia, South Africa and Tanzania, suggesting pathogen movement between the UK and these countries (Smith *et al.*, 2011). The origin of both African clonal complexes is still unknown.

## Bovine tuberculosis in African wildlife

In Africa, the first cases of BTB in free-ranging wildlife were described in the early 20th century in Uganda and South Africa (Paine and Martinaglia, 1929; Gallagher *et al.*, 1972; Woodford, 1982a,b). Later, the African buffalo and the lechwe (*Kobus leche*) were found to be BTB reservoir hosts in Southern Africa (de Vos *et al.*, 2001; Caron *et al.*, 2003; Munyeme and Munang'andu, 2011). Greater kudus (*Tragelaphus strepsiceros*) and warthogs (*Phacochoerus africanus*) are also thought to be potential reservoirs (Michel *et al.*, 2006; Renwick *et al.*, 2007; Bengis, 2012). All wildlife mammals are susceptible to BTB. So far, BTB in sub-Saharan Africa has been described in at least two dozen wildlife species including carnivores, omnivores and herbivores (Woodford, 1982a,b; Tarara *et al.*, 1985; Keet *et al.*, 2000; Cleaveland *et al.*, 2005; Michel *et al.*, 2009; Katale *et al.*, 2012). The number of species hosting BTB is increasing and the disease is thus referred to as a dynamic multi-species-host–pathogen system (Renwick *et al.*, 2007). Prevalence studies at the continental level, however, are still lacking and confirmed cases originate from only five countries in Southern and Eastern Africa. According to the World Organisation for Animal Health (OIE), 33 out of 54 (61%) countries have no data at all on wildlife BTB (de Garine-Wichatitsky *et al.*, 2013).

## Bovine tuberculosis in humans

BTB cases reported in humans are few despite the disease being endemic in livestock, the often close relationship between people and livestock in rural Africa, and the lack of milk pasteurization and meat inspection. A meta-analysis by Müller *et al.* (2013) showed that a median 2.8% of all TB cases in humans were attributable to *M. bovis* in Africa, with significant country variations. In Ethiopia, Firdessa *et al.* (2013) found a minimal *M. bovis* involvement in human TB (4 out of 964 patients) despite high BTB prevalence in livestock. Transmission to humans through raw milk consumption seems also to be rare, probably due to inactivation of *M. bovis* through rapid fermentation processes commonly used (Kazwala *et al.*, 1998; Mariam, 2009). In a simultaneous human and cattle study in a pastoralist area of south-eastern Ethiopia, out of 163 human mycobacterium tuberculosis complex isolates three were *M. bovis*. One of them had the same spacer spoligotype as strains isolated from cattle in the same study area (Gumi *et al.*, 2012).

To date there are no published reports of direct BTB transmission from wildlife to humans in Africa (de Garine-Wichatitsky *et al.*, 2013). The direct risks are likely to be similar to those originating from livestock with the exception of raw milk consumption. Hence people at risk would include game-meat consumers, veterinarians, taxidermists, hunters and park staff. However, it is most likely that human cases are under-reported due to the lack of data gathered on human disease burden, the lack of diagnostic facilities and poor disease knowledge, particularly from the wildlife side.

## The Human–Livestock–Wildlife Interface

The concept of human–livestock–wildlife interface and One Health has been discussed extensively in the last decade, with various definitions of One Health given. Here the definition by Zinsstag (2012) is used: 'any added value in terms of human and animal health, financial savings or environmental benefits from closer cooperation of human and animal health sectors at all levels of organization'. It will be shown hereafter that a human–livestock–wildlife interface is not a standard concept but rather one that varies tremendously across sub-Saharan Africa depending on human, livestock and wildlife densities and their movements (e.g. migration, transhumance), wildlife species, environmental factors and anthropogenic land-use change. Detailed knowledge of the epidemiology and ecology at a particular interface is therefore essential before embarking on a One Health programme.

### Cattle densities

Domestication of livestock is believed to date back 10,000 years in the Levant and Near East (Prins, 2000). The history of the origin of the current African cattle breeds is still unclear and complex despite various theories (Hanotte *et al.*, 2000; Ibeagha-Awemu *et al.*, 2004). Exotic to sub-Saharan Africa, livestock are thought to have invaded habitats abounding with native locally adapted wild ungulates around 4000–5000 BC and moved southwards, probably on an eastern route (Prins, 2000; Hanotte *et al.*, 2002). Subsequent waves of *Bos indicus* cattle immigration from the east, European *B. taurus* more recently during the colonial era, and indigenous *B. taurus* breeds originating probably in northern Africa (Hanotte *et al.*, 2002) further contributed to the current genetic make-up, and probably the disease pool of the current African cattle population.

Sub-Saharan Africa has very diverse ecosystems, climates, vegetation and endemic diseases such as trypanosomiasis and theileriosis that are either conducive or not for agriculture and livestock keeping. Hence, diseases and agro-ecological zones have helped shape the agricultural landscape of Africa, leading to various livestock distributions and stocking densities. The pattern has been further shaped in recent decades by climate change with population declines in some arid areas (Lunde and Lindtjorn, 2013). East Africa holds over half of the total livestock population of sub-Saharan Africa, followed by West Africa (26.3%), Central Africa (5.8%) and Southern Africa (1.6%) (Ibrahim and Olaloku, 2000). Ethiopia and Sudan hold the largest share of the cattle population per country (FAOStat, 2014). These various livestock densities across the continent are thus likely to be an influencing factor for the livestock–wildlife contact dynamics and infection pressure at the interface.

### Cattle competition with wildlife

The co-existence between livestock, people and wildlife over millennia changed dramatically in the last half century as population growth exploded in Africa, leading to inevitable habitat and diet overlaps and hence competition between wild and domestic animals. The contact interface between animals and humans intensified rapidly and continues to do so, as natural resources become scarcer. Natural habitats continue to be changed into agricultural land (Patz *et al.*, 2004; Hibert *et al.*, 2010) and wildlife was extirpated as it became a competitor to livestock, a pest (e.g. crop damage) or a threat (e.g. predation), leading to a general dramatic wildlife population decline all over the continent (Grootenhuis and Olubayo, 1993; Norton-Griffiths, 2000; Prins, 2000; Gordon, 2009; Maisels *et al.*, 2013). Taxons related to the domestic bovid are particularly affected due to their similarity regarding physiology, ecology and biology (Gordon, 2009), which is consistent with the potential of disease sharing between the domestic cattle and their wild counterparts. In general, disease transmission from domestic animals to wildlife affects wildlife more severely than vice versa (Prins, 2000).

## Role of Wildlife/Importance of Wildlife

In past decades, a lot of research has been done on BTB prevalence in livestock, wildlife and humans in Africa. Interestingly, very little considered the interface of epidemiology and ecology and even less looked at the disease prevalence simultaneously in livestock, humans and wildlife in the same areas (Munyeme *et al.*, 2009; Tschopp *et al.*, 2010a).

In many sub-Saharan countries, wildlife plays a minor role in the economy of the countries, which is often reflected in low national budgets allocated for conservation and the country's priorities regarding their economy. A quarter of all people living below US$1/day are found in sub-Saharan Africa and a high proportion of the continent's human population is food insecure (Kock, 2005). Hence, the livestock sector remains the economic priority for many African countries, where 80% of rural farmers and pastoralists are directly dependent on their animals for daily subsistence and livelihood (Cartin-Rojas, 2012). Livestock are kept for meat, milk, blood, hides, manure and as economic assets. In countries like Ethiopia, cattle as draught animal are also intimately linked with agriculture (Tschopp *et al.*, 2010b). Livestock population growth in sub-Saharan Africa is projected to be 1.2% in the next few decades, with the main drivers believed to be increased demand for animal products, an increased economic status and achievement of food security (Thornton, 2010; Lunde and Lindtjorn, 2013). As seen in the rinderpest epidemic in the late 19th century, the wiping out of livestock throughout Africa led to severe famines due to direct loss of animal protein and also because of the loss of agricultural production due to the absence of draught animals.

Nevertheless, wildlife remains an important player in sub-Saharan Africa, for economic, animal and human health and conservation reasons.

Wildlife has important nutritional and economic value. For many African communities, bush-meat remains a major source of animal protein (Chardonnet *et al.*, 2002; Timah *et al.*, 2008). Live animals and bush-meat are also traded worldwide as a multi-billion US dollar per year industry. For the most part, the international wildlife trade is illegal and thus uncontrolled, putting people, livestock and ecosystems at risk (Chomel *et al.*, 2007; Karesh *et al.*, 2007, 2012; Ogun *et al.*, 2010; Smith *et al.*, 2013). The estimated consumption and trade in bush-meat from Central Africa alone is over 1 billion kg/year, which is equivalent to an estimated 200 million animals (Wilkie and Carpenter, 1999; Karesh *et al.*, 2012). A wide range of wildlife is hunted both legally and illegally, but in many places the African buffalo – a known reservoir for BTB – remains the favourite species for meat consumption due to its taste and price (Ndibalema and Songorwa, 2008; Alexander *et al.*, 2012). The public food safety concern originating from wildlife products not only includes bushmeat, but also legal wildlife exploitation. In Southern Africa, the wildlife meat industry is booming. Up to a quarter of farmland in Namibia has been converted into commercial game farms (Turpie *et al.*, cited in Magwedere *et al.*, 2012). Namibia produces between 16,000 and 26,000 t of game meat for national and international markets (Lindsey, 2011), thus putting wildlife in an important niche for foodborne zoonosis (Magwedere *et al.*, 2012). In Zimbabwe, game ranching is becoming more profitable than cattle ranching and game meat is often more expensive than beef (Chardonnet *et al.*, 2002). In Zambia, there is rising concern about the utilization of the lechwe antelope, an economically high profile species in the country due to its BTB status, as it is estimated that around 80% of the hunted lechwe carcasses are BTB infected (Siamudaala *et al.*, 2005; Malama *et al.*, 2013). So far, no cases of BTB in humans originating from wildlife have been described in sub-Saharan Africa. However, this may reflect more a lack of disease assessment at the human–wildlife interface rather than true absence of disease transmission. Hence, in sub-Saharan Africa, the increasing exploitation of wildlife for human consumption will necessitate stricter meat examination protocols. There is likely a negligible risk of BTB to be transmitted directly from wildlife to humans. However, it is possible that BTB may spill back from wildlife to cattle and consequently affect cattle production (Meisinger, 1970; Cosivi *et al.*, 1998). Future BTB control programmes may be an additional economic burden on such countries. For instance, the resurgence of BTB in cattle in the UK due to an uncontrolled reservoir in badgers cost the government £100 million/year (control, trade and market loss) (Matthews *et al.*, 2006). In sub-Saharan Africa, a spill-back scenario has not been described so far.

Finally, the existence of BTB in wildlife can have serious conservation issues and impacts on a nation's wildlife-related tourism. The example of the BTB south–north spread through Krueger National Park, South Africa (KNP), starting in 1990 shows the extent of the problem if uncontrolled. BTB acquired from cattle in the southern part of the park spread amongst the buffalo population that maintained the infection and also to at least 13 other spill-over species including lions preying on sick buffaloes. This puts the carnivore population at risk (Michel *et al.*, 2009; Maas *et al.*, 2012; Bengis, 2012). BTB has also recently spread from KNP to the neighbouring buffalo populations in Gonarezhou National Park in Zimbabwe (de Garine-Wichatitsky *et al.*, 2013). The scenario highlights the threat of BTB in sub-Saharan Africa to tourism, to biodiversity, to the viability of endangered species and to the anticipated sustainable ecological and economic benefits of the Transfrontier National Parks initiative (Bengis, 2005).

## Poorly Studied Livestock–Wildlife Interface

Although protected areas have been created to provide biodiversity protection, still a large proportion of wildlife lives outside these areas, particularly when unfenced (Prins and Grootenhuis, 2000; Mworia *et al.*, 2008). Some species need a bigger territory to live in than that provided by the national parks and some species need to migrate regularly (Woodroffe *et al.*, 2005). Humans encroach into protected habitats with their livestock in search of grazing areas and water, particularly during the drought season (Plate 7), and in arid and semi-arid areas, wildlife share the same water points with pastoralist livestock (de Leeuw *et al.*, 2001; Mizutani *et al.*, 2005; Sitters *et al.*, 2009).

The contact interface is therefore not restricted to protected areas and buffer zones but exists also in agriculture and rangeland.

Overall, with some exceptions, the epidemiology and ecology at the wildlife–livestock interface are still poorly known in terms of spatial and temporal livestock–wildlife relations, animal behaviour and between-species dynamics, ecology and socio-economic dynamics. We also do not know how pastoralists view all the factors influencing the potential transmission of diseases in general and BTB in particular. Risk factors for disease transmission between wildlife and livestock have rarely been described in sub-Saharan Africa (de Garine-Wichatitsky *et al.*, 2013).

### Contact interface at water points

Rainfall and water shortages are the main drivers and constraining factors for the distribution and abundance of wildlife species and thus for contact opportunity between species (Gereta *et al.*, 2004; Martin, 2005; Epaphras *et al.*, 2008). Interaction between different wildlife species around natural and artificial water sources have been described (Valeix *et al.*, 2007; Epaphras *et al.*, 2008) but how wildlife and livestock interact is poorly known. Generally, wildlife tend to avoid livestock, but this is species specific and dependent on prevailing environmental conditions (de Leeuw *et al.*, 2001; Zvidai *et al.*, 2013). Negative associations in terms of animal displacement, between the presence of livestock and the biodiversity and distribution of wildlife have been described (Prins, 2000). Herders tend to chase wildlife away from water points so that wildlife use times of the day when human disturbance is at its lowest (Zvidzai *et al.*, 2013). Zvidzai *et al.* (2013) studied livestock–wildlife at water points located within Gonarezhou National Park (Zimbabwe), at the park boundaries and in the agricultural area. The authors concluded that BTB transmission was unlikely to be caused by direct contact at the interface around water sources. However, intermediate species such as impala, kudu and warthog (*Phacochoerus africanus*), which are less affected by livestock presence (Prins, 2000; Zvidzai *et al.*, 2013), could play a role as disease 'vector' by having close physical contact with BTB buffalo reactors, that stay within the park, and with livestock in the agricultural land outside the park.

### Contact interface on grazing land

Common use of pasture land is another potential risk for BTB transmission between wildlife and livestock. Mainly wildlife grazer species (as opposed to browser species) are likely to compete with cattle. There seems to be a species-specific tolerance level for cattle presence (Young *et al.*, 2005). Hartebeest and cattle compete directly for pasture in Kenya (Ego *et al.*, 2003) and Ethiopia (Tschopp, personal observation) (Plate 8).

Lechwe and cattle are regularly seen grazing together in Zambia (Malama *et al.*, 2013). On the other hand, no mountain nyalas (*Tragelaphus buxtoni*) (an endemic endangered species) have been observed in The Bale Mountain National Park (Ethiopia), when there is high livestock pressure (Stephens *et al.*, 2001).

Many grazer species favour grazing in old pastoral places where grass cover is rich due to the cattle manure (Reid *et al.*, 2004). As *M. bovis* can be excreted in cattle manure and survive in the environment over days and months (Tanner and Michel, 1999; Courtenay *et al.*, 2006; Jha *et al.*, 2007), it is worth remembering that disease transmission can still occur even with a temporally asymmetric interface (with no direct animal contact).

Presence and abundance of wildlife species is also affected by the vegetation cover (Mosugelo *et al.*, 2002). If the latter is altered naturally or anthropogenetically, wild animals will move elsewhere (Hibert *et al.*, 2010), likely shifting the existing dynamics of the interface.

## Added Value of a One Health Approach

Control of zoonoses in the domestic animal reservoir is likely to reduce human disease burden and is, in general, much cheaper than controlling the disease in the human population (Roth *et al.*, 2003; Knobel *et al.*, 2005). The One Health concept has so far, primarily, only included domestic animals and humans in its equation, rarely considering wildlife and, even less often, the ecosystem. However, as described above, livestock, human and wildlife health are as intimately linked with each other as they are with ecosystem ecology and health. Interventions strategies regarding BTB would therefore benefit from a synergy of two movements, One Health and ecohealth, that have tended to work separately so far. The One Health movement includes various sectors but its main focus remains the management of health risks to humans and animals (Zinsstag, 2012), whereas the more recent ecohealth movement has its core focus on ecosystem health, and how this eventually impacts human–animal health (Charron, 2012). Regarding BTB in particular, the One Health concept – although much discussed – is still weakly used despite the lessons learned from the UK, New Zealand and KNP for instance. In sub-Saharan Africa, information on the role of BTB in wildlife at the interface with people and livestock is still lacking. This reflects a low priority given to wildlife but also lack of infrastructure (e.g. diagnostic laboratory), remoteness of sites, lack of a good diagnostic test for wildlife, and cost and difficult logistics of testing wildlife in the field (e.g. cost of drugs, elaborate equipment, number of staff required) (de Garine-Wichatitsky *et al.*, 2013).

## Control of bovine tuberculosis

So far, BTB control, similar to foot and mouth disease control in wildlife in Southern Africa, has included culling, fencing, corridors kept free of animals, as well as a combination of these or a do nothing strategy (Caron *et al.*, 2003). All approaches have drawbacks, ranging from inefficiency to interference with wildlife migration leading to decreased wildlife population, and even mass mortality (Prins, 2000; Martin, 2005). In sub-Saharan Africa, BTB vaccination research in livestock (Ameni *et al.*, 2010) as well as in buffaloes (de Klerk *et al.*, 2010) is ongoing but has shown various successes so far.

In New Zealand, brushtail possums are considered an exotic species and pest and are thus extirpated as a mean of controlling BTB (Nugent, 2011). However, African wildlife has an economic and environmental value, is an integral part of the African heritage and many species are nowadays threatened or endangered and in need of protection. Wildlife auctions in RSA reflect true economic value for wildlife (Chardonnet *et al.*, 2002). BTB is widespread amongst African wildlife and its eradication is therefore impossible. This reinforces the importance of close collaboration between the agriculture and wildlife sectors to avoid spill-overs from domestic livestock into the naive wildlife populations, and spill-backs into the livestock population. The collaboration should not only include disease management but also habitat and land-use management, so wildlife and livestock can continue to co-exist without posing a health threat to each other and community livelihoods continue to be secured.

Few cost analyses of BTB control options have been performed for the livestock sector (Bernues *et al.*, 1997; Tschopp *et al.*, 2012; Mwacalimba *et al.*, 2013). In Ethiopia, Tschopp *et al.* (2012) showed that there was neither loss of asset value, nor cost of disease due to BTB in rural and urban livestock systems. In Zambia, the cost of control was shown to outweigh the benefits from controlling BTB (Mwacalimba *et al.*, 2013). However, the results of both studies have to be seen purely from a monetary point of view. The quantification of benefits resulting from a BTB control programme is difficult and its sectoral ramifications have so far not been studied in sub-Saharan Africa. This represents an important knowledge gap. An additional reason why this assessment must include wildlife is to assess cost-sharing schemes between the public health, livestock and wildlife sectors. This would include the economic value and return from wildlife. There is an urgent need for research at the contact interface throughout the continent, integrating epidemiology and habitat/species ecology, in particular to gain a better understanding of the interactions between species and also the impacts of co-infections on BTB prevalence in wildlife (Caron *et al.*, 2003; Maas *et al.*, 2012; Beechler, 2013). Therefore, research has to go beyond mere BTB prevalence studies.

## Synergies and added values

The BTB example shows the important added value of an implementation of intersectoral collaboration between public health, the agricultural and the wildlife sectors. However, it should also include the educational and sanitation sectors as well as ecologists, veterinarians and biologists. BTB directly impacts livestock health and thus indirectly public health and people's livelihoods. BTB also directly impacts biodiversity and wildlife conservation, hence the need for synergy between the One Health and the ecohealth movements. The information collected at the interface, reported and analysed, should be shared by the health, agriculture and wildlife ministries. Further added value can include sharing knowledge and expertise between the sectors, conducting common disease surveillance, and sharing laboratory facilities and transport.

Local communities, including pastoral communities, also have to be empowered and included in disease control strategies. Similarly, they must benefit from disease awareness programmes and socio-economic returns from wildlife (Sindiga, 1995; Kock *et al.*, 2002; Molyneux *et al.*, 2011; Homewood *et al.*, 2012).

## Future and Conclusions

The One Health approach in controlling BTB in sub-Saharan Africa is still in its infancy and has many gaps, in particular concerning wildlife. Human–livestock–wildlife interfaces are variable, fluid and dynamic in nature. They will continue to change as population growth continues and more natural resources are used. Further factors influencing the interface include climate change, intensification of animal husbandry and the different conservation choices made by countries (e.g. agricultural expansion versus wildlife conservation/tourism or game industry) (Bulte and Horan, 2003). All will influence the future interfaces and BTB transmission.

There is interdependence between people–livestock–wildlife and the environment that requires intersectoral collaboration in BTB control, so that it benefits livestock and wildlife-related economies, people's health and livelihoods, as well as biodiversity conservation. A merging of One Health and ecohealth approaches would likely strengthen any intervention strategies on BTB. Future research and development agenda should encompass the establishment of diagnostic capacity, ecological studies at the interfaces, the extension of cross-sectorial economic analysis, the development of locally adapted control strategies through participatory approaches, and further research on vaccine development.

## References


Alexander, K.A., Blackburn, J.K., Vandewalle, M.E., Pesapane, R. and Baipoledi, E.K. (2012) Buffalo, bush meat, and the zoonotic threat of brucellosis in Botswana. *PLoS One* 7(3), e32842. doi:10.1371

Ameni, G., Vordermeier, M., Aseffa, A., Young, D.B. and Hewinson, R.G. (2010) Field evaluation of the efficacy of *Mycobacterium bovis* Bacillus Calmette-Guerin against bovine tuberculosis in neonatal calves in Ethiopia. *Clinical and Vaccine Immunology* 17(10), 1533–1538.

Ayele, W.Y., Neill, S.D., Zinsstag, J., Weiss, M.G. and Pavlik, I. (2004) Bovine tuberculosis: an old disease but a new threat to Africa. *International Journal of Tuberculosis and Lung Disease* 8, 924–937.

Beechler, B. (2013) Rift Valley fever in African buffalo (*Syncerus caffer*): basic epidemiology and the role of bovine tuberculosis coinfection. PhD thesis, Oregon State University.

Bengis, R.G. (2005) Transfrontier conservation area initiatives in Sub-Saharan Africa: some animal health challenges. In: Osofsky, S.A., Cleaveland, S., Karesh, W.B. *et al.*, (eds) *Conservation and Development Interventions at the Wildlife/Livestock Interface: Implications for Wildlife, Livestock and Human Health*. IUCN, Gland, Switzerland, pp. 15–19.

Bengis, R.G. (2012) *Bovine tuberculosis in free-ranging wildlife: a review of global occurrence, pathology and epidemiology of this disease, and potential conservation implications*. International Wildlife TB Conference, Skukuza, Kruger National Park.

Berg, S., Garcia-Pelayol, M.C., Mueller, B., Hailu, E., Asiimwe, B., Kremer, K. *et al.* (2011) African 2: a clonal complex of *Mycobacterium bovis* epidemiologically important in East Africa. *Journal of Bacteriology* 193, 670–678.

Bernues, A., Manrique, E. and Maza, M.T. (1997) Economic evaluation of bovine brucellosis and tuberculosis eradication programmes in a mountain area of Spain. *Preventive Veterinary Medicine* 30, 137–149.

Boukary, A.R., Thys, E., Abatih, E., Gamatié, D., Ango, I., Yenikoye, A. and Saegerman, C. (2011) Bovine tuberculosis prevalence survey on cattle in the rural livestock system of Torodi (Niger). *PLoS ONE* 6, e24629.

Brosch, R., Gordon, S.V., Marmiesse, M., Brodin, P., Buchrieser, C., Eiglmeier, K., Garnier, T., Gutierrez, C., Hewinson, G., Kremer, K., Parsons, L.M., Pym, A.S., Samper, S., Van Soolingen, D. and Cole, S.T. (2002) A new evolutionary scenario for the Mycobacterium tuberculosis complex. *Proceedings of the National Academy of Sciences USA* 99, 3684–3689.

Bulte, E.H. and Horan, R.D. (2003) Habitat conservation, wildlife extraction and agricultural expansion. *Journal of Environmental Economics and Management* 45(1), 109–127.

Caron, A., Cross, P.C. and du Toit, J.T. (2003) Ecological implications of bovine tuberculosis in African Buffalo herds. *Ecological Applications* 13, 1338–1345.

Cartin-Rojas, A. (2012) Transboundary animal diseases and international trade. In: Bobek, V. (ed.) *International Trade from Economic and Policy Perspective*. InTech Publishing, pp. 143–166; DOI: 10.5772/2726. Available from: http://www.intechopen.com/books/international-trade-from-economic-and-policy-perspective/transboundary-animal-diseases-and-international-trade.

Chardonnet, Ph., des Clers, B., Fischer, J., Gerhold, R., Jori, F. and Lamarque, F. (2002) The value of wildlife. *Revue Scientifique et Technique (International Office of Epizootics)* 21(1), 15–51.

Charron, D.F. (2012) Ecosystem approaches to health for a global sustainability agenda. *EcoHealth* 9, 256–266.

Chomel, B.B., Belotto, A. and Meslin, F.-X. (2007) Wildlife, exotic pets, and emerging zoonoses. *Emerging Infectious Diseases* 13(1), 6–11.

Cleaveland, S., Mlengeya, T., Kazwala, R.R., Michel, A., Kaare, M.T., Jones, S.L., Eblate, E., Shirima, G.M. and Packer, C. (2005) Tuberculosis in Tanzanian wildlife. *Journal of Wildlife Disease* 41, 446–453.

Coleman, J.D. and Cooke, M.M. (2001) *Mycobacterium bovis* infection in wildlife in New Zealand. *Tuberculosis* 81, 191–202.

Cosivi, O., Grange, J.M., Daborn, C.J., Raviglione, M.C., Fujikura, T., Cousins, D., Robinson, R.A., Huchzermeyer, H.F., de Kantor, I. and Meslin, F.X. (1998) Zoonotic tuberculosis due to *Mycobacterium bovis* in developing countries. *Emerging Infectious Diseases* 4, 59–70.

Courtenay, O., Reilly, L.A., Sweeney, F.P., Hibberd, V., Bryan, S., Ul-Hassan, A., Newman, C., Macdonald, D.W., Delahay, R.J. , Wilson, G.J. and Wellington, E.M.H. (2006) Is *Mycobacterium bovis* in the environment important for the persistence of bovine tuberculosis? *Biology Letters* 2, 460–462.

Daszak, P., Cunningham, A.A. and Hyatt, A.D. (2001) Anthropogenic environmental change and the emergence of infectious diseases in wildlife. *Acta Tropica* 78, 103–116.

De Garine-Wichatitsky, M., Caron, A., Kock, R., Tschopp, R., Munyeme, M., Hofmeyr, M. and Michel, A. (2013) A review of bovine tuberculosis at the wildlife-livestock-human interface in sub-Saharan Africa. *Epidemiology and Infection* 141, 1342–1356.

De Jong, B.C., Antonio, M. and Gagneux, S. (2010) *Mycobacterium africanum* – Review of an important cause of human tuberculosis in West Africa. *PLoS Neglected Tropical Diseases* 4(9), e744. doi:10.1371/journal.pntd.0000744.

De Klerk, L.M., Michel, A., Bengis, R., Kriek, N. and Godfroid, J. (2010) BCG vaccination failed to protect yearling African buffaloes (*Syncerus caffer*) against experimental intratonsilar challenge with *Mycobacterium bovis*. *Veterinary Immunology and Immunopathology* 137, 84–92.

De Leeuw, J., Waweru, M.N., Okello, O.O., Maloba, M., Ngutu, P., Said, M.Y., Aligula, H.M., Heitkoenig, I.M.A. and Reid, R.S. (2001) Distribution and diversity of wildlife in Northern Kenya in relation to livestock and permanent water points. *Biological Conservation* 100, 297–306.

De Lisle, G.W., Bengis, R.G., Schmitt, S.M. and O'Brien, D.J. (2002) Tuberculosis in free-ranging wildlife: detection, diagnosis and management. *Revue Scientifique et Technique (International Office of Epizootics)* 21(2), 317–334.

De Vos, V., Bengis, R.G., Kriek, N.P., Michel, A., Keet, D.F., Raath, J.P. and Huchzermeyer, H.F. (2001) The epidemiology of tuberculosis in free-ranging African buffalo (*Syncerus caffer*) in the Kruger National Park, South Africa. *Onderstepoort Journal of Veterinary Research* 68, 119–130.

Diguimbaye-Djaibé, C., Hilty, M., Ngandolo, R., Mahamat, H.H., Pfyffer, G.E., Baggi, F., Hewinson, G., Tanner, M., Zinsstag, J. and Schelling, E. (2006) *Mycobacterium bovis* isolates from tuberculous lesions in Chadian zebu carcasses. *Emerging Infectious Diseases* 12(5), 769–771.

Ego, W.K., Mbuvi, D.M. and Kibet, P.F.K. (2003) Dietry composition of wildebeest (*Connochaetes taurinus*) kongoni (*Alcephalus buselaphus*) and cattle (*Bos indicus*), grazing on a common ranch in south-central Kenya. *African Journal of Ecology* 41, 83–92.

Epaphras, A.M., Gereta, E., Lejora, I.A., Ole Meing'ataki, G.E., Ng'umbi, G., Kiwango, Y., Mwangomo, E., Semanini, F., Vitalis, L., Balozi, J. and Mtahiko, M.G.G. (2008) Wildlife water utilization and importance of artificial waterholes during dry season at Ruaha National Park, Tanzania. *Wetlands Ecology and Management* 16, 183–188.

FAOStat (2014) Available at: http://faostat.fao.org (accessed 15 January 2014).

Firdessa, R., Tschopp, R., Wubete, A., Sombo, M., Hailu, E., Erenso, G., Kiros, T., Yamuah, L., Vordermeier, M., Hewinson, G., Young, D., Gordon, S.V., Sahile, M., Aseffa, A. and Berg, S. (2012) High prevalence of bovine tuberculosis in dairy cattle in central Ethiopia: implications for the dairy industry and public health. *PlosOne* 7(12), e52851.

Firdessa, R., Berg, S., Hailu, E., Schelling, E., Gumi, B., Erenso, G., Gadisa, E., Kiros, T., Habtamu, M., Hussein, J., Zinsstag, J., Robertson, B., Ameni, G., Lohan, A.J., Loftus, B., Comas, I., Gagneux, S., Tschopp, R. *et al.* (2013) Mycobacterial lineages causing pulmonary and extrapulmonary tuberculosis, Ethiopia. *Emerging Infectious Diseases* 9(3), 4 pp.

Fofana, M. (2003) Bovine tuberculosis in Mali; results of an epidemiological survey of dairy farms from periurban areas in Bamako district. *Revue d'Elevage et de Médecine Vétérinaire des Pays Tropicaux* 56, 115–120.

Gallagher, J., Macadam, I., Sayer, J. and Van Lavierens, L.P. (1972) Pulmonary tuberculosis in free-living lechwe antelope in Zambia. *Tropical Animal Health and Production* 4, 204–213.

Gereta, E., Mwangomo, E. and Wolanski, E. (2004) The influence of wetlands in regulating water quality in the Seronera River, Serengeti National Park, Tanzania. *Wetlands Ecology and Management* 12, 301–307.

Gordon, I.J. (2009) What is the future for wild, large herbivores in human-modified agricultural landscapes? *Wildlife Biology* 15, 1–9.

Griffin, J.M., Williams, D.H., Kelly, G.E., Clegg, T.A., O'Boyle, I., Collins, J.D. and Morea, S.J. (2005) The impact of badger removal on the control of tuberculosis in cattle herds in Ireland. *Preventive Veterinary Medicine* 67, 237–266.

Grootenhuis, J.G. and Olubayo, R.O. (1993) Disease research in the wildlife–livestock interface in Kenya. *Veterinary Quarterly* 15(2), 55–59.

Gumi, B., Schelling, E., Berg, S., Firdessa, R., Erenso, G., Mekonnen, W., Hailu, E., Melese, E., Hussein, J., Aseffa, A. and Zinsstag, J. (2012) Zoonotic transmission of tuberculosis between pastoralists and their livestock in South-East Ethiopia. *EcoHealth* 9(2), 139–149.

Hanotte, O., Tawah, C.L., Bradley, D.G., Okomo, M., Verjee, Y., Ochieng, J. and Rege, J.E.O. (2000) Geographic distribution and frequency of a taurine *Bos taurus* and an indicine *Bos indicus Y* specific allele amongst sub-Saharan African cattle breeds. *Molecular Ecology* 9, 387–396.

Hanotte, O., Bradley, D.G., Ochieng, J.W.,Verjee, Y., Hill, E.W. and Rege, J.E.O. (2002) African pastoralism: genetic imprints of origins and migrations. *Science* 296, 336.

Hibert, F., Calenge, C., Fritz, H., Maillard, D., Bouche, P., Ipavec, A., Convers, A., Ombredane, D. and de Visscher, M.-N. (2010) Spatial avoidance of invading pastoral cattle by wild ungulates: insights from using point process statistics. *Biodiversity and Conservation* 19, 2003–2024.

Homewood, K.M., Chenevix Trench, P. and Brockington, D. (2012) Pastoralist livelihoods and wildlife revenues in East Africa: a case for coexistence? *Research, Policy and Practice* 2, 19.

Ibeagha-Awemu, E.M., Jann, O.C., Weimann, C. and Erhardt, G. (2004) Genetic diversity, introgression and relationships among West/Central African cattle breeds. *Genetics Selection Evolution* 36, 673–690.

Ibrahim, H. and Olaloku, E. (2000) Improving cattle for milk, meat and traction. *ILRI Manual 4*. ILRI (International Livestock Research Institute), Nairobi, Kenya, 135 pp.

Jha, V.C., Monta, Y., Dhakal, M., Besnet, B., Sato, T., Nagai, A., Kato, M., Kozawa, K., Yamamoto, S. and Kimura, H. (2007) Isolation of *Mycobacterium* spp. in milking buffaloes and cattle in Nepal. *Journal of Veterinary Medical Science* 69(8), 819–825.

Jones, K.E., Patel, N.G., Levy, M.A., Storeygard, A., Balk, D., Gittleman, J.L. and Daszak, P. (2008) Global trends in emerging infectious diseases. *Nature* 451(21), 990–994.

Karesh, W.B., Cook, R.A., Gilbert, M. and Newcomb, J. (2007) Implications of wildlife trade on the movement of influenza and other infectious diseases. *Journal of Wildlife Diseases* 43(3), 55–59.

Karesh, W.B., Loh, E. and Machalaba, C. (2012) Food safety: a view from the wild side. In: Institute of Medicine (US). *Improving Food Safety Through a One Health Approach*: Workshop Summary. National Academies Press, Washington, DC.

Katale, B.Z., Mbugi, E.V., Kendal, S., Fyumagwa, R.D., Kibiki, G.S., Godfrey-Faussett, P., Keyyu, J.D., Van Helden, P. and Matee, M.I. (2012) Bovine tuberculosis at the human-livestock-wildlife interface: is it a public health problem in Tanzania? A review. *Onderstepoort Journal of Veterinary Research* 79(2), 463.

Kazwala, R.R., Daborn, C.J., Kusiluka, L.J., Jiwa, S.F., Sharp, J.M. and Kambarage, D.M. (1998) Isolation of *Mycobacterium* species from raw milk of pastoral cattle of the Southern Highlands of Tanzania. *Tropical Animal Health and Production* 30(4), 233–239.

Keet, D.F., Kriek, N.P., Bengis, R.G., Grobler, D.G. and Michel, A. (2000) The rise and fall of tuberculosis in a free-ranging chacma baboon troop in the Kruger National Park. *Onderstepoort Journal of Veterinary Research* 67(2), 115–122.

Knobel, D.L., Cleaveland, S., Coleman, P.G., Fèvre, E.M., Meltzer, M.I., Miranda, M.E.G., Shaw, A., Zinsstag, J. and Meslin, F.-X. (2005) Re-evaluating the burden of rabies in Africa and Asia. *Bulletin of the World Health Organization* 83, 360–368.

Kock, R., Kebkiba, B., Heinonen, R. and Bedane, B. (2002) Wildlife and pastoral society – Shifting paradigms in disease control. *Annals of the New York Academy of Sciences* 969, 24–33.

Kock, R.A. (2005) What is this infamous 'wildlife/livestock disease interface?' A review of current knowledge for the African continent. In: Osofsky, S.A., Cleaveland, S., Karesh, W.B. *et al.* (eds) *Conservation and Development Interventions at the Wildlife/Livestock Interface: Implications for Wildlife, Livestock and Human Health*. IUCN, Gland, Switzerland, pp. 1–13.

Lindsey, P. (2011) An analysis of game meat production and wildlife based land uses on freehold land in Namibia: links with food security. TRAFFIC East/Southern Africa, Harare, Zimbabwe. Available from: http://www.trafficj.org/publication/11_An_Analysis_of_Game_Meat.pdf (accessed 5 February 2013).

Lunde, T.M. and Lindtjorn, B. (2013) Cattle and climate in Africa: how climate variability has influenced national cattle holdings from 1961–2008. *PeerJ* 1:e55

Maas, M., van Kooten, P.J.S., Schreuder, J., Morar, D., Tijhaar, E., Michel, A.L. and Rutten, V.P.M.G. (2012) Development of a lion-specific interferon-gamma assay. *Veterinary Immunology and Immunopathology* 149(3–4), 292–297.

Magwedere, K., Hemberger, M.Y., Hoffman, L.C. and Dziva, F. (2012) Zoonoses: a potential obstacle to the growing wildlife industry of Namibia. *Infection Ecology and Epidemiology* 2, 18365.

Maisels, F., Strindberg, S., Blake, S., Wittemyer, G., Hart, J., *et al.* (2013) Devastating decline of forest elephants in Central Africa. *PloS One* 8(3), e59469.

Malama, S., Muma, J.B. and Godfroid, J. (2013) A review of tuberculosis at the wildlife-livestock-human interface in Zambia. *Infectious Diseases of Poverty* 2, 13.

Mariam, S.H. (2009) Interaction between lactic acid bacteria and *M. bovis* in Ethiopian fermented milk. *Applied Environmental Microbiology* 75, 1790–1792.

Martin, R.B. (2005) The influence of veterinary control fences on certain wild large mammal species in the Caprivi, Namibia. In: Osofsky, S.A., Cleaveland, S., Karesh, W.B. *et al.* (eds) *Conservation and Development Interventions at the Wildlife/Livestock Interface: Implications for Wildlife, Livestock and Human Health*. IUCN, Gland, Switzerland, pp. 27–39.

Matthews, F., MacDonald, D.W., Taylor, G.M., Gelling, M., Norman, R.A., Honess, P.E., Foster, R., Gower, C.M., Varley, S., Harris, A., Palmer, S., Hewinson, G. and Webster, J.P. (2006) Bovine tuberculosis (*Mycobacterium bovis*) in British farmland wildlife: the importance to agriculture. *Proceedings of the Royal Society of Biological Sciences Series B* 273, 357–365.

Meisinger, G. (1970) Economic effects of the elimination of bovine tuberculosis on the productivity of cattle herds. 2. Effect on meat production. *Monatshefte für Veterinärmedizin* 25, 7–13.

Michel, A.L., Bengis, R.G., Keet, D.F., Hofmeyr, M., De Klerk, L.M., Cross, P.C., Jolles, A.E., Cooper, D., Whyte, I.J., Buss, P. and Godfroid, J. (2006) Wildlife tuberculosis in South African conservation areas: implications and challenges. *Veterinary Microbiology* 112, 91–100.

Michel, A.L., Coetzee, M.L., Keet, D.F., Maré, L., Warren, R., Cooper, D., Bengis, R.G., Kremer, K. and van Helden, P. (2009) Molecular epidemiology of *Mycobacterium bovis* isolates from free-ranging wildlife in South African game reserves. *Veterinary Microbiology* 133, 335–343.

Mizutani, F., Muthiani, E., Kristjanson, P. and Recke, H. (2005) Impact and value of wildlife in pastoral livestock production systems in Kenya: possibilities for healthy ecosystem conservation and livestock development for the poor. In: Osofsky, S.A., Cleaveland, S., Karesh, W.B. *et al.* (eds) *Conservation and Development Interventions at the Wildlife/Livestock Interface: Implications for Wildlife, Livestock and Human Health*. IUCN, Gland, Switzerland, pp. 121–132.

Molyneux, D., Hallaj, Z., Keusch, G.T., McManus, D.P., Ngowi, H., Cleaveland, S., Ramos-Jimenez, P., Gotuzzo, E., Kar, K., Sanchez, A., Garba, A., Carabin, H., Bassili, A., Chaignat, C.L., Meslin, F.-X., Abushama, H.M., Willingham, A.L. and Kioy, D. (2011) Zoonoses and marginalised infectious diseases of poverty: where do we stand? *Parasites and Vectors* 4, 106.

Mostowy, S., Inwald, J., Gordon, S., Martin, C., Warren, R., Kremer, K., Cousins, D. and Behr, M.A. (2005) Revisiting the evolution of *Mycobacterium bovis*. *Journal of Bacteriology* 187, 6386–6395.

Mosugelo, D.K., Moe, S.R., Ringrose, S. and Nellemann, C. (2002) Vegetation changes during a 36-year period in northern Chobe National Park, Botswana. *African Journal of Ecology* 40, 232–240.

Müller, B., Steiner, B., Bonfoh, B., Fané, A., Smith, N.H. and Zinsstag, J. (2008) Molecular characterisation of *Mycobacterium bovis* isolated from cattle slaughtered at the Bamako abattoir in Mali. *BMC Veterinary Research* 4, 26.

Müller, B., Hilty, M., Berg, S., Garcia-Pelayo, M.C., Dale, J., Boschiroli, M.L., *et al.* (2009) African 1, an epidemiologically important clonal complex of *Mycobacterium bovis* dominant in Mali, Nigeria, Cameroon, and Chad. *Journal of Bacteriology* 191, 1951–1960.

Müller, B., Duerr, S., Alonso, S., Hattendorf, J., Laisse, C.J.M., Parsons, S.D.C., van Helden, P.D. and Zinsstag, J. (2013) Zoonotic *Mycobacterium bovis*-induced tuberculosis in humans. *Emerging Infectious Diseases* 19(6), 899–908.

Munyeme, M. and Munang'andu, H.M. (2011) A review of bovine tuberculosis in the Kafue Basin ecosystem. *Veterinary Medicine International*, DOI: 10.4061/2011/918743

Munyeme, M., Muma, J.B., Samui, K.L., Skjerve, E., Nambota, A.M., Phiri, I.G., Rigouts, L. and Tryland, M. (2009) Prevalence of bovine tuberculosis and animal level risk factors for indigenous cattle under different grazing strategies in the livestock/wildlife interface areas of Zambia. *Tropical Animal Health and Production* 41, 345–352.

Mwacalimba, K.K., Mumba, C. and Munyeme, M. (2013) Cost benefit analysis of tuberculosis control in wildlife–livestock interface areas of Southern Zambia. *Preventive Veterinary Medicine* 110, 274–279.

Mworia, J.K., Kinyamario, J.I. and Githaiga, J.M. (2008) Influence of cultivation, settlements and water sources on wildlife distribution and habitat selection in south-east Kajiado. *Kenya Environmental Conservation* 35(2), 117–124.

Naranjo, V., Gortazar, C., Vicente, J. and de la Fuente, J. (2008) Evidence of the role of European wild boar as a reservoir of *Mycobacterium* tuberculosis complex. *Veterinary Microbiology* 127, 1–9.

Ndibalema, V.G. and Songorwa, A.N. (2008) Illegal meat hunting in Serengeti: dynamics in consumption and preferences. *African Journal of Ecology* 46, 311–319.

Norton-Griffiths, M. (2000) Wildlife losses in Kenya: an analysis of conservation policy. *Natural Resource Modeling* 13(1), 1–6.

Nugent, G. (2011) Maintenance, spillover and spillback transmission of bovine tuberculosis in multi-host wildlife complexes: a New Zealand case study. *Veterinary Microbiology* 151, 34–42.

Ogun, A.A., Okonko, I.O., Udeze, A.O., Shittu, I., Garba, K.N., Fowotade, A., Adewale, O.G., Fajobi, E.A., Onoja, B.A., Babalola, E.T. and Adedeji, A.O. (2010) Feasibility and factors affecting global elimination and possible eradication of rabies in the world. *Journal of General and Molecular Virology* 2(1), 001–027.

Paine, R. and Martinaglia, G. (1929) Tuberculosis in wild buck living under natural conditions. *Journal of Comparative Pathology and Theriology* XLII(1), 1–8.

Patz, J.A., Daszak, P., Tabor, G.M., Alonso Aguirre, A., Pearl, M., Epstein, J., Wolfe, N.D., Kilpatrick, A.M., Foufopoulos, J., Molyneux, D. and Bradley, D.J. (2004) Unhealthy landscapes: policy recommendations on land use change and infectious disease emergence. *Environmental Health Perspectives* 112(10), 1092–1098.

Phillips, C.J.C., Foster, C.R.W., Morris, P.A. and Teverson, R. (2003) The transmission of *Mycobacterium bovis* infection to cattle. *Research in Veterinary Science* 74, 1–15.

Prins, H.H.T. (2000) Competition between wildlife and livestock in Africa. In: Prins, H., Grootenhuis, J.G. and Dolan, T. (eds) *Wildlife Conservation by Sustainable Use*. Kluwer Academic Publishers, Boston, Massachusetts.

Prins, H.H.T. and Grootenhuis, J.G. (2000) Introduction: the value of priceless wildlife. In: Prins, H., Grootenhuis, J.G. and Dolan, T. (eds) *Wildlife Conservation by Sustainable Use*. Kluwer Academic Publishers, Boston, Massachusetts.

Reid, R.S., Thornton, P.K. and Kruska, R.L. (2004) Loss and fragmentation of habitat for pastoral people and wildlife in east Africa: concepts and issues. *African Journal of Range and Forage Science* 21(3), 171–181.

Renwick, A.R., White, P.C. and Bengis, R.G. (2007) Bovine tuberculosis in southern African wildlife: a multi-species hostpathogen system. *Epidemiology and Infection* 135, 529–540.

Rodwell, T.C., Kriek, N.P., Bengis, R.G., Whyte, I.J., Viljoen, P.C., De Vos, V. and Boyce, W.M. (2001) Prevalence of bovine tuberculosis in African buffalo at Kruger National Park. *Journal of Wildlife Diseases* 37, 258–264.

Roth, F., Zinsstag, J., Orkhon, D., Chimed-Ochir, G., Hutton, G., Cosivi, O., Carrin, G. and Otte, J. (2003) Human health benefits from livestock vaccination for brucellosis: case study. *Bulletin of the World Health Organization* 81, 867–876.

Siamudaala, V.M., Muma, J., Munang'andu, H.M. and Mulumbu, M. (2005) Disease challenges concerning the utilization of the Kafue lechwe (*Kobus leche kafuensis*) in Zambia. In: Osofsky, S.A., Cleaveland, S.,

Karesh, W.B. *et al.* (eds) *Conservation and Development Interventions at the Wildlife/Livestock Interface: Implications for Wildlife, Livestock and Human Health.* IUCN, Gland, Switzerland, pp. 75–80.
Sindiga, I. (1995) Wildlife-based tourism in Kenya: land use conflicts and government compensation policies over protected areas. *The Journal of Tourism Studies* 6(2), 45–55.
Sitters, J., Heitkoenig, I.M.A., Holmgren, M. and Ojwang, G.S.O. (2009) Herded cattle and wild grazers partition water but share forage resources during dry years in East African savannas. *Biological Conservation* 142, 738–750.
Smith, K.F., Behrens, M., Schloegel, L.M., Marano, N., Burgiel, S. and Daszak, P. (2013) Reducing the risks of the wildlife trade. *Science* 324, 594–595.
Smith, N., Berg, B., Dale, J., Allen, A., Rodriguez, S., Romero, B., Matos, F., Ghebremichael, S., Karoui, C. *et al.* (2011) European 1: a globally important clonal complex of *Mycobacterium bovis*. *Infection, Genetics and Evolution* 11, 1340–1351.
Smith, N.H., Gordon, S.V., de la Rua-Domenech, R., Clifton-Hadley, R.S. and Hewinson, R.G. (2006) Bottlenecks and broomsticks: the molecular evolution of *Mycobacterium bovis*. *Nature Revues Microbiology* 4, 670–681.
Stephens, P.A., d'Sa, C.A., Sillero-Zubiri, C. and Leader-Williams, N. (2001) Impact of livestock and settlement on the large mammalian wildlife of Bale Mountains National Park, southern Ethiopia. *Biological Conservation* 100, 307–322.
Swai, E.S. and Schoonman, L. (2012) Differences in prevalence of tuberculosis in indigenous and crossbred cattle under extensive and intensive management systems in Tanga region of Tanzania. *Tropical Animal Health and Production* 44(3), 459–465.
Tanner, M. and Michel, A.L. (1999) Investigation of the viability of *M. bovis* under different environmental conditions in the Kruger National Park. *Onderstepoort Journal of Veterinary Research* 66, 185–190.
Tarara, R., Suleman, M.A., Sapolsky, R., Wabomba, M.J. and Else, J.G. (1985) Tuberculosis in wild olive baboons, *Papio cynocephalus anubis* (Lesson), in Kenya. *Journal of Wildlife Diseases* 21(2), 137–140.
Thornton, P.K. (2010) Livestock production: recent trends, future prospects. *Philosophical Transactions of the Royal Society* 365, doi: 10.1098/rstb.2010.0134.
Timah, E.A., Ajaga, N., Tita, D.F., Ntonga, L.M. and Bongsiysi, I.B. (2008) Demographic pressure and natural resources conservation. *Ecological Economics* 64, 475–483.
Tschopp, R., Aseffa, A., Schelling, E., Berg, S., Hailu, E., Gadisa, E., Habtamu, M., Argaw, K. and Zinsstag, J. (2010a) Bovine tuberculosis at the wildlife-livestock-human interface in Hamer Woreda, South Omo, Southern Ethiopia. *PloSOne* 5(8), e12205.
Tschopp, R., Aseffa, A., Schelling, E. and Zinsstag, J. (2010b) Perception of farmers towards agriculture, livestock and natural resources in Ethiopia. *Journal of Mountain Research and Development* 30(4), 381–390.
Tschopp, R., Schelling, E., Hattendorf, J., Young, D., Aseffa, A. and Zinsstag, J. (2010c) Repeated representative cross-sectional skin testing for bovine tuberculosis in cattle in traditional husbandry system in Ethiopia. *Veterinary Record* 167, 250–256.
Tschopp, R., Hattendorf, J., Roth, F., Choudhoury, A., Shaw, A., Aseffa, A. and Zinsstag, J. (2012) Cost estimate of bovine tuberculosis to Ethiopia. *Current Topics in Microbiology and Immunology* 365, 249–268.
Valeix, M., Chamaille-Jammes, S. and Fritz, H. (2007) Interference competition and temporal niche shifts: elephants and herbivore communities at waterholes. *Oecologia* 153, 739–748.
Vordermeier, M., Ameni, G., Berg, S., Bishop, R., Robertson, B.D., Aseffa, A., Hewinson, R.G. and Young, D.B. (2012) The influence of cattle breed on susceptibility to bovine tuberculosis in Ethiopia. *Comparative Immunology, Microbiology and Infectious Diseases* 35(3), 227–232.
Wilkie, D.S. and Carpenter, J.F. (1999) Bushmeat hunting in the Congo Basin: an assessment of impacts and options for mitigation. *Biodiversity and Conservation* 8, 927–955.
Woodford, M.H. (1982a) Tuberculosis in wildlife in the Ruwenzori National Park Uganda (Part I). *Tropical Animal Health and Production* 14(2), 81–88.
Woodford, M.H. (1982b) Tuberculosis in wildlife in the Ruwenzori National Park, Uganda (Part II). *Tropical Animal Health and Production* 14(3), 155–160.
Woodroffe, R., Lindsey, P., Romanach, S., Stein, A. and Ole Ranah, S.M.K. (2005) Livestock predation by endangered African wild dogs (*Lycaon pictus*) in northern Kenya. *Biological Conservation* 124, 225–234.
Young, T.P., Palmer, T.M. and Gadd, M.E. (2005) Competition and compensation among cattle, zebras, and elephants in a semi-arid savanna in Laikipia, Kenya. *Biological Conservation* 122, 351–359.
Zinsstag, J. (2012) Convergence of Ecohealth and One Health. *EcoHealth* 9, 371–373.
Zvidzai, M., Murwira, A., Caron, A. and de Garine Wichatitsky, M. (2013) Waterhole use patterns at the wildlife/livestock interface in a semi-arid savanna of Southern Africa. *International Journal of Development and Sustainability* 2(2), 455–471.

# 16 Integrated Rabies Control

**Monique Léchenne,[1]* Mary Elizabeth Miranda[2] and Jakob Zinsstag[1]**
[1]*Swiss Tropical and Public Health Institute, Basel and University of Basel, Switzerland;* [2]*Research Institute for Tropical Medicine, Department of Health, the Philippines*

## Introduction

Rabies is a classic zoonotic disease, infecting all mammal species. It is generally transmitted through an invasive manner from saliva to a bite wound, leading to encephalitis with distinct, severe symptoms followed by death. Since the earliest descriptions of this ancient disease, animals, and especially dogs, have been recognized as the source and cause of rabies in humans (Rosset, 1985). To this day, rabies provides an exemplar of a One Health problem requiring an understanding of the linkages between human and animals and an integrated approach to disease control.

In 1882, shortly before discovering the first rabies vaccine for humans, aided by experiments on rabbits and dogs, Louis Pasteur wrote in his third correspondence to the Academy of Science:

> ...l'homme ne contractant jamais la rage qu'à la suite d'une morsure par un animal enragé, il suffira de trouver une méthode propre à s'opposer à la rage du chien pour préserver l'humanité du terrible fléau. [People contract rabies only after a bite of a rabid animal; it would be enough to find a proper method to fight rabies in the dog to protect humanity from this terrible scourge.][1]

Although this statement by Pasteur simplifies the epidemiology of rabies by ignoring sylvatic rabies in wildlife reservoirs and lyssavirus transmission by bats, it describes the very essence of the prevention of rabies in humans. Even now, the domestic dog is the main vector for transmission of rabies to people, being responsible for more than nine out of ten cases worldwide. An estimated 7 million people per year come into contact with a rabid dog (Knobel *et al.*, 2005) and should receive post-exposure prophylaxis (PEP). This treatment is the only measure available to prevent onset of the disease, but it is often inaccessible for various reasons, including lack of knowledge about where to seek help, lack of money to pay for it or simply lack of the vaccine itself in local health facilities.

Despite exploration of different protocols, no consistently effective treatment exists against rabies encephalitis and the disease is almost always fatal (Jackson, 2013). Although PEP is highly effective in terms of prevention, many hundreds of thousands of people across Africa and Asia do not have access to prompt and appropriate PEP. As a result, it is estimated that at least 55,000 people die of rabies each year, which represents an under-reporting of human rabies cases by a

*E-mail: monique.lechenne@unibas.ch

factor of from 20 (Asia) to 160 times (Africa) (Knobel *et al.*, 2005).

Rabies can also be effectively prevented in both human and animal hosts through pre-exposure vaccination, with several highly immunogenic and effective vaccines available. The availability of effective vaccines raises the prospect for effective control and elimination of rabies, and several other features of rabies further meet the criteria for a disease that can be eliminated (Klepac *et al.*, 2013). The virus cannot persist in the environment, no carrier state has been identified, and the infectious period lasts only a few days until the host invariably dies (Warrell and Warrell, 2004). Furthermore, the basic reproductive ratio ($R_0$) of canine rabies transmission is consistently below 2, regardless of dog density and demographic setting (Hampson *et al.*, 2009; Morters *et al.*, 2013), which suggests that elimination should be epidemiologically feasible. This is supported by empirical evidence demonstrating the success of canine rabies elimination in Europe (Aikimbayev *et al.*, 2014), North America and recently in Latin America, where human and dog rabies cases have declined considerably following dog mass vaccination campaigns (Streicker *et al.*, 2010; Vigilato *et al.*, 2013).

The main burden from this disease is now found in Asia and Africa, where rabies continues to be neglected in many regions, and too often its public health impact is overshadowed by other priority diseases like HIV/AIDS, malaria and avian influenza (Knobel *et al.*, 2005; Shwiff *et al.*, 2013). This situation typifies the inequities in health investments that are directed to the prevention of emerging zoonoses (perceived as a threat to high-income countries) in comparison to the prevention and control of neglected endemic zoonoses (predominantly affecting low-income communities) (De Balogh *et al.*, 2013; Zinsstag, 2013). Although the number of lives lost and the estimated costs (Shwiff *et al.*, 2013) may be viewed as less compelling than other public health priorities, several studies have demonstrated the cost-effectiveness of canine rabies control for preventing human rabies deaths (Zinsstag *et al.*, 2011b; Fitzpatrick *et al.*, 2014). The threshold immunization coverage of a reservoir species required to interrupt transmission has been estimated at 70% (Coleman and Dye, 1996). For canine rabies, vaccination campaigns have successfully achieved this level (Kayali *et al.*, 2003; Kaare *et al.*, 2009), but challenges remain for reaching and maintaining sufficient coverage in some rural and urban low-income settings, where dog populations are both dynamic and poorly supervised. Awareness is also growing about the importance of ensuring completeness of vaccination campaigns among communities, in order to prevent gaps in coverage which can severely jeopardize control efforts (Townsend *et al.*, 2013b). For human rabies prevention, poor access to pre- and post-exposure vaccines remains a problem for remote and marginalized communities (Warrell, 2003; Hampson *et al.*, 2011). A major challenge also relates to surveillance for both human and animal rabies, which are very poor or non-existent in many parts of Africa and Asia (Banyard *et al.*, 2013; Nel, 2013).

The described obstacles to rabies control can be addressed by an integrated approach based on the 'One Medicine' concept, which is extended to One Health and to a broader systemic understanding of ecological (ecohealth) and social systems (health in social-ecological systems, HSES; Zinsstag *et al.*, 2011a). The resulting 'equity effectiveness' approach aims towards an approach for the control of dog rabies that considers disadvantaged groups in order to reach the whole population equitably (Zinsstag *et al.*, Chapter 12, this volume). Even when a vaccine is highly effective, as is the case for dog rabies vaccine, use in the field is often limited by a number of factors in a multiplicative way. As a result, the effectiveness of an intervention, assessed here as the proportion of dogs protected from transmission, may be well below the actual biological efficacy of the vaccine. A vaccine's effectiveness is determined, among other factors, by availability, accessibility and affordability (Zinsstag *et al.*, 2011b). To understand better these determinants of intervention effectiveness, we move from 'One Medicine' to a HSES approach, and discuss in detail their involvement in a sustainable, cost-effective elimination of rabies in domestic animals.

## One Medicine

More than a century ago, Austin Peters, veterinarian and contemporary to Louis Pasteur, addressed the following words on the subject of combatting rabies to the Cattle Commission of the United States (Peters, 1891):

> I merely offer the suggestion, would it not be better to merge matters pertaining to the public health in one bureau, this board not only to do what the present Cattle Commission does, but also to act in a broader scope, considering contagious animal diseases in their relation to the public health, as well as a menace to our live-stock interests. (...) Before we can ever have a system of protection to the public health approaching perfection, it will be necessary to place the contagious and infectious diseases of animals in the same category with those of man, and have the same authorities exercise supervision over both.

Such a system would truly be preferable for the surveillance of rabies. Reliable incidence data on animal and human rabies, brought together in one shared database, would significantly enhance communication with decision makers on the different national and international levels, as well as with the public as a whole (Lembo *et al.*, 2011; Banyard *et al.*, 2013; Meslin and Briggs, 2013; Taylor and Partners for Rabies, 2013). In reality, even separate reliable surveillance systems do not currently exist for either the veterinary or the public health sector. An online database created by WHO, the Rabnet website, was discontinued due to inconsistent reporting and poor response (Nel, 2013). In many countries, rabies is not even included as a reportable disease (Nel, 2013). This dire situation is best illustrated by the low figure of financial resources allocated to rabies diagnostics and the very small percentage of animal tests performed, compared to PEP numbers (Townsend *et al.*, 2013a). In Bhutan over 10,000 PEP treatments were reported between 2001 and 2008. In the same period only a little over 200 animals were tested by a laboratory (Tenzin *et al.*, 2012), which means that the infectious status of the source was ascertained for less than 2% of all exposed cases. Lack of knowledge about rabies leads to extreme under-reporting of cases both in animals and humans, and can also lead to misdiagnosis in humans as another encephalitic infection, particularly malaria (Mallewa *et al.*, 2007). This might be due to differential diagnosis of rabies being considered only when typical symptoms, hydrophobia in humans and aggressive behaviour in animals, are present. Therefore other less frequent syndromes, for example paralytic progression, might not be thoroughly investigated particularly in situations with a lack of history of an animal bite.

Good surveillance is not only an important prompt for the international community to recognize rabies as a public health tragedy, but is also indispensable for control and especially elimination attempts (Klepac *et al.*, 2013). Diagnostic capacity and surveillance are essential to promote vaccination campaigns and to demonstrate the effectiveness of interventions. During and after mass vaccination campaigns, surveillance sensitivity must increase considerably in order to continue detecting cases once they become rare (Klepac *et al.*, 2013; Townsend *et al.*, 2013a).

Such an improvement can be achieved by close communication between animal- and human-health workers (Meslin and Briggs, 2013). The advantage of sharing information is clear: related to each human rabies case, there is an animal rabies case; connected to each animal rabies case, there are possible human exposures. From information about incidence of bites to humans, the veterinary sector can draw conclusions about rabies incidence in animals. Conversely, starting from a known rabid animal, human exposure can be explored by a contact tracing approach (Hampson *et al.*, 2009; Banyard *et al.*, 2013). Such a tracking method is in line with the concept of risk-based surveillance, which is economically advantageous for both sectors (Stark *et al.*, 2006). In Bohol in the Philippines, contact tracing has been successfully applied (Lapiz *et al.*, 2012).

Because a common sign of rabies in dogs is unusual aggressiveness, one rabid individual can expose several victims. The average number of bite victims per rabid animal from 2011 to 2014 was 2.5, as derived from the database of the rabies laboratory in N'Djamena, Chad. A retrospective study in Senegal on human rabies cases revealed that for each victim who died at a hospital, there were four non-reported people exposed to the same initial source of infection (Diop *et al.*, 2007).

Arguably the greatest advantage of close cooperation of human and animal health services is the avoidance of unnecessary, costly PEP delivery resulting from the unknown status of a biting animal and uncertainty about the epidemiological situation in an area. Examples of over-use of vaccine are frequent, and are partly a direct consequence of poor cooperation but also a result of the understandable anxiety associated with consequences of mistakenly withholding PEP. In Bhutan, a whole region continued PEP treatment to bite-patients despite elimination of rabies from this particular district because in the southern part of the country frequent introduction of rabies from India still occurred. Due to these introductions, Bhutan did not acquire rabies-free status from WHO (Tenzin *et al.*, 2011, 2012). Similarly in Tunisia, Thailand and Sri Lanka, the demand for PEP increased after dog vaccination campaigns, presumably due to increasing awareness of rabies, but contrary to the expectations (Mitmoonpitak *et al.*, 1998; Kumarapeli and Awerbuch-Friedlander, 2009; Touihri *et al.*, 2011).

For India, Dr M.J. Mahendra described a phenomenon that grew among people with public awareness that he called the 'hydrophobia phobia', and Cleaveland *et al.* (2006) found that in Tanzania rabies was more feared than malaria, despite being less prevalent. In France where the rabies-free status is repeatedly threatened by imported rabid dogs from endemic countries, media warnings of such a reintroduction increase the demand for PEP and rabies immunoglobulin (RIG) (Lardon *et al.*, 2010; Gautret *et al.*, 2011).

Wasting valuable products, which are indispensable in the event of an actual exposure, can lead to shortages as described in Europe and the USA (Bourhy *et al.*, 2009). In low-income countries, where post-exposure vaccines are rare and RIG is virtually non-existent, each injudiciously used dose can potentially result in a fatality for another exposed rabies victim. Clearly, it is not ethical to deny treatment to those with uncertain exposure history because the consequences could be grave, but this uncertainty could in many cases be avoided through 'One Medicine' thinking and close collaboration between physicians and veterinarians. Simple questions about the circumstances of the bite incident or potential exposure (e.g. provoked or unprovoked attack), the whereabouts of an aggressive animal (free-roaming or confined), ownership status (owner known or not known), animal vaccination and health status (symptoms of rabies observed) and, most importantly, its fate (dead or missing versus alive and well) can guide the initial inquiry step. Only when an animal has a valid immunization certificate and can be clearly identified, is it possible to know with certainty that it has been correctly immunized. But often this information is not available. In Turkey, only 17% of suspect dogs which were investigated after a bite had a valid vaccination certificate (Kilic *et al.*, 2006). Compulsory dog registration would facilitate this identification and decrease the amount of PEP due to uncertain vaccination status. Where doubt exists, veterinary services can observe and follow up animals that inflicted a bite for 2 weeks. If the animal is still alive after that period of time, there is no risk of rabies and PEP for the respective victim can be discontinued. This simple but evidence-based method is still used in many regions, particularly where diagnostic facilities are not in place (Mitmoonpitak *et al.*, 1998).

To prevent unnecessary, expensive PEP after bites from negative animals or undetected exposures from a truly rabid case, each human presenting at any health facility for the treatment of a bite wound should trigger a contact to the veterinary service to notify the case. Thus, information on vaccination status of the animal and the result of diagnostic tests, if performed, can be shared and an investigation on the occurrence of other exposures (human or animal) or additional cases in the same area can jointly be undertaken.

Ideally, as suggested by Peters in 1891, a One Health rabies surveillance system should automatically involve such direct communication between public and animal health sectors and involve well-trained specialized personnel who are able to engage in timely dog rabies diagnosis and human PEP. Even if human and animal health facilities remain separated, scarce infrastructure and equipment, such as microscopes and refrigerators, as well as resources such as electricity, could potentially be shared for rabies surveillance and control (Schelling *et al.*, 2005). Savings from such sharing of resources in developing countries should not be underestimated, where the most basic infrastructure can be hard to find, especially for public institutions.

A recent study in Tanzania showed that even if only 1% of all PEP administered are given to people truly exposed, it remains cost effective (Hampson *et al.*, 2011). Critics might therefore argue why bother to put in place a common surveillance system, when the prevention of human cases can be cost effectively achieved by extensive, widely available PEP treatment alone? Such reasoning ignores the fact that concentrating on human PEP will never interrupt transmission. Ultimately, only an intervention in the reservoir host can lead to dog rabies elimination, and this approach will be more cost-effective than human PEP (Zinsstag *et al.*, Chapter 12, this volume). The next step to sustainable control should be a joint effort of veterinary and human medicine, enhancing intersectoral communication and controlling rabies at its animal source. The detailed benefits of such a One Health approach are discussed in the following section.

## One Health

While 'One Medicine' has a clinical and curative connotation, the term One Health emphasizes the added value of preventive action from closer cooperation between public and animal health (Zinsstag *et al.*, Chapters 2 and 5, this volume). The WHO's recommended and well-proven threshold to interrupt rabies transmission in a given population is 70%, owing to the generally low reproductive number being close to 1 (Coleman and Dye, 1996), irrespective of dog density (Hampson *et al.*, 2009). In low-income countries, this coverage can often only be achieved by providing the vaccine free of charge (Durr *et al.*, 2008, 2009). It is usually recommended that freedom from dog rabies is considered a public good, and that in low-income settings, dog rabies vaccination should be free of charge to the owner. Comparative cost-effectiveness analyses of dog mass vaccination compared to human PEP alone informs authorities and decision makers considering whether to engage in dog rabies mass vaccination. While government veterinary services remain committed to mechanisms for cost recovery, it is unlikely that any fees recoverable during a mass dog vaccination campaign would offset the additional costs involved (i.e. an extra person involved in handling cash during vaccination campaigns). There are many reasons why charging a fee at the point of vaccine delivery could be counter-productive, for example, if vaccine is refused to dogs brought by children who are without the means to pay for vaccination. None the less, other mechanisms may exist for supporting dog vaccination campaigns through owner payments, for example through charging dog registration fees, as has been introduced successfully in the Philippines, or through establishing community insurance schemes.

WHO promotes mass canine vaccination as part of a cost-effective approach to human rabies prevention, and estimates that in areas where the dog population is the only driver of epidemiology, this approach becomes more cost effective than PEP alone after a period of 15 years (Bogel and Meslin, 1990). Many successful dog vaccination campaigns have been undertaken in the last decades, and led to the control of rabies and marked declines of human rabies in Latin America and several regional settings in Africa and Asia (Belotto *et al.*, 2005; Lucas *et al.*, 2008; Davlin and Vonville, 2012). The cost-effectiveness of such campaigns has occasionally been assessed (Cleaveland *et al.*, 2006; Zinsstag *et al.*, 2009; Tenzin *et al.*, 2012). In N'Djaména, Chad, the cost of dog vaccination compared to PEP alone breaks even after 5 years, provided there is no reintroduction after the successful elimination occurs (Zinsstag *et al.*, 2009; Zinsstag *et al.*, Chapter 12, this volume). An equal time period to achieve similar cost-effectiveness has been reported for vaccination campaigns in Bhutan (Tenzin *et al.*, 2012).

This clear advantage of canine vaccination is due to the very high costs of human PEP vaccine and immunoglobulin. Vaccinated, rabies-free domestic dog populations can considerably lower the demand for PEP, but as discussed in the previous section, this does not always occur. Figure 16.1 shows a projection of possible worst and best case scenarios for the progress of PEP demand after a vaccination campaign. The rise of awareness for rabies in the course of interventions is closely linked to a rise in PEP numbers. Closer contact between veterinary and human medicine can buffer this impact. In parallel, studies to find new, less expensive vaccines and regimens demanding smaller and less frequent vaccine doses, like the recent WHO accepted intradermal administration, must be maintained to constantly improve cost-effectiveness of PEP itself (Verma *et al.*, 2011; Warrell, 2012).

If one area has successfully eradicated rabies, there will always be a danger of reintroduction so long as the disease persists in other regions. Even if natural barriers block the free movement of dogs, human behaviour can transmit the disease over long distances (Talbi *et al.*, 2010). In the same speech cited above, Austin Peters also pointed out the necessity for the local authorities to enforce the law and supress outbreaks of the disease, but regretted that neighbouring authorities do not cooperate together well enough (Peters, 1891):

> ... last summer the town of Framingham ordered that all dogs within its limits must be muzzled. Now the town of Brookline orders all dogs muzzled or chained for sixty days, while most of our cities and towns take no action whatever in regard to the matter; but it is very doubtful if such erratic and independent action has any marked influence upon the prevalence of the disease.

For successful elimination of rabies, concerted joint measures and common efforts are needed across many different administrative zones within a country, and even between countries. Unfortunately, the dog falls into an administrative gap in developing countries. The veterinary sector is focused on livestock health, and companion animals are ignored because they lack value for the economy, whereas most public health ministries will only deal with human aspects, rarely being

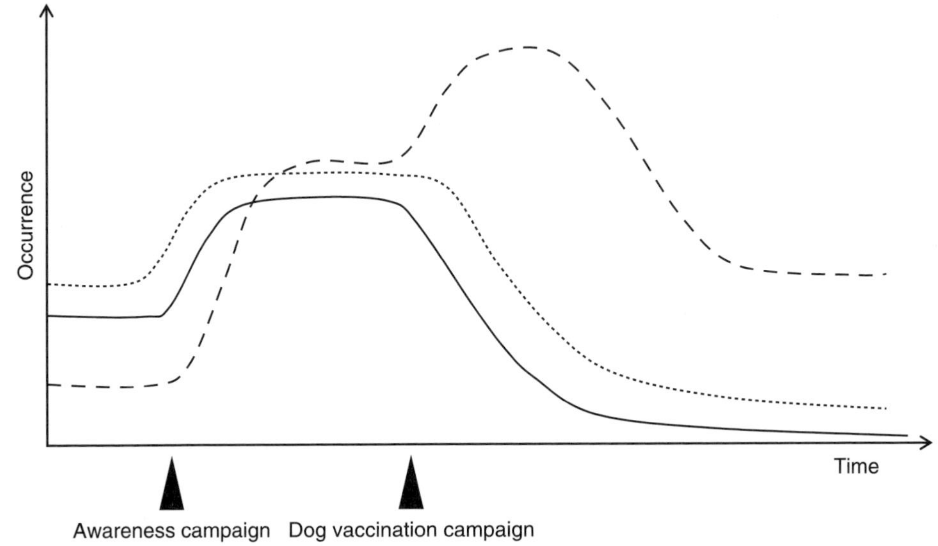


**Fig. 16.1.** Scenarios for the influence of dog vaccination campaigns on the demand for human post-exposure prophylaxis (PEP). Trend of rabies incidence (continuous line); possible rise in PEP due to elevated rabies awareness (broken line) and the decline of PEP hoped for following the decrease of rabies risk (dotted line).

motivated (or trained) to tackle problems in other species.

Meanwhile, a simple calculation illustrates financial advantages for actions at the source of rabies transmission. If an unvaccinated dog contracts rabies and bites two people, these two victims each have to take three to five doses, depending on the post-exposure regimen applied. If treatment is not sought, not available or properly administered, each victim faces a 20% probability of death from rabies (Shim *et al.*, 2009). As a practical example, dog owners in N'Djaména are shown the advantage of vaccination with the help of very clear figures: it is their choice to spend the equivalent of US$5 for dog vaccination now, to spend US$100 per victim in the event that their dog becomes rabid and bites, or to pay for the death of a person when no PEP is administered. What is evident in this micro-relationship from case to case also holds as a broad picture for the macro-level of rabies economics. If money is not allocated to prevention at the source of infection, the spending that occurs farther on for PEP treatment of all possible victims to prevent human rabies is considerably higher (Fig. 16.2). Ultimately, the loss of lives, if sufficient resources for good access to PEP are lacking, will cost the economy of a country 100 times more than an investment in dog vaccination. Millions of dollars are therefore lost worldwide. Expressed in disability adjusted life years (DALYs), rabies accounts for 1.74 million life years lost, a figure that considers the number of deaths but also the fact that most victims are children, resulting in the lost potential of tens of thousands of productive years (Knobel *et al.*, 2005).

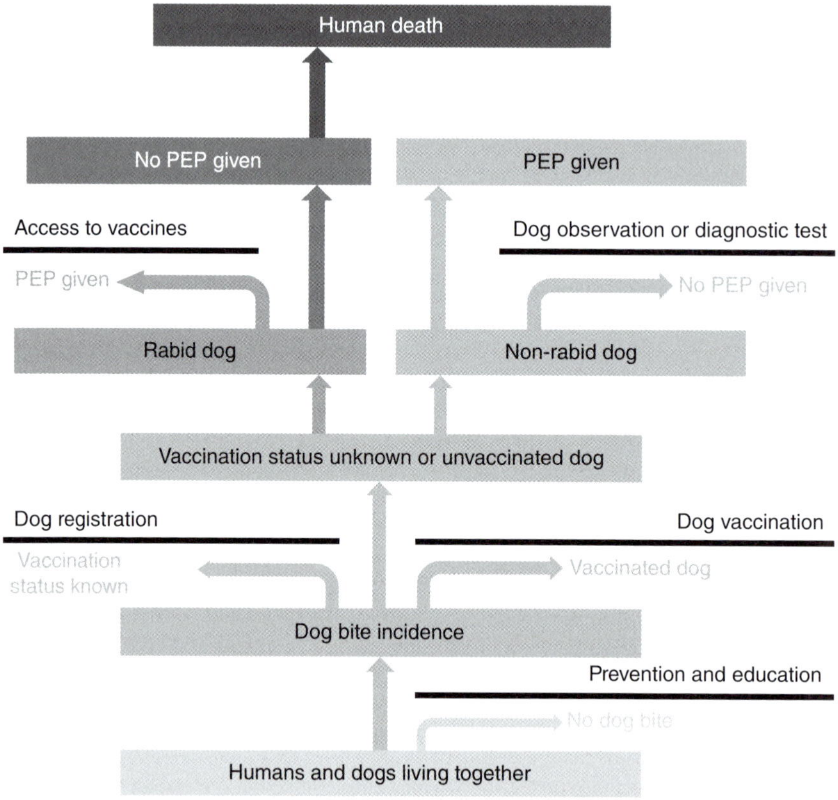


**Fig. 16.2.** Possible progress from a dog bite to post-exposure prophylaxis (PEP) or human death. Black bars show intervention possibilities to prevent further economic impact and harm.

A substantial part of the economic burden to a country can also be livestock losses due to rabies, especially in Asia where the highest numbers are reported (Shwiff *et al.*, 2013). This provides an additional incentive to take action against dog rabies. In some areas, e.g. Botswana, cattle are the species for which most rabies cases are reported. Because they are kept on farms far from settled areas, it is suspected that jackals rather than dogs could be the vector for rabies transmission to livestock (Moagabo *et al.*, 2010). Such additional disease reservoirs might only become apparent during the last phase of disease elimination (Klepac *et al.*, 2013). Others are already identified and may undermine attempts to control rabies by repeatedly re-infecting previously rabies-free domestic populations. The ecological perspective of rabies control and the problem of complex epidemiological settings for the elimination of rabies will be discussed in the next section.

## Ecosystem Approaches to Health

One Health focuses on the closer cooperation of human and animal health. As such it is embedded in the broader concept of ecosystem approaches to health (Zinsstag, 2012). Because in the Americas the majority of domestic animals are vaccinated, bats became apparent as the second most important source of rabies in humans (Belotto *et al.*, 2005). Particularly in the USA, where rabies has been eliminated in domestic animals, the epidemiology has shifted to wildlife species like foxes, raccoons and skunks (Rupprecht *et al.*, 1995). A very valuable source of information to establish the background relationships in rabies epidemiology in a given region is the molecular study of identified viral strains. With this method, it has been shown that mongoose rabies in Southern Africa forms an independent cycle (Nel *et al.*, 2005). The same reservoir function is being disputed for the bat-eared fox (Nel, 1993; Sabeta *et al.*, 2007). These examples show that in certain environments the control of rabies through dog vaccination should be complemented by the control of rabies in wildlife reservoirs (Muller *et al.*, 2012). Close communication among biologists and wildlife veterinarians is required to detect these changes and patterns.

As rabies leads inevitably to death, outbreaks of the disease in small, vulnerable species populations can potentially lead to extinction. In the 1980s, domestic dogs were most probably responsible for an outbreak of rabies in the African wild dog (*Lycaon pictus*) (Gascoyne *et al.*, 1993), listed as an endangered species. Domestic dogs are also blamed for repeated outbreaks of rabies in the Ethiopian wolf (*Canis simensis*) (Mebatsion *et al.*, 1992), a distinct canid species, endemic only to the Ethiopian Highlands. These examples show how rabies and other diseases transmitted from an abundant vector species like the domestic dog can have devastating impacts on small, endangered populations. This kind of local or worldwide extinction is not only an irrevocable loss for biodiversity, but often also results in a downgrading of the affected national parks and conservation areas (Cumming *et al.*, Chapters 4 and 21, this volume).

An example where the epidemiology of rabies is driven by a domestic reservoir is the Serengeti and Ngorongoro region (Lembo *et al.*, 2008), where dog vaccination can be of great value to wildlife and ecosystems. Mass dog vaccination campaigns conducted in a *cordon sanitaire* around the Serengeti National Park (Kaare *et al.*, 2009) have resulted in the elimination of canine rabies from pastoral and wildlife-protected areas of the ecosystem, despite the presence of abundant and diverse wildlife populations (Lembo *et al.*, 2010). While much emphasis has been given to achieving sufficient levels of vaccination coverage, with 70% coverage considered a critical threshold, recent studies have also highlighted the importance of 'completeness' of coverage. Even small areas of low coverage, involving <0.5% of dog population, could have a significant impact on the effectiveness of rabies control and time to elimination as shown for Bali (Townsend *et al.*, 2013b).

## Health in Social-ecological Systems

Finally, the One Health idea can be extended to systemic approaches of health and well-being known as health in social-ecological systems (HSES) (Zinsstag *et al.*, 2011a). In complement to ecological determinants, systemic social determinants are emphasized, such as the functioning of health systems and, arguably the most important actor in the fight against rabies, the dog owners. In addition to affordability, other critical determinants of a successful dog vaccination campaign must be considered: accessibility, adequacy, acceptability and adherence. These factors are related in a multiplicative way and depend on the social and cultural context. Lack of understanding of these effectiveness factors prevents mass vaccination campaigns from reaching sufficient coverage (Matter *et al.*, 2000; Kaare *et al.*, 2009; Thomas *et al.*, 2013). Even when vaccination teams work well and the logistics are guaranteed, if there is low accessibility of vaccination posts or facilities, performance will be low. Polo *et al.* (2013) defines accessibility in this context as the sum of: (i) supply (vaccination sites); (ii) demand (dog densities); (iii) geographical barriers between supply and demand; and (iv) people's awareness of the benefit. The first three points are closely linked: the locations of vaccination points should be carefully chosen based on dog density, as determined by prior dog demographic studies, or as estimated on the basis of human density and dog to human ratio as well as geographical distances and barriers. These location choices can only be optimized with the help of geographers and local people who know the current setting well. In special cases where there are only a few small far apart settlements or where mobile populations are involved, mobile vaccination teams might be a better option than poorly performing fixed posts (Kaare *et al.*, 2009).

Stakeholders, including dog owners, municipal authorities, community health and veterinary workers, should be involved in planning interventions from the beginning. Community ownership and participation are part of a transdisciplinary approach (Matter *et al.*, 2000; Catley and Leyland, 2001; Lapiz *et al.*, 2012; Schelling and Zinsstag, Chapter 30, this volume). In Grenada, willingness to bring a dog to vaccination facilities was low, because people feared that their animal might be infected by ectoparasites from other animals (Thomas *et al.*, 2013). In such cases, rabies vaccination could be combined with a treatment against parasites or hygiene measures, to increase the perceived benefits of participation (Catley and Leyland, 2001; Kaare *et al.*, 2009; Thomas *et al.*, 2013). Another cause for low participation can be misconception about the vaccine itself (Belsare and Gompper, 2013). For instance, fear that it might cause rabies, weakness or aggressive behaviour or that the vaccine is a poison (M. Léchenne, personal observation, Chad). A recent dog mass vaccination campaign in N'Djaména showed that dog owner participation markedly affects cost per vaccinated dog. The cost per vaccinated dog varied between US$0.6 and US$130 per dog, depending on whether 300 dogs or only one were vaccinated per day.

A further aspect of effectiveness is the willingness of the dogs to be handled (Plate 9). The human–dog relationship is determined by socio-cultural factors, with differences in the tameness of dogs observed between different religious backgrounds in Chad and in Tanzania; dogs in predominantly Moslem communities were more difficult to handle than in others (Cleaveland *et al.*, 2003), whereas in a Buddhist setting, it may be possible to handle even stray dogs (Bogel and Joshi, 1990). In certain contexts, dogs in wealthy households are more likely to be vaccinated (Awoyomi *et al.*, 2008). Consideration of social and ecological determinants provides the key for locally adapted and effective approaches towards dog rabies elimination in a given context. Such systemic approaches contribute to a science of dog rabies elimination (Zinsstag, 2013).

Cultural practices and low income may lead to poor supervision of dogs in developing countries. The majority of people in Africa for example do not allocate resources for their dogs. Dogs are fed with leftovers from the table and left to forage when the quantity is insufficient. A false conclusion that the majority of dogs roaming in the street are ownerless is often drawn in low income countries. This false supposition is then followed by another wrong conclusion that getting rid of these ownerless dogs equals getting rid of rabies. Despite substantial scientific evidence against the culling of dogs as a control for rabies (Windiyaningsih *et al.*, 2004; Morters *et al.*, 2013; Putra *et al.*, 2013), the practice continues. There are several reasons for failure of this method. Among others, due to fear of culling, people may relocate dogs to an area where rabies is not currently prevalent or may seek a replacement dog from a rabies-prevalent area and reintroduce the disease (Davlin and Vonville, 2012). But one of the most important undesirable effects of culling interventions is that the fight against rabies is negatively perceived in society, and results in lack of community support.

To confront the problems of low awareness, low motivation and low possibility of handling dogs, participatory community engagement, information, education and communication are central elements of successful rabies control. Education can help to prevent dog bites and human rabies exposure. Children, the most vulnerable group for exposure, can be taught right from the beginning how to behave to avoid conflicts with animals (Mitmoonpitak *et al.*, 2000; Kilic *et al.*, 2006). In addition, by teaching owners responsible dog ownership, a healthier more stable dog population could be attained – one that is less susceptible to rabies (Davlin and Vonville, 2012). In the Bohol Provincial Rabies Elimination Programme, the Department of Education is mandated to integrate lessons on responsible pet ownership, and rabies and its prevention into the elementary school curriculum. During a 2-year adaptation process, teaching modules on rabies were incorporated into diverse subjects, including mathematics, science, health, social science, English and Filipino. The key to this successful assimilation was the involvement and ownership of Bohol teachers, educators and provincial officials from the Department of Education, and their work in adapting the national prototype teacher's manual on rabies curriculum integration (Lapiz *et al.*, 2012). Initially, roundtable discussions with teachers, intensive planning and workshops to develop lesson plans, and orientation and training of the teachers who would use the tool were conducted. A pre-test of the first developed lesson plan was carried out for 6 months in one municipal school in Corella. The following school year, the teacher's textbook was published and distributed to all 982 public elementary schools in the province, with the target that every teacher should have a personal copy. The orientation and training of the teachers were done by those who had pre-tested the curriculum in the previous school year. The province-wide rollout by 2009 reached over 182,000 children between 5 and 12 years old, representing about 20% of the provincial population. A complement to this effort was the creation of Rabies Scouts. These were boy and girl scouts who had successfully completed a rabies and responsible pet ownership training programme. They were engaged as peer advocates and served as examples of positive action for other children. Throughout the school year, fun educational events for children were also undertaken, such as poster-making contests and pet shows to celebrate the bond between children and pets. The main programme limitation is that the intervention only reaches children who are enrolled in school, and does not include those who are likely at higher risk of being exposed to rabid dogs. Nevertheless, this education component of a comprehensive One Health approach is important to long-term sustainability of the programme, since the children continue to have higher awareness and are a source of accurate information about the disease, its prevention and responsible pet ownership.

## Conclusion

Integrated approaches to rabies control based on One Health thinking have clear advantages towards the elimination of dog rabies. For example, integrated surveillance of dog rabies and human exposure, by closer cooperation between public and animal health, increases the sensitivity of surveillance and should avoid unnecessary or overuse of PEP. One Health approaches further provide the evidence for:

**1.** The feasibility of elimination of dog rabies by mass vaccination at high coverage which cannot be achieved by dog culling or the prevention in humans alone.

**2.** A higher cost-effectiveness of dog mass vaccination and PEP versus PEP alone, after 5 to 15 years, and the interruption of dog rabies transmission.

**3.** The importance of understanding rabies ecology, and community engagement, for the development of locally effective and equitable dog mass vaccination campaigns.

To reach the goal of elimination of rabies by the year 2025, set by the Global Alliance for Rabies Control (GARC) (Lembo *et al.*, 2011), we will have to reach further than veterinary and human medicine and also include biologists, cultural scientists, sociologists and geographers. Some might say that the goal of elimination is a far reach, but more than 100 years ago in his letter to the Academy of Science, Pasteur continued the above cited text regarding the control of rabies:

Ce but est encore éloigné, mais, en présence de faits qui précédent, n'est–il pas permit d'espérer que les efforts de la science actuelle l'atteindront un jour? [This goal is still far away, but in light of the facts that precede, is it not permitted to hope that the efforts of modern science will achieve it one day?]

## Acknowledgement

Sarah Cleaveland is gratefully acknowledged for her critical comments and contributions to this chapter.

## Note

[1] Louis Pasteur; 3rd communication of Pasteur regarding rabies; 'New facts to serve the knowledge of rabies'; 11 December 1882; letter to the academy of science cited in Rosset, R. (1985).

## References

Aikimbayev, A., Briggs, D., Coltan, G., Dodet, B., Farahtaj, F., Imnadze, P., Korejwo, J., Moiseieva, A., Tordo, N., Usluer, G., Vodopija, R. and Vranjes, N. (2014) Fighting rabies in Eastern Europe, the Middle East and Central Asia - experts call for a regional initiative for rabies elimination. *Zoonoses and Public Health* 61(3), 219–226.

Awoyomi, O., Adeyemi, I. and Awoyomi, F. (2008) Socioeconomic factors associated with non-vaccination of dogs against rabies in Ibadan, Nigeria. *Nigerian Veterinary Journal* 28, 59–63.

Banyard, A.C., Horton, D.L., Freuling, C., Muller, T. and Fooks, A.R. (2013) Control and prevention of canine rabies: the need for building laboratory-based surveillance capacity. *Antiviral Research* 98, 357–364.

Belotto, A., Leanes, L., Schneider, M., Tamayo, H. and Correa, E. (2005) Overview of rabies in the Americas. *Virus Research* 111, 5–12.

Belsare, A.V. and Gompper, M.E. (2013) Assessing demographic and epidemiologic parameters of rural dog populations in India during mass vaccination campaigns. *Preventive Veterinary Medicine* 111, 139–146.

Bogel, K. and Joshi, D.D. (1990) Accessibility of dog populations for rabies control in Kathmandu valley, Nepal. *Bulletin of the World Health Organization* 68, 611–617.

Bogel, K. and Meslin, F.X. (1990) Economics of human and canine rabies elimination: guidelines for programme orientation. *Bulletin of the World Health Organization* 68, 281–291.

Bourhy, H., Goudal, M., Mailles, A., Sadkowska-Todys, M., Dacheux, L. and Zeller, H. (2009) Is there a need for anti-rabies vaccine and immunoglobulins rationing in Europe? *Eurosurveillance* 14.

Catley, A. and Leyland, T. (2001) Community participation and the delivery of veterinary services in Africa. *Preventive Veterinary Medicine* 49, 95–113.

Cleaveland, S., Kaare, M., Tiringa, P., Mlengeya, T. and Barrat, J. (2003) A dog rabies vaccination campaign in rural Africa: impact on the incidence of dog rabies and human dog-bite injuries. *Vaccine* 21, 1965–1973.

Cleaveland, S., Kaare, M., Knobel, D. and Laurenson, M.K. (2006) Canine vaccination – providing broader benefits for disease control. *Veterinary Microbiology* 117, 43–50.

Coleman, P.G. and Dye, C. (1996) Immunization coverage required to prevent outbreaks of dog rabies. *Vaccine* 14, 185–186.

Davlin, S.L. and Vonville, H.M. (2012) Canine rabies vaccination and domestic dog population characteristics in the developing world: a systematic review. *Vaccine* 30, 3492–3502.

De Balogh, K., Halliday, J. and Lubroth, J. (2013) Integrating the surveillance of animal health, foodborne pathogens and foodborne diseases in developing and in-transition countries. *Revue Scientifique et Technique* 32, 539–548.

Diop, S.A., Manga, N.M., Dia, N.M., Ndour, C.T., Seydi, M., Soumare, M., Diop, B.M. and Sow, P.S. (2007) [The point on human rabies in Senegal from 1986 to 2005]. *Médecine et Maladies Infectieuses* 37, 787–791.

Durr, S., Meltzer, M.I., Mindekem, R. and Zinsstag, J. (2008) Owner valuation of rabies vaccination of dogs, Chad. *Emerging Infectious Diseases* 14, 1650–1652.

Durr, S., Mindekem, R., Kaninga, Y., Doumagoum Moto, D., Meltzer, M.I., Vounatsou, P. and Zinsstag, J. (2009) Effectiveness of dog rabies vaccination programmes: comparison of owner-charged and free vaccination campaigns. *Epidemiology and Infection* 137, 1558–1567.

Fitzpatrick, M.C., Hampson, K., Cleaveland, S., Mzimbiri, I., Lankester, F., Lembo, T., Meyers, L.A., Paltiel, A.D. and Galvani, A.P. (2014) Cost-effectiveness of canine vaccination to prevent human rabies in rural Tanzania. *Annals of Internal Medicine* 160, 91–100.

Gascoyne, S.C., King, A.A., Laurenson, M.K., Borner, M., Schildger, B. and Barrat, J. (1993) Aspects of rabies infection and control in the conservation of the African wild dog (*Lycaon pictus*) in the Serengeti region, Tanzania. *Onderstepoort Journal of Veterinary Research* 60, 415–420.

Gautret, P., Labreuil, C., Seyni, M., Delmont, J., Parola, P. and Brouqui, P. (2011) Effect of media warnings on rabies postexposure prophylaxis, France. *Emerging Infectious Diseases* 17, 1131–1132.

Hampson, K., Dushoff, J., Cleaveland, S., Haydon, D.T., Kaare, M., Packer, C. and Dobson, A. (2009) Transmission dynamics and prospects for the elimination of canine rabies. *PLoS Biol* 7, e53.

Hampson, K., Cleaveland, S. and Briggs, D. (2011) Evaluation of cost-effective strategies for rabies post-exposure vaccination in low-income countries. *PLoS Neglected Tropical Diseases* 5, e982.

Jackson, A.C. (2013) Current and future approaches to the therapy of human rabies. *Antiviral Research* 99, 61–67.

Kaare, M., Lembo, T., Hampson, K., Ernest, E., Estes, A., Mentzel, C. and Cleaveland, S. (2009) Rabies control in rural Africa: evaluating strategies for effective domestic dog vaccination. *Vaccine* 27, 152–160.

Kayali, U., Mindekem, R., Yemadji, N., Vounatsou, P., Kaninga, Y., Ndoutamia, A.G. and Zinsstag, J. (2003) Coverage of pilot parenteral vaccination campaign against canine rabies in N'Djamena, Chad. *Bulletin of the World Health Organization* 81, 739–744.

Kilic, B., Unal, B., Semin, S. and Konakci, S.K. (2006) An important public health problem: rabies suspected bites and post-exposure prophylaxis in a health district in Turkey. *International Journal of Infectious Diseases* 10, 248–254.

Klepac, P., Metcalf, C.J.E., Mclean, A.R. and Hampson, K. (2013) Towards the endgame and beyond: complexities and challenges for the elimination of infectious diseases. *Philosophical Transactions of the Royal Society B: Biological Sciences* 368.

Knobel, D.L., Cleaveland, S., Coleman, P.G., Fevre, E.M., Meltzer, M.I., Miranda, M.E., Shaw, A., Zinsstag, J. and Meslin, F.X. (2005) Re-evaluating the burden of rabies in Africa and Asia. *Bulletin of the World Health Organization* 83, 360–368.

Kumarapeli, V. and Awerbuch-Friedlander, T. (2009) Human rabies focusing on dog ecology – A challenge to public health in Sri Lanka. *Acta Tropica* 112, 33–37.

Lapiz, S.M., Miranda, M.E., Garcia, R.G., Daguro, L.I., Paman, M.D., Madrinan, F.P., Rances, P.A. and Briggs, D.J. (2012) Implementation of an intersectoral program to eliminate human and canine rabies: the Bohol Rabies Prevention and Elimination Project. *PLoS Neglected Tropical Diseases* 6, e1891.

Lardon, Z., Watier, L., Brunet, A., Bernede, C., Goudal, M., Dacheux, L., Rotivel, Y., Guillemot, D. and Bourhy, H. (2010) Imported episodic rabies increases patient demand for and physician delivery of anti-rabies prophylaxis. *PLoS Neglected Tropical Diseases* 4, e723.

Lembo, T., Hampson, K., Haydon, D.T., Craft, M., Dobson, A., Dushoff, J., Ernest, E., Hoare, R., Kaare, M., Mlengeya, T., Mentzel, C. and Cleaveland, S. (2008) Exploring reservoir dynamics: a case study of rabies in the Serengeti ecosystem. *Journal of Applied Ecology* 45, 1246–1257.

Lembo, T., Hampson, K., Kaare, M.T., Ernest, E., Knobel, D., Kazwala, R.R., Haydon, D.T. and Cleaveland, S. (2010) The feasibility of canine rabies elimination in Africa: dispelling doubts with data. *PLoS Neglected Tropical Diseases* 4, e626.

Lembo, T., Attlan, M., Bourhy, H., Cleaveland, S., Costa, P., De Balogh, K., Dodet, B., Fooks, A.R., Hiby, E., Leanes, F., Meslin, F.X., Miranda, M.E., Muller, T., Nel, L.H., Rupprecht, C.E., Tordo, N., Tumpey, A., Wandeler, A. and Briggs, D.J. (2011) Renewed global partnerships and redesigned roadmaps for rabies prevention and control. *Veterinary Medicine International* 2011, 923149.

Lucas, C.H., Pino, F.V., Baer, G., Morales, P.K., Cedillo, V.G., Blanco, M.A. and Avila, M.H. (2008) Rabies control in Mexico. *Journal of Development Biology (Basel)* 131, 167–175.
Mallewa, M., Fooks, A.R., Banda, D., Chikungwa, P., Mankhambo, L., Molyneux, E., Molyneux, M.E. and Solomon, T. (2007) Rabies encephalitis in malaria-endemic area, Malawi, Africa. *Emerging Infectious Diseases* 13, 136–139.
Matter, H.C., Wandeler, A.I., Neuenschwander, B.E., Harischandra, L.P. and Meslin, F.X. (2000) Study of the dog population and the rabies control activities in the Mirigama area of Sri Lanka. *Acta Tropica* 75, 95–108.
Mebatsion, T., Sillero-Zubiri, C., Gottelli, D. and Cox, J.H. (1992) Detection of rabies antibody by ELISA and RFFIT in unvaccinated dogs and in the endangered Simien jackal (*Canis simensis*) of Ethiopia. *Zentralblatt Veterinärmedizin B* 39, 233–235.
Meslin, F.X. and Briggs, D.J. (2013) Eliminating canine rabies, the principal source of human infection: what will it take? *Antiviral Research* 98, 291–296.
Mitmoonpitak, C., Tepsumethanon, V. and Wilde, H. (1998) Rabies in Thailand. *Epidemiology and Infections* 120, 165–169.
Mitmoonpitak, C., Tepsumethanon, V., Raksaket, S., Nayuthaya, A.B. and Wilde, H. (2000) Dog-bite injuries at the Animal Bite Clinic of the Thai Red Cross Society in Bangkok. *Journal of the Medical Association of Thailand* 83, 1458–1462.
Moagabo, K.T., Monyame, K.B., Baipoledi, E.K., Letshwenyo, M., Mapitse, N. and Hyera, J.M.K. (2010) A retrospective longitudinal study of animal and human rabies in Botswana 1989–2006. *Onderstepoort Journal of Veterinary Research* 76(4), 399.
Morters, M.K., Restif, O., Hampson, K., Cleaveland, S., Wood, J.L. and Conlan, A.J. (2013) Evidence-based control of canine rabies: a critical review of population density reduction. *Journal of Animal Ecology* 82, 6–14.
Muller, T., Batza, H.J., Freuling, C., Kliemt, A., Kliemt, J., Heuser, R., Schluter, H., Selhorst, T., Vos, A. and Mettenleiter, T.C. (2012) Elimination of terrestrial rabies in Germany using oral vaccination of foxes. *Berliner und Münchener tierärztliche Wochenschrift* 125, 178–190.
Nel, J.A. (1993) The bat-eared fox: a prime candidate for rabies vector? *Onderstepoort Journal of Veterinary Research* 60, 395–397.
Nel, L.H. (2013) Discrepancies in data reporting for rabies, Africa. *Emerging Infectious Diseases* 19, 529–533.
Nel, L.H., Sabeta, C.T., Teichman, B.V., Jaftha, J.B., Rupprecht, C.E. and Bingham, J. (2005) Mongoose rabies in southern Africa: a re-evaluation based on molecular epidemiology. *Virus Research* 109, 165–173.
Peters, A. (1891) Rabies: its prevalence and suppression. *Journal of the Massachusetts Association of Boards of Health* 1, 102–108.
Polo, G., Acosta, C.M. and Dias, R.A. (2013) Spatial accessibility to vaccination sites in a campaign against rabies in Sao Paulo city, Brazil. *Preventive Veterinary Medicine* 111, 10–16.
Putra, A.A., Hampson, K., Girardi, J., Hiby, E., Knobel, D., Mardiana, I.W., Townsend, S. and Scott-Orr, H. (2013) Response to a rabies epidemic, Bali, Indonesia, 2008–2011. *Emerging Infectious Diseases* 19, 648–651.
Rosset, R. (ed.) (1985) *Pasteur et la rage*. Informations techniques des Services Vétérinaries, Ministère de l' Agriculture, Paris.
Rupprecht, C.E., Smith, J.S., Fekadu, M. and Childs, J.E. (1995) The ascension of wildlife rabies: a cause for public health concern or intervention? *Emerging Infectious Diseases* 1, 107–114.
Sabeta, C.T., Mansfield, K.L., Mcelhinney, L.M., Fooks, A.R. and Nel, L.H. (2007) Molecular epidemiology of rabies in bat-eared foxes (*Otocyon megalotis*) in South Africa. *Virus Research* 129, 1–10.
Schelling, E., Wyss, K., Chir, M., Daugla, D. and Zinsstag, J. (2005) Synergy between public health and veterinary services to deliver human and animal health interventions in rural low income settings. *British Medical Journal* 331, 1264–1267.
Shim, E., Hampson, K., Cleaveland, S. and Galvani, A.P. (2009) Evaluating the cost-effectiveness of rabies post-exposure prophylaxis: a case study in Tanzania. *Vaccine* 27, 7167–7172.
Shwiff, S., Hampson, K. and Anderson, A. (2013) Potential economic benefits of eliminating canine rabies. *Antiviral Research* 98, 352–356.
Stark, K.D., Regula, G., Hernandez, J., Knopf, L., Fuchs, K., Morris, R.S. and Davies, P. (2006) Concepts for risk-based surveillance in the field of veterinary medicine and veterinary public health: review of current approaches. *BMC Health Services Research* 6, 20.
Streicker, D.G., Turmelle, A.S., Vonhof, M.J., Kuzmin, I.V., Mccracken, G.F. and Rupprecht, C.E. (2010) Host phylogeny constrains cross-species emergence and establishment of rabies virus in bats. *Science* 329, 676–679.

Talbi, C., Lemey, P., Suchard, M.A., Abdelatif, E., Elharrak, M., Jalal, N., Faouzi, A., Echevarría, J.E., Morón, S.V. and Rambaut, A. (2010) Phylodynamics and human-mediated dispersal of a zoonotic virus. *PLoS Pathogens* 6, e1001166.

Taylor, L. and Partners for Rabies Prevention (2013) Eliminating canine rabies: the role of public-private partnerships. *Antiviral Research* 98, 314–318.

Tenzin, Dhand, N.K. and Ward, M.P. (2011) Human rabies post exposure prophylaxis in Bhutan, 2005–2008: trends and risk factors. *Vaccine* 29, 4094–4101.

Tenzin, Wangdi, K. and Ward, M.P. (2012) Human and animal rabies prevention and control cost in Bhutan, 2001–2008: the cost-benefit of dog rabies elimination. *Vaccine* 31, 260–270.

Thomas, D., Delgado, A., Louison, B., Lefrancois, T. and Shaw, J. (2013) Examining dog owners' beliefs regarding rabies vaccination during government-funded vaccine clinics in Grenada to improve vaccine coverage rates. *Preventive Veterinary Medicine* 110, 563–569.

Touihri, L., Zaouia, I., Elhili, K., Dellagi, K. and Bahloul, C. (2011) Evaluation of mass vaccination campaign coverage against rabies in dogs in Tunisia. *Zoonoses and Public Health* 58, 110–118.

Townsend, S.E., Lembo, T., Cleaveland, S., Meslin, F.X., Miranda, M.E., Putra, A.a.G., Haydon, D.T. and Hampson, K. (2013a) Surveillance guidelines for disease elimination: a case study of canine rabies. *Comparative Immunology, Microbiology and Infectious Diseases* 36, 249–261.

Townsend, S.E., Sumantra, I.P., Pudjiatmoko, Bagus, G.N., Brum, E., Cleaveland, S., Crafter, S., Dewi, A.P., Dharma, D.M., Dushoff, J., Girardi, J., Gunata, I.K., Hiby, E.F., Kalalo, C., Knobel, D.L., Mardiana, I.W., Putra, A.A., Schoonman, L., Scott-Orr, H., Shand, M., Sukanadi, I.W., Suseno, P.P., Haydon, D.T. and Hampson, K. (2013b) Designing programs for eliminating canine rabies from islands: Bali, Indonesia as a case study. *PLoS Neglected Tropical Diseases* 7, e2372.

Verma, R., Khanna, P., Prinja, S. and Rajput, M. (2011) Intra-dermal administration of rabies vaccines in developing countries: at an affordable cost. *Human Vaccines and Immunotherapeutics* 7, 792–794.

Vigilato, M.A., Cosivi, O., Knobl, T., Clavijo, A. and Silva, H.M. (2013) Rabies update for Latin America and the Caribbean. *Emerging Infectious Diseases* 19, 678–679.

Warrell, M.J. (2003) The challenge to provide affordable rabies post-exposure treatment. *Vaccine* 21, 706–709.

Warrell, M.J. (2012) Intradermal rabies vaccination: the evolution and future of pre- and post-exposure prophylaxis. *Current Topics in Microbiology and Immunology* 351, 139–157.

Warrell, M.J. and Warrell, D.A. (2004) Rabies and other lyssavirus diseases. *The Lancet* 363, 959–969.

Windiyaningsih, C., Wilde, H., Meslin, F.X., Suroso, T. and Widarso, H.S. (2004) The rabies epidemic on Flores Island, Indonesia (1998–2003). *Journal of the Medical Association of Thailand* 87, 1389–1393.

Zinsstag, J. (2012) Convergence of Ecohealth and One Health. *EcoHealth* 9(4), 371–373.

Zinsstag, J. (2013) Towards a science of rabies elimination. *Infectious Diseases of Poverty* 2, 22.

Zinsstag, J., Durr, S., Penny, M.A., Mindekem, R., Roth, F., Menendez Gonzalez, S., Naissengar, S. and Hattendorf, J. (2009) Transmission dynamics and economics of rabies control in dogs and humans in an African city. *Proceedings of the National Academy of Sciences USA* 106, 14996–15001.

Zinsstag, J., Bonfoh, B., Cissé, G., Nguyen-Viet, H., Silué, B., N'guessan, T.S., Weibel, D., Schertenleib, R., Obrist, B. and Tanner, M. (2011a) Towards equity effectiveness in health interventions. In: Weismann, U. and Hurni, H. (eds) *Research for Sustainable Development: Foundations, Experiences, and Perspectives.* Perspectives of the Swiss National Centre of Competence in Research (NCCR) North-South, Geographica Bernensis, Berne, Switzerland, 6, pp. 623–640.

Zinsstag, J., Schelling, E., Waltner-Toews, D. and Tanner, M. (2011b) From 'one medicine' to 'one health' and systemic approaches to health and well-being. *Preventive Veterinary Medicine* 101, 148–156.

# 17 Leptospirosis: Development of a National One Health Control Programme in Fiji

**Simon Reid[1]* and Mike Kama[2]**
[1]*School of Population Health, University of Queensland, Australia;*
[2]*Fiji Centre for Communicable Disease Control, Suva, Republic of Fiji*

## Introduction

This case study examines the complex associations between reservoir hosts, the environment and the human communities involved in transmission cycles of *Leptospira* spp. and show how this information can be used in the design of research and policy interventions to reduce the impact of leptospirosis. The output of recent activities in Fiji to draft a national strategy for the control of leptospirosis will be used to highlight key issues required to successfully develop a multi-sectoral programme. The scope of the case study will not include issues related to the clinical management of cases of leptospirosis. This has been done to allow the text to focus on the intersectoral components of a control programme because clinical management falls within the direct responsibility of the health system with little involvement of other sectors. One Health has been defined as 'the collaborative effort of multiple disciplines – working locally, nationally, and globally – to attain optimal health for people, animals and our environment' (American Veterinary Medical Association, 2008). The intersectoral management of leptospirosis in Fiji clearly demonstrates the need for this type of approach. This is because the close collaboration between public health, animal health and agricultural sectors is required to identify local environmental drivers (including animal reservoirs) and to develop sustainable programmes to manage risks in the community.

## Leptospirosis – an Introduction

Leptospirosis is a globally important zoonotic disease that occurs mainly in tropical or subtropical countries in both urban and rural settings (Victoriano *et al.*, 2009). It is generally accepted that rodents (rats and mice) and domestic mammals, such as cattle, pigs and possibly dogs are the major reservoir hosts (World Health Organization, 2003). Leptospirosis is caused by spirochetes of the genus *Leptospira*. To date over 200 pathogenic serovars divided into 25 serogroups have been described (World Health Organization, 2003). Serovars have proven to be a useful classification system because of the observed associations between individual serovars and epidemiological aspects of leptospirosis. The most obvious traits are pathogenicity and adaptation to reservoir hosts. Approximately half of the

*E-mail: simon.reid@uq.edu.au

pathogenic serovars belong to *L. interrogans* or *L. borgpetersenii* (Victoriano *et al.*, 2009). Whilst humans are susceptible to infection with all serovars the severity of clinical disease induced by different serovars appears to differ. For example, Merien and Perolat (1996) showed that whilst serovar Icterohaemorrhagiae was only implicated in 20% of 192 human cases in New Caledonia, it was associated with over 50% of severe clinical cases requiring intensive care.

The annual incidence of human leptospirosis is highest in tropical regions where it may reach 100 cases per 100,000 in outbreaks and communities at risk of high levels of exposure (Victoriano *et al.*, 2009). The magnitude of the problem in tropical and subtropical regions is largely attributed to climatic and environmental conditions and the increased risks of transmission associated with factors such as local agricultural practices, recreational activities (e.g. swimming and fishing) and poor housing and waste disposal (World Health Organization, 2003). In addition, leptospirosis is a major cause of economic loss to the livestock industry as a result of abortion and early calf mortality (i.e. infertility/poor productivity) of farmed animals and disease in people associated with livestock (Faine *et al.*, 1999).

The exclusive sources of human infection, direct or indirect, are animal carriers and shedders of *Leptospira* spp., because humans are a 'dead-end' host and pathogenic leptospires are unable to replicate outside a mammalian host (Babudieri, 1958). The importance of different mammalian hosts in the epidemiology of human leptospirosis depends on their ability to act as long-term carriers and their ability to contaminate the environment associated with humans with urine containing viable leptospires (Babudieri, 1958).

## Leptospirosis in Fiji

Fiji is one of the larger Pacific island countries with a population of 837,271 (in 2007), comprising 57% iTaukei (predominantly Melanesian), 37% Indians of Fijian descent (Indo-Fijian) and the remainder from other ethnic groups (Fiji Bureau of Statistics, 2007). The two largest islands, Viti Levu and Vanua Levu, account for approximately 87% of the total land area and 90% of the population (Fiji Bureau of Statistics). Indigenous Fijians (iTaukei) own 87.9% of the land with the remainder divided between Freehold (7.9%), State Land (3.9%) and Rotuman land (0.3%) (Fiji Bureau of Statistics). There has been significant change in land use in Fiji as a result of the non-renewal of leases on agricultural land over the past 10 years or more, which has resulted in a gradual reduction in the land used for cultivation of sugarcane (Narayan, 2005) as well as a reduction in the national beef herd (Mcfarlane, 2009).

Fiji's climate is affected by the South Pacific convergence zone rainfall patterns, which creates a 'dry zone' on the north-western side of both main islands with a 'wet zone' on the south-eastern side of each main island. The effect of this rainfall pattern is significant differences in the types of land use and vegetation cover in the two zones. The 'dry zone' is characterized by more open grassland with significant agriculture, mostly sugarcane growing. The 'wet zone' has significantly greater forest cover with larger livestock enterprises such as dairy farming. The smaller islands are more homogeneous with regards to their climate. Regular flooding occurs in low-lying coastal as well as urban areas located near the four main rivers: the Rewa, Sigatoka, Ba and Navua. Flooding is usually associated with the passage of slow-moving tropical cyclones, storm tides and heavy tropical downpours.

There is a dearth of published reports on leptospirosis in Fiji. The pattern of disease occurrence since the first report in 1952 (Ram, 1977b) has been a slight increase in numbers during the rainy season, mostly seen in men with a majority of cases attributed to Icterohaemorrhagiae (45%), Australis (24%) and Canicola (13%) (Ram, 1977a). Data from the Ministry of Health indicates a steady increase of leptospirosis incidence in Fiji with 20–100 cases per year being reported over the past 15 years until 2009, after which the number of cases increased significantly with over 500 cases and 52 deaths reported in 2012 (Ministry of Health, unpublished data). However, there has been no systematic evaluation of serovars from more recent cases. Two separate unpublished reviews of data from cases of human leptospirosis from 1991 to 2001 (Kubuabola, 2003) and 1998 to 2009 (Fiji School of Medicine and Fiji Ministry of Health, 2009) showed that Australis,

Copenhageni, Canicola and Cynoptera were the serovars most commonly isolated.

There have been few reports of animal leptospirosis in Fiji, which reflects the lack of investigation of its presence and impact rather than its absence. Surveys conducted in 1966–1967 showed a significant prevalence of antibodies to serovar Pomona in healthy cattle at slaughter and serovar Canicola and Icterohaemorrhagiae in dogs showing signs of nephritis and hepatitis (Ram, 1977b). A survey in 1981 showed that the sero-prevalence, using a complement fixation test, was 27.5%, 17.1%, 10.3%, 10.0%, 57.0%, 55.8%, 53.1% and 40.0% in cattle, sheep, goats, pigs, dogs, rats (*Rattus* spp.), mongooses (*Herpestes auropunctatus*) and mice (species unknown) (Collings, 1984).

## The Cycle of *Leptospira* Species Transmission

The transmission cycles of pathogenic *Leptospira* spp. can be conceptualized as a number of smaller self-sustaining cycles within separate mammalian species that 'spill-over' into other species when environmental and epidemiological factors permit (Plate 10). The most significant cycles from a public health point of view are associated with rodents and livestock species because they are ecologically associated with humans and hence more likely to contaminate the environment inhabited by human communities. This is important because human infection nearly always occurs through indirect exposure to water, mud or food contaminated with urine from an animal infected with *Leptospira* spp. (Babudieri, 1958).

There is insufficient information to characterize accurately the transmission cycles in Fiji. However, reviews of data from reported cases in Fiji tend to draw similar conclusions regarding the likely types of exposure patterns. Ram and Collings (1982) drew the following conclusions from a review of data from reported cases of leptospirosis from 1969 to 1981:

- The low prevalence in the 0–9-year-old age group suggested that rodents in the home environment were not important reservoirs of infection. This is possibly due to the reduced likelihood that rodent (or other animal) urine is present in the home or that children in the home have less access to mud and water bodies, which are most commonly associated with adolescent and adult leptospirosis.
- The high prevalence of infection in young (20–29) indigenous Fijian (iTaukei) males, compared to the low rates in Indo-Fijians, strongly suggested a link with the place and nature of work and recreation activities that were associated with specific risk factors such as time spent in water (e.g. fishing or swimming) or walking barefoot (e.g. gardening and other land-based agriculture).

However, this generalized pattern of exposure variables may change as Fiji's agricultural sector undergoes structural changes that can be seen in the increasing rate of urbanization, which is associated with the changing land-use patterns, especially in the Indo-Fijian populations that were previously leasehold farmers (Storey, 2006).

## The Domestic Cycle of Transmission

### Domestic animals

The domestic cycle of leptospirosis involves infection of mainly cattle and pigs and, to a lesser extent, sheep, goats and dogs. Domestic animals are maintenance hosts of specific serovars: cattle usually maintain serovars Hardjo, Pomona and Grippotyphosa; pigs harbour serovars Pomona, Tarassovi or Bratislava; sheep may harbour Hardjo and Pomona; and dogs may harbour Canicola (Levett, 2001).

The domestic cycle is largely driven by factors associated with the management of each livestock species by humans. In general, livestock are relatively intensively managed in Fiji along a continuum from smallholder village-based settings to larger commercially focused enterprises that have significant economic investment in infrastructure and agricultural inputs such as feed and veterinary drugs. In similar setting in Papua New Guinea (PNG) *Leptospira* spp. infection in beef cattle does not become prevalent until animals are maintained in larger (>200 head) commercially focused herds (Wai'in, 2007). In these settings, surveys of village livestock (including cattle, pigs and dogs) showed a low prevalence of infection compared to the larger commercial farms. This was most likely due in part to the increased stocking densities employed on larger farms. In addition, commercial farms tend to actively manage cattle, which create opportunities for young uninfected cohorts to be mixed with older, actively shedding cattle or exposed to mud in handling facilities that is contaminated with leptospires. This situation is generally not a feature of the management of cattle in small semi-commercial herds that are usually maintained as a single cohort.

Leptospirosis can be a significant cause of production loss in cattle and pig production enterprises as a result of abortion, fetal/neonatal mortality and prolonged infertility (Higgins *et al.*, 1980; Faine *et al.*, 1999; Ramos *et al.*, 2006). However, there are no data on the burden of disease or associated economic costs in humans. There is a need for cross-sectoral studies in humans and animals to gather data that would enable the calculation of impact in all species. Similar studies have been performed for brucellosis (Bonfoh *et al.*, 2012).

There is less information about transmission cycles in dogs. Dogs are considered 'spillover' hosts in that infection with serovar Icterohaemorrhagiae (presumably from rodents) can cause severe disease similar to classical Weil's disease, with high mortality (Weekes *et al.*, 1997). Furthermore, dogs have been shown to be a source of infection in human cases of leptospirosis (Weekes *et al.*, 1997). This may be because dogs fed a vegetable-based diet have more-alkaline urine compared to a meat-based diet, which may enable leptospires to survive longer and hence present a greater risk to humans (Babudieri, 1958). This may be important because dogs are usually kept in loosely or unmanaged groups in rural communities in Fiji that mostly scavenge for food or are fed left-over food from household meals that is usually low in protein.

## Drivers of human infection

Human infection with *Leptospira* spp. of domestic animal origin is largely associated with occupational exposure. Some examples of risky activities include: managing domestic and farm animals; milking cattle; assisting in births, removing stillbirths or removal of abortion products; dressing carcases; cleaning urine spills from dogs; and practising as veterinarians and meat inspectors (Blackmore and Schollum, 1982; Faine *et al.*, 1999). In addition, rodents are synonymous with livestock production systems. Recent studies in American Samoa have demonstrated the high risk of human leptospirosis as a result of the proximity of housing to piggeries, especially those enterprises at higher points in a watershed (Lau *et al.*, 2012). However, this study was not able to discriminate the role of pigs or rodents as reservoir species because no animal sampling was undertaken.

## Interventions and responses

An optimal programme to control leptospirosis in domestic livestock should be designed to prevent clinical disease and urinary shedding of leptospires. The most effective control programmes in livestock are based on the prevention of exposure, which includes measures such as isolation, herd management and vaccination. Isolation and herd management involve strategies to prevent direct and indirect transmission of leptospires from infected adults to susceptible young stock, because active infection often persists in older animals. For this programme to be successful, successive cohorts of animals have to remain isolated to remain free from infection, until all the infected cohorts have passed through the population. In addition, adult carriers in the herd should be identified and culled (removed) and procedures implemented to vaccinate all animals introduced on to the property (Little *et al.*, 1992a,b). Vaccination is the most important method of preventing leptospirosis in livestock (Little *et al.*, 1992b). Depending on the degree of exposure or the level of risk, vaccinating the herd one to two times a year may be warranted (Faine *et al.*, 1999).

In PNG, the geographic separation of young cattle on one property and the aggressive identification and removal of infertile cows (i.e. those that did not produce a calf) accompanied by annual vaccination significantly reduced the transmission of *Leptospira* spp. in the livestock (Wai'in, 2007). This was presumably accompanied by a concomitant reduction in risk for farm workers, although this was not evaluated in the studies. Further research is required to evaluate this hypothesis because *in silico* models of livestock vaccination for brucellosis have demonstrated the likelihood of health benefits from a reduction in human brucellosis for communities associated with ruminant livestock (Roth *et al.*, 2003).

Bi- and quadrivalent (serovars Icterohaemorrhagiae, Canicola, Grippotyphosa and Pomona) vaccines are available for the prevention of canine leptospirosis (Sykes *et al.*, 2011). Whilst the widespread use of these vaccines would significantly reduce the risk of zoonotic transmission there is insufficient evidence to recommend dog vaccination in Fiji as a way of reducing the incidence of human leptospirosis. Further cross-sectoral research is required to understand the role of dogs as reservoirs for human leptospirosis in Fiji and other Pacific island countries.

### Summary of key points

- Leptospirosis in livestock is a significant cause of production loss and risk of human infection.
- Leptospirosis in cattle and pigs is driven by management practices used in their production.
- Dogs may suffer severe fatal or mild subclinical leptospirosis.
- The role of dogs in human leptospirosis is unclear but may be significant under certain circumstances.
- Livestock are a significant source of *Leptospira* spp. infection for associated occupational groups.
- Cheap and effective vaccines are available for the major economically significant serovars that infect cattle and pigs.
- The impact of leptospirosis on commercial cattle can be reduced through improved management to avoid infection of young animals.
- Vaccines are also available for serovars that cause severe disease in dogs.
- There are no human vaccines for domestic animal-associated leptospiral serovars.

## Sylvatic (Rodent) Transmission Cycles

Rodents are closely associated with human habitation and human agriculture principally because they provide food and shelter for the animals. The transmission of *Leptospira* spp. in rodent populations is governed by a complex interplay of rodent population dynamics, depending on available feed, climatic conditions and endemic status. In some circumstances the occurrence of leptospirosis is strongly seasonal with peaks of transmission occurring synchronously with the seasonal increase in rainfall in tropical and subtropical areas (i.e. the wet season). This pattern of human disease has been associated with increases in the size of the rodent population and increases in the prevalence of carriage (shedding) of leptospires (Holt *et al.*, 2006; Perez *et al.*, 2011). This association has been explained in terms of increases in survival of leptospires in environmental media, which increased the rate of infection in rodents at the same time as the increase in rodent population (presumably due to increases in available food and shelter) generated a larger pool of naive individuals (Holt *et al.*, 2006; Perez *et al.*, 2011).

The epidemiology and in particular the seasonality of leptospirosis differs in the different agroecological zones in Fiji. There is a more apparent seasonal pattern in the north-west of the main island that is associated with a strong seasonal rainfall and frequent flooding events. The pattern of disease occurrence in the south-eastern part of the main island is less seasonal, which may be due to the more even rainfall distribution or due to a different set of reservoir hosts. Rodents are also a significant source of economic loss for agricultural communities through the damage to crops and stored food.

### Drivers of human infection

Human behaviour and activity drive exposure to leptospire-contaminated environments. The main source of risk in Fiji is agricultural activities that expose people to mud and surface water, such as sugarcane harvesting (Ram, 1977a). In addition, recreational use of water also poses a risk (World Health Organization, 2003). It appears that higher levels of knowledge of leptospirosis are protective with regards to the risk of infection (Keenan *et al.*, 2010), which shows the importance of effective health promotion in control programmes for leptospirosis.

### Potential interventions and responses

The results of the studies by Holt *et al.* (2006) and Perez *et al.* (2011) suggest that environmental modification by removal of standing water and rodent control may be effective interventions to reduce the size of the reservoir of *Leptospira* spp. in rodents. This would be achieved by reducing the rate of replication of rodents, removal of an environmental source of leptospires and stabilizing the herd immunity in the existing population.

Ecologically based rodent management is based on the principles of integrated pest management. These principles include gaining an understanding of the biology of the rodent populations with regards to their species, local drivers of population dynamics and the cultural and social environment that exists (Singleton *et al.*, 1999). Methods to manage rodents are based on removing or limiting sources of food and shelter accompanied by physical removal of animals by trapping (Singleton *et al.*, 1999). The limitation of food and shelter is achieved by practices such as exclusion of food sources (i.e. stored and household food) and changes to cropping and vegetation control practices to reduce habitat that provides shelter and food.

Prophylaxis in humans is a contentious issue and considered to be of use under specific circumstances (World Health Organization, 2003). Once-weekly doxycycline prophylaxis has been shown to be effective at reducing the number of clinical cases. However, its widespread use requires careful consideration of logistical issues and its overall role in the prevention of leptospirosis. Vaccination of high-risk populations (sewer workers) to prevent infection with the single serovar Icterohaemorrhagiae has been successfully used in France to prevent an occupational disease for almost 25 years (Nardone *et al.*, 2004).

### Summary of key points

- Rodents are the major source of infection for humans, especially for serovar Icterohaemorrhagiae, which is the most important cause of severe leptospirosis.
- The dynamic of transmission in rodents is associated with climatic factors in some circumstances as a result of increased rodent numbers and an associated increase in carriage rates.
- Reducing rodent populations before the wet season and removing sources of standing water may reduce the incidence of leptospirosis.
- Rodent control will also provide indirect economic benefits to agricultural communities.
- Increasing the knowledge of 'at risk' populations is an essential part of a programme to reduce the incidence of leptospirosis.
- Chemo- and immune-prophylaxis in humans may have a role in specific situations.

## The Process to Develop a National Strategy for the Control of Leptospirosis in Fiji

The Fiji Ministry of Health (MoH) initiated a process to develop a national strategy for the control of leptospirosis in 2011 that was facilitated by Secretariat of the Pacific Community (SPC). This process has involved two consultation workshops and an experts meeting to develop a consensus set of goals and objectives for implementation by the different government and partner agencies involved. The authors worked collaboratively as co-facilitators of the process with Dr Reid providing overall facilitation (as part of SPC and then University of Queensland) and Dr Kama providing local leadership.

### Initial consultations

The process began with two 1-day consultation meetings that initiated discussion on the topic of leptospirosis amongst representatives from six government ministries (Health, Agriculture, Environment, Labour, Planning and Local Government), local government (Suva City Council), non-government organizations (NGOs), international agencies (WHO, SPC) and industry bodies representing the meat, dairy and pest control industries.

The workshops were structured to enable discussion on four broad thematic areas that were considered to be the core areas required within the strategy:

- agriculture;
- clinical management;
- environmental health and health promotion; and
- laboratory.

Broadly, the common themes that emerged from the discussions in the first consultation were:

- multi-sectoral collaboration (internal/external);
- communication/feedback/reporting;
- early detection and treatment and investigation when case presented;
- behaviour change communication to improve early presentation of cases; and
- health promotion.

### Diagnosis and case management

The consultations identified that current systems of diagnosis and clinical management were effective when the index of suspicion was high, resulting in good management of acute cases of leptospirosis. In general, the response to an outbreak was relatively good with adequate provision of medical care and good public awareness activities implemented by environmental health officers (EHOs). However, a number of areas for improvement were noted that became the major focus of the discussions.

It was identified that there was a need to improve the diagnostic processes in Fiji to increase the sampling rate in cases of febrile illness and to enhance the follow-up and investigation of negative results by re-sampling and testing with a diagnostic panel for fevers. In addition, the logistics of sample submission were identified as contributing to delays in diagnosis because of batching at subdivisional and laboratory level. Furthermore, a more formal allocation of funding was required to establish dedicated systems to refer samples for diagnostic confirmation and serovar determination because these capacities do not currently exist in Fiji. A major gap that was identified was the lack of animal health laboratory capacity with regards to detection of leptospirosis. This was identified as an urgent need because the current system of specimen referral was considered to be unsustainable. Opportunities for collaboration between the public and animal health laboratories was highlighted as an urgent need but further discussion is required to establish mechanisms for obtaining dedicated resources to enable this. This is a complicated issue because the protocols for testing of animal samples by the public health laboratory do not exist and it is possible that this would not be permitted under existing laboratory management policies. Short-term alternatives, such as the molecular testing of blood/kidney samples from animals at the public health laboratory, were identified.

The groups identified that there was a need for tools to improve early detection and treatment of cases (tests/case definition), standardization of treatment protocols, improved feedback from clinical departments, better understanding of risk factors to provide evidence for index of suspicion, clinical studies to improve understanding of clinical complications and burden of disease and improved coverage of communication campaigns. In terms of capacity building, they identified education of clinicians in clinical symptoms to improve early presentation and research on the cause of fevers to improve differential diagnosis.

### Intersectoral collaboration and communication

The groups felt that there was good information sharing in the human health sector but that there is no collaboration across the sectors. The need to evaluate success of public awareness campaigns and health promotion activities was considered an immediate priority for the people involved in these activities. In terms of the agricultural sector there was a consensus that the country needed a more structured approach to rodent management. This would include monitoring/surveillance of rodent populations and improved approaches to reduce populations of rodents in high-risk areas. The need for enhanced collaboration/communication across the sectors (Ministry of Primary Industries and MoH) was also highlighted. The final item was the need for resources to enable enforcement of existing legislation as well as a review and possible revision of this legislation.

### Outcomes of initial consultations

The outcome of the two workshops was a list of the goals and objectives for each of the four core areas and a broad range of proposed activities that participants of the second workshop believed were necessary to achieve these objectives. The overall goal of the Plan was to reduce the burden attributable to leptospirosis in Fiji by reducing the incidence of and mortality due to leptospirosis in Fijian communities. The component objectives set after the initial consultations were the following.

**1.** Reduce the mortality rate in the human population.
**2.** Strengthen laboratory capacity.
**3.** Implement a structured programme to reduce leptospirosis in livestock.
**4.** Strengthen community-based programmes to control reservoir species and exposure to leptospires.

### Experts meeting on leptospirosis

A meeting of international experts was convened to identify knowledge gaps with regards to leptospirosis in Fiji and solutions to address those gaps. In addition to identifying critical knowledge gaps, the experts meeting was designed to focus on Fiji-specific leptospirosis control strategies, based on the currently available knowledge. The meeting aimed to provide the following three outputs.

**1.** Strategies to reduce the burden (incidence and mortality) of leptospirosis in Fiji based on existing knowledge/information.
**2.** Identification of gaps in knowledge and strategies to address these gaps.
**3.** Finalization of the National Strategic Plan for Leptospirosis.

The overwhelming outcome of the experts meeting was the identification of the urgent need for data on the serovars involved in human disease and their likely reservoir hosts. Leptospirosis has a highly variable epidemiology in Fiji and is likely to involve multiple different reservoir hosts and transmission cycles. Current attempts to develop rational interventions are hampered by the absence of this information. To achieve this Fiji needs to improve its current surveillance system for communicable diseases to increase the capture of epidemiologically relevant data, improve case management and increase diagnostic capacity. In addition, there was an urgent identified need to evaluate health promotion activities to ensure a strong foundation for the design of a future programme.

### A short workshop on ecological rodent control

A 1-day workshop was run for 40 staff of the MoH (Public Health and Environmental Health) and the Ministry of Primary Industries (MPI) with the following objectives.

**1.** Identification of current knowledge and practices of rodent management in Fiji.
**2.** Consider impacts and management across agriculture, peri-urban, urban.
**3.** Provide knowledge and access to resources.
**4.** Consider agricultural and health impacts.
**5.** Identify major gaps in knowledge and possible actions for the future.

The major gaps in knowledge and possible actions identified related to the need for more information on the temporal dynamics of rodent population and their role in the epidemiology of leptospirosis. There is a need to assess cultural beliefs because rats are a totem in some areas, which may curtail efforts to manage them. The workshop suggested gathering evidence to support the current management plans developed by the Environmental Health Unit and to determine the losses caused by rodents to agriculture to support more widespread activities. A key outcome of the meeting was the identification that there is a need for a cross-sector task force and a 'stakeholder learning alliance', which includes the pest control sector. This would then enable an increase in the capacity and transfer of technology to improve rodent management.

## A One Health Approach to Controlling Leptospirosis in Fiji

We are now left with two questions. The first is, 'What should a multi-sectoral programme to reduce the impact of leptospirosis in Fiji look like?' To answer this question, we move back to the transmission cycles to examine the individual components and key drivers and interactions. We must also examine the institutional domains that govern the activities that form part of a multi-sectoral response. The key institutions involved are the MPI and MoH. There are multiple units in the MPI that would be involved, including: crop protection, animal health, animal production and land use/planning. Within the MoH, the units responsible include the public health, health promotion and environmental health units.

Further information is needed on the impact of leptospirosis on Fijian society in terms of its public and animal health impacts and their resultant economic burdens. This information can only be obtained through well-designed research studies that involve assessment of causal pathways for the development of human and animal leptospirosis using incident human cases as a focus. This would involve a multi-disciplinary research team to disentangle the different components (social, cultural, economic and biological) of the causal web and construct bio-economic simulations to determine the outcome of different control scenarios.

Table 17.1 shows the major components according to the institutional domain of a suggested programme to reduce the incidence of leptospirosis in Fiji through a reduction in the reservoir of infection and in the risk of transmission.

The second question is, 'How does Fiji manage a multi-sectoral process?' The MoH in Fiji has formed the National Task Force for the Control of Outbreak Prone Diseases (NTCOPD) to provide the best evidence-based prevention and control strategy and the relevant policies for the different outbreak-prone communicable diseases, including leptospirosis. The prevention and control strategies are based on five thematic areas, which are: Coordination & Collaboration, Surveillance & Research, Clinical Management, Prevention and Control & Communication. The NTCOPD is an ideal vehicle for the coordination of an intersectoral programme to manage leptospirosis because its core membership includes the major technical and operational units in the MoH and it will be expanded to include representatives from the Ministry of Primary Industries, in particular members of the veterinary services.

A key enabling document for the NTCOPD will be the National Strategy for Leptospirosis. This document is important for two reasons. First, it enables the NTCOPD to clearly identify the roles and responsibilities of the different sectors involved in the management of leptospirosis. It also describes the main activities and their resource requirements. This provides the NTCOPD with the ability to gain commitment from senior ministry officers who are able to provide the resources required. The second reason is that it provides a powerful advocacy tool for the ministries involved to argue for an allocation of funding for activities in the agricultural sector to provide a public health benefit.

**Table 17.1.** Key objectives, outcomes and rationale for potential interventions to reduce the incidence of leptospirosis in Fiji.

| Ministry of Primary Industries Strategy | | |
|---|---|---|
| Objectives | Outcome | Rationale |
| Implement a structured programme to reduce leptospirosis in livestock and other domestic animals | Reduction in the prevalence of leptospirosis in domestic animals in Fijian communities | This will reduce the overall risk of transmission to humans and decrease the economic losses to the livestock sector |
| Determine the impact of leptospirosis on livestock enterprise and the broader agricultural community in Fiji (i.e. cross-sector economic impact) | Information on the economic impact of leptospirosis on livestock enterprise and human health in Fiji that provides evidence for rational control programmes to reduce the prevalence (i.e. vaccination) | Initial research required to gather evidence to justify a programme |
| Strengthen stray dog management in urban and rural communities | Stray dog populations are significantly reduced in Fijian communities in a welfare-sensitive way | Reduced stray dogs may decrease a reservoir of infection whilst also preventing animal welfare issues associated with leptospirosis in these dogs |
| Develop and implement a structured communication programme for agricultural communities in high-risk areas | Agricultural communities understand better the risks related to leptospirosis and strategies to minimize environmental transmission | Increased knowledge is protective with regards to the risk of leptospirosis |
| Develop and implement strategies to ensure joint case and outbreak investigation is undertaken | Improved epidemiological data collection and increased knowledge of risk factors associated with clinical disease | Human serovar data alone are insufficient to provide information on reservoir species |

## References


American Veterinary Medical Association (2008) One Health: A New Professional Imperative. Available at: https://www.avma.org/KB/Resources/Reports/Pages/One-Health.aspx (accessed 16 January 2015).

Babudieri, B. (1958) Animal reservoirs of leptospires. *Annals of the New York Academy of Sciences* 70, 393–413.

Blackmore, D.K. and Schollum, L.M. (1982) Risks of contracting leptospirosis on the dairy farm. *The New Zealand Medical Journal* 95, 649–652.

Bonfoh, B., Kasymbekov, J., Durr, S., Toktobaev, N., Doherr, M.G., Schueth, T., Zinsstag, J. and Schelling, E. (2012) Representative seroprevalences of brucellosis in humans and livestock in Kyrgyzstan. *EcoHealth* 9, 132–138.

Collings, D.F. (1984) *Leptospira interrogans* infection in domestic and wild animals in Fiji. *New Zealand Veterinary Journal* 32, 21–24.

Faine, S., Adler, B., Bolin, C. and Perolat, P. (1999) *Leptospira and Leptospirosis*. MediSci, Melbourne, Australia.

Fiji Bureau of Statistics (2007) Population and Housing Census, Fiji. Available at: http://www.statsfiji.gov.fj/index.php/2007-census-of-population (accessed 28 March 2014).

Fiji School of Medicine and Fiji Ministry of Health (2009) Fiji's unrelenting plagues: Dengue, Leptospirosis and Typhoid. Phase I: Disease profile. Fiji School of Medicine and Fiji Ministry of Health , Project report.

Higgins, R.J., Harbourne, J.F., Little, T.W. and Stevens, A.E. (1980) Mastitis and abortion in dairy cattle associated with *Leptospira* of the serotype hardjo. *The Veterinary Record* 107, 307–310.

Holt, J., Davis, S. and Leirs, H. (2006) A model of Leptospirosis infection in an African rodent to determine risk to humans: seasonal fluctuations and the impact of rodent control. *Acta Tropica* 99, 218–225.

Keenan, J., Ervin, G., Aung, M., McGwin, G., Jr and Jolly, P. (2010) Risk factors for clinical leptospirosis from Western Jamaica. *The American Journal of Tropical Medicine and Hygiene* 83, 633–636.

Kubuabola, I. (2003) Leptospirosis in Fiji: Serology confirmed leptospirosis data analysis, 1991–2000. Masters in Applied Epidemiology Bound Volume, Australian National University.

Lau, C.L., Dobson, A.J., Smythe, L.D., Fearnley, E.J., Skelly, C., Clements, A.C.A., Craig, S.B., Fuimaono, S.D. and Weinstein, P. (2012) Leptospirosis in American Samoa 2010: epidemiology, environmental drivers, and the management of emergence. *The American Journal of Tropical Medicine and Hygiene* 86, 309–319.

Levett, P.N. (2001) Leptospirosis. *Clinical Microbiology Reviews* 14, 296–326.

Little, T.W., Hathaway, S.C., Boughton, E.S. and Seawright, D. (1992a) Development of a control strategy for *Leptospira hardjo* infection in a closed beef herd. *The Veterinary Record* 131, 383–386.

Little, T.W., Hathaway, S.C., Broughton, E.S. and Seawright, D. (1992b) Control of *Leptospira hardjo* infection in beef cattle by whole-herd vaccination. *The Veterinary Record* 131, 90–92.

Mcfarlane, D.C. (2009) Country Pasture/Forage Resource Profiles; Fiji. Available at: http://www.fao.org/ag/AGP/AGPC/doc/Counprof/southpacific/fiji.htm (accessed 28 March 2014).

Merien, F. and Perolat, P. (1996) Public health importance of human leptospirosis in the South Pacific: a five-year study in New Caledonia. *The American Journal of Tropical Medicine and Hygiene* 55, 174–178.

Narayan, P.K. (2005) Economic importance of the sugar industry for Fiji. *Review of Urban & Regional Development Studies* 17, 104–114.

Nardone, A., Capek, I., Baranton, G., Campese, C., Postic, D., Vaillant, V., Lienard, M. and Desenclos, J.C. (2004) Risk factors for leptospirosis in metropolitan France: results of a national case-control study, 1999–2000. *Clinical Infectious Diseases: an official publication of the Infectious Diseases Society of America* 39, 751–753.

Perez, J., Brescia, F., Becam, J. and Goarant, C. (2011) Deciphering leptospirosis eco-epidemiology in New Caledonia. *BMC Proceedings* 5, P110.

Ram, P. (1977a) Epidemiology of leptospirosis in Fiji. *Medical Journal of Australia* Suppl. 3, 70–72.

Ram, P. (1977b) History of leptospirosis in Fiji. *Medical Journal of Australia* Suppl. 3, 68–69.

Ram, P. and Collings, D.F. (1982) Further observations on the epidemiology of leptospirosis in Fiji. *Fiji Medical Journal* May/June, 71–75.

Ramos, A.C.F., Souza, G.N. and Lilenbaum, W. (2006) Influence of leptospirosis on reproductive performance of sows in Brazil. *Theriogenology* 66, 1021–1025.

Roth, F., Zinsstag, J., Orkhon, D., Chimed-Ochir, G., Hutton, G., Cosivi, O., Carrin, G. and Otte, J. (2003) Human health benefits from livestock vaccination for brucellosis: case study. *Bulletin of the World Health Organization* 81, 867–876.

Singleton, G.R., Hinds, L.A., Leirs, H. and Zhang, Z. (eds) (1999) *Ecologically-based Management of Rodent Pests*. Australian Centre for International Agricultural Research, Canberra, Australia.

Storey, D. (2006) State, Society and Governance in Melanesia Project – Urbanisation in the Pacific. Available at: http://www.unescap.org/EPOC/documents/R3.12_Study_2.pdf (accessed 28 March 2014).

Sykes, J.E., Hartmann, K., Lunn, K.F., Moore, G.E., Stoddard, R.A. and Goldstein, R.E. (2011) 2010 ACVIM small animal consensus statement on leptospirosis: diagnosis, epidemiology, treatment, and prevention. *Journal of Veterinary Internal Medicine/American College of Veterinary Internal Medicine* 25, 1–13.

Victoriano, A., Smythe, L., Gloriani-Barzaga, N., Cavinta, L., Kasai, T., Limpakarnjanarat, K., Ong, B., Gongal, G., Hall, J., Coulombe, C., Yanagihara, Y., Yoshida, S.-i. and Adler, B. (2009) Leptospirosis in the Asia Pacific region. *BMC Infectious Diseases* 9, 147.

Wai'in, P.M. (2007) Epidemiology of infection with Leptospira species in livestock in Papua New Guinea. PhD thesis, Murdoch University, Perth, Australia.

Weekes, C.C., Everard, C.O. and Levett, P.N. (1997) Seroepidemiology of canine leptospirosis on the island of Barbados. *Veterinary Microbiology* 57, 215–222.

World Health Organization (2003) Human leptospirosis: guidance for diagnosis, surveillance and control. Available at: http://whqlibdoc.who.int/hq/2003/WHO_CDS_CSR_EPH_2002.23.pdf (accessed 28 March 2014).

# 18 Human and Animal African Trypanosomiasis

**Susan C. Welburn[1]* and Paul Coleman[2]**
[1]*Division of Infection and Pathway Medicine, School of Biomedical Sciences, College of Medicine & Veterinary Medicine, The University of Edinburgh, Edinburgh, UK;*
[2]*Department of Disease Control, Faculty of Infectious and Tropical Diseases, London School of Hygiene & Tropical Medicine, London, UK*

## Introduction

Management of zoonotic disease risk arising from interactions between animals, humans and the environment, demands integrated action from both human and animal health sectors, support from other sectors or industries with a stake in health governance and key inputs from the environmental sector (Cook *et al.*, 2004; Okello *et al.*, 2011; Welburn, 2011; Zinsstag *et al.*, 2012).

In this chapter, we describe evidence that the evolution of a One Health (OH) approach has been key to the sustainability of control of human African trypanosomiasis (HAT) or 'sleeping sickness' in Uganda. We summarize critical elements of design, events and outcomes of the Stamp Out Sleeping Sickness campaign (SOS), a One Health approach to management of an emerging zoonotic disease in Uganda, and look at the possibility of sustainable long-term disease management. Prevention of disease outbreaks is preferable and less costly in the long term but this requires long-term financial commitments that become difficult to sustain when the health impact, or consequences of emerging neglected zoonoses, are not recognized in global terms (Maudlin *et al.*, 2009).

## Human African Trypanosomiasis

### A re-emerging disease

HAT is a neglected tropical zoonotic disease, which is of significant public health importance across much of sub-Saharan Africa. HAT is an expensive and difficult disease to diagnose and treat. It is fatal in the absence of treatment. Today, HAT is considered as a re-emerging disease, but for much of the last century HAT was a pandemic with major epidemics emerging across the African continent. A fearful narrative developed, which described an untreatable disease, with serious social and economic consequences, not unlike current fears of pandemic influenza, but one for which unique One Health solutions have evolved (Okello *et al.*, 2014).

Transmitted by a number of species of tsetse flies, HAT exists in two forms: (i) *Trypanosoma*

*E-mail: sue.welburn@ed.ac.uk

*brucei rhodesiense*, an acute disease that causes death within 6 months; and (ii) the more prevalent chronic form caused by infection with *Trypanosoma brucei gambiense*, in which death may take several years and may cause serious damage to the central nervous system even before symptoms emerge. Across the tsetse fly belts of sub-Saharan Africa the two forms of HAT are separated by the Great Rift Valley, with acute *T. b. rhodesiense* lying to the east and chronic *T. b. gambiense* found to the west (Welburn *et al.*, 2001a). The site of disease acquisition plays an important role in determining approaches to diagnosis, treatment and control (Wastling and Welburn, 2011) (see Plate 11).

## Uganda's unique position

Uganda is the only country in Africa that has disease foci for both acute and chronic forms of human sleeping sickness, harbouring *T. b. rhodesiense* in the south-east and *T. b gambiense* in the north-west, close to the Sudanese border (Welburn *et al.*, 2001a). HAT (the 'colonial disease') emerged in Busoga, around the shores of Lake Victoria in 1896 followed by emergence in West Nile in 1905 (Maudlin, 2006). Rapid, medical and scientific breakthroughs identified the trypanosome as the disease agent and tsetse flies as the vector of transmission, suggesting that infection could be passed between animals and humans, but at the time there were no drugs available to contain the epidemic. In both regions, sleeping sickness was assumed to be caused by infection with a haemoflagellate pathogen (named *T. ugandense* at the time). By 1908, at least 300,000 people had died and in 1909 Governor Bell evacuated the lakeshore area. Castellani had, however, noted two clinical forms in Uganda – one that was rapidly fatal and one that was not (Maudlin, 2006). Re-analysis of sleeping sickness records from 1900 to 1920 in Uganda clearly confirmed that there were two diseases present in Uganda at this time and that acute HAT was responsible for the epidemic around the shores of Lake Victoria (Koerner *et al.*, 1995; Févre *et al.*, 2004).

HAT is characterized by periodic large-scale outbreaks separated by periods of lower transmission. Although we are currently in an inter-epidemic period with WHO highlighting a decline in the numbers of new cases of sleeping sickness in recent years (Simarro *et al.*, 2008), data on sleeping sickness cases in Uganda are subject to significant under-reporting, and the potential for the disease to return in epidemic proportions is high (see Fig. 18.1).

While HAT foci expand and contract, HAT tends not to move far with cases of disease largely limited to localized sleeping sickness foci. For over a century, the two forms of human disease in Uganda were confined to separate geographical foci facilitating surveillance, diagnosis, treatment and control (Welburn *et al.*, 2001a; Welburn and Maudlin, 2012). There was concern in the 1970s that the Gambian form would spread southwards within the tsetse fly belt with human population movements, particularly mass movements of people to and from internally displaced person (IDP) refugee camps.

Today, 50 districts of Uganda are at risk from one or the other form of sleeping sickness, mostly in poor, rural areas. Gambian sleeping sickness is a chronic illness that is transmitted from person to person via infected tsetse flies. Rhodesian sleeping sickness is the acute form of the disease, with cattle acting as the main reservoir for the human infective parasite, which is also transmitted via tsetse flies and threatens 9 million people in Uganda.

## Under-reporting and the hidden burden of disease

Data on sleeping sickness deaths are also subject to gross errors since people affected are often beyond the reach of health-care systems and are not reported in any health metrics (Odiit *et al.*, 2004b). Both forms of HAT are difficult to diagnose and largely under-reported (Odiit *et al.*, 2005; Févre *et al.*, 2008a,b) leading to fears of a 'silent epidemic' (Wastling *et al.*, 2011). Under-reporting is as high as 40% in some *T. b. rhodesiense* foci; for every reported sleeping sickness case, 12 are undetected. In Uganda, it is estimated that 92% of HAT deaths are unreported due to confusion with malaria and other infectious diseases (Odiit *et al.*, 2005).

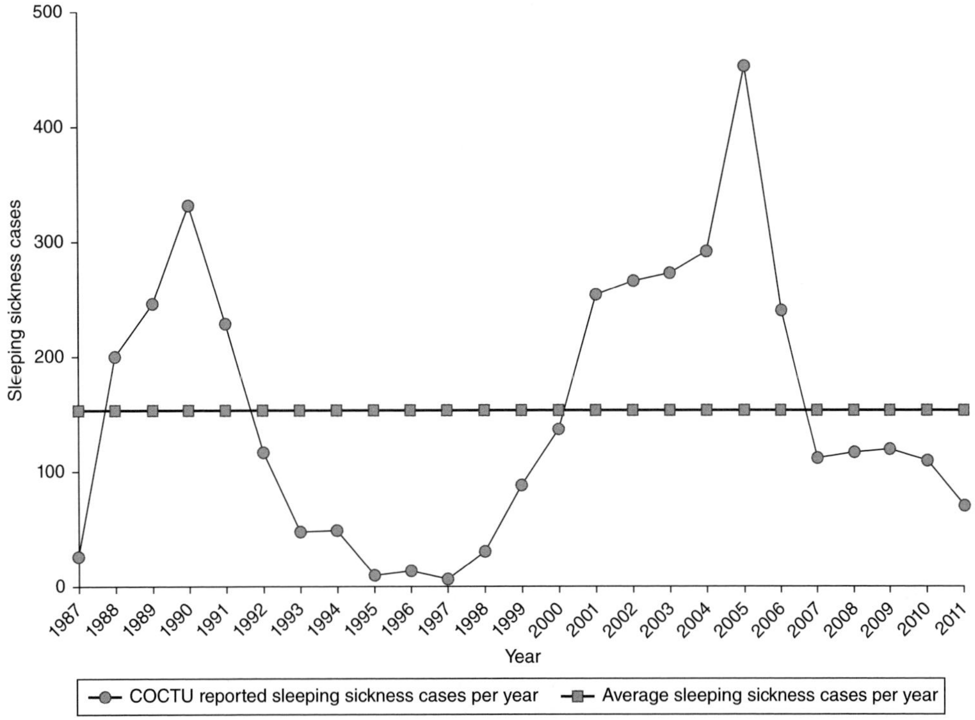


**Fig. 18.1.** Incidence of HAT in Uganda from 1987 to 2011, characterized by periodic large-scale outbreaks separated by periods of lower transmission (COCTU, 2014).

To estimate the current burden of disease, official figures for zoonotic sleeping sickness have been used to calculate a baseline average number of human cases per year; from this an average DALY burden can be calculated using standard WHO/World Bank methodologies. Preliminary calculations conservatively place this number at around 900 human cases per year. This is based on COCTU records from 1987 to 2011 and conversion factors from the published literature (see Fig. 18.1). Medical services are estimated to be identifying less than 10% of cases using the present means of surveillance.

## HAT as a zoonosis – animal reservoirs of infection

*Trypanosoma b. gambiense* and *T. b. rhodesiense* which infects humans co-exist in HAT foci with a suite of other trypanosome infections that cause African animal trypanosomiasis (nagana) in both wild and domestic animals. *Trypanosoma b. rhodesiense*, the agent that causes acute sleeping sickness, is a significant zoonosis which infects a wide range of non-human wild and domestic animal hosts (Anderson *et al*., 2011; Auty *et al*., 2012). The presence of human infective parasites in non-human animal blood has been known for some time after confirmation from work with human volunteers who were infected with parasites derived from wild and domestic animal hosts (Onyango *et al*., 1966). However, although wild animals have been found to form part of the parasite reservoir in Zambia (Anderson *et al*., 2011) and Tanzania (Auty *et al*., 2012), in south-east Uganda today, where game animals are no longer common, cattle have been shown to act as the major reservoir for Rhodesian sleeping sickness (Welburn *et al*., 2001b; von Wissmann *et al*., 2014).

*Trypanosoma b. gambiense* HAT is transmitted predominantly from person to person via infected tsetse fly–man–fly–man transmission.

Although there are reports of identification of *T. b. gambiense* in pigs in some HAT foci in West Africa, they are not considered to play a major role in disease epidemiology (Jamonneau *et al.*, 2004).

Until recently, measuring the extent of the domestic animal reservoir of zoonotic *T. b. rhodesiense* was not possible as cattle could also be infected with non-human-infective *T. b. brucei*, morphologically indistinguishable from *T. b. rhodesiense* by microscopy. In 2000, a single gene was identified that can differentiate human infectivity in *T. brucei* s.l. parasites. However, with the identification of a molecular marker (SRA – serum-resistance-associated gene) for *T. b.* rhodesiense (Xong *et al.*, 1998), differentiation of human infective parasites in animals became possible. The SRA gene can be used as a genetic marker to distinguish between *T. b. brucei* and *T. b. rhodesiense* (Welburn *et al.*, 2001b). Using the SRA marker, up to 18% of cattle in Soroti District were found to be infected with *T. b. rhodesiense* (Welburn *et al.*, 2001b), compared with 1% using previous methods (Hide *et al.*, 1994), and it is clear that infections in animals had been missed using field methods then available. Tsetse exhibit a strong feeding preference for cattle (Waiswa *et al.*, 2006) and the risk of becoming infected by a fly infected from an infected cow is five times more likely than from a human (Hide *et al.*, 1996).

## Risk and consequences of overlap of two forms of HAT

Identification of HAT and the type of treatment given is at present simply based on knowing which type of sleeping sickness focus the patient originated from and the stage of the disease (Welburn *et al.*, 2001a; Wastling and Welburn; 2011). For stage I *T. b. rhodesiense* HAT, patients are treated with Suramin (discovered in 1921) and for *T. b. gambiense* with pentamidine (discovered in 1941). For both forms of late stage HAT, patients can be treated with Melarsoprol (discovered in 1949) but there is considerable resistance of *T. b. gambiense* to this drug and patients are more often treated with Eflornothine (registered in 1990).

Traditionally the two forms of HAT in Uganda have been confined to separate geographical foci facilitating surveillance and differential treatment. Historically, sleeping sickness did not move far; areas affected by *T. b. gambiense* expanded and contracted, but the disease largely remained in localized sleeping sickness foci. In Uganda, there was concern that the Gambian form would spread southwards within the tsetse fly belt, with human population movements, particularly via mass movements of people to and from refugee camps. The public health consequences of convergence of the two forms of HAT have significant cost implications. If the two forms of the disease were to coexist in the same area then diagnosis and treatment of sleeping sickness, already problematic, would become almost impossible. Overlap would make disease management complex in terms of diagnosing the parasite responsible, applying the different recommended treatments and selecting appropriate control policies.

## The spread of HAT

Historical data show HAT to be characterized by periodic large-scale outbreaks separated by periods of lower transmission, but the potential for the disease to recur is high. Cases of acute HAT were limited to the south-east of the country until 1985, when the disease began migrating northwards at a rate of one district per year. By 2005, the two diseases were only 150 km apart (Picozzi *et al.*, 2005), and concern grew among researchers and policy makers that the two forms would overlap in Uganda. There was significant risk of convergence of the two strains by 2015.

This movement northwards was unexpected, since between 1985 and 2005 there had been significant investment in vector control (tsetse fly trapping) and active human disease surveillance supported by a series of large-scale EU control programmes. Active disease surveillance screening is considered highly effective for both forms of HAT. Trapping tsetse flies is far less effective in Uganda for *T. b. rhodesiense* than in regions where transmission is predominantly man–fly–man. This is because infected tsetse flies are rare; flies can only become infected if they are susceptible (Welburn and Maudlin, 1991), being co-infected with a symbiotic bacterium (*Sodalis glossinidius*) and if they take in the infection at their first meal (Welburn and Maudlin, 1992, 1999; Soumana *et al.*, 2012). Furthermore, even if susceptible flies do feed on an infected host, development of the infection and progression from the fly gut to develop into mammalian infected forms is not a certainty; cyclical transmission is sex-linked with male flies transmitting significantly more infections than females (Milligan *et al.*, 1995; Welburn *et al.*, 1995). Most parasites ingested by tsetse flies die in the midgut and are not transmitted (Welburn *et al.*, 1996). Even at the height of an epidemic of *T. b. rhodesiense* in Tororo, only 1:1000 flies were found to be infected, with typical daily trap catches ranging between 0 and 5 flies per trap (or per km$^2$).

For animal surveillance, microscopy-based techniques are not useful for detecting low-level infections. When parasite numbers are low, as is often the case in cattle in HAT endemic regions, positive diagnoses can be often be missed by microscopy (Picozzi *et al.*, 2002; Magona *et al.*, 2003). Furthermore, microscopy is labour intensive, requires a skilled microscopist and can be difficult to manage in a field situation without a reliable power source. While newer methods are available for best practice to assess prevalence of trypanosomes in cattle (Cox *et al.*, 2010; Ahmed *et al.*, 2011, 2013), the methods used by the veterinary screening teams in this period failed to indicate the extent of the risk from domestic livestock.

In December 1998, a case of human sleeping sickness was reported in Soroti District, which was north-west of the documented extent of the *T. b. rhodesiense* focus; this was the first case in areas north of Lake Kyoga, and 70 additional cases presented over the following 18 months. Limited tsetse control measures were implemented, but the outbreak was not contained, and by June 2000, 119 cases had been recorded. New cases of sleeping sickness were still being reported in Soroti in 2005, bringing the total reported cases to over 400 and, by extrapolation, total reported and unreported cases to over 700 (Févre *et al.*, 2005). The disease subsequently spread across Lake Kyoga into Kaberamaido District (Batchelor *et al.*, 2009; Wardrop *et al.*, 2013).

## Disease drivers – infected livestock – infected people

A case-controlled study showed a strong association between the early sleeping sickness cases in Soroti District and proximity to the cattle market known as Brookes Corner (Févre *et al.*, 2001). Distance from Brookes Corner was a highly significant risk factor ($p < 0.001$) but as time progressed distance from the market become less of a risk factor. It was estimated that more than 50% of the cattle being traded at this market had come from the *T. b. rhodesiense* endemic zone to the south, making cattle the most likely cause of the outbreak. Surveys confirmed that the domestic animal reservoir was the primary source of human infective trypanosomes for tsetse, with up to 40% of cattle carrying *T. b. rhodesiense* in south-east Uganda (Welburn *et al.*, 2001b). While pigs (Okuna *et al.*, 1986) and dogs can also be infected, pigs are relatively short lived and do not present long-term disease reservoirs while dogs are quickly killed by the disease. In Uganda, treating only cattle would, therefore, significantly reduce *T. b. rhodesiense* infection (Welburn *et al.*, 2006). Between 1998 and 2006, uncontrolled movements of infected cattle resulted in zoonotic HAT being introduced to eight new districts in Uganda (Févre *et al.*, 2005; Picozzi *et al.*, 2005) (see Fig. 18.2).

## The politics of restocking and disease instability

In the late 1970s, Karamojong pastoralists intensified their traditional practice of cattle raiding (Epelu-Opio, 2009), which devastated farming systems and led to depopulation of Teso and thus fallow land providing a favourable tsetse habitat (Hutchinson *et al.*, 2003). The ensuing 'Teso War' (1986–1992) caused widespread disruption in Soroti and Kaberamaido districts (Epelu-Opio, 2009). Stability returned in the late 1990s, and the population began to return to the area, assisted by government and donor-driven large-scale cattle restocking programmes (Hutchinson *et al.*, 2003; Selby *et al.*, 2014). However, in June 2003 a brutal insurgency by the Lord's Resistance

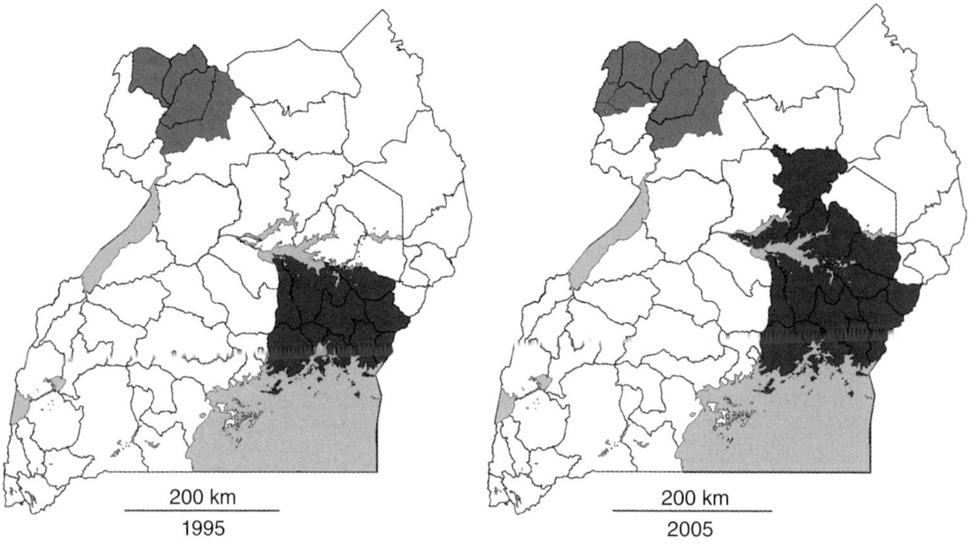


**Fig. 18.2.** Convergence of HAT foci 1995–2005 (adapted from Picozzi *et al.*, 2005).

Army (LRA) spread south-east towards Lira, Apac, Kaberamaido, Katakwi and Soroti districts. Much of the population was displaced to refugee camps, and in some cases people slept in the camps and travelled back to their villages to farm by day. Lira and Apac districts were subject to large-scale restocking interventions, from NGOs and the World Bank/government of Northern Uganda Social Action Fund (NUSAF), implemented by the government through District Veterinary Officers (under the AfDB-funded National Livestock Productivity Improvement Programme (NLPIP)). Many cattle purchased for restocking were sourced from Kamuli, Palissa, Tororo and Mbare districts in south-eastern Uganda, which were endemic for *T. b. rhodesiense*. These restocking programmes and a large proportion of independent restocking failed to comply with strict disease controls that had previously been imposed on cattle moving between districts (Selby *et al.*, 2014).

Insecurity and its resolution in Southern Sudan have also impacted on trypanosomiasis risk in Uganda. In 2008 there were reports of livestock traders and agents from Southern Sudan buying cattle as far south as the Ochero market in Kaberamaido District to supply meat in Juba, which contributed to the northward flow of cattle increasing trypanosomiasis transmission risk. Uncontrolled movement around Lake Kyoga of infected cattle, which were not treated with trypanocides at the point of sale, resulted in zoonotic HAT being introduced to eight new districts of Uganda, communities that were unaware of the disease and risk, between 1998 and 2006.

## One Health Approaches to HAT

### The emergence of a One Health platform – COCTU

Uganda is unique in its early development of a One Health framework for coordination of trypanosomiasis control that cuts across human health, animal health and the environment. The Coordinating Office for Control of Trypanosomiasis in Uganda (COCTU) is the governmental body responsible for coordinating and monitoring sleeping sickness interventions in Uganda, providing a concrete example of a One Health platform that is working in practice (Okello *et al.*, 2014). Establishment of this One Health platform was in part driven by the resurgence of a major *T. b. rhodesiense* epidemic in the late 1980s, where significant human and financial inputs necessitated a change from the disaggregated silo approach of past control programmes.

COCTU is the formal Secretariat of the Ugandan Trypanosomiasis Control Council (UTCC) formed by a parliamentary act in 1992. This permanently funded inter-ministerial platform coordinates policy for all stakeholders involved in tsetse and trypanosomiasis control in Uganda. Seated within Uganda's Ministry of Agriculture, Animal Industries and Fisheries (MAAIF) and endorsed by the Office of the Prime Minister for two decades, COCTU is an example of Uganda's foresight and commitment to One Health, established long before this approach became fashionable. COCTU coordinates sleeping sickness policies, provides linkages to work and research in the field and collates data. The statute established a Technical Committee, which is composed of heads of relevant Ministry departments represented in UTCC and can co-opt experts. The Technical Committee advises on technical interventions and work plans and, through COCTU, makes recommendations to UTCC.

The existence of COCTU also offered some continuity for HAT and animal trypanosomiasis control during the disruptive processes of decentralization and recentralization. Under the Uganda Constitution of 1995, local government became responsible for the planning and administration of health and agriculture and the function of line ministries was reduced to inspection, monitoring and technical support (Asiimwe and Katorobo, 2007). Previously, district government staff reported to the Commissioner for Livestock Health and Entomology; after decentralization the Commissioner could propose work on particular diseases, and channel funds but could not compel work to be undertaken. The subsequent 're-centralization' of veterinary services in October 2008 meant that costs for government veterinary work would be paid from the Centre and that the Centre would manage veterinary staff between districts.

## The genesis of Stamp Out Sleeping Sickness – WHO Round Table

As a response to the fact that by 2005 the two forms of sleeping sickness were only 150 km apart, COCTU asked WHO for technical support to address the threat of the merger of *T. b. gambiense* and *T. b. rhodesiense*. A meeting, supported by WHO/TDR (the Special Programme for Research and Training in Tropical Diseases), was held during the 28th ISCTRC in Addis Ababa, Ethiopia in 2005 and a resolution (WHO/AFRO Regional Committee resolution – AFR/RC55/R3) recommended that WHO/AFRO should support implementation of the regional strategy for HAT control and prevent further spread of the disease (Morton, 2009).

It was proposed that trypanocidal drugs would be used to eliminate the reservoir of *T. b. rhodesiense* infection in domestic cattle within the newly affected districts and that this would be followed up with application of deltamethrin spray to cattle to prevent re-infection by tsetse. Acute HAT would be rolled back through south-eastern Uganda to prevent the merger of the two forms of sleeping sickness while building up sustainable animal African trypanosomiasis (AAT) control at the local level. The shortage of veterinary human resources following downsizing of the civil service was identified as a constraint and the option of using final-year veterinary students was seen as a way of addressing this. This action was viewed as an open-ended process, involving an emergency intervention followed by interventions taken by farmers themselves to provide sustainability.

## Stamp Out Sleeping Sickness – a public–private partnership for human African trypanosomiasis

On 1 June 2006, a Memorandum of Understanding (MoU) was drafted and signed by the Chairman of UTCC and by representatives of the pharmaceutical company Ceva and Industri Kapital (IK), a private equity firm with a charitable arm (IKARE). Ceva/IK agreed to contract Makerere University and the University of Edinburgh to implement block treatment and related activities and to work through their local distributors to introduce insecticidal treatment of cattle. This laid the foundations for what was to become the Stamp Out Sleeping sickness campaign (SOS) – a public–private partnership (PPP).

SOS focused on the use of trypanocidal drugs to eliminate human infective parasite infection in the animal reservoir and application of insecticides to the tsetse predilection sites of cattle to prevent reinfection. Stakeholder interests included cattle owners, district veterinary officers, Faculty of Veterinary Medicine (FVM) at Makerere University, Uganda, The University of Edinburgh, the corporate sector, local private sector companies, donors and national regulatory authorities. Prior to the launching of the SOS campaign, members of COCTU and their technical committee met in Kaberamaido with the entire District Council, plus council staff and members of the public and visited IDP camps and villages.

The primary aim of SOS was to treat 85% of the cattle in five districts in northern Uganda that were at risk of disease overlap (Welburn *et al.*, 2006). Modelling indicated that treating at least 85% of cattle population could eliminate human-infective parasites, given that half of all tsetse feeds were taken from cattle. Over a period of 8 weeks approximately 250,000 cattle were treated across five districts. In the higher risk districts of Dokolo and Kaberamaido, cattle were treated with isometamidium chloride (Veridium ®), which has a prophylactic effect against trypanosome infections for up to 3 months. Cattle in Lira, Amolatar and Apac were treated with diminazene aceturate (Veriben B12®), which is curative, but offers no prophylactic effect against new trypanosome infections.

To prevent reinfection after treatment, cattle were to be protected using deltamethrin-based insecticides. When applied to a sufficiently large proportion of cattle, insecticides can provide a sufficiently even level of treated cattle per hectare to control tsetse flies at a population level (Hargrove *et al.*, 2002). However, either all-over treatment of cattle or the use of pour-on applications had proven cost-prohibitive. Since tsetse flies preferentially feed on the legs and belly of cattle, treating only these areas proved more cost-effective than whole-body treatment (Torr *et al.*, 2007). This Restricted Application Protocol (RAP) can reduce the cost of product for treatment to as little as US$0.02 per head of cattle (Kabasa, 2007). RAP uses cattle as live baits through application of insecticide at normal dip concentration to predilection sites at a fraction of the cost of a whole-body treatment. Modelling indicates that only 1.1% or 1.6% of village cattle need to be treated per day, equating to 21% herd whole-body application or 27% RAP for $R_0 < 1$ (Kajunguri *et al.*, 2014).

Cattle in the SOS treatment zones were sprayed with the deltamethrin-based insecticide (Vectocid®) using RAP – spraying only the legs and belly of the cow, as well as spraying the ears for ticks, in order to prevent reinfection by tsetse (Fig. 18.3). Spraying needs to be repeated at least monthly to provide protection against reinfection. Monthly application of RAP after trypanocidal treatment was shown to maintain prevalence <1% of all trypanosomes in Tororo District, which is

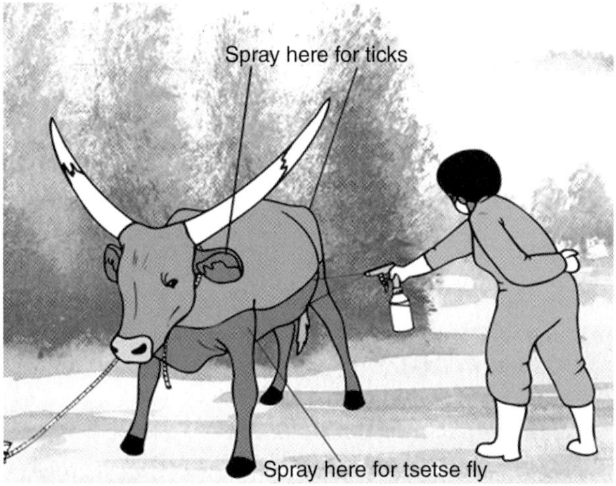


**Fig. 18.3.** Restricted Application Proctocol (RAP) for insecticide treatment on cattle.

endemic for both HAT and AAT (Brownlow, 2009). RAP also protects against a range of tick-borne diseases such as theileriosis, anaplasmosis and cowdriosis and tick damage that are endemic to this region (Magona *et al.*, 2008, 2011; Muhanguzi *et al.*, 2014a).

SOS engaged in building a One Health platform for sustainability, educating farmers and key stakeholders about the close links between animal health and human health and economic development. SOS turned to Makerere University for human resources to support the SOS campaign, and this opened the opportunity to engage final-year veterinary students in development activity. Makerere University needed to prepare graduates for private veterinary practice and addressed the need for alternative private sector mechanisms to deliver field-level services in the SOS districts. The Veterinary Faculty at Makerere University revised their curriculum to accommodate lecture-free periods and launched the MinTracs programme; students were deployed to work with communities to undertake treatment, spraying, sampling and interviews as part of their final year of study (Schelling and Zinsstag, Chapter 30, this volume).

After the initial treatment, insecticide was left with district veterinary officers for them to undertake a second and third free spraying, and communities were supported by a thorough educational and awareness campaign – through radio messages and posters on the importance of continuing to administer the treatment on a regular basis in the districts concerned.

## Outcomes from the Stamp Out Sleeping Sickness public–private partnership

At the inception of SOS, spatial analysis showed that *T. b. brucei* and *T. b. rhodesiense* were distributed throughout four of the five districts of the SOS target area in cattle (see Plate 12a, c). The initial phase resulted in a reduction of the prevalence of the sleeping sickness parasite in the cattle by close to 70% and human cases of HAT by 90% and a 75% reduction of all trypanosomes in cattle (human and cattle pathogens) (see Plate 12b, d) and halted the northerly expansion of *T. b. rhodesiense* HAT focus. The impact of the intervention was greater in *T. b. rhodesiense* since there is a fitness cost to being human infective (Coleman and Welburn, 2004; Welburn *et al.*, 2008). The amount of *T. brucei* in cattle is related to risk of human infection (von Wissmann *et al.*, 2014); reductions in *T. b. rhodesiense* in cattle are reflected in a reduction in the number of sleeping sickness cases recorded within the SOS target area. From 1:100 cattle infected with *T. b. rhodesiense*, SRA by analysis before treatment samples showed a reduction to 1:1000 post-treatment.

Over the period in which the SOS campaign has been in operation, the number of reported sleeping sickness cases has fallen in four out of the five SOS target districts, with no cases reported from Apac. Post-treatment human cases were only observed clustered near to cattle markets (Batchelor *et al.*, 2009; Selby *et al.*, 2014) and a second phase of cattle treatments was introduced. The reduction of cases in Lira indicates that the barrier between the two forms of sleeping sickness has been maintained. The northerly movement of *T. b. rhodesiense* and sleeping sickness had been halted 18 months post-treatment.

Sleeping sickness is a disease of rural areas that are remote and poorly serviced by health facilities. By increasing awareness of disease among rural and remote populations, as well as health staff and decision makers, the SOS campaign has the potential to increase access to sleeping sickness treatment. Reducing the incidence of sleeping sickness in remote populations has the potential to contribute to reducing regional inequality and inequality caused by remoteness.

## A sustainable community-based spray network

Relatively modest levels of treatment (~20% of animals, even where tsetse numbers are not reduced by the intervention) have been predicted to result in elimination of HAT in south-east Uganda (Hargrove *et al.*, 2012). Furthermore, treating a reasonable proportion of cattle with insecticides can lead to total eradication of the disease; only 1.6% of village cattle need to be treated with RAP per day equating to 27% maintained coverage of RAP for $R_0 < 1$ (Kajunguri *et al.*, 2014). It follows that if a sustainable spray market can be developed, tsetse-transmitted trypanosomiasis will cease to be a problem and sleeping sickness will be eliminated. Farmers must protect their cattle from tick-borne diseases, and these RAP coverage targets were achievable and affordable.

Initiatives put in place by the private sector SOS partners (IKARE and Ceva Sante Animale), including mobile spray teams and the start-up of private veterinary practices and drug shops in previously unserved areas of the SOS districts, aim to develop a sustainable network. The 3 V Vet Initiative that followed the mass intervention was seen as: increasing awareness about trypanosomiasis and HAT; promoting interaction with government and NGOs; maintaining high visibility at main markets; developing contact and sales through local traders in agro-veterinary products; engaging in community work (demonstrations of spraying and training of community sprayers) and working with local media. Individual sprayers were recruited to form a community-based network. Sprayers operate as independent micro-entrepreneurs with support and training provided by their local veterinarian. Price per spray is currently decided by the individual spray person and depends on the size of the animals and number of animals to be treated. The average price per spray ranges from 200 to 300 Ugandan Shillings (about US$0.10), yielding about a 50% profit margin for the spray person. Ensuring reliable and affordable access to quality drugs is a key part of developing a commercially sustainable network. Farmers are encouraged to spray their cattle every 2 weeks or more frequently for tick control and at least once a month for tsetse flies using RAP methods.

It is estimated that at least 100,000 animals are being regularly sprayed using RAP in the SOS districts. A similar number are being treated with whole-body application of deltamethrin-based products, which is sufficient to control both animal and human trypanosomiasis at the village level. Farmers report that treated animals are healthier, more productive and better nourished, and animals are also protected against a range of other tick-borne diseases such as theileriosis, anaplasmosis and cowdriosis. For insecticide-treated cattle targets to be achieved, however, farmers need to use products that work against both ticks and tsetse flies rather than products that are only active against ticks (Bardosh *et al.*, 2013) and some farmers are still using tick-only products. There is a case to be made for putting in place acaricide zoning in HAT affected and HAT at-risk zones.

The establishment of a network of community-based spray teams in Uganda provides a model for the long-term prevention of parasite reinfection and should ensure the gains of mass treatment campaigns are maintained. Ensuring reliable and affordable access to quality drugs is a key to developing a commercially sustainable network.

## Added Value of a One Health Approach

### Socio-economic impact of the Stamp Out Sleeping Sickness campaign on sleeping sickness – an 'averted disaster'

Estimations of *total societal burden* of emerging and endemic zoonoses (defined as the combined human and animal +/− environmental costs of disease for the public and private sectors including indirect impacts on food security of smallholder farmers and micro- and macroeconomic impacts of disease on livestock productivity losses and health) can provide compelling evidence for the value of operationalizing One Health (Narrod *et al.*, 2012), but these estimates are generally not available for most neglected zoonotic diseases.

A number of calculations were made to assess the economic impact of the scenario where the two forms of HAT came to overlap – the 'averted disaster'. Human-health gains as a result of reduced parasite prevalence can be quantified from this in terms of: (i) sleeping sickness cases averted; (ii) DALYs averted (with US$ value); and (iii) care costs averted. Calculations were made based on a series of assumptions: levels of non-reporting, numbers of patients reporting at first and second stage, survival rates of the disease and patterns of spread using available evidence.

Assumptions about the rate at which an unchecked epidemic would expand are based on previous experience and expert opinion. In 2009, without the SOS intervention, it is likely that we would have experienced some 4000 new cases (majority under-reported). WHO suggest these would triple annually; in our projection, we conservatively assume they may double. The figures of between 0.4 and 1.6 million DALYs averted (or extra life years gained) are realistic. In addition, between US$15 million and US$60 million of health-care expenditure for patients and the health services have been saved (Shaw, 2009a). These figures provide a first-level assessment of how much the averted disaster might have cost and indicate the large range of values that highlight the difficulties of this type of 'what if' calculation. They show that the SOS programme has resulted in savings to the health services, protecting rural livelihoods and saving people's lives (Shaw, 2009a) (Table 18.1).

For animal health, cost is a major issue, not just for livestock keepers but also for policy makers in the field of tsetse control. Recent estimates of how insecticide-treated cattle (ITC) and particularly the restricted application (RAP) version of ITC compare with other methods of tsetse control indicate that it can be substantially cheaper (Shaw *et al.*, 2014). Animal productivity gains as a result of reduced parasite prevalence can be quantified in terms of sleeping sickness parasite-free cattle and tick-free cattle. The application of RAP to maintain AAT animals can result in average gains of US$20 per bovine per year (maximum US$30–40 per fertile female or working bull). Combining this with costs of tick-borne diseases in traditionally managed cattle (Minjauw and McLeod, 2003) indicates that benefits would be in the range of US$34 per head per year. This translates into approximately US$9–10,000 gained per square km 'productive land' per year while animals are protected (Shaw, 2009b).

The loss of an animal in these communities will increase vulnerability in these households, but many consider animal health as a private good which therefore should be paid for by the beneficiary, in contrast to state support, which is seen as justified for human health. The fact that animal health is linked to human welfare as a route out of poverty needs continual reinforcement. In the model adopted by the SOS campaign, it is recognized that the curative elements of the programme – the mass treatment of cattle to remove trypanosomes – should be free of charge to cattle keepers. However, spray treatment to maintain reduced levels of Rhodesian sleeping sickness are largely the financial responsibility of cattle keepers. To be accepted by cattle keepers, the latter has to be affordable to purchase, easy to acquire and demonstrate a rapid benefit (Butcher, 2009).

### Scaling the Stamp Out Sleeping Sickness One Health approach

SOS oversaw the mass treatment of 250,000 cattle in five high-risk areas undertaken in 2006–2007. In 2010–2012 the programme was extended to cover an additional 175,000 cattle in market hotspots and in two additional districts (see Fig. 18.4). These treatments demonstrated significant reductions in both human

**Table 18.1.** Health implications in terms of human life and money for a 20-year cycle can be saved by SOS approaches for four scenarios regarded as likely by WHO experts (Shaw, 2009a).

| Maximum annual number of new cases | Year reached | What happens thereafter | Million DALYs averted | US$ million health costs saved | Economic[a] total: US$ million saved |
|---|---|---|---|---|---|
| 30,000 | 2012 | Reduce by 1/3 each year | 1.55 | 57.63 | 367.25 |
| 20,000 | 2012 | Reduce by 1/4 each year | 1.14 | 42.53 | 275.47 |
| 20,000 | 2012 | Reduce by 1/2 each year | 0.75 | 28.17 | 194.88 |
| 10,000 | 2011 | Reduce by 1/2 each year | 0.39 | 14.50 | 103.25 |

[a]Discounted at 5% per annum and valuing 1 DALY at US$340

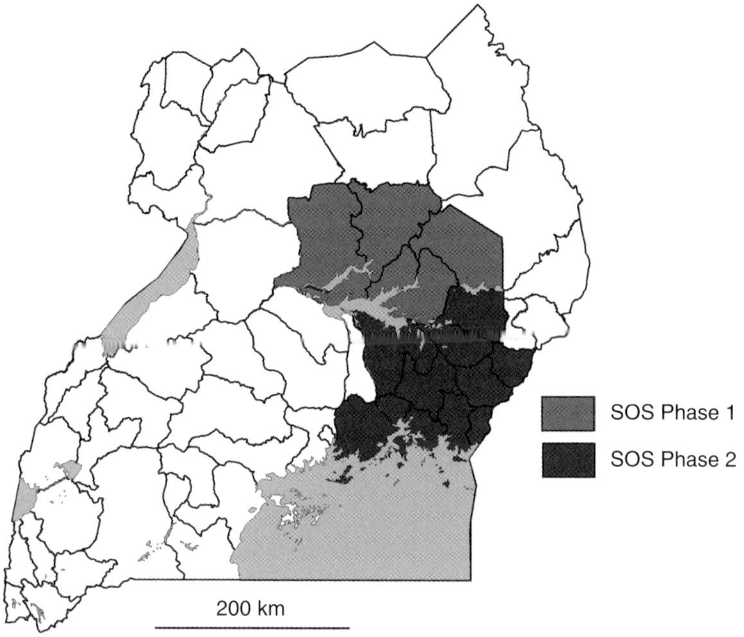


**Fig. 18.4.** Districts treated by the Stamp Out Sleeping Sickness campaign.

and animal pathogens. However, to eliminate the threat of Rhodesian sleeping sickness in Uganda the reservoir of infection must be eliminated at scale.

Fifty districts of Uganda are at risk from one or the other form of sleeping sickness mostly in poor, rural areas (see Fig. 18.5). Nine of these districts account for 80% of all cases of zoonotic *T. b. rhodesiense* HAT recorded over the last 25 years (see Fig. 18.6).

Following on from the demonstrated success of the SOS approach to disease control, the aim is to follow this up to reduce *T. b. rhodesiense* HAT across high- and lower-risk districts in Uganda. The high-risk zone includes districts historically affected by *T. b. rhodesiense* HAT and districts in which humans are currently at risk of infection. The lower risk zone includes districts in which there have not been any reported cases of *T. b. rhodesiense* sleeping sickness but from which reinfection and/or overlap of the two strains of disease is a potential risk. These include the districts currently affected by *T. b. gambiense* HAT and the contiguous districts (highlighted in Fig. 18.7).

The One Health approach proposed is an initial 3-year mass-cattle treatment programme – injection and spray – to quickly reduce human-infective parasite prevalence in cattle. Community-based spray teams will sustain gains achieved through mass treatment by delivering insecticide treatment to cattle in high-risk areas. The impact of the proposed intervention will be evaluated in terms of effective delivery of the mass treatment programme in years 1–3 and a consequent reduction in the human-infective parasite prevalence rate in cattle in years 4–8. To achieve this, interventions trialled under SOS need to be implemented rapidly and at scale with significant up-front loading of investment.

We have calculated that mass treatment should comprise an annual drug treatment for three annual cycles followed by an insecticide RAP spray. The aim is for these treatments to be delivered by mobile treatment teams on a parish-level basis, with additional resources to deliver treatments in markets. In the high-risk districts, mass treatment will apply isometamidium/diminazine (alternated yearly) and insecticide spray. It is anticipated that the treatment will be repeated annually for a 3-year period (approx. 2.6 million cattle) – continuous monitoring will be undertaken to inform precise delivery of treatment. In the lower risk districts, it is anticipated that a preventative

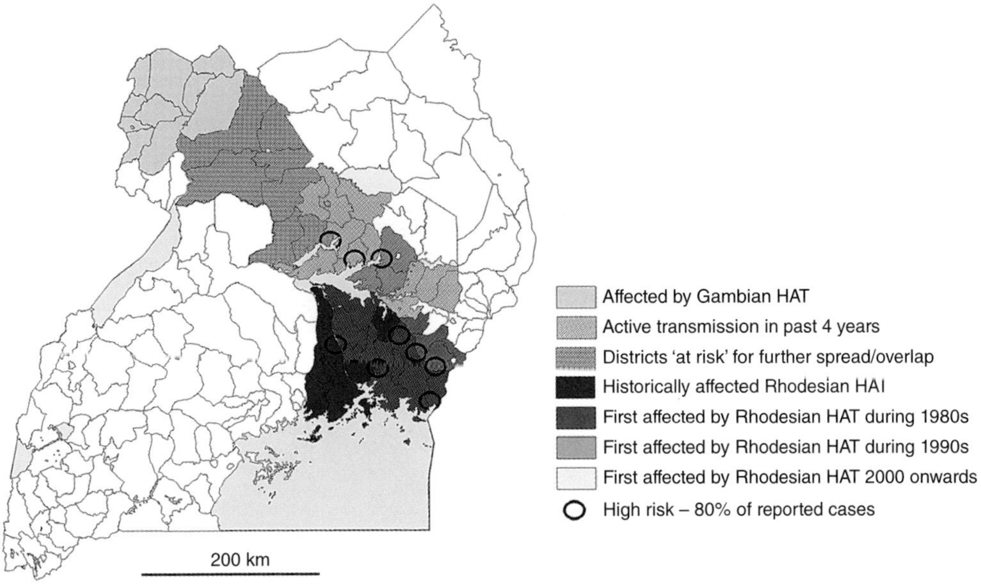


**Fig. 18.5.** Sleeping sickness status for districts of Uganda.

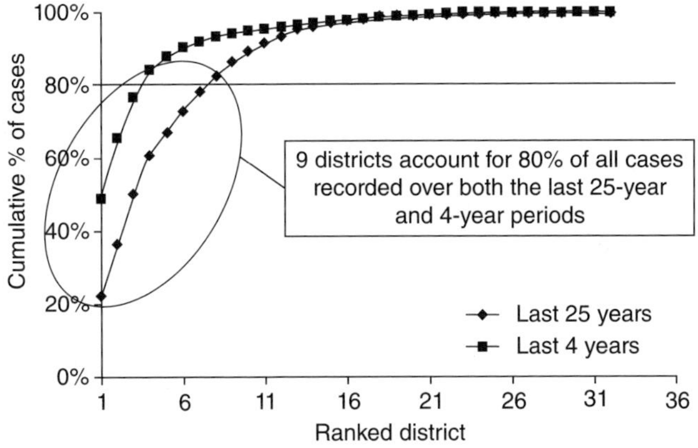


**Fig. 18.6.** Case incidence for HAT, by district.

treatment will be undertaken in year 1 only (approx. 1.8 million cattle), reflecting the lower risk posed to humans in this area.

### Development Impact Bonds – a new approach to funding disease control

The campaign has the potential to contribute towards development in northern Uganda; those districts in which SOS is operating have higher than average percentages of the population below the poverty line. Prevention of disease outbreaks is preferable and less costly in the long term but requires long-term financial commitments that become difficult to sustain when the health impact, or consequences of emerging zoonoses, is not realized in global terms, as for HAT.

There is significant and growing interest among traditional development donors (such as DFID, USAID and the World Bank), philanthropic institutions (such as the Bill & Melinda Gates Foundation and Rockefeller Foundation) and the emerging class of impact investors in the use of Development Impact

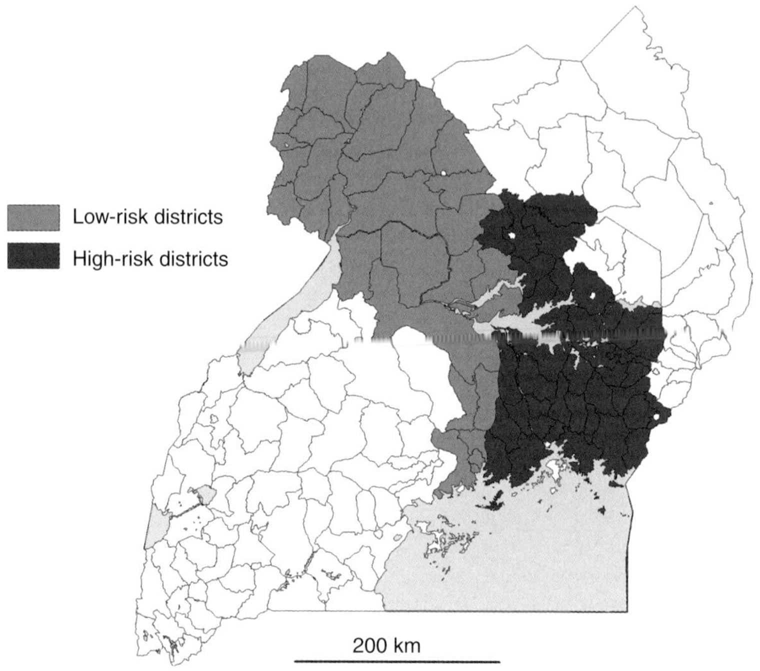


**Fig. 18.7.** Districts under consideration for mass intervention.

Bonds (DIBs) to more effectively deliver impacts in developing countries. DIBs use private investment to provide upfront risk capital for development programmes, only calling on donor funding to repay capital, plus a potential return (i.e. premium), once clearly defined and measured development outcomes are achieved. DIBs are seen as having the potential to attract new capital from impact investors motivated by both social and financial returns. By transferring the risk of programme failure to these investors, DIBs bring a greater focus on implementation and delivery of successful results. In this way, DIBs also satisfy the growing demands for publicly funded aid (Centre for Global Development and Social Finance, 2013). If the outcomes are not met, the investors absorb the loss, but if they are met, international donors repay the investors, with interest. Investors therefore have a strong incentive to manage their risk by bringing rigour and discipline to the DIB process. This should increase both the likelihood of achieving the social outcome and financial return. A sleeping sickness DIB could help provide the investment which Uganda lacks to tackle HAT at scale.

## A framework for exploring the economic benefits of scaling disease control

In order to design a DIB, it is necessary to understand the dynamic links between control activities at scale and economic benefits unlocked by controlling zoonotic HAT in Uganda. A framework was developed to simulate the effects of the proposed interventions (mass deployment of drug therapy and insecticide spraying of cattle followed by the expansion of routine spraying of cattle) on changes in parasite prevalence in cattle (the main outcome indicator) and to link it to the impact, quantified as a reduction in human health burden (expressed as DALYs), reduced healthcare costs (expressed as US$) and improvement in animal health (expressed as US$). This framework needed to be flexible enough to allow us to examine a variety of different intervention structures and all possible treatment coverages, predict the temporal dynamics of changes in prevalence and thus impact, describe the quantitative relationship between the outcome indicator (changes in *T. brucei* prevalence in cattle) and impact (DALYs plus

US$) over the long-term period of the DIB and, therefore, provide a robust basis for payment triggers based on changes in the outcome indicator.

The core of the framework is a detailed epidemiological model of *T. b. rhodesiense* transmission by tsetse flies among cattle and humans (based on Kajunguri *et al*., 2014). This model allows the different control interventions to be modelled with costs associated with different levels of coverage achieved. The intervention assumptions feed into the epidemiological model that in turn predicts the dynamic changes in parasite prevalence in cattle (*T. b. brucei* and *T. b. rhodesiense* – although we could also extend the model to track the more cattle pathogenic trypanosome species of *T. congolense* and *T. vivax* for completeness) and also incidence of sleeping sickness in humans. The epidemiological model outputs are translated to human cases and health-care costs averted, estimated from the literature and adjusting for the proportion of case reporting to the health-care system rates (Odiit *et al*., 2005; Févre *et al*., 2008b; Shaw, 2009a; Zinsstag *et al*., Chapter 12, this volume).

For animal health benefits, the model permits calculation of the number of cattle days free of trypanosomes (relative to the baseline equilibrium prevalence), which are translated into dollars gained, estimated from published literature on the burden of cattle trypanosomiasis (see Shaw, 2009b; Shaw *et al*., 2014). Similarly, the model allows us to work out the cattle days covered with insecticide, which can be linked to an improvement in animal health through reducing tick-borne disease (estimated from Shaw *et al*., 2014).

The model framework can be used to design an epidemiological outcome measure and sampling system that monitors changes in *T. brucei* prevalence in cattle and links these to DIB outcome payments triggered at agreed levels of impact. The outcomes, specifically DALYs averted, health-care costs avoided and economic gains due to improved animal health and productivity, are dynamically driven by the epidemiological model, so the model framework can be used to examine the costs and benefits associated with all possible coverage levels of drugs and insecticides delivered in a variety of different scenarios. An example of the model outputs is shown in Fig. 18.8 and Tables 18.2 and 18.3.

Moreover, the framework allows us to quantify the relationship between prevalence of *T. brucei* in cattle (a tractable, verifiable indicator that can be measured with pre-agreed statistical accuracy) and the impact of the interventions (DALYs averted and US$ saved, which are difficult and costly to measure directly). In this way, the framework can be used to design an epidemiological outcome measure and sampling system that monitors changes in *T. brucei* prevalence in cattle and links these to DIB outcome payments triggered at agreed levels of impact. The framework developed here, in which the economics of disease control is dynamically linked to the epidemiological changes resulting from control efforts, is essential in exploring the non-linear relationships between outcomes and inputs. The approach avoids the unsatisfactory alternative approach taken in much of the health economics literature of defining, a priori, an arbitrary, limited subset of intervention scenarios and assumed outcomes. This approach is essential in fully exploring the One Health costs and benefits associated with scaling disease control efforts and is applicable to other zoonotic disease systems that will behave in a highly non-linear manner when interventions are implemented.

## Discussion and Conclusions

The SOS Campaign has played a major role to date, in terms of halting the northerly movement of *T. b. rhodesiense* and averting the potential crisis of the two forms of HAT overlapping. SOS is based on sound science that clearly relates the presence of human sleeping sickness to the animal reservoir, in this case, domestic cattle, and thus significantly reduced the prevalence in the animal reservoir using improved diagnostics and new application techniques. Studies have confirmed the potential of the methodology in maintaining a low prevalence of disease by spraying cattle and treating with appropriate drugs (Brownlow, 2009; Muhanguzi *et al*., 2014b).

The fearful narrative that had developed of HAT as an untreatable disease, with serious social and economic consequences, which led to the establishment of COCTU, was

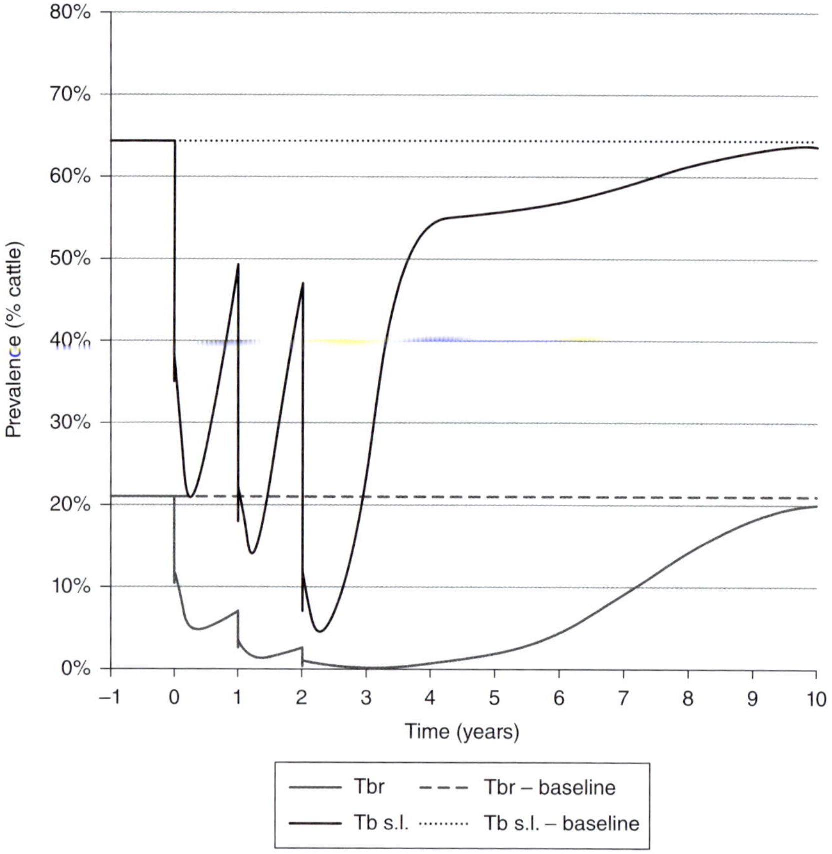


**Fig. 18.8.** Outputs from the framework linking the epidemiology and economics of disease control. Simulated changes in the prevalence of *T. b. rhodesiense* 'Tbr' and *T. brucei sensu latu* 'Tb s.l.' in cattle with (solid lines) and without (broken lines) intervention. The intervention assumes three rounds of mass treatment of cattle with trypanocidal drugs and insecticide spray with coverage levels of 50% (time=0 year), 65% (time=1 year) and 85% (time=2 years) of all cattle.

**Table 18.2.** Model predicted health-care benefits expressed as the number of sleeping sickness cases averted, the DALYs averted and health-care costs averted, assuming a baseline of 800 cases per year and 80% under-reporting (which gives ~18 DALYs and ~US$200 health-care cost per case).

| Year | Sleeping sickness cases averted | DALYs averted | Care US$ averted |
|---|---|---|---|
| 1 | 584 | 10,956 | 116,856 |
| 2 | 737 | 13,816 | 147,354 |
| 3 | 790 | 14,819 | 158,051 |
| 4 | 783 | 14,687 | 156,648 |
| 5 | 756 | 14,178 | 151,217 |
| 6 | 691 | 12,963 | 138,261 |
| 7 | 561 | 10,528 | 112,288 |
| 8 | 371 | 6,965 | 74,285 |
| 9 | 191 | 3,588 | 38,264 |
| 10 | 80 | 1,509 | 16,089 |
| Total | 5,545 | 104,009 | 1,109,313 |
| Discounted total (20% discount rate) | 2,661 | 49,919 | 532,420 |

**Table 18.3.** The animal health-care benefits resulting from cattle days free of trypanosome infections, assuming an average ~US$15 per cow per year free of trypanosomes, and cattle protected from tick infestation from insecticide treatment, assuming an average of ~US$8 per cow per year protected with insecticide treatment. Health-care costs averted and animal benefits unlocked can be discounted.

| Year | Trypanosome-free cattle years | Tryps US$ benefit | ITC years | Tick US$ benefit | Total US$ benefit |
|---|---|---|---|---|---|
| 1 | 725,441 | 10,973,522 | 53,652 | 401,617 | 11,375,139 |
| 2 | 798,079 | 12,072,301 | 69,748 | 522,102 | 12,594,403 |
| 3 | 1,204,087 | 18,213,861 | 91,209 | 682,749 | 18,896,611 |
| 4 | 289,976 | 4,386,378 | 0 | 0 | 4,386,378 |
| 5 | 6,855 | 103,693 | 0 | 0 | 103,693 |
| 6 | 98 | 1,483 | 0 | 0 | 1,483 |
| 7 | 1 | 21 | 0 | 0 | 21 |
| 8 | 0 | 0 | 0 | 0 | 0 |
| 9 | 0 | 0 | 0 | 0 | 0 |
| 10 | 0 | 0 | 0 | 0 | 0 |
| Total | 3,024,537 | 45,751,260 | 214,609 | 1,606,469 | 47,357,729 |
| Discounted total (20% discount rate) | 1,998,195 | 30,226,092 | 145,929 | 1,092,362 | 31,318,454 |

not dissimilar to fears of the rapid spread of avian influenza (H5N1) virus, responsible for HPAI that caused huge losses in poultry production with a direct negative impact on the livelihoods of the global poor (Vandermissen and Welburn, 2014). The potentially disastrous overlap of the two types of sleeping sickness was clear to decision-makers, both specialist and non-specialist alike. Strong institutional networks, amenable to a One Health approach, were in place in Uganda, which allowed for an effective response to a crisis situation that would impact on the livelihood of poor rural communities (Okello and Welburn, 2014). Without these established networks and mutual trust, backed up by a supportive coordination body at a high level within government, it is difficult to envision the mobilization of resources and the overcoming of legal and logistical hurdles in time to respond effectively to the northerly progress of the disease. Expressed as a crisis, there was a need for urgent decision making and imperatives to use available science.

Several factors were key to the evolution of SOS (http://www.stampoutsleepingsickness.org), including the patterns of insecurity and responses that led to migration of HAT a sense of urgency to prevent overlap of acute and chronic HAT, the existence of strong intersectoral mechanisms for coordination on AAT and HAT control (COCTU), a realization of the consequences of decentralization of government services for animal health work and strong research evidence to support intervention and private sector support.

The narrative used with farmers to deliver the impact focused on reducing tick burden and prevention of animal trypanosomiasis (nagana), bringing benefits to farmers in the short term. Coping with vulnerability depends on different social strata, from the household to the district, provincial and, finally, national level, and their interactions. Dialogue between livestock keepers, communities and authorities to identify interventions that are acceptable, affordable and adequate will embed One Health at local, district and national levels (Butcher, 2009). Interventions that translate gender, knowledge, cultural practices and risk perceptions into disease control involving human behaviour, supported by measures to improve acceptance are invaluable and can be underpinned by a One Health approach.

The primary objective of COCTU is to strengthen and optimize HAT surveillance and control practices for improved livelihoods, ecosystems management and human and animal health. The institutional vision required to initiate and subsequently sustain OH platforms such as the COCTU secretariat should not be underestimated, but is not without its challenges. Under Ugandan law, any permanent platform must be housed within a single ministry and the decision to house COCTU in MAAIF resulted from the major drive for trypanosomiasis control in farm animals. Roles and responsibilities must be agreed upon and understood by all stakeholders involved in One Health approaches, particularly regarding financial resource allocation. Ministerial ownership related to long-term financial support of the initiative presents an ongoing challenge to the secretariat. Since the MAAIF budget only allows for administrative activities undertaken by the secretariat, control interventions in the animal reservoir still require funding from a separate budget line. Despite ongoing financial challenges, the Ugandan ownership and high-level political endorsement of COCTU and SOS demonstrates how One Health success is likely to be much more sustainable and appropriate when owned nationally (Okello and Welburn, 2014).

## References

Ahmed, H.A., MacLeod, E.T., Hide, G., Welburn, S.C. and Picozzi, K. (2011) The best practice for preparation of samples from FTA cards for diagnosis of blood borne infections using African trypanosomes as a model system. *Parasites & Vectors* 4, 68.

Ahmed, H., Picozzi, K., Welburn, S.C. and MacLeod, E.T. (2013) Evaluation of two PCR reactions in use for trypanosome diagnosis. *Parasites & Vectors* 6, 316.

Anderson, N.E., Mubanga, J., Fevre, E.M., Picozzi, K., Eisler, M., Thomas, R. and Welburn, S.C. (2011) Characterisation of the wildlife reservoir community for human and animal trypanosomiasis in the Luangwa Valley, Zambia. *PLoS Neglected Tropical Diseases* 5(6), e1211.

Asiimwe, D. and Katorobo, J. (2007) Introduction. In: Asiimwe, D. and Musisi, B.M. (eds) *Decentralisation and Governance in Uganda*. Fountain Publishers, Kampala, Uganda, pp. xvii–xx.

Auty, H., Anderson, N.E., Picozzi, K., Lembo, T., Mubanga, J., Hoare, R., Fyumagwa, R.D., Mable, B., Hamill, L., Cleaveland, S. and Welburn, S.C. (2012) Trypanosome diversity in wildlife species from the Serengeti and Luangwa Valley ecosystems. *PLoS Neglected Tropical Diseases* 6(10), e1828.

Bardosh, K., Waiswa, C. and Welburn, S.C. (2013) Conflict of interest: use of pyrethroids and amidines against tsetse and ticks in zoonotic sleeping sickness endemic areas of Uganda. *Parasites & Vectors* 6, 204.

Batchelor, N.A., Atkinson, P.M., Gething, P.W., Picozzi, K., Fèvre, E.M., Kakembo, A. and Welburn, S.C. (2009) Spatial predictions of Human African Trypanosomiasis prevalence in Kaberamaido and Dokolo, two newly affected districts of Uganda. *PLoS Neglected Tropical Diseases* 15;3(12), e563.

Brownlow, A. (2009) Evaluation of a novel method for controlling bovine trypanosomiasis. PhD thesis, University of Edinburgh, UK.

Butcher, C. (2009) Poverty and Poverty Reduction Strategies in Uganda, a Brief review. Working Paper 5.

Center for Global Development and Social Finance Development Impact Bonds Working Group Report (2013).

COCTU (2014) Records from 1987 to 2011. The Government of Uganda. Available at: http://www.agriculture.go.ug/index-page-bodies-id-104.htm (accessed 18 April 2014).

Coleman, P.G. and Welburn, S.C. (2004) Are fitness costs associated with resistance to human serum in *Trypanosoma brucei rhodesiense*? *Trends in Parasitology* 20, 311–315.

Cook R.A., Karesh, W.B. and Osofsky, S.A. (2004) Comments from Conference Summary One World One Health: Building Interdisciplinary Bridges to Health in a Globalised World, 29 September 2004, Rockefeller University. Wildlife Conservation Society, New York. *EcoHealth* 9(4), 371–373.

Cox, A., Tosas, O., Tilley, A., Picozzi, C.K., Coleman, P.G., Hide, G. and Welburn, S.C. (2010) Constraints to estimating the prevalence of trypanosome infections in East African Zebu Cattle. *Parasites & Vector.* 3(1), 82.

Epelu-Opio, J. (2009) *Teso War 1986–1992: Causes and Consequences*. Fountain Publishers, Kampala, Uganda.

Févre, E.M., Coleman, P.G., Odiit, M.D., Magona, J., Welburn, S.C. and Woolhouse, M.E.J. (2001) The origins of a new sleeping sickness outbreak (caused by *Trypanosoma brucei* infection) in eastern Uganda. *Lancet* 358, 625–628.

Févre, E.M., Coleman, P.G., Welburn, S.C. and Maudlin, I. (2004) Reanalyzing the 1900–1920 sleeping sickness epidemic in Uganda. *Emerging Infectious Diseases* 10(4), 567–573.

Févre, E.M., Picozzi, K., Fyfe, J., Waiswa, C., Odiit, M., Coleman, P.G. and Welburn, S.C. (2005) A burgeoning epidemic of sleeping sickness in Uganda. *Lancet* 366, 747.

Févre, E.M., Wissmann, B.V., Welburn, S.C and Lutumba, P. (2008a) The burden of human African trypanosomiasis. *PLoS Neglected Tropical Diseases* 2(12), e333.

Févre, E.M., Odiit, M., Coleman, P.G., Woolhouse, M.E.J. and Welburn, S.C. (2008b) Estimating the burden of rhodesiense sleeping sickness during an outbreak in Serere, eastern Uganda. *BMC Public Health* 26(8), 96.

Hargrove, J.W., Torr, S.J. and Kindness, H.M. (2002) Factors affecting the efficacy of using insecticide-treated cattle to control tsetse. *Bulletin of Entomological Research* 93, 203–217.

Hargrove, J.W., Ouifki, R., Kajunguri, D., Vale, G.A. and Torr, S.J. (2012) Modeling the control of trypanosomiasis using trypanocides or insecticide-treated livestock. *PLoS Neglected Tropical Diseases* 6(5), e1615.

Hide, G., Welburn, S.C., Tait, A. and Maudlin, I. (1994) Epidemiological relationships of *Trypanosoma brucei* stocks from South East Uganda: evidence for different population structures in human infective and non-human infective isolates. *Parasitology* 109, 95–111.

Hide, G., Tait, A., Maudlin, I. and Welburn, S.C. (1996) The origins, dynamics and generation of *Trypanosoma brucei rhodesiense* epidemics in East Africa. *Parasitology Today* 12(2), 50–55.

Hutchinson, O.C., Fèvre, E.M., Carrington, M. and Welburn, S.C. (2003) Lessons learnt from the emergence of a new *Trypanosoma brucei rhodesiense* sleeping sickness focus in Uganda. *Lancet Infectious Diseases* 3, 42–45.

Jamonneau, V., Ravel, S., Koffi, M., Kaba, D., Zeze, D.G., Ndri, L., Sane, B., Coulibaly, B., Cuny, G. and Solano, P. (2004) Mixed infections of trypanosomes in tsetse and pigs and their epidemiological significance in a sleeping sickness focus of Côte d'Ivoire. *Parasitology* 129, 693–702.

Kabasa, J.D. (2007) Public-private partnership works to stamp out sleeping sickness in Uganda. *Trends in Parasitology* 23(5), 191–192.

Kajunguri, D., Hargrove, J.W., Ouifki, R., Mugisha, J.Y.T., Coleman, P.G. and Welburn, S.C. (2014) Modelling the control of tsetse and *Trypanosoma brucei rhodesiense* in a multi-host population through insecticide-treated cattle. *Bulletin of Mathematical Biology* (in press).

Koerner, T., de Raadt, P. and Maudlin, I. (1995) The 1901 Uganda sleeping sickness epidemic revisited – a case of mistaken identity? *Parasitology Today* 11, 303–306.

Magona, J.W., Mayende, J.S., Olaho-Mukani, W., Coleman, P.G., Jonsson, N.N., Welburn, S.C. and Eisler, M.C. (2003) A comparative study on the clinical, parasitological and molecular diagnosis of bovine trypanosomosis in Uganda. *Onderstepoort Journal of Veterinary Research* 70(3), 213–218.

Magona, J.W., Walubengo, J., Olaho-Mukani, W., Jonsson, N.N., Welburn, S.C. and Eisler, M.C. (2008) Clinical features associated with sero-conversion to *Anaplasma marginale*, *Babesia bigemina* and *Theileria parva* infections in African cattle under natural tick challenge. *Veterinary Parasitology* 155, 273–280.

Magona, J.W., Walubengo, J., Olaho-Mukani, W., Jonsson, N.N., Welburn, S.C. and Eisler, M.C. (2011) Spatial variation of tick abundance and seroconversion rates of indigenous cattle to *Anaplasma marginale*, *Babesia bigemina* and *Theileria parva* infections in Uganda. *Experimental and Applied Acarology* 55(2), 203–213.

Maudlin, I. (2006) African Trypanosomiasis. *Annals of Tropical Medicine & Parasitology* 100(8), 679–701.

Maudlin, I., Eisler, M.C. and Welburn, S.C. (2009) Neglected and endemic zoonoses. *Philosophical Transactions of the Royal Society B* 364, 2777–2787.

Milligan, P.J., Maudlin, I. and Welburn, S.C. (1995) Trypanozoon: infectivity to humans is linked to reduced transmissibility in tsetse. II. Genetic mechanisms. *Experimental Parasitology* 81, 409–415.

Minjauw, B. and McLeod, A. (2003) Tickborne diseases and poverty. The impact of ticks and tick-borne diseases on the livelihood of small-scale and marginal livestock owners in India and eastern and southern Africa. Research report, DFID Animal Health Programme, Centre for Tropical Veterinary Medicine, University of Edinburgh, UK.

Morton, J. (2009) The Stamp Out Sleeping Sickness Campaign in Uganda: an Institutional and Policy Study. Available at: http://www.au-ibar.org/isctrc/28Meeting/en/annex/002a.html (accessed 16 May 2014).

Muhanguzi, D., Picozzi, K., Hatendorf, J., Thrusfield, M., Kabasa, J.D., Welburn, S.C. and Waiswa, C. (2014a) Spatial distribution of *Theileria parva* in cattle under crop-livestock farming systems in Tororo District, Eastern Uganda. *Parasites & Vectors* doi: 10.1186/1756-3305-7-91.

Muhanguzi, D., Picozzi, K., Hattendorf, J., Thrusfield, M., Welburn, S.C., Kabasa, J.D. and Waiswa, C. (2014b) Improvements on restricted insecticide application protocol for control of Human and Animal African Trypanosomiasis in eastern Uganda. *PLoS Neglected Tropical Diseases 10/2014*; doi: 10.1371/journal.pntd.0003284.

Narrod, C., Zinsstag, J. and Tiongco, M. (2012) A one health framework for estimating the economic costs of zoonotic diseases on society. *EcoHealth* 9(2), 150–162.

Odiit, M., Coleman, P.G., McDermott, J.J., Fevre, E.M., Welburn, S.C. and Woolhouse, M.E.J. (2004a) Spatial and temporal risk factors for the early detection of *Trypanosoma brucei rhodesiense* sleeping sickness patients in Tororo and Busia districts, Uganda. *Transactions of the Royal Society of Tropical Medicine and Hygiene* 98(10), 569–576.

Odiit, M., Shaw, A., Welburn, S.C., Fevre, E.M., Coleman, P.G. and McDermott, J.J. (2004b) Assessing the patterns of health-seeking behaviour and awareness among sleeping-sickness patients in eastern Uganda. *Annals of Tropical Medicine and Parasitology* 98(4), 339–348.

Odiit, M., Coleman, P.G., Liu, W.C., McDermott, J.J., Fèvre, E.M., Welburn, S.C. and Woolhouse, M.E. (2005) Quantifying the level of under-detection of *Trypanosoma brucei rhodesiense* sleeping sickness cases. *Tropical Medicine and International Health* 10, 840–849.

Okello, A.L. and Welburn, S.C. (2014) The importance of veterinary policy in preventing the emergence and re-emergence of zoonotic disease: examining the case of Human African Trypanosomiasis in Uganda. *Frontiers in Public Health* 11/2014; 2 (218).

Okello, A.L., Gibbs, E.P.J., Vandersmissen, A. and Welburn, S.C. (2011) One Health and the neglected zoonoses: turning rhetoric into reality. *Veterinary Record* 169, 281–285.

Okello, A.L., Bardosh, K., Smith, J. and Welburn, S.C. (2014) One Health: past successes and future challenges in three African contexts. *PLoS Neglected Tropical Diseases* (in press).

Okuna, N.M., Mayende, J.S. and Guloba, A. (1986) *Trypanosoma brucei* infection in domestic pigs in a sleeping sickness epidemic area of Uganda. *Acta Tropica* 43(2), 183–184.

Onyango, R.J., Van Hoeve, K. and De Raadt, P. (1966) The epidemiology of *Trypanosoma rhodesiense* sleeping sickness in Alego location, Central Nyanza, Kenya. I. Evidence that cattle may act as reservoir hosts of trypanosomes infective to man. *Transactions of the Royal Society of Tropical Medicine and Hygiene* 60(2), 175–182.

Picozzi, K., Tilley, A., Fèvre, E.M., Coleman, P.G., Odiit, M., Magona, J., Eisler, M.C. and Welburn, S.C. (2002) The diagnosis of trypanosome infections: applications of novel technology for reducing disease risk. *African Journal of Biotechnology* 1(2), 39–45.

Picozzi, K., Fevre, E.M., Odiit, M., Carrington, M., Eisler, M.C., Maudlin, I. and Welburn, S.C. (2005) Sleeping sickness in Uganda: a thin line between two fatal diseases. *British Medical Journal* 331(7527), 1238–1241.

Selby, R., Bardosh, K., Waiswa, C. and Welburn, S.C. (2014) Cattle movements and trypanosomes: Restocking efforts and the spread of Rhodesian sleeping sickness in post-conflict Uganda. *Parasites & Vectors* 6, 281.

Shaw, A.P.M. (2009a) The Socio-economic Impact of the SOS Programme on Human African Trypanosomiasis (HAT). The cost of the averted disaster. DfID Research Into Use Monitoring & Evaluation of a Public–Private Partnership: Stamp out Sleeping Sickness Case Study Working Paper 9. Available at: http://www.researchintouse.com/resources/riu09sos-synth-mon-butcher.pdf (accessed 23 January 2015).

Shaw, A.P.M. (2009b) Understanding the Burden of Human African Trypanosomiasis: DALYs, Under-reporting and the Cost to Communities. DfID Research Into Use Monitoring & Evaluation of a Public–Private Partnership: Stamp out Sleeping Sickness Case Study Working Paper 8. Available at: http://www.researchintouse.com/resources/riu09sos-synth-mon-butcher.pdf (accessed 23 January 2015).

Shaw, A.P., Cecchi, G., Wint, G.R., Mattioli, R.C. and Robinson, T.P. (2014) Mapping the economic benefits to livestock keepers from intervening against bovine trypanosomosis in Eastern Africa. *Preventive Veterinary Medicine* 113(2), 197–210.

Simarro, P.P., Jannin, J. and Cattand, P. (2008) Eliminating human African trypanosomiasis: where do we stand and what comes next? *PLoS Medicine* 5: e55.

SOS http://www.stampoutsleepingsickness.com (accessed 1 May 2014).

Soumana, I.H., Simo, G., Njiokou, F., Tchicaya, B., Abd-Alla, A.M., Cuny, G. and Geiger, A. (2012) The bacterial flora of tsetse fly midgut and its effect on trypanosome transmission. *Journal of Invertebrate Pathology* 112(Suppl.), S89–93.

Torr, S.J., Maudlin, I. and Vale, G.A. (2007) Less is more: restricted application of insecticide to improve the cost and efficacy of tsetse control. *Medical and Veterinary Entomology* 21, 53–64.

Vandersmissen, A. and Welburn, S.C. (2014) Current Initiatives in One Health. In: *OIE Scientific and Technical Review* 33(2), August 2014.

von Wissmann, B., Fyfe, J., Picozzi, K., Hamill, L., Waiswa, C. and Welburn, S.C. (2014) Quantifying the association between human and bovine trypanosomiasis in newly affected sleeping sickness areas of Uganda. *PLoS Neglected Tropical Diseases* 8(6): e2931.

Waiswa C., Picozzi, K., Katunguka-Rwakishaya, E., Olaho-Mukani E. and Welburn, S.C. (2006) *Glossina fuscipes fuscipes* in the trypanosomiasis endemic areas of south eastern Uganda: apparent density, trypanosome infection rates and host feeding preferences. *Acta Tropica* 99(1), 23–29.

Wardrop, N., Fevre, E.M., Atkinson, P. and Welburn, S.C. (2013) The dispersal ecology of Rhodesian sleeping sickness following its introduction to a new area. *Plos Neglected Tropical Diseases* 7(10), e2485.

Wastling, S.L. and Welburn, S.C. (2011) New techniques for old diseases I. Diagnostics for human sleeping sickness – Sense and senstivity. *Trends in Parasitology* 27(9), 394–402.

Wastling, S.L., Picozzi, C.L., Wamboga, C., von Wissmann, B., Wardrop, N.A., Stothard, R., Kakembo, A.S. and Welburn, S.C. (2011) Latent *Trypanosoma brucei gambiense* foci in Uganda: a silent epidemic in children and adults? *Parasitology* 18, 1–8.

Welburn, S. (2011) One Health: the 21st century challenge. *Veterinary Record* 168(23), 614–615.

Welburn, S.C. and Maudlin, I. (1991) Rickettsia-like organisms, puparial temperature and susceptibility to trypanosome infection in *Glossina morsitans*. *Parasitology* 102, 201–206.

Welburn, S.C. and Maudlin, I. (1992) The nature of the teneral state in *Glossina* and its role in the acquisition of trypanosome infection in tsetse. *Annals of Tropical Medicine and Parasitology* 86, 529–536.

Welburn, S.C. and Maudlin, I. (1999) Tsetse trypanosome interactions: rites of passage. *Parasitology Today* 15, 399–403.

Welburn, S.C. and Maudlin, I. (2012) Priorities for the elimination of sleeping sickness. *Advances in Parasit ology* 79, 299–337.

Welburn, S.C., Maudlin, I. and Milligan, P.J. (1995) *Trypanozoon*: infectivity to humans is linked to reduced transmissibility in tsetse. I. Comparison of human serum resistant and human serum sensitive field isolates. *Experimental Parasitology* 81, 404–408.

Welburn, S.C., Dale, C., Ellis, D., Beecroft, R., Pearson, T.W. and Maudlin, I. (1996) Apoptosis in procyclic *Trypanosoma brucei rhodesiense in vitro*. *Cell Death and Differentiation* 3, 229–236.

Welburn, S.C., Coleman, P.G., Fevre, E. and Maudlin, I. (2001a) Sleeping sickness – a tale of two diseases. *Trends in Parasitology* 17, 19–24.

Welburn, S.C., Picozzi, K., Fevre, E.M., Coleman, P.G., Odiit, M., Carrington, M. and Maudlin, I. (2001b) Identification of human infective trypanosomes in animal reservoir of sleeping sickness in Uganda by means of serum-resistance-associated (*SRA*) gene. *Lancet* 358, 2017–2019.

Welburn, S.C., Coleman, P.G., Fevre, E.M., Odiit, M., Maudlin, I. and Eisler, M.C. (2006) Crisis, what crisis? Control of Rhodesian sleeping sickness. *Trends in Parasitology* 22, 123–128.

Welburn, S.C., Picozzi, K., Coleman, P.G. and Packer, C. (2008) Patterns in age-seroprevalence consistent with acquired immunity against *Trypanosoma brucei* in Serengeti Lions. *PLOS Neglected Infectious Diseases* 2(12), e347.

Xong, H.V., Vanhamme, L., Chamekh, M., Chimfwembe, C.E., Van Den Abbeele, J., Pays, A., Van Meirvenne, N., Hamers, R., De Baetselier, P. and Pays, E. (1998) A VSG expression site-associated gene confers resistance to human serum in *Trypanosoma rhodesiense*. *Cell* 95, 839–846.

Zinsstag, J., Mackenzie, J.S., Jeggo, M., Heymann, D.L., Patz, J.A. and Daszak, P. (2012) Mainstreaming One Health. *EcoHealth* 9(2), 107–110.

# 19 Non-communicable Diseases: How Can Companion Animals Help in Connection with Coronary Heart Disease, Obesity, Diabetes and Depression?

**Dennis C. Turner***
*Institute for Interdisciplinary Research on the Human–Animal Relationship (IEMT), Basel, Switzerland*

## Non-communicable Diseases

According to the World Health Organization (WHO, 2014a), non-communicable diseases (NCDs) kill more than 36 million people each year, with nearly 80% of the NCD deaths occurring in low- and middle-income countries. Further, four groups of diseases account for around 80% of all NCD deaths: cardiovascular diseases, 17.3 million per year; cancers, 7.6 million; respiratory diseases, 4.2 million; and diabetes, 1.3 million. One risk factor in all four groups is physical inactivity, associated with about 3.2 million deaths annually (WHO, 2014a). Certain behaviours lead to four key metabolic/physiological changes that increase NCD risk: raised blood pressure, overweight/obesity, hyperglycaemia and hyperlipidaemia.

The numbers of young and older overweight people have increased at an alarming rate in recent years. Globally, ca. 35% of adults aged 20 and over were overweight in 2008; ca. 12% were obese by definition (WHO, 2014b). The mean body mass index (BMI) of the world's population increased dramatically between 1980 and 2008. According to the Global Health Observatory of WHO at least 2.8 million people die each year as a result of being overweight or obese and ca. 35.8 million of global DALYs (disability-adjusted life years, or lost 'healthy' life years) are caused by these problems (WHO, 2014c).

Depression is also considered in this chapter on non-communicable diseases and companion animals. Globally, some 350 million people of all ages suffer from depression, more women than men; it is the leading cause of disability worldwide (WHO, 2012a). Thus it is a major contributor to the global burden of disease.

## Companion Animals: More Than Just Companions

Many people consider the keeping of animals as companions, or pets, as status symbols of wealth and, in general, a useless by-product of affluent societies. This view, however, ignores the facts that: (i) at least for the two most common domesticated species of pets, dogs and cats, the animals first fulfilled utilitarian

*E-mail: dennis@turner-iet.ch

tasks; and (ii) that such animals are found in practically all cultures of the world, irrespective of economic status (Serpell, 1986).

Further, over the last three decades research has provided much evidence of positive effects of animals, in particular dogs, cats and horses, on the health and well-being of people of all ages (Turner *et al.*, 2013). No doubt pets, especially exotic species, can be the source of zoonotic diseases; but a number of studies have now concluded that a healthy, immunized and parasite-free domestic animal can bring more health benefits to the owner (or a patient, in the case of an animal-assisted intervention) than health risks (CALLISTO Strategy Report, 2013). Raina *et al.* (1999) further demonstrated that dog-ownership was associated with decreased health-care costs in people over 65 years old living in their own homes, particularly during times of stress. Indeed, the role that companion animals can (or might) play in combating a number of NCDs will be elucidated below.

## Coronary Heart Disease

Friedmann and Thomas (1995) reported that both high social support by humans (which was already known at the time) and rather unexpectedly, pet ownership, predicted 1-year survival rates after hospitalization for acute myocardial infarction independently of physiological severity, demographic and other psychosocial factors. Dog owners were significantly less likely to die within 1 year than non-owners. Friedmann and Lockwood (1993) found the same result for non-dog pet owners versus non-pet owners. Friedmann *et al.* (2011) later summarized the physiological correlates of the health benefits from pets. Based on research on adults, the presence of companion animals is associated with reductions in chronic levels of physiological stress indicators and reductions in stress response to mild to moderate stressors. Although there are fewer studies on children, the conclusions are in the same direction. However, no studies have been conducted to date on the impact of companion animals on major stressors.

Early studies showed a reduction in systolic and diastolic blood pressure as well as heart rate while stroking an animal (a dog) and a stronger effect if the study participants – all dog owners – were able to stroke their own animal as opposed to an unknown dog (Baun *et al.*, 1984). More importantly, pet ownership is associated with lower levels of accepted cardiovascular disease risk factors in men (and women over 40) such as high systolic blood pressure, plasma cholesterol and plasma triglyceride levels, whereas BMI, tobacco use and other potential factors were the same in the pet owners ($n$=784) and non-owners ($n$=4957) (Anderson *et al.*, 1992). However, the pet owners were more likely to be physically active.

## Obesity

Physical inactivity has been identified as the fourth leading risk factor for global mortality causing an estimated 3.2 million deaths a year (WHO, 2014d). WHO concludes that regular, moderate intensity physical activity – such as walking, cycling, or participating in sports – has significant health benefits; it can reduce the risk of cardiovascular diseases, diabetes, colon and breast cancer and depression (WHO, 2014d). Interestingly, companion animals, especially dogs and cats, have been shown to reduce the risk of cardiovascular diseases (Anderson *et al.*, 1992) and increase survival after myocardial infarction (Friedmann and Thomas, 1995), as well as reduce depression. Are the former related to dog walking? Although both dog and cat owners have significantly improved survival rates 1 year after a heart attack, usually only dogs are walked by their owners. Indeed, in Anderson *et al.* (1992), pet owners reported qualitatively that they were walking more, and Serpell (1991) quantitatively demonstrated this during a 10-month prospective study of owners after acquiring a new pet. WHO (2014e), in its Global Strategy on Diet, Physical Activity and Health, aims to reduce risk factors for chronic diseases that stem from unhealthy diets and physical inactivity through public health actions that are sustainable, comprehensive and actively engage all sectors. Owned dogs live many years and require daily movement outside of the home. It is therefore not surprising that a number of studies presented at the recent triennial conferences of the International Association of Human-Animal Interaction Organizations (IAHAIO, 2014) as well as the conferences jointly organized by the US National Institute of Child Health and Human Development (NICHD) and Mars Corp./WALTHAM® Centre in the UK, have investigated the link between dog ownership and physical exercise. These are summarized below.

Johnson *et al.* (2011) provide the most recent and comprehensive review of the health benefits of dog walking to people and their dogs. Findings from at least six studies indicate that dog owners are more physically active and more likely to meet the recommended level of physical activity than non-dog owners (Thorpe *et al.*, 2011). Because physical activity levels appear to be different for dog and cat owners, there might be differences in their respective health status. However, Turner and Gutzwiller (2004) found in Switzerland significantly lower expenditures for health and medication in cat-owning households than non-animal-owning households, as well as a tendency for such in dog-owning households, but no reduction in households with other pet species. Various potentially confounding variables such as overall income, household size and expenditures for the pets in this Swiss national random sample were taken into account.

A further study called the OPET (Owners and Pets Exercising Together) is currently attempting to assess the metabolic benefits of 'walking the dog' and whether physical activity counselling for the dog provided by a speciality-care veterinarian impacts the metabolic status of owners and their dogs (Stephens *et al.*, 2011).

Johnson and McKenney (2011) in their 'Walk a hound, lose a pound' community dog walking programme match behaviourally tested shelter dogs with non-dog-owning families. It is hypothesized that the dog may be a social lubricant for participants and their families to communicate while walking and afterward. Further, dog walking may have potential for improving long-term physical activity adherence through increasing readiness to engage in physical activity even beyond the dog walking (Johnson and Meadows, 2010). It has recently been shown that dogs motivate obese children for physical activity (Wohlfahrt *et al.*, 2013).

Lastly, dog walking appears to be a catalyst for strengthening the social fabric of the community (Wood and Christian, 2011). Dog walking has been shown to facilitate social interactions, social support and sense of community, benefiting not only the dog walkers themselves, but also having a ripple effect into the broader community.

Of course, under most circumstances, the dog also benefits from being walked. Canine obesity is widespread in dogs today, with an estimated 44% of US dogs being overweight or obese (i.e. ca. 33 million dogs in the USA alone) (Stregowski, 2014). The main causes are improper diet and lack of sufficient exercise. As with humans the health risks of obesity in dogs are well known and include cardiac disease, hypertension, orthopedic problems, various forms of cancer, and diabetes. Obviously, weight problems in humans and their companion animals fit well within the realm of One Health.

## The Diagnostic Value of Companion Animals

Although both humans and their companion dogs and cats can suffer from diabetes as well as other NCDs such as various cancers and epilepsy, and research on these ailments in the one species can help the other, in this section I would like to point out another role that companion dogs have taken on to assist their human partners: medical detection dogs. Medical detection dogs are usually divided into two broad categories, namely medical alert dogs and cancer and bio-detection dogs (Medical Detection Dogs, 2014). Dr Clair Guest in the UK is the pioneer in this field, which is rapidly expanding to other countries. Although some reports exist indicating a natural ability of dogs with their excellent olfactory sense to detect medical problems and change their behaviour in a way noticed by their owners, a number of programmes now exist to train dogs to reliably notify their owners of such problems.

One survey study indicated that behavioural reactions to hypoglycemic episodes in owners with type I diabetes commonly occur in untrained dogs (Wells *et al.*, 2008).

Case reports indicating this ability have also been published in the medical literature (Chen *et al.*, 2000; O'Connor *et al.*, 2008). Dog-training programmes now exist to channel the dog's sensitivity and train specific reactions, e.g. fetching glucose tablets, barking near a comatose owner to gain attention of neighbours or pedestrians. But the reliability of hypoglycaemia-alerting dogs remains to be tested.

Similarly, (epileptic) seizure-alert dogs, capable of warning their owners of an oncoming seizure in time to take medication, have been reported in the popular literature but less often, or with mixed results, in the professional literature. An early report was quite promising (Strong *et al.*, 1999). Dogs trained to alert their owners of an oncoming seizure were able to provide overt signals 15–45 min prior to a seizure and, in each case, the owner's seizure frequency was reduced. Authors of a later study in the same journal stated that the success of such dogs depends largely on the handler's awareness and response to the dog's alerting behaviour (Dalziel *et al.*, 2003). Two case reports found poor, misleading alerting behaviour within a clinical setting; in this case the setting was acknowledged to be part of the problem, at least for the dogs (Ortiz and Liporace, 2005). Finally, Brown and Goldstein (2011) suspect that such dogs can detect subtle behaviour changes, but might even be sensitive to heart rate or olfactory cues. Nevertheless, rigorous studies are needed to determine whether seizure prediction by such dogs is better than chance and what the false positive and negative prediction rates might be.

There is a fair amount of good evidence for the detection of various cancers by trained 'medical detection dogs'. In most cases the tests utilize the extreme sensitivity of the dog's olfactory ability after an initial training period. On average, the dog is able to detect, e.g. a small concentration of butyric acid (10,000 molecules/$cm^3$ air), whereas humans require a concentration a million times higher for initial detection (Feddersen-Petersen, 1986). Volatile chemicals are probably released by the cancerous cells either on the skin surface or into the blood and urine of afflicted persons. With respect to melanoma detection in an early experimental test with two dogs, the animals demonstrated reliable localization of melanoma tissue samples hidden on the skin of healthy volunteers (Pickel *et al.*, 2004).

McCulloch *et al.* (2006) examined the accuracy of canine scent detection in early- and late-stage lung and breast cancers. A food reward-based training method was employed on five ordinary household dogs to distinguish by scent alone exhaled breath samples of 55 lung and 31 breast cancer patients from those of 83 healthy controls. The dogs were taught to sit/lie in front of positive samples upon detection; a correct response to the control samples was to ignore them. The dog handlers and experimental observers were blinded to the identity of the breath samples. Concerning the lung cancer patients and controls, overall sensitivity of canine scent detection compared to biopsy-confirmed conventional diagnosis was 0.99 and overall specificity 0.99. For the breast cancer patients and controls, sensitivity was 0.88 and specificity 0.98. Sensitivity and specificity remained similar across all four stages of both diseases. The authors concluded that the dog training was efficient and cancer identification of exhaled breath samples was accurate.

Ovarian carcinomas have been detected by a trained dog in double-blind tests with 100% sensitivity and 97.5% specificity (Horvath *et al.*, 2008). Colorectal cancer screening with odour material (exhaled breath and watery stool samples) by one trained labrador yielded a sensitivity of canine scent detection of breath samples compared with conventional colonoscopy diagnosis of 0.91 with a specificity of 0.99 (Sonoda *et al.*, 2011). Sensitivity of detection of the stool samples was 0.97 with a specificity of 0.99. Olfactory detection of human bladder cancer by dogs trained to distinguish patients with this ailment on the basis of urine odour was more successful than expected by chance alone, although taken as a group, the dogs had a mean success rate of (only) 41% (Willis *et al.*, 2004).

In conclusion, these discussions are summarized well with a fitting citation from an editorial by McCulloch *et al.* (2012) on lung cancer detection by canine scent:

> In both the literal and the metaphorical sense, with the publication of these papers on canine scent detection of lung cancer, dogs are once again demonstrating their ability to serve as protectors and guides. People worldwide feel a close affinity with the dog as a friend and protector. Whether or not sniffer dogs actually make it into the continuum of diagnostic evaluation has yet to be seen; their image could be employed in public health outreach for cancer screening, and may encourage people with worrisome symptoms to take earlier action. This would be a case of the dog acting as a shepherd; Lassie and Rin Tin Tin are still out there looking out for our health.

## Depression

By all accounts and sources, depression is on the increase in modern societies. According to the World Health Organization at least 350 million people live with depression and it is the leading cause of disability worldwide (WHO, 2012b): 'Depression is treatable, but most people with depression do not receive the care and support they need. . . . Lack of access to treatment and stigma associated with depression are major obstacles to people seeking help.' Perhaps this is where companion animals can help – not in the sense of replacing classical therapies or medical treatment, but by providing additional support for the depressed person in the home setting. Several studies (Rieger and Turner, 1999; Turner and Rieger, 2001; Turner *et al.*, 2003) have demonstrated that both the presence of a cat in the private home, even more so interacting with it in the right moment, decreases negative mood-sets (fear, depression, introversion) significantly, which is explicable by changes in the cat's behaviour when close to a person in such a mood. It should not surprise us that many psychiatric clinics and psychotherapeutic practices maintain cats on their premises. But the aforementioned studies were not conducted on clinically depressed persons, indicating a salutogenic effect of the presence of animals in the home setting. Rieger and Turner (1999) proposed why the cat might be an ideal co-therapist for clinically depressed persons. Psychiatrist Daniel Hell found that in human–human relationships the depressed person increasingly dissociates him/herself, the more (s)he feels misunderstood by the partner, who often attempts to help (Hell, 1994). The cat accepts the level of 'interactivity' the (depressed) owner wants to have and is present when the owner desires that contact without forcing itself on the human partner. Rieger and Turner (1999) found that the influence of a cat on human mood is similar to its behaviour: either neutral or positive, but not negative. To some degree, cats can be more pleasant partners for depressed people than humans. This might make cats the better co-therapists than dogs for depressed patients (as dogs constantly seek contact and approval of their pack leader), but this remains to be tested directly.

There have been many studies purporting to examine the effects of dogs and cats on depression/depressed clients of psychotherapists, but many have been fraught with design problems and are inconclusive. A more rigorous study design with larger sample sizes would help. Nevertheless, Souter and Miller (2007) conducted a meta-analysis of the data in five very strictly controlled studies and found a significant positive effect of the animals, more importantly, of moderate size on top of the other therapies still being applied to the depressive persons.

Again in connection with One Health it is interesting to note that ever more veterinarians with training in animal behaviour believe that dogs and cats can also suffer from depression ('believe', simply because they cannot be asked and 'only' show behaviour patterns similar to humans suffering from depression) (Eckstein, 2014; Veterinary Pet Insurance, 2014). A further indication that this is indeed the case is reduction of the symptoms after prescription of antidepressants usually developed for humans in the pet-appropriate dosage (Schöning and Turner, 2011; Turner and Mertens, 2015).

## Conclusion

This chapter demonstrates that companion animals are more than just companions, and that they contribute significantly toward our health in one way or the other. The human–animal relationship is in fact an ideal topic to illustrate the added value that the One Health concept has to offer (IEMT, 2014). Not only is public health affected, but also increasingly, the health of individually challenged persons through animal-assisted interventions, which is the focus of a number of international organizations today (IAHAIO, 2014; ISAAT, 2014). But only when we look after the health and welfare of those companion animals can we expect to benefit from their company – either in the private setting, in special settings such as hospitals, rehabilitation centres and schools, or in public society. That is truly One Health.

## References

Anderson, W., Ried, C. and Jennings, G. (1992) Pet ownership and risk factors for cardiovascular disease. *Medical Journal of Australia* 157, 298–301.

Baun, M., Bergstrom, N., Longston, N. and Thoma, L. (1984) Physiological effects of human/companion animal bonding. *Nursing Research* 50, 126–129.

Brown, S. and Goldstein, L. (2011) Can seizure-alert dogs predict seizures? *Epilepsy Research* 97, 236–242.

CALLISTO Strategy Report (2013) Sociological and Human Welfare Aspects of Keeping Companion Animals. CALLISTO project, EU, Federation of Veterinarians of Europe (ed.), Brussels, pp. 21–27. Available at: http://www.callistoproject.eu/joomla/attachments/article/77/strategy_report_first_cycle.pdf (accessed 9 October 2014).

Chen, M., Daly, M. and Williams, G. (2000) Non-invasive detection of hypoglycaemia using a novel fully biocompatible and patient friendly alarm system. *British Medical Journal* 321, 1565–1566.

Dalziel, D., Uthman, B., McGorray, S. and Reep, R. (2003) Seizure-alert dogs: a review and preliminary study. *Seizure* 12, 115–120.

Eckstein, S. (2014) Depression in dogs. WebMD Pet Health Feature. Available at: http://pets.webmd.com/dogs/features/depression-in-dogs (accessed 21 March 2014).

Feddersen-Petersen, D. (1986) *Hundepsychologie. Wesen und Sozialverhalten*. Kosmos Verlag, Stuttgart, Germany.

Friedmann, E. and Lockwood, R. (1993) Perception of animals and cardiovascular responses during verbalisation with an animal present. *Anthrozooös* 6, 115–134.

Friedmann, E. and Thomas, S.A. (1995) Pet ownership, social support, and one-year survival after acute myocardial infarction in the Cardiac Arrhythmia Suppression Trial (CAST). *American Journal of Cardiology* 76, 1213–1217.

Friedmann, E., Barker, S.C. and Allen, K.M. (2011) Physiological correlates of health benefits from pets. In: McCardle, P., McCune, S., Griffin, J. and Maholmes, V. (eds) *How Animals Affect Us*. American Psychological Association, Washington, DC, pp. 163–182.

Hell, D. (1994) *Welche Sinn macht Depression? Ein integrativer Ansatz*. Rohwolt, Reinbeck bei Hamburg, Germany.

Horvath, G., af Klinteberg Järverud, G., Järverud, S. and Horvath, I. (2008) Human ovarian carcinomas detected by specific odor. *Integrative Cancer Therapies* 7(2), 76–80.

IAHAIO, the International Association of Human-Animal Interaction Organizations (2014) See www.iahaio.org (accessed 21 March 2014).

IEMT-Switzerland. (2014) See Weissbuch Nr. 6 (German)/ Lievre Blanc numero 6 (French). http://www.iemt.ch/deu/publikationen/109-fundierte-hintergrundinformationen-zu-ausgewaehlten-themen-der-mensch-tier-beziehungen (accessed 21 March 2014).

ISAAT, the International Society for Animal-Assisted Therapy (2014) Available at: http://www.aat-isaat.org (accessed 21 March 2014).

Johnson, R.A. and McKenney, C.A. (2011) 'Walk a hound, lose a pound': a community dog walking program for families. In: Johnson, R.A., Beck, A.M. and McCune, S. (eds) *The Health Benefits of Dog Walking for People and Pets*. Purdue University Press, West Lafayette, Indiana, pp. 89–104.

Johnson, R.A. and Meadows, R.L. (2010) Dog-walking: motivation for adherence to a walking program. *Clinical Nursing Research* 19(4), 387–402.

Johnson, R.A., Beck, A.M. and McCune, S. (eds) (2011) *The Health Benefits of Dog Walking for People and Pets*. Purdue University Press, West Lafayette, Indiana.

McCulloch, M., Jezierski, T., Broffman, M., Hubbard, A., Turner, K. and Janecki, T. (2006) Diagnostic accuracy of canine scent detection in early- and late-stage lung and breast cancers. *Integrative Cancer Therapies* 5(1), 1–10.

McCulloch, M., Turner, K. and Broffman, M. (2012) Lung cancer detection by canine scent: will there be a lab in the lab (Editorial). *European Respiratory Journal* 39, 511–512.

Medical Detection Dogs (2014) Available at: http://www.medicaldetectiondogs.org.uk (accessed 20 March 2014).

O'Connor, M., O'Connor, C. and Walsh, C. (2008) A dog's detection of low blood sugar: a case report. *Irish Journal of Medical Science* 177, 155–157.

Ortiz, R. and Liporace, J. (2005) 'Seizure-alert dogs': Observations from an inpatient video/EEG unit. *Epilepsy & Behavior* 6, 620–622.

Pickel, D., Manucy, G., Walker, D., Hall, S. and Walker J. (2004) Evidence for canine olfactory detection of melanoma. *Applied Animal Behaviour Science* 89(1), 107–116.

Raina, P., Waltner-Toews, D., Bonnett, B., Woodward, W. and Abernathy, T. (1999) Influence of companion animals on the physical and pyschological health of older people: an analysis of 1-year longitudinal study. *Journal of American Geriatric Society* 47, 323–329.

Rieger, G. and Turner, D.C. (1999) How depressive moods affect the behavior of singly living persons toward their cats. *Anthrozoös* 12(4), 224–233.

Schöning, B. and Turner, D. (2011) Verhaltensprobleme und Verhaltensstörungen. In: Schwarz, G., Kohn, B. and Suter, P. (eds) *Peraktikum der Hundeklinik, 10. Auflage*. Enke Ferdinand, Stuttgart, Germany.

Serpell, J. (1986) *In the Company of Animals*. Basil Blackwell, Oxford, UK.

Serpell, J. (1991) Beneficial effects of pet ownership on some aspects of human health and behaviour. *Journal of the Royal Society of Medicine* 84, 717–720.

Sonoda, H., Kohnoe, S., Yamazato, T., Satoh, Y., Morizono, G., Shikata, K., Morita, M., Watanabe, A., Morita, M., Kakeji, Y., Inoue, F. and Maehara, Y. (2011) Colorectal cancer screening with odour material by canine scent detection. *British Medical Journal* doi: 10.1136/gut.2010.218305.

Souter, M.A. and Miller, M.D. (2007) Do animal-assisted activities effectively treat depression? A meta-analysis. *Anthrozoös* 20(2), 167–180.

Stephens, M.B., Wilson, C.C., Goddie, J.L., Netting, E., Olsen, C., Byers, C.G. and Yonemura, M.E. (2011) Owners and pets exercising together: the metabolic benefits of 'walking the dog'. In: Johnson, R.A., Beck, A.M. and McCune, S. (eds) *The Health Benefits of Dog Walking for People and Pets*. Purdue University Press, West Lafayette, Indiana, pp. 147–162.

Stregowski, J. (2014) Obesity in Dogs. Available at: http://dogs.about.com/od/caninediseases/p/obesity.htm (accessed 10 February 2014).

Strong, V., Brown, S. and Walker, R. (1999) Seizure-alert dogs – fact or fiction? *Seizure* 8, 62–65.

Thorpe, R.J. Jr, Christian, H.E. and Baumann, A. (2011) Dog walking as physical activity for older adults. In: Johnson, R.A., Beck, A.M. and McCune, S. (eds) *The Health Benefits of Dog Walking for People and Pets*. Purdue University Press, West Lafayette, Indiana, pp. 75–88.

Turner, D.C. and Gutzwiller, F. (2004) Hundehaltung und Gesundheit, Gesundheitskosten. In: Kotrschal, K., Bromundt, V. and Foeger, B. (eds) *Faktor Hund. Eine sozio-ökonosmische Bestandesaufnahme der Hundehaltung in Österreich*. Czernin Verlag, Vienna, Austria, pp. 45–46.

Turner, D. and Mertens, P. (2015) Verhalten, störendes Verhalten und Verhaltensstörungen. In: Lutz, H., Kohn, B. and Forterre, F. (eds) *Krankheiten der Katze, 5. Aufl.* Enke Verlag, Stuttgart, Germany.

Turner, D.C. and Rieger, G. (2001) Singly living people and their cats: a study of human mood and subsequent behavior. *Anthrozoös* 14(1), 38–46.

Turner, D.C., Rieger, G. and Gygax, L. (2003) Spouses and cats and their effects on human mood. *Anthrozoös* 16(3), 213–228.

Turner, D.C., Waiblinger, E. and Meslin, F.-X. (2013) Benefits of the human-dog relationship. In: Macpherson, C.N.L., Wandeler, A. and Meslin, F.-X. (eds) *Dogs, Zoonoses and Public Health*, 2nd edn. CAB International, Wallingford, UK, pp. 13–23.

Veterinary Pet Insurance (2014) Feline depression. Available at: https://www.petinsurance.com/healthzone/pet-articles/pet-behavior/Feline-Depression.aspx (accessed 21 March 2014).

Wells, D., Lawson, S. and Niroshan Siriwardena, A. (2008) Canine responses to hypoglycemia in patients with Type I diabetes. *Journal of Alternative and Complementary Medicine* 14(10), 1235–1241.

Willis, C., Church, S., Guest, C., Cook, W., McCarthy, N., Bransbury, A., Church, M. and Church, J. (2004) Olfactory detection of human bladder cancer by dogs: proof of principle study. *British Medical Journal* 329, 712.

Wohlfahrt, R., Mutschler, B., Beetz, A., Kreuser, F. and Korsten-Reck, U. (2013) Dogs motivate obese children for physical activity: key elements of a motivational theory of animal-assisted interventions. *Frontiers in Psychology* 4, 796.

Wood, L.J. and Christian, H.E. (2011) Dog walking as a catalyst for strengthening the social fabric of the community. In: Johnson, R.A., Beck, A.M. and McCune, S. (eds) *The Health Benefits of Dog Walking for People and Pets*. Purdue University Press, West Lafayette, Indiana, pp. 51–74.

World Health Organization (2012a) Media center, Depression. Fact sheet Nr. 369. Available at: http://www.who.int/mediacentre/factsheets/fs369/en (accessed 6 March 2014).

World Health Organization (2012b) Global strategy on diet, physical activity and health. Available at: http://www.who.int/dietphysicalactivity/goals/en/index.html (accessed 6 March 2014).

World Health Organization (2014a) Noncommunicable diseases. Fact sheet 355. Available at: http://www.who.int/mediacentre/factsheets/fs355/en (accessed 6 March 2014).

World Health Organization (2014b) Global Health Observatory, Overweight and obesity. Available at: http://www.who.int/gho/ncd/risk_factors/overweight/en (accessed 6 March 2014).

World Health Organization (2014c) Global Health Observatory, Obesity. Available at: http://www.who.int/gho/ncd/risk_factors/obesity_text/en (accessed 6 March 2014).

World Health Organization (2014d) Health topics. Physical activity. Available at: http://www.who.int/topics/physical_activity/en (accessed 6 March 2014).

World Health Organization (2014e) Depression, a hidden burden. Available at: http://www.who.int/mental_health/management/depression/flyer_depression_2012.pdf (accessed 6 March 2014).

# 20 Integrated One Health Services

**Esther Schelling,[1]* Mahamat Béchir Mahamat,[2] Jakob Zinsstag[1] and Marcel Tanner[1]**
[1]*Swiss Tropical and Public Health Institute, Basel and University of Basel, Switzerland;* [2]*Ministère de la Santé Publique, N'Djaména and Centre de Support en Santé Internationale, N'Djaména, Chad*

## Health Services in Remote and Rural Zones

This chapter describes the added value of One Health making use of synergies in delivery of health services that were perceived as disconnected. Both One Health and ecohealth approaches seek a broader understanding of health beyond the biomedical realm (Zinsstag, 2012) and thus also include health delivery systems. Health and well-being relates to individuals (people, animals, plants and, in a broader sense, ecosystems) and to populations or communities embedded in their cultures, customs and livelihood systems. Health of ecosystems is difficult to define as ecosystems are inherently dynamic and changing. We consider an ecosystem as 'healthy' when it provides high quality services (e.g. clean water) continuously. Thereby the provision of services is dynamic and often has a cyclical behaviour. The organization of service delivery systems for humans, animals and the environment show similarities but also differences. In the first part of this chapter, we summarize these services as a foundation for the chapter. The focus is on rural and remote zones in resource-poor countries because new integrated ways to deliver health services seem to have most potential and leverage in these zones.

### Human health systems service delivery and inequities in health

An equitable human health system delivers quality services to all people, when and where they are needed. Inequity refers to unnecessary and avoidable differences, which are in addition considered unfair and unjust, reflecting its normative dimension (Whitehead *et al.*, 2001). Health inequality is a distinct aspect regarding the performance of a health system and may be defined as measurable variations in health status across individuals of a population. An equitable health system is challenged to ensure that interventions benefit the disadvantaged. Effective responses to inequalities in health often require actions outside the health sector such as poverty alleviation. Without an explicit assessment of the impact of population health interventions on health inequalities, policies and public or private programmes run the risk of benefiting only the more privileged and better-off without improving the health of the poor – despite national averages indicating overall

*E-mail: esther.schelling@unibas.ch

improvements (Tugwell *et al.*, 2006; Welch *et al.*, 2008; WHO, 2013).

Improving access, coverage and quality of services, particularly primary health care, depends on availability of key resources such as trained professionals and equipment. Improvements also depend on the organization and management of services, the incentives influencing providers and users (WHO, 2013), and the availability of reliable information. WHO recognizes that integrated health services are critical for reaching universal health coverage within the continuum of health promotion, disease prevention, diagnosis, treatment, disease-management, rehabilitation and palliative care services. Evidence-based guidelines and best practices of integrated services can be tailored to various country settings. Studies show that rather than taking a traditional approach, i.e. initially serving those who are easiest to reach, approaches designed to first increase coverage among disadvantaged groups show most progress towards universal health coverage (Gwatkin and Ergo, 2011).

Health service delivery to 'hard-to-reach populations' is difficult, in particular due to logistical, organizational and financial constraints. Increasing numbers of displaced people, mobile, migratory populations and remote rural communities are unable to benefit equally from governmental or private health services, compared to those in urban centres. Health inequities in these zones owe their existence to factors that also exist in rural zones of, for example, Australia and Europe: lower access to new diagnostic and treatment techniques; unpredictable socio-economic and ecological circumstances, an out-migration and ageing population, rural families being poorer and attaining lower levels of education. Additional factors for developing countries are vulnerability to exclusion from markets and absence of outreach services. The latter is also important for services requiring multiple service contacts, such as antenatal care and tuberculosis treatment. The ability of health and veterinary systems to deliver services is constrained by a number of strong factors: declining public-sector budgets, loss of confidence by the community as a result of unmet demand, a severe shortage of human resources, especially qualified personnel (Wyss *et al.*, 2003), inadequate infrastructure and equipment, and weak monitoring and information systems (Schelling *et al.*, 2007b). Approximately one-half of the global population lives in rural areas, but these areas are served by only 38% of the total nursing workforce and by less than 25% of the total physician workforce (WHO, 2010). The increased number of people being forced to leave rural zones and live in urban slums leads to emerging health inequities in urban centres.

### Veterinary services and rural zones

In animal health, collective interests of disease control are frequently discussed (Johnston, 2013). Highly contagious animal diseases and epidemics pose an economic threat to livestock producers, the entire agricultural sector and national economies. Animal disease control and elimination is therefore considered a public good. Animal health officials worldwide coordinate their disease control strategies with the World Organisation for Animal Health (OIE). Typically, national veterinary services are responsible for ensuring the protection of animal health, for the safety of food products of animal origin and for the control of major animal diseases, as well as the quality control of veterinary pharmaceuticals. Most veterinary services may enforce animal welfare standards, and in some countries, the veterinary service is also responsible for monitoring and controlling wildlife diseases (World Bank, 2010). Authors such as Riviere-Cinnamond (2005) and Ahuja (2004) have used excludability principles to separate animal health services into groups. Private good services cover endemic disease control and prevention, sales of drugs and vaccines and clinical services, because the user captures all benefits. Common or public good services cover diagnosis, surveillance, movement control and quarantine services for epidemic or zoonotic disease control, control of foodborne diseases and tsetse control. Thus the control of zoonoses is considered to be a public good in that it protects human and animal public health and thus benefits society as a whole. The 'public good' nature of some services does not necessarily imply that the government must take direct responsibility for their delivery. These services may be subcontracted to private organizations (e.g. non-governmental or research organizations) and private veterinarians (Stephen and Waltner-Toews, Chapter 32, this volume).

Animal-health systems have been neglected in many parts of the world, leading to institutional weaknesses and information gaps as well as inadequate investments in animal-health-related public goods (FAO, 2009). This is particularly evident in remote and rural zones, where between 46 and 82% of rural households in Asia, Africa and Latin America keep livestock (Zezza *et al.*, 2007).

### Wildlife health services

Issues that touch the health of wildlife generally fall under the jurisdiction of environment ministries, whose involvement in wildlife is largely limited to management of parks and related matters concerning biodiversity conservation (Cumming *et al.*, Chapter 21, this volume). In most developing countries, these services are greatly underfunded. They are generally not allowed to use the revenues generated by parks for their own operation and management costs (World Bank, 2010).

Although the majority of newly discovered zoonotic diseases originate in wildlife (Cleaveland *et al.*, 2001), there is much more emphasis on diseases at the human–livestock interface. The latter seems justified, because the most frequent zoonoses in people are those with livestock or pet transmission cycles. Still, a more systematic approach to surveillance and control would be more inclusive, and would expand to agencies and institutions concerned with environmental health, and to wildlife health in particular (Rabinowitz *et al.*, 2013). Such efforts could lead to a more robust understanding of the human health impacts of accelerating environmental change and inform decision making in the land-use planning, environmental conservation and public health policy realms (Myers *et al.*, 2013; Cumming *et al.*, Chapter 21, this volume).

## Potential of Integrated One Health Services

The vertical organization of work, in which institutions operate independently of one another and strictly from the perspective of their own discipline or sector, leads to gaps and sometimes to overlaps (Fig. 20.1). Integrated approaches can be depicted as a reorientation along horizontal lines in which regular communication takes place between practitioners in different disciplines and sectors, revising questions like 'Is this my job?' into statements of 'This work needs to be done'. With regard to

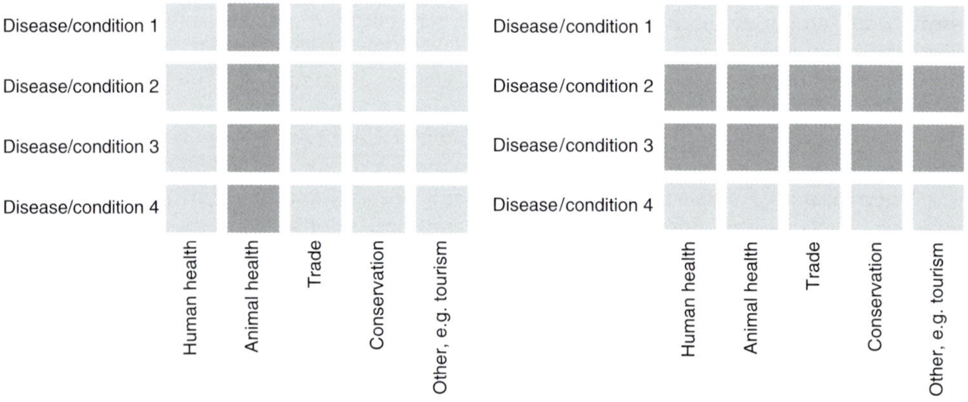


**Fig. 20.1.** Vertical (left) versus horizontal (right) orientation of work for disease prevention and control. Note that two disease groups are highlighted in the horizontal approach, because single disease programmes can also be regarded as vertical approaches (adapted from World Bank, 2010).

integrated One Health services, there is overlap between sectors in infectious disease control, targeted populations and in organization of services.

Note that 'integrated' used in relation to One Health services is largely 'integrated surveillance'. However, we use it here with reference to cross-sectoral integrated health service delivery. This means that the service needs of communities are identified jointly by at least two health sectors, and cross-sector planning occurs to identify ways to make services more community-effective. Thus interventions and services work better when applied in communities (Tanner *et al.*, 1993; Tugwell *et al.*, 2006), including joint monitoring of health outcomes and possibly the added value of shared resources. We exclude here other health services, such as laboratories and registries, as well as surveillance and monitoring of diseases, referred to in other chapters (for example, Schelling and Hattendorf, Chapter 10, this volume). Research on adapted social services (e.g. health and education) requires social scientists and the social science perspective is an integral part of One Health as described in Whittaker (Chapter 6, this volume).

Ministries of health in resource-poor countries give priority to primary health care and diseases with the highest burden, such as the reduction of mother and child mortality, and control of HIV/AIDS, malaria and tuberculosis. Veterinary services often give the highest priority to the 'diseases of trade', such as foot-and-mouth disease (FMD), classical swine fever and contagious bovine pleuropneumonia (CBPP). Wildlife agencies are mainly concerned with conservation of threatened and endangered species (World Bank, 2010). Zoonotic diseases, therefore, tend to be neglected among these priorities.

Veterinarians are not allowed to treat human patients, and paraprofessionals often are not allowed to handle certain human and animal drugs or to perform simple interventions. These restrictions also apply in remote areas, where neither physicians nor veterinarians are available. With a proper legal framework and appropriate training, however, certain selected public health activities could be shared – for instance, in surveillance. Patient care would, of course, remain the sole responsibility of the human health agents (Catley *et al.*, 2004; Kahn *et al.*, 2007). While the animal health sector lacks institutional focus, such as conceiving long-term community animal health systems, human health lacks participatory rural appraisal methods to increase community involvement in implementation (Riviere-Cinnamond, 2005). Public health and veterinary programmes should more widely share their knowledge and their different approaches – and explore local priorities and perceived needs. They can then develop joint implementation arrangements to improve services to remote and rural communities.

Both sectors face difficulties in establishing private health providers in rural zones, which is constrained by low affordability for potential clients from poor areas. Numerous incentive schemes were designed to stimulate the privatization of veterinary services to improve the animal health systems' effectiveness while reducing public expenditure. The World Bank released privatization guidelines for the livestock sector in 1991–1992. Two decades later, however, the effectiveness of the system still could not be increased as expected (Riviere-Cinnamond, 2005). Newly established private veterinarians in remote zones quickly give up due to insufficient clients who are able and willing to pay for clinical services. Private veterinary services are currently rarely viable in remote and sparsely populated areas.

## The role of vaccination in public health and veterinary medicine

Vaccination remains a key community-effective health intervention in human and animal health and is increasingly an important tool in wildlife health management. Small pox and rinderpest eradication programmes benefited from committed financial and personnel investments. There are poliomyelitis- and contagious bovine pleuropneumonia (CBPP)-eradication programmes that need to deal with vaccines requiring a cold chain. This necessitates innovations and adaptation to successfully reach all communities and remaining pockets of disease transmission.

Although the poliomyelitis and CBPP-eradication programmes have achieved huge progress, the expected outputs could not be met within their targeted timeframe, e.g. polio was to be eradicated by the year 2000, but transmission was still ongoing in 2012 and 2013 (Fig. 20.2). The new targeted time-frame for final wild polio virus transmission is now the end of 2014. Similarly, national CBPP control programmes were to be implemented at the end of the PACE (Pan African Programme for the Control of Epizootics) programme in 2007, but an African-continent-wide implementation is further postponed.

Mobile pastoralists may play a special role in a disease eradication programme. Although the numbers of nomadic or semi-nomadic populations are relatively small and there is no hard evidence that, for example, the burden of polio disease is higher in these populations compared with others, there is genetic and epidemiological evidence that pastoralists play a critical role in transmitting wild polio virus between different regions of a country and across borders. Also, their general vaccination coverage level tends to be lower because they are often not reached by national Expanded Programmes on Immunization. The last pockets of rinderpest were among pastoralists, and only participatory approaches allowed for reaching these remote communities (Jost *et al.*, 2007).

Human and animal health vaccination programmes may experience both periodic lack of vaccination-related supplies and limited or not well-maintained infrastructure in the governmental services. Poor implementation or inferior quality of animal vaccines not only causes economic losses in the livestock sector but can also be a human health threat when vaccines against zoonoses are not efficacious. There are, for example, animal vaccines against zoonoses: anthrax, rabies, brucellosis and Rift Valley fever, as well as a very new vaccine against porcine cysticercosis. Livestock vaccine production could benefit from the more stringent and internationally coordinated quality control applied to human vaccines. On the other hand, public health practitioners sometimes envy their veterinary colleagues who have a public-good mandate to vaccinate against epidemic and zoonotic diseases. Veterinary authorities may declare a livestock vaccine as compulsory given the economic and societal interests to better control these diseases. Vaccination programmes rooted either in the public health and veterinary sectors have hardly exchanged in the past, despite the fact to a large extent they target the same populations, those vulnerable to exclusion from any health services.

## Tuberculosis control for remote livestock-keeping communities

Brosch *et al.* (2002) showed that the popular hypothesis of human tuberculosis (TB) deriving

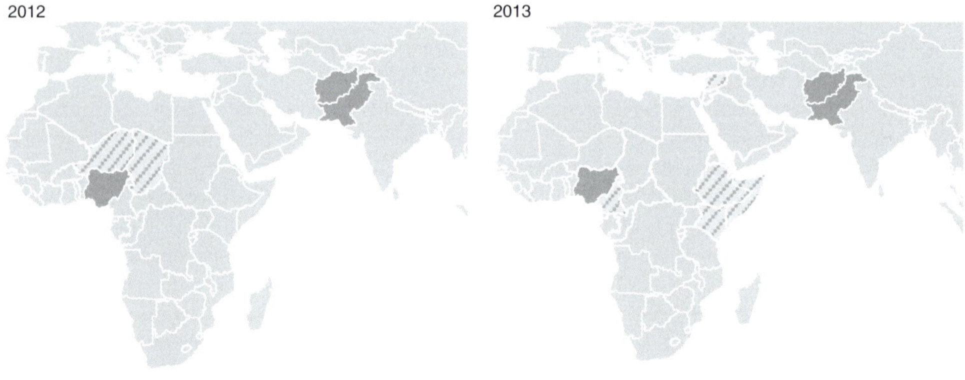


**Fig. 20.2.** Wild polio virus endemic and importation countries in 2012 and 2013 (http://www.polioeradication.org/Dataandmonitoring/Poliothisweek/Poliocasesworldwide.aspx). Solid dark grey fill are 'endemic countries'; shaded countries are 'importation countries'. Almost all of these countries have child vaccination coverages <80%.

from domestication of cattle was incorrect, since ancestral human tuberculosis complex strains were evolutionarily older than *Mycobacterium bovis*. It also seems that the proportion of human tuberculosis due to *M. bovis* is lower than was generally thought two decades ago (Muller *et al.*, 2013), but *M. bovis* causes considerable losses, especially to peri-urban dairy production (Tschopp *et al.*, 2013). In Ethiopia, *M. bovis* in human TB infection was very low. Among 1000 *M. tuberculosis* isolates from clinical suspects of pulmonary and extra-pulmonary TB, only four isolates were *M. bovis* (Firdessa *et al.*, 2013). Interestingly, *M. tuberculosis* was isolated from several cattle and from one camel (Gumi *et al.*, 2012).

Tuberculosis patients in remote and rural zones have less access to information and diagnostic resources and have higher dropout rates in treatment, all of which lead to higher TB incidences (Khogali *et al.*, 2014). Among Mauritanian pastoralists, TB was part of different illness concepts, according to different causes and different stages of the disease. Tuberculosis was perceived either as due to spiritual or biomedical causes, it could also be stigmatizing. Diagnosis was usually made by people in the local vicinity of the patient, such as a faith healer and/or traditional healer but could also be made by community members. This means the patient may not seek health facility care until the later stage of the disease (Ould Taleb, 2007). After information campaigns emphasizing availability of a treatment against TB and including livestock health messages, markedly more pastoralists were registered at the diagnostic centre of the zone (M. Ould Taleb, 2011, National TB Programme, Mauritania, personal communication). The WHO-recommended 6-month directly observed treatment short course (DOTs) is not adaptable to the mobile pastoralist lifestyle if only offered at a health facility. As a consequence, treatment adherence is poor (Khogali *et al.*, 2014). Innovations in TB service delivery to remote and rural zones are warranted and integrated services seem promising. For example, animal health services can be an incentive for TB patients in rural zones to adhere to treatment, because livestock services increase the often desperately needed additional income of families with a TB patient. Prophylactic treatment against livestock trypanosomiasis or deworming of animals increase their productivity. A full cost analysis of tuberculosis treatment in Mauritania showed that the bulk of treatment costs (44%) are attributed to improved nutrition for the patient (Bonfoh *et al.*, 2011). Animal health staff could also be enrolled as DOTs supervisors, thereby increasing the number of service delivery points for mobile pastoralists.

## Integrated One Health information delivery

Animal health problems are sometimes perceived by livestock-keeping communities with more straightforward local concepts than are human illness concepts (Krönke, 2004). Perceived human illness categories, which do not necessarily correspond to biomedical disease categories, are based on the illness experience and meaning, and influences health-seeking behaviour and health-care practices (Whittaker, Chapter 6, this volume). One Health services can play a role in providing appropriate health information in rural zones. People who work with animals may understand human health concepts better when linked to their experiential knowledge of animal health and diseases.

Communities do often demand more health information. Health messages that are disseminated in Information, Education and Communication (IEC) and social marketing approaches should be adapted to cultural background and should accommodate the high levels of illiteracy of rural communities. How to make effective health communications and social marketing is understood (Maibach *et al.*, 2007) but rather often is not done because of resourcing or concerns about how to provide understandable concepts to low-literacy populations. Findings regarding the absence of an illness concept for zoonotic diseases among pastoralists in Chad were confirmed in northern Cameroon by a recent ethno-veterinary study (Moritz *et al.*, 2013). Anthropological studies on diseases among livestock-keeping communities, however, are still sparse and limited (Whittaker, Chapter 6, this volume).

## Possible additional actors in One Health service delivery

McCorkle (1996) argues that, especially for remote or rural people in developing countries, an intersectoral approach, partly modelled along the lines of traditional patterns for human and animal health joint service delivery, would be more feasible than attempting to impose a dualistic Western-style structure on services. Formal and informal and traditional and modern medical sectors could be joined by including traditional/local practitioners. Effective ethno-medical practices and traditional health-care networks could be an integral part of such a delivery system (Last, 1990; McCorkle, 1994). However, the issue of how to integrate the two systems of medicine without complete structural and cultural subordination of traditional medicines remains unresolved (McCorkle, 1996). Livestock often contribute to multiple livelihood objectives, where food production is only one objective. Focusing on Western technology to maximize individual animal production is a solution that is too often inappropriately put in the foreground (Randolph *et al.*, 2007).

Community health and community animal health workers can provide primary health care in remote zones. After the initial training, key activities for long-term provision of both human and animal health community services include continued exchange on quality services and supervision by the health systems, as well as patient referral systems (Catley *et al.*, 2004; Jaskiewicz and Tulenko, 2012). The advantage of community workers is that they are more accessible to community members who may face difficulties to access services further away. Also, strong producer organizations or farmer cooperative structures can offer logistics for delivering human and animal health services, although care is needed regarding the fact that mixing marketing and service functions may lead to an undesirable confounding of both functions and responsibilities of the public and private sectors (capacity.org, 2008). We believe that all possible actors, including also those of non-governmental organizations, should be included to identify opportunities of closer cooperation, which may lead to synergies.

## Joint human and animal vaccination campaigns

Different authors have proposed joining veterinary and health services to increase the level of coverage to communities in remote zones, to reduce costs and to increase acceptance (reviewed in Swift *et al.*, 1990). Wherever single-sector approaches cannot be achieved, mainly due to financial constraints, all potentially multi-use resources could be actively shared including facilities, personnel and outreach activities of animal and human vaccination, education, water and environmental services. When pastoral and other livestock-keeping families in remote zones can be reached, maximal use should be made of each visit (Ward *et al.*, 1993; Majok and Schwabe, 1996). In conflict situations, animal health services are sometimes still active when health services already have broken down (B. Peterhans, personal communication). Organizations such as the International Committee of the Red Cross (ICRC) have – in situations of humanitarian crises such as droughts or armed conflicts – implemented joint human and livestock vaccinations, however, such approaches are rarely documented.

Based on findings of a simultaneous assessment of human and health service needs in Chad, a broad agreement was reached with national and local authorities as well as communities to test joint human and animal vaccination services (Schelling *et al.*, 2008). Together with authorities, such joint vaccination campaigns were evaluated from 2000 through 2005, and showed the feasibility of combining vaccination programmes for mobile pastoralists and their livestock. Sharing of transport logistics and equipment between physicians and veterinarians reduced total costs (15% of the public health sector) (Schelling *et al.*, 2007a). The Chad Ministry of Health's Expanded Programme on Immunization (EPI), together with the veterinary services, continue to implement such joint vaccination campaigns in priority zones, particularly in regions with frequent cross-border movements of pastoralists, representing ~20% of all pastoralist zones in Chad. More information exchange with neighbouring countries is envisioned to establish cross-country campaigns. Agronomes et Vétérinaires sans Frontières, which faced difficulties with absent private veterinarians, have facilitated joint health delivery systems in Niger and Mali (Agronomes et Vétérinaires sans Frontières, 2010). These joint campaigns also helped improve understanding of how to set up a system that alternates between mobile and static health services, because outreach and mobile services alone are not sustainable if they operate independently from static health facilities (Brenzel and Claquin, 1994).

## Costs and cost-saving potential of integrated service delivery

One outcome of a cost assessment for a measles vaccination campaign in Ghana was additional costs for insecticide-treated bednets (ITN) delivered during the campaign. The vaccination campaign contributed to ITN distribution in terms of programme planning, social mobilization, salaries for some health workers and transportation and supervision costs. The marginal costs of ITN distribution were those costs that occurred in addition to the costs of measles vaccination (Grabowsky *et al.*, 2005). This is an example of an evaluated integrated service that was demanded by WHO and UNICEF in their joint immunization strategy 2006–2015. Such integrated approaches should lead to more equity-effective planning (WHO and UNICEF, 2005).

The cost assessment of joint human and livestock vaccination campaigns in Chad (Schelling *et al.*, 2007a) was based on a health and veterinary service perspective to determine the proportion of shared costs between the public health and veterinary sectors; household costs were excluded. The same unit costs were used for the joint campaigns, the dispensary-based approaches and the stand-alone veterinary vaccination campaigns. Wherever possible, unit costs were based on detailed local prices (e.g. replacement and maintenance costs of vehicles) as opposed to annual or aggregate costs (Gold *et al.*, 1996). Costs were divided into variable (recurrent) costs, such as personnel and supplies, and fixed (non-recurrent) costs, such as buildings. The costs were taken from literature, field data or from interviews with medical and veterinary staff. The questionnaire followed the Partnerships for Health Reform guidelines for cost evaluation of the EPI at the facility level (Partnerships for Health Reform, 2000). Vaccine costs included storage and supplies (e.g. syringes and needles) and a vaccine wastage proportion of 10% for human and 5% for livestock vaccines.

The proportion of public health costs saved due to sharing with veterinary services was calculated on the basis of single campaigns of the public health sector, compared to joint vaccination campaigns that achieved equal numbers of fully immunized children and women. Human vaccination costs were assessed for static vaccination service and for outreach activities for the same period as joint vaccinations, and it was assumed that they also began with zero fully immunized children and women. Follow-up rates for the second and third rounds were based on national averages for rural Chad. The approach used to allocate the costs to the two sectors for jointly used resources distributed the costs of the vehicle(s), fuel and guides according to the number of personnel in the field. The costs of the cold chain, programme coordination/administration, information campaigns (social mobilization) and the car and fuel used for preparation were distributed according to the number of vaccination rounds in each sector. Cold-chain costs were only charged to the livestock sector when vaccines against contagious bovine pleuropneumonia (CBPP) vaccines were used (the only livestock vaccines that needed a cold chain). Costs could only be shared during four joint rounds, from a total of 12 vaccination rounds; sharing was further limited when two vehicles were used, as opposed to one car for all professionals. Since the livestock sector deployed more personnel, they had a higher share of the vehicle costs. Other resources used by both sectors were guides, transportation and personnel for information campaigns, as well as administration costs (Schelling, 2002; Zinsstag *et al.*, Chapter 12, this volume).

## Can plant health services be integrated with extension services from other sectors?

Plants serve as feed for animals and food for humans in mixed crop/livestock smallholder production systems (Wright *et al.*, 2012). Plant diseases and pests jeopardize health and lead to increased food/feed insecurity and decreased income (Boa *et al.*, Chapter 22, this volume). Extension services for preventive interventions and treatment of acute problems may exist, but they are separated into crop, animal and human health services, and access to them is limited for many rural populations. Agricultural and human health extension services have both technical and educational components and can, in a broader context, be regarded as possible tools for community empowerment and development. Extensions should be close to the end-users and remain flexible in order to react to the real needs. However, a tripartite approach incorporating all three fields has not yet been tested (Fletcher *et al.*, 2009). One should indeed assess whether the combination of human, animal and plant health services would improve quantitative (e.g. time and costs) and qualitative access to services, when compared to single-sector approaches.

### Integration of human and environmental health services

In Madagascar in the early 1990s, in response to the lack of access to both health and environmental/agricultural extension services and the lack of family planning services in conservation zones, different groups began experimenting with joint population, health and environmental initiatives. By the late 1990s, implementation strategies from both the environmental and health sectors supported joint activities such as social marketing. By focusing on small, achievable actions at the community level, the population, health and environmental (PHE) movement began to grow. Activities were implemented by local health and environment NGOs and a strategy of 'Champion Communities' was adopted in four of the six provinces in Madagascar. By 2005, a national consortium with 29 member groups was formed to link PHE efforts. Progress was measured by local monitoring that tracked the increased use of essential health services. Key health indicators and land-use practices have improved over a 3-year period among integrated versus non-integrated communities. Use of preventive health services such as vaccination and modern family planning, home-based prevention measures (e.g. use of ITNs) as well as participation in reforestation efforts and vector control increased in PHE project zones, surpassing national norms. In addition, malnutrition prevalence dropped, and access to safe water improved (Ribaira and Rossi, 2007). Synergies between sectors manifested themselves in improved capacity at the programme and organizational levels and in the communities' progress towards self-determined and sustainable development. The integrated approach resulted in greater effectiveness of interventions and achieved relatively better outcomes for low incremental costs compared with single-sector vertical approaches (Kleinau *et al.*, 2005). The PHE programme serves as a flagship example of integrating health, population and environment services (Kleinau *et al.*, 2005; Gaffikin *et al.*, 2007; Ribaira and Rossi, 2007). This programme combining health and environment services has similar goals, evaluation approaches and conclusions as the good practices described for delivery of health services to remote populations (Schelling *et al.*, 2009).

## The Way Forward with One Health Services

After a broad literature review and expert interviews, a panel in the UK identified conditions necessary to successfully scale up innovation across the public sector (Capability Building Programme of Civil Service and National School of Goverment, 2011). We present the conditions here because we think there are the same issues when scaling up innovative cross-sector health service delivery approaches.

**1.** Build a culture that rewards and encourages scaling up innovation.
**2.** Make the business case and demonstrate the social return.
**3.** Embed skills needed for scaling up and understand that skills to innovate and to scale up are different.
**4.** Develop and use networks to make connections, provide advice, share knowledge and create dialogue.
**5.** Embed processes and mechanisms that facilitate scaling up.

**6.** Recognize that a feeling of ownership acts as an incentive to share learning about what works; manage resources, funding, expertise and support to actively encourage scaling up.
**7.** Credibility, endorsement and reputation provide the business case for scaling up.

There are barriers in establishing cross-sector integrated approaches. Some of these barriers are imposed by the bureaucratic division of responsibility between institutions. Others relate to budgetary constraints, unequal institutional capabilities and differing cultures, limited communication of information, the absence of a shared vision and disincentives to work horizontally (World Bank, 2010). Although public health is underfunded in relation to curative health care, the human health sector more often has greater human and financial resources available for disease control activities than have environmental or animal health agencies. In Kenya, the Ministry of Health deployed five times more staff in response to Rift Valley fever than could be deployed by veterinary services (Schelling and Kimani, 2007). Further incentives for collaboration and resource sharing could be created. For example, budget lines could be shared between different agencies, directed by the Ministry of Finance. Also, equity analyses based on the geographical deployment of new programmes and strategies can help assess whether the programmes are reaching those who need them most (Victora *et al.*, 2006).

Our conclusions from the examples in remote and rural zones described above are as follows.

**1.** There is a seemingly high potential in remote and rural areas to combine health services for joint delivery of human and animal health, plant and environmental care; integrated health services have become a prime example of added value of One health (World Bank, 2010). However, to date, few documented studies exist that illustrate the feasibility, acceptability and potential gains/savings of sharing of logistics and personnel, and increased accessibility, coverage and chances for sustainability.
**2.** The inclusion of different stakeholders in the conceptual and planning phase is crucial, as it increases ownership among the concerned populations and authorities (Schelling and Zinsstag, Chapter 30, this volume).
**3.** As much as possible, one must avoid establishing parallel structures and instead make use of existing health systems, infrastructure and human resources that are well linked into the service provision systems of their countries – but have so far not benefited from cross-over synergies such as transportation, information and management of cases of illness in their communities.
**4.** The evaluation of community effectiveness should be designed and carried out with multiple stakeholders, including communities, national and local services, international organizations and standards.
**5.** Integrated services should try to meet communities' health priorities – both felt and measured needs.
**6.** Health systems and traditional institutional arrangements must be carefully examined to identify opportunities to join public health and veterinary services. Case studies and demonstrating feasibility are recommended before gradually expanding to other zones.

## References

Agronomes et Vétérinaires sans Frontières (2010) Mixed service of human and animal health in pastoral zones: An innovative and promising experience. Available at: http://de.slideshare.net/copppldsecretariat/mixed-service-ofhumanandanimalhealthavsfinnovativeexperience (accessed 10 October 2014).

Ahuja, V. (2004) The economic rationale of public and private sector roles in the provision of animal health services. *Revue Scientifique et Technique OIE* 23, 33–45.

Bonfoh, B., Keita, M., Ould Taleb, M. and Schelling, E. (2011) Nourriture: facteur d'adhésion des patients tuberculeux au traitement. Policy Brief NCCR North-South. Available at: http://www.nccr-north-south.unibe.ch/publications/Infosystem/On-line%20Dokumente/Upload/Regional_Policy_Brief_01_West_Africa_Nutrition_TB_treatment.pdf (accessed 10 October 2014).

Brenzel, L. and Claquin, P. (1994) Immunization programs and their costs. *Social Science and Medicine* 39, 527–536.

Brosch, R., Gordon, S.V., Marmiesse, M., Brodin, P., Buchrieser, C., Eiglmeier, K., Garnier, T., Gutierrez, C., Hewinson, G., Kremer, K., Parsons, L.M., Pym, A.S., Samper, S., Van Soolingen, D. and Cole, S.T. (2002) A new evolutionary scenario for the *Mycobacterium tuberculosis* complex. *Proceedings of the National Academy of Sciences USA* 99, 3684–3689.

Capability Building Programme of Civil Service and National School of Goverment (2011) Scaling Up Innovation in the Public Sector. Final report of the Capability Building Programme Project Group. Available at: http://webarchive.nationalarchives.gov.uk/+/http://blogs.bis.gov.uk/publicsectorinnovation/files/2011/07/Scaling-Up-Innovation-in-the-Public-Sector-Full-Report.pdf (accessed 10 October 2014).

capacity.org (2008) Producer organisations and value chains. A gateway for capacity development. Available at: http://www.capacity.org/capacity/opencms/en/index.html (accessed 10 October 2014).

Catley, A., Leyland, T., Mariner, J.C., Akabwai, D.M., Admassu, B., Asfaw, W., Bekele, G. and Hassan, H.S. (2004) Para-veterinary professionals and the development of quality, self-sustaining community-based services. *Revue Scientifique et Technique OIE* 23, 225–252.

Cleaveland, S., Laurenson, M.K. and Taylor, L.H. (2001) Diseases of humans and their domestic mammals: pathogen characteristics, host range and the risk of emergence. *Philosophical Transactions of the Royal Society B: Biological Sciences* 356, 991–999.

FAO (2009) The State of Food and Agriculture: Livestock in the Balance. FAO, Rome. Available at: http://www.fao.org/docrep/012/i0680e/i0680e00.htm (accessed 10 October 2014).

Firdessa, R., Berg, S., Hailu, E., Schelling, E., Gumi, B., Erenso, G., Gadisa, E., Kiros, T., Habtamu, M., Hussein, J., Zinsstag, J., Robertson, B.D., Ameni, G., Lohan, A.J., Loftus, B., Comas, I., Gagneux, S., Tschopp, R., Yamuah, L., Hewinson, G., Gordon, S.V., Young, D.B. and Aseffa, A. (2013) Mycobacterial lineages causing pulmonary and extrapulmonary tuberculosis, Ethiopia. *Emerging Infectious Diseases* 19, 460–463.

Fletcher, J., Franz, D. and LeClerc, J.E. (2009) Healthy plants: necessary for a balanced 'One Health' concept? *Veterinaria Italiana* 45, 79–95.

Gaffikin, L., Ashley, J. and Blumenthal, P.D. (2007) Poverty reduction and Millennium Development Goals: recognizing population, health, and environment linkages in rural Madagascar. *Medscape General Medicine* 9, 17.

Gold, M.R., Siegel, J.E., Russell, L.B. and Weinstein, M.C. (1996) *Cost-effectiveness in Health and Medicine.* Oxford University Press, New York.

Grabowsky, M., Nobiya, T., Ahun, M., Donna, R., Lengor, M., Zimmerman, D., Ladd, H., Hoekstra, E., Bello, A., Baffoe-Wilmot, A. and Amofah, G. (2005) Distributing insecticide-treated bednets during measles vaccination: a low-cost means of achieving high and equitable coverage. *Bulletin of the World Health Organization* 83, 195–201.

Gumi, B., Schelling, E., Berg, S., Firdessa, R., Erenso, G., Mekonnen, W., Hailu, E., Melese, E., Hussein, J., Aseffa, A. and Zinsstag, J. (2012) Zoonotic transmission of tuberculosis between pastoralists and their livestock in South-East Ethiopia. *EcoHealth* 9, 139–149.

Gwatkin, D.R. and Ergo, A. (2011) Universal health coverage: friend or foe of health equity? *Lancet* 377, 2160–2161.

Jaskiewicz, W. and Tulenko, K. (2012) Increasing community health worker productivity and effectiveness: a review of the influence of the work environment. *Human Resources for Health* 10, 38.

Johnston, C. (2013) Lessons from medical ethics. In: Wathes, C.M., Corr, S.A., May, S.A., McCulloch, S.P. and Whiting, M.C. (eds) *Veterinary & Animal Ethics*. Wiley-Blackwell, New Jersey.

Jost, C.C., Mariner, J.C., Roeder, P.L., Sawitri, E. and Macgregor-Skinner, G.J. (2007) Participatory epidemiology in disease surveillance and research. *Revue Scientifique et Technique OIE* 26, 537–549.

Kahn, L.H., Kaplan, B. and Steele, J.H. (2007) Confronting zoonoses through closer collaboration between medicine and veterinary medicine (as 'one medicine'). *Veterinaria Italiana* 43, 5–19.

Khogali, M., Zachariah, R., Reid, T., Alipon, S.C., Zimble, S., Mahama, G., Etienne, W., Veerman, R., Dahmane, A., Weyeyso, T., Hassan, A. and Harries, A. (2014) Self-administered treatment for tuberculosis among pastoralists in rural Ethiopia: how well does it work? *International Health* Epub ahead of print.

Kleinau, E., Randriamananjara, O. and Rosensweig, F. (2005) Healthy People in a Healthy Environment: Impact of an Integrated Population, Health, and Environment Program in Madagascar. Washington, DC/USAID: Environmental Health Project. Available at: http://www.ehproject.org/PDF/phe/madagascar-phe.pdf (accessed 10 October 2014).

Krönke, F. (2004) Zoonosen bei pastoralnomadischen FulBe im Tschad. *Zeitschrift für Ethnologie* 129.

Last, M. (1990) Professionalization of indigenous healers. In: Johnson, T.M. and Sargent, C.F. (eds) *Medical Anthropology: Contemporary Theory and Method.* Praeger, New York, pp. 349–366.

Maibach, E.W., Abroms, L.C. and Marosits, M. (2007) Communication and marketing as tools to cultivate the public's health: a proposed 'people and places' framework. *BMC Public Health* 7, 88.

Majok, A.A. and Schwabe, C.W. (1996) *Development Among Africa's Migratory Pastoralists*. Greenwood Publishing Group, Westport, Connecticut.

McCorkle, C.M. (1994) Intersectoral action and policy directions in traditional health systems for humans and animals. Paper presented to the International workshop on Traditional Health Systems and Public Policy. International Development Research Centre, Ottawa.

McCorkle, C. (1996) Intersectoral Healthcare Delivery. In: Chesworth, J. (ed.) *The Ecology of Health*. Sage Publications, Thousand Oaks, California, pp. 187–200.

Moritz, M., Ewing, D. and Garabed, R.B. (2013) On not knowing zoonotic diseases: pastoralists' ethnoveterinary knowledge in the far north region of Cameroon. *Human Organization* 72, 1–11.

Muller, B., Durr, S., Alonso, S., Hattendorf, J., Laisse, C.J., Parsons, S.D., van Helden, P.D. and Zinsstag, J. (2013) Zoonotic *Mycobacterium bovis*-induced tuberculosis in humans. *Emerging Infectious Diseases* 19, 899–908.

Myers, S.S., Gaffikin, L., Golden, C.D., Ostfeld, R.S., Redford, K.H., Ricketts, T.H., Turner, W.R. and Osofsky, S.A. (2013) Human health impacts of ecosystem alteration. *Proceedings of the National Academy of Sciences USA* 110, 18753–18760.

Ould Taleb, M. (2007) Santé, vulnérabilité et tuberculose en milieu nomade sahélien: étude des représentations sociales de la tuberculose chez les populations nomades de la Mauritanie et du Tchad. Thèse unique en sociologie, Université de Cocody, Abidjan, Côte d'Ivoire.

Partnerships for Health Reform (2000) Outil d'évaluation du financement des services de vaccinations. Abt Accociates Inc. Bethesda, Maryland. Available at: http://www.path.org/vaccineresources/files/Fin_Assess_Tool_Fr.pdf (accessed 10 October 2014).

Rabinowitz, P.M., Kock, R., Kachani, M., Kunkel, R., Thomas, J., Gilbert, J., Wallace, R., Blackmore, C., Wong, D., Karesh, W., Natterson, B., Dugas, R. and Rubin, C. (2013) Toward proof of concept of a one health approach to disease prediction and control. *Emerging Infectious Diseases* 19(12).

Randolph, T.F., Schelling, E., Grace, D., Nicholson, C.F., Leroy, J.L., Cole, D.C., Demment, M.W., Omore, A., Zinsstag, J. and Ruel, M. (2007) Invited review: Role of livestock in human nutrition and health for poverty reduction in developing countries. *Journal of Animal Science* 85, 2788–2800.

Ribaira, G.Y. and Rossi, E.E. (2007) Scaling Up Across Sectors: The Growth of the Population-Health–Environment Program JSI Best Practices in Scaling Up. John Snow, Inc., Boston. Available at: http://www.jsi.com/JSIInternet/Inc/Common/_download_pub.cfm?id=10164&lid=3 (accessed 10 October 2014).

Riviere-Cinnamond, A. (2005) Animal Health Policy and Practice: Scaling-up Community-based Animal Health Systems, Lessons from Human Health. PPLPI Working Paper No. 22. Available at: http://www.fao.org/ag/againfo/programmes/en/pplpi/docarc/wp22.pdf (accessed 10 October 2014).

Schelling, E. (2002) Human and animal health in nomadic pastoralist communities of Chad: zoonoses, morbidity and health services. University of Basel, Switzerland. Available at: http://edoc.unibas.ch/57 (accessed 10 October 2014).

Schelling, E. and Kimani, T. (2007) Human and animal health response capacity and costs: a rapid appraisal of the 2007 Rift Valley fever outbreak in Kenya. International Livestock Research Institute.

Schelling, E., Bechir, M., Ahmed, M.A., Wyss, K., Randolph, T.F. and Zinsstag, J. (2007a) Human and animal vaccination delivery to remote nomadic families, Chad. *Emerging Infectious Diseases* 13, 373–379.

Schelling, E., Grace, D., Willingham, A.L. and Randolph, T. (2007b) Research approaches for improved pro-poor control of zoonoses. *Food and Nutrition Bulletin* 28, S345–S356.

Schelling, E., Wyss, K., Diguimbaye, C., Bechir, M., Ould Taleb, M., Bonfoh, B., Tanner, M. and Zinsstag, J. (2008) Towards integrated and adapted health services for nomadic pastoralists and their animals: a North-South partnership. In: Hirsch Hadorn, G., Hoffmann-Riem, H., Biber-Klemm, S., Grossenbacher, W., Joye, D., Pohl, C., Wiesmann, U. and Zemp, E. (eds) *Handbook of Transdisciplinary Research*. Springer, Heidelberg, pp. 277–291.

Schelling, E., Weibel, D. and Bonfoh, B. (2009) Learning from the delivery of social services to pastoralists: Elements of good practice. IUCN World Initiative for Sustainable Pastoralism. Available at: http://www.iucn.org/wisp/resources/?4133 (accessed 10 October 2014).

Swift, J., Toulmin, C. and Chatting, S. (1990) UNICEF staff working papers number 8. UNICEF, New York.

Tanner, M., Lengeler, C. and Lorenz, N. (1993) From the efficacy of disease control tools to community effectiveness: case studies from the biomedical and health systems research activities of the Swiss Tropical Institute in Africa. *Transactions of the Royal Society of Tropical Medicine and Hygiene* 87, 518–523.

Tschopp, R., Hattendorf, J., Roth, F., Choudhoury, A., Shaw, A., Aseffa, A. and Zinsstag, J. (2013) Cost estimate of bovine tuberculosis to Ethiopia. *Current Topics in Microbiology and Immunology* 365, 249–268.
Tugwell, P., de, S.D., Hawker, G. and Robinson, V. (2006) Applying clinical epidemiological methods to health equity: the equity effectiveness loop. *British Medical Journal* 332, 358–361.
Victora, C.G., Huicho, L., Amaral, J.J., Armstrong-Schellenberg, J., Manzi, F., Mason, E. and Scherpbier, R. (2006) Are health interventions implemented where they are most needed? District uptake of the integrated management of childhood illness strategy in Brazil, Peru and the United Republic of Tanzania. *Bulletin of the World Health Organization* 84, 792–801.
Ward, D.E., Ruppaner, R., Marchot, P.J. and Hansen, J.W. (1993) One medicine - practical application for non-sedentary pastoral populations. *Nomadic Peoples* 32, 55–63.
Welch, V., Tugwell, P. and Morris, E.B. (2008) The equity-effectiveness loop as a tool for evaluating population health interventions. *Revista de salud publica (Bogota, Colombia)* 10(Suppl.), 83–96.
Whitehead, M., Dahlgren, G. and Evans, T. (2001) Equity and health sector reforms: can low-income countries escape the medical poverty trap? *Lancet* 358, 833–836.
WHO (2010) Increasing access to health workers in remote and rural areas through improved retention. Available at: http://www.ncbi.nlm.nih.gov/books/NBK138618/pdf/TOC.pdf (accessed 10 October 2014).
WHO (2013) Handbook on Health Inequality Monitoring - With a special focus on low- and middle-income countries. WHO, Geneva, Switzerland. Available at: http://www.who.int/gho/health_equity/handbook/en (accessed 10 October 2014).
WHO and UNICEF (2005) Global Immunization Vision and Strategy 2006–2015 WHO/IVB/05.05. Available at: http://www.who.int/immunization/givs/en (accessed 10 October 2014).
World Bank (2010) *People, Pathogens and Our Planet.*Vol. 1: Towards a One Health Approach for Controlling Zoonotic Diseases. Report No. 50833-GLB. The World Bank, Agriculture and Rural Development Health, Nutrition and Population, Washington, DC.
Wright, I.A., Tarawali, S., Blummel, M., Gerard, B., Teufel, N. and Herrero, M. (2012) Integrating crops and livestock in subtropical agricultural systems. *Journal of the Science of Food and Agriculture* 92, 1010–1015.
Wyss, K., Moto, D.M. and Callewaert, B. (2003) Constraints to scaling-up health related interventions: the case of Chad, Central Africa. *Journal of International Development* 15, 87–100.
Zezza, A., Winter, P., Banjamin, D., Carletto, G., Covarrubias, K., Quiñones, E., Stamoulis, K., Tasciotti, L. and Di Giuseppe, S. (2007) Rural Household Access to Assets and Agrarian Institutions: A Cross Country Comparison. Working Paper No. 07-17 Agricultural and Development Economics Division, FAO, Rome. Available at: http://www.fao.org/fileadmin/user_upload/riga/pdf/aj303e.pdf (accessed 10 October 2014).
Zinsstag, J. (2012) Convergence of EcoHealth and One Health. *EcoHealth* 9, 371–373.

# 21 Beyond Fences: Wildlife, Livestock and Land Use in Southern Africa

**David H.M. Cumming,[1]* Steven A. Osofsky,[2] Shirley J. Atkinson[2] and Mark W. Atkinson[2]**

[1]*Percy FitzPatrick Institute, University of Cape Town, South Africa and Tropical Resource Ecology Programme, University of Zimbabwe, Harare, Zimbabwe;* [2]*Wildlife Conservation Society, New York*

## Introduction

The formerly open rangelands and savannahs of the world are increasingly being enclosed by boundaries that demarcate smaller and smaller parcels of land. The resulting changes in the scales at which these landscapes are managed have impacts on both ecological and social processes, and ultimately on system health and human health and well-being. A One Health approach provides a novel conceptual framework within which to examine the issue of fragmentation in southern African rangelands.

Fences of one sort or another now dominate southern Africa's landscapes. Veterinary cordon fences, separating domestic livestock and large wild mammals, are a major feature in many parts of the region (Gadd, 2012). The rapid transition from vast open landscapes with few natural barriers to ones fragmented by roads, railways and multiple boundaries demarcated by fences is, in evolutionary terms, a very recent development. Wire fences first appeared in the region less than 140 years ago. In South Africa, fences demarcating farm boundaries became a legal requirement in 1912 (Salomon *et al.*, 2013); however, in the last two decades there have been moves to dismantle fences in order to re-establish wildlife migration routes in several larger conservation landscapes. Groups of farmers on private land have formed conservancies and removed intervening fences that once demarcated internal farm boundaries (e.g. Lindsey *et al.*, 2009). Southern Africa is now tentatively experimenting with a return to open rangelands in selected areas, the most prominent example being the development of transfrontier conservation areas (Osofsky *et al.*, 2005; Andersson *et al.*, 2013).

A move to more open rangelands will require developing a range of social, policy and legal instruments (i.e. institutions) to effectively manage large open landscapes. New methods and approaches will be needed to manage what are essentially common property regimes with varying forms of land tenure, property and resource access rights. Managing the transmission of infectious diseases at a potentially more open human–livestock–wildlife interface will also be a challenge. These issues arise whether it involves a few farmers joining properties to develop a conservancy, or a transfrontier conservation area (TFCA) that encompasses state, private and communal land.

*E-mail: cummingdhm@gmail.com

Managing diseases across international boundaries is also an important consideration in the development of transfrontier conservation areas.

This chapter outlines the context and explores the implications of these transitions from open to closed, and closed to open, landscapes in relation to human health and livelihoods, animal and ecosystem health, and disease management.

## Ecological and Historical Context

Southern Africa[1] is predominantly a semi-arid to arid region with some 60% of its 3.4 million km$^2$ receiving less than 600 mm of rainfall a year, with high spatial and temporal variability. The result is that extensive domestic animal production systems, rather than cultivation, predominate in more than half of southern Africa. Most of southern Africa's protected wildlife areas occur in the drier parts of the region.

The region carried a rich diversity of large mammals for millions of years, with localized areas carrying 20 or more species of ungulates, ranging in size from the diminutive dik-dik weighing about 5 kg to elephant bulls weighing as much as 5000 kg. This assemblage formed an important component of the livelihoods of autochthonous Khoi-San hunter-gatherers. Approximately 2000–2500 years ago, Bantu migrants from the north brought cattle, sheep and goats to southern Africa (e.g. Denbow and Wilmsen, 1986). Multispecies systems of ungulates, a mixture of wild and domestic herds, shaped the region's open rangelands for about 2000 years. However, substantial areas where tsetse flies, the vectors of trypanosomiasis, occurred were not accessible to domestic stock. The advent of European exploration, settlement and colonial occupation between 1600 and 1900 resulted in the introduction of alien human and animal diseases along with excessive exploitation of wildlife. Introduced human diseases included measles and smallpox, while introduced animal diseases included rinderpest, bovine tuberculosis and canine distemper. The rinderpest pandemic that swept through the region in the 1890s decimated herds of domestic livestock and the remaining, overhunted wildlife populations (Mack, 1970).

The switch from open multispecies systems to closed single-species animal production systems began with the establishment of colonial boundaries and land apportionment based on race. Land reserved for European settlers was divided into farms of varying sizes with freehold title. Reserves under traditional common property regimes were established for Bantu and Khoi-San people. Boundaries between these land tenure regimes shifted with time and changing political dispensations as elaborated, for example, by Murphree and Cumming (1993) for Zimbabwe. With the advent of private ownership of farms, and the subdivision of what were formerly open common-property grazing lands, came the erection of fences to establish farm boundaries and paddocks within farms to control predators. Subdividing and fragmenting formerly open rangelands to manage domestic species (cattle, sheep and goats) inevitably altered ecological processes and plant–herbivore interactions, resulting in long-term implications for biodiversity, ecosystem health and sustainability. Dean and Macdonald (1994) examined the long-term changes that occurred in semi-arid rangelands in the Cape Province of South Africa under livestock farming between 1911 and 1981. In many areas livestock carrying capacity declined by more than 50% during this period. Declines in rangeland productivity for livestock, often accompanied by severe bush encroachment and loss of grazing for cattle and sheep, have occurred elsewhere in the region (Scholes, 2009; Eldridge *et al.*, 2011). These changes represented losses of ecosystem services and system health in ecological, social and economic terms with inevitable impacts on human health and well-being in rural areas.

## Enclosed Landscapes, Fences and Disease Management

Following the rinderpest pandemic of the late 1800s, there was a slow recovery of wild and domestic ungulates. Game reserves began to be established for wildlife (Cumming, 2004) and livestock were imported into the region to boost the recovery of domestic animal populations. As recovery gained momentum, so did the incidence of animal diseases and their spread from wild to domestic animals and vice versa. The inevitable next step of using fences to separate wild and domestic ungulates soon followed (D'Amico Hales *et al.*, 2004). By the 1960s game-proof cordon fences to control the movements of wildlife and livestock in southern Africa spanned nearly the entire subcontinent from west to east (Fig. 21.1). Formerly open systems were closed and fragmented. Fences were used, in combination with game elimination, to control the spread of tsetse fly (*Glossina* sp.), the vector of trypanosomiasis of livestock and humans, and as a means of separating wildlife from livestock in order to control foot and mouth disease (FMD) and protect subsidized commercial beef export markets. The control measures used are examples of decisions that were made to protect a single sector, with consequences for alternative land uses and the environment, as the following examples from three countries in southern Africa illustrate.

## Large-scale game elimination and pesticide applications to control tsetse fly

The most prolific use of fences for the control of tsetse fly and trypanosomiasis, which causes nagana of domestic stock, occurred in Southern Rhodesia (now Zimbabwe). The rinderpest pandemic in the 1890s resulted in the decimation of large mammal populations on which tsetse fly feed. As a result, tsetse fly populations collapsed and only survived in a few isolated pockets in Zimbabwe (e.g. Jack, 1914). By the 1920s, however, tsetse began to spread into their former range and threaten cattle production in both commercial and traditional farming areas. Based on the drastic effect of rinderpest on the wild hosts of tsetse fly, the government introduced a programme of game elimination to contain the

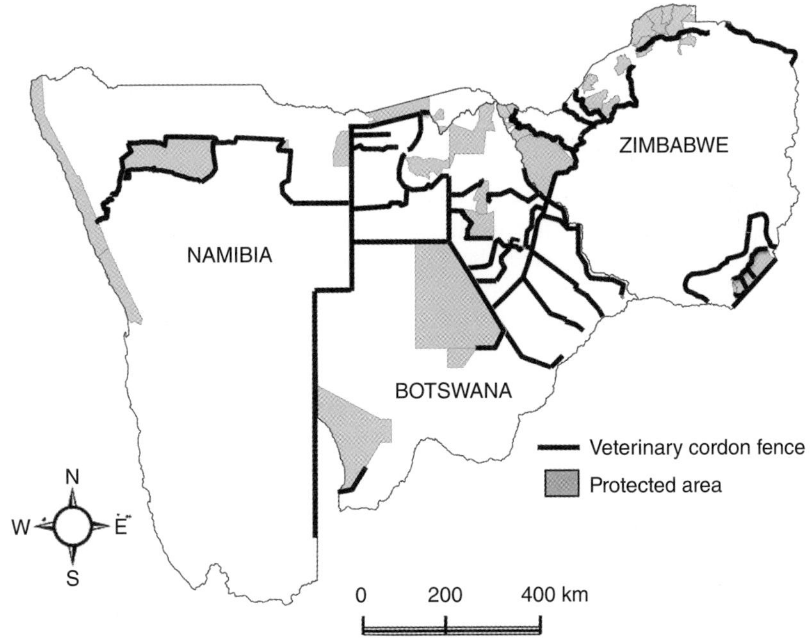


**Fig. 21.1.** Map of the major veterinary cordon fences used in southern Africa between 1950 and 2010. Some fences in Botswana have been decommissioned. Fences used in tsetse control operations in Zimbabwe have been removed and those used to control FMD have mostly fallen into disrepair (redrawn and modified from maps developed by R.B. Martin).

spread of the fly (Jack, 1923). Child and Riney (1987) provided an analysis of the numbers and species of animals killed on hunting operations between 1919 and 1961. A total of some 660,000 animals of 36 species were killed. Early hunting was directed at the full spectrum of large mammals, including black rhinoceros and elephant, in the designated areas. Tsetse control hunting and the use of game fences also occurred in Botswana[2] between 1942 and 1967 in the southern parts of the Okavango Delta to prevent tsetse fly spreading southwards to Maun (Child *et al.*, 1970).

Once techniques had been developed to identify the species on which recently engorged tsetse flies had fed (Weitz, 1963), hunting in Zimbabwe could be restricted to the six primary hosts of tsetse flies, namely warthog (*Phacochoerus africanus*), bushpig (*Potamochoerus porcus*), bushbuck (*Tragelaphus scriptus*), kudu (*Tragelaphus strepciceros*), buffalo (*Syncerus caffer*) and elephant (*Loxodonta africana*). A second phase of selective hunting to halt the spread of tsetse fly began in the 1960s. Fenced corridors, approximately 20 km wide, were established along the advancing fly front. The six primary host species of tsetse fly were eliminated from these corridors. The game elimination corridors, together with adjacent cattle-free buffer zones, served to separate tsetse-infested areas in the Zambezi and Limpopo valleys from livestock farming areas.

In the early 1970s tsetse control switched from elimination of their hosts to the selective application of DDT to resting sites of the fly (e.g. Pilson and Pilson, 1967; Robertson *et al.*, 1972), followed by aerial spraying of endosulfan, and the very successful use of odour-baited traps known as targets (Vale *et al.*, 1988). Despite site-selective application of DDT, the overall amounts used were high and the pesticide found its way into rivers and the food chain. High levels of DDT and its derivatives were recorded, for example, in the eggs and eggshells of fish eagles nesting on Lake Kariba, and in mothers' milk.

In terms of its objectives, the tsetse and trypanosomiasis control programme in Zimbabwe was very successful. More than 25,000 km$^2$ of land was reclaimed in order to protect commercial livestock production. Remote and sparsely populated areas of the country were opened for smallholder agriculture and livestock keeping and were rapidly settled by immigrants from elsewhere in the country (Cumming and Lynam, 1997). However, whether these agriculturally marginal areas can now sustain ecosystem health and human well-being, avoid desertification and cope with climate change remains to be seen.

## Subsidized beef markets and foot and mouth disease control

Botswana,[2] a semi-arid country of some 600,372 km$^2$, was mostly an open system almost devoid of fences, but since the building of the first veterinary cordon fences in 1954 and 1955, and the 300 km Kuke fence in 1958, the management of FMD in the country has been dominated by fences. The fences serve to control animal movements and so create and maintain FMD-free areas to meet the requirements of a subsidized beef export industry (Osofsky *et al.*, 2008; Gadd, 2012). Whilst successfully meeting the requirements of the beef industry, the fences contributed to the collapse of populations of wild ungulates by interfering with their seasonal movements and blocking access to water in dry years (Osofsky *et al.*, 2008; Gadd, 2012). For example, between 1978 and 2003, formerly abundant mobile populations of wildebeest and red hartebeest in the Kalahari system in western Botswana declined by an order of magnitude (Perkins, 2010). Wildebeest declined from 315,000 to 16,000 and hartebeest from 293,000 to 45,000 as a result of fragmentation of their range by game fences. Similar impacts occurred in the Makgadikgadi system as a result of cordon fencing (Perkins, 2010). Fencing around the western, southern and south-eastern edges of the Okavango Delta presently constrains seasonal dispersal of wild ungulates from the delta at the onset of the rainy season. The result is increased pressure on habitats within the delta that may be contributing to the decline of several antelope species (e.g. Mbaiwa and Mbaiwa, 2006; Hamandawana, 2012). However, without those fences inroads by cattle would likely exacerbate degradation.

The impacts of veterinary cordon fences on wildlife populations and their habitats have resulted in a foreclosing of options to diversify land uses involving wildlife and nature-based tourism. As Perkins (2010) has stated:

> The network of veterinary cordon fences in Botswana means that the protected areas have not maintained ecosystem integrity and functioning such that the Government is now locked into expensive and risky forms of manipulative wildlife management ... such as fencing and borehole provision. Ironically, the spectacular loss of wildlife in the Kalahari and Makgadikgadi ecosystems, precipitated by the requirements for disease control fencing by the EU beef subsidy, has in turn given rise to a number of often donor-assisted projects to seek ways to try and improve rural livelihoods and achieve sustainable development.

In other words, system health and human well-being have been compromised. Gadd (2012) provides a comprehensive assessment of the wide range of ecological impacts that have resulted from veterinary cordon fencing in southern Africa.

## Moving Beyond Fences to Open Systems?

The last two decades have seen a rise in nature-based tourism as an economic driver in land-use change, new potential approaches to disease control and ongoing shifts in subsidized beef export markets that have affected the financial returns from livestock. These changes, combined with increasing conservation concerns, have resulted in a reconsideration of the value of wildlife-based land use and the need to re-establish large, open landscapes. One result has been the creation of private conservancies by amalgamating properties, dismantling internal fences and jointly managing wildlife resources. Notable examples are the development of the Save Valley and Bubye Valley conservancies in south-eastern Zimbabwe, each of which covers more than 3000 $km^2$ (Lindsey *et al.*, 2009). New developments in conservation planning have provided a sound scientific basis for examining trade-offs between alternative land uses to meet conservation and other targets in larger landscapes (e.g. Margules and Pressey, 2000). Progress in conserving areas of exceptionally high biodiversity in the Eastern and Western Cape Provinces of South Africa provides good examples of the application of sound conservation planning to establish large conservation landscapes (e.g. Knight *et al.*, 2006; Rouget *et al.*, 2006). However, the most ambitious 'beyond fences' initiative in southern Africa is the development of transfrontier national parks and conservation areas.

## Developing Transfrontier Conservation Areas

A primary conservation reason for developing Transfrontier Conservation Areas (TFCAs) is to re-establish ecological processes such as large mammal migrations and historical dispersal routes across environmentally artificial national boundaries. Larger conservation areas are also able to conserve a greater number of plant and animal species and are likely to be more resilient to changing climates.

TFCAs include national parks, game reserves, hunting areas and conservancies, embedded within a matrix of land under traditional communal tenure (Osofsky *et al.*, 2008; Andersson *et al.*, 2013). As a result, TFCAs provide opportunities for biodiversity conservation and sustainable development (e.g. Cumming *et al.*, 2013a) and ten terrestrial TFCAs are presently being developed within southern Africa or along the Kunene–Zambezi Rivers (Fig. 21.2). Most of them face resource management issues associated with human well-being (Cumming *et al.*, 2013b), as well as disease problems at the interface between wild animals, domestic animals and people (Table 21.1).

The economic rationale for developing TFCAs is based on the realization that southern Africa's charismatic large mammal fauna provides a major local and international tourist attraction. Nature-based tourism is an area in which southern Africa has a high comparative advantage and it contributes as much, if not more, to gross domestic product (GDP) than the livestock industry (Cumming, unpublished data). With a livestock industry growing at about 2% per annum and a tourism industry growing at between 5 and 15%

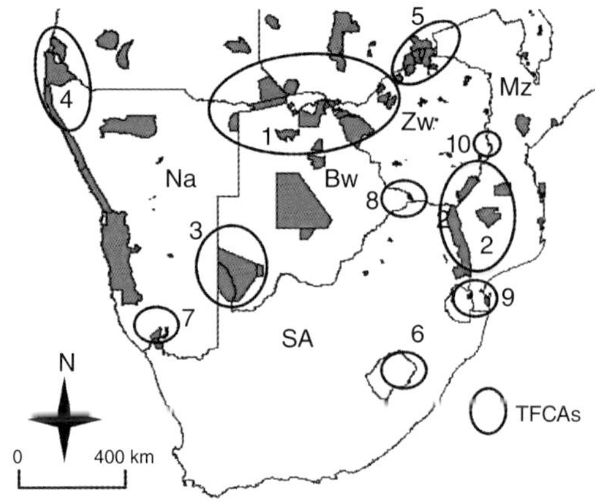


**Fig. 21.2.** Map of southern Africa showing the location of terrestrial transboundary conservation areas presently being developed. The names of the TFCAs, in order of declining size, are as follows: 1, Kavango Zambezi; 2, Great Limpopo; 3, Kgalagadi Transfrontier National Park; 4, Iona-Skeleton Coast; 5, Mana Pools-Lower Zambezi; 6, Drakensberg-Maloti; 7, Ai-Ais-Richtersveld; 8, Greater Mapungubwe; 9, Lebombo; 10, Chimanimani (see Table 21.1).

per annum, increasing interest is being shown in wildlife-based land use throughout the region.

## Open landscapes and the wildlife/ livestock interface

Given southern Africa's long history of investment in fences as a means of separating wild and domestic animals to control disease, it is not surprising that shifting from closed to open landscapes and removing fences is a major issue in implementing TFCAs. It was in this context that the Wildlife Conservation Society's AHEAD (Animal & Human Health for the Environment And Development) initiative convened a 2-day multi-disciplinary forum in partnership with IUCN at the World Parks Congress in Durban, South Africa, in September 2003. The full proceedings of the forum (Osofsky *et al.*, 2005) included abstracts, papers and outputs of working groups. The AHEAD programme recognized from its inception that developing an integrated One Health approach[3] (Osofsky *et al.*, 2008; Barrett and Osofsky, 2013) in practice is constrained by: (i) the challenges of obtaining funding support for broadly based exploratory and innovative research and development initiatives that might lead to science-based approaches to managing system health; (ii) markedly different policies and practices between countries; (iii) narrow disciplinary training of professionals and limited resources and outlets for interdisciplinary research and collaboration; (iv) competing single resource policies and decisions (e.g. between livestock production and wildlife conservation/tourism); and (v) severe constraints on transboundary research, including movement of researchers between countries.

## The AHEAD-GLTFCA Initiative

One of the working groups formed at the 2003 AHEAD launch meeting focused on interdisciplinary research and development issues associated with the interface between wildlife, livestock and human health and well-being in the Great Limpopo Transfrontier Conservation Area (GLTFCA). The GLTFCA straddles the Limpopo River and includes parts of Mozambique, South Africa and Zimbabwe. It covers an area of approximately 90,000 km$^2$ and includes, within its still ill-defined boundaries, national parks, game reserves, safari areas, private conservancies, commercial farms, communal lands occupied by small-scale farmers, and a biosphere reserve. The landscape is thus highly fragmented, resulting in an extensive interface between

**Table 21.1.** Important diseases of wildlife, domestic animals and humans and their distribution in the transfrontier conservation areas (TFCAs) being developed in southern Africa (revised from Cumming and Atkinson, 2012).

| | | Disease | | | | | | | | | | | | | | |
|---|---|---|---|---|---|---|---|---|---|---|---|---|---|---|---|---|
| | | Foot and mouth disease | Bovine tuberculosis | Brucellosis | Canine distemper virus | Contagious bovine pleuropneumonia | African trypanosomiasis[a] | Malignant catarrhal fever | Anthrax | Rabies | Rift Valley fever | African Swine fever | African horse sickness | Theileriosis | Heartwater | Echinococcosis and cysticercosis |
| TFCA | Area km$^2$ | WD | WDH | WDH | WD | D | WDH | WD | WDH | WDH | WDH | WD | WD | WD | WD | WDH |
| 1. Kavango Zambezi | 444,000 | + | + | + | + | ? | + | + | + | + | + | + | + | + | + | + |
| 2. Great Limpopo | 87,000 | + | + | + | + | – | + | + | + | + | + | + | + | + | + | + |
| 3. Kgalagadi TFP | 37,256 | ? | – | + | + | – | – | + | + | – | + | + | + | – | – | + |
| 4. Iona-Skeleton Coast | 32,000 | + | – | – | – | – | – | – | + | – | + | ? | ? | – | – | ? |
| 5. Lower Zambezi-Mana Pools | 25,000 | + | – | + | + | – | + | – | + | – | ? | + | ? | + | + | + |
| 6. Drakensberg-Maloti | 13,000 | – | – | + | – | – | – | – | + | + | ? | ? | ? | – | – | ? |
| 7. Ai-Ais-Richtersveld | 6,681 | ? | – | – | – | – | – | – | + | – | ? | – | ? | – | – | + |
| 8. Greater Mapungubwe | 4,872 | + | – | + | + | – | – | + | + | + | + | + | + | + | + | + |
| 9. Lubombo | 4,195 | + | + | + | – | – | – | + | + | + | ? | ? | + | + | + | + |
| 10. Chimanimani | 2,056 | + | ? | ? | ? | – | – | – | ? | + | ? | + | ? | + | + | ? |

[a]In southern Africa two *Trypanosoma* subspecies are involved, one of which causes nagana of domestic stock and the other causes human sleeping sickness

W, may infect wildlife; D, may infect domestic animals; H, may infect humans; +, reported from one or more countries involved in the TFCA and likely to be present in the TFCA; –, not reported from the countries involved in the TFCA and unlikely to be present; ?, status uncertain.

people, livestock and wildlife (Cumming *et al.*, 2007; Andersson and Cumming, 2013). Several contagious and vector-borne diseases, both introduced and indigenous (Table 21.1), are present. The northward spread of bovine tuberculosis through Kruger National Park across the Limpopo River and into Gonarezhou National Park in Zimbabwe is of particular concern because of its potential spread to livestock and people in areas where HIV-AIDS is prevalent (Caron *et al.*, 2003; Osofsky *et al.*, 2008; De Garine-Wichatitsky *et al.*, 2010).

Internal and external constraints to change in the status of health (human, animal and environmental) in the GLTFCA exist. The main internal constraints identified include: (i) the complex patterns of land tenure and land use, with overlapping jurisdictions governing both resources and human and animal health; (ii) the high ethnic diversity, historical displacements and population growth; (iii) little consultation with people at local levels; (iv) a lack of baseline information against which to measure progress; and (v) no generally agreed development objectives that are shared across spatial scales and institutional levels by governments, districts, villages, and/or households.

## The AHEAD Kavango Zambezi TFCA Initiative

The importance of the Kavango Zambezi (KAZA) TFCA to the region was reaffirmed in August 2011 when the presidents of Angola, Botswana, Namibia, Zambia and Zimbabwe signed a binding Implementation Treaty formally and legally establishing a transboundary area spanning over 444,000 km$^2$. The KAZA TFCA, located in the Okavango and Zambezi river basins includes, for example, the Caprivi Strip, Chobe National Park, the Okavango Delta (the largest Ramsar site in the world) and the Victoria Falls World Heritage Site. KAZA is also home to many of the world's most charismatic mega-vertebrates, including the largest contiguous population of elephants (approximately 250,000) on the continent. A key economic driver behind TFCAs like KAZA is nature-based tourism, a sector in which southern Africa enjoys a global comparative advantage, as noted.

The WCS-AHEAD programme extended its activities to the KAZA TFCA in 2010. The programme has been focused on facilitating interdisciplinary communication and policy reform relating to transboundary animal diseases within SADC and across agencies responsible for developing the TFCA. Key developments have been the recognition by the SADC Livestock Technical Committee of the potential importance of multispecies systems in relation to the development of TFCAs, and promulgation of the:

> Resolution by the Southern African Development Community (SADC) Calling for Adoption of Commodity-Based Trade and Other Non-Geographic Approaches for Foot and Mouth Disease Management as Additional Regional Standards for Trade in Animal Products

which includes 'The Phakalane Declaration on Adoption of Non-Geographic Approaches for Management of Foot and Mouth Disease' (http://www.wcs-ahead.org/phakalane_declaration.html).

The final section of the three-page declaration is as follows:

> Now, therefore, be it resolved that the Southern African Development Community hereby:
>
> *Recommends* the adoption of commodity-based trade and other non-geographic approaches such as compartmentalization for foot and mouth disease control as additional regional standards for the livestock and wildlife sectors, where applicable;
>
> *Recommends* to Member States that they utilize commodity-based trade and other non-geographic approaches as needed to bolster trade, first and foremost, within the region itself, and with other African partners;
>
> *Recommends* that Member States identify and address their needs to implement non-geographic approaches in terms of institutional, infrastructural, and human capacity;
>
> *Recommends* that SADC work together with the OIE, FAO and other international organizations to formalize the implementation guidance needed for certification, auditing

and thus wider international acceptance of appropriately prepared livestock-derived commodities by potential importing countries within the SADC region and around the world. This needs to be done in partnership with the private sector and with national veterinary services, the latter having both official responsibility and expertise critical for safe and successful deployment of any animal disease control strategies;

*Recommends* that SADC Member States and their appropriate government agencies responsible for livestock agriculture, veterinary services, and wildlife conservation and production work together and in partnership with the private sector and civil society organizations to promulgate context-appropriate approaches to transboundary animal disease management and wildlife utilization policies that mitigate conflicts at the wildlife/livestock interface.

*Recommends* that Member States seize upon the socioeconomic as well as conservation opportunities offered by SADC's collective vision for transfrontier conservation areas as facilitated by strategic alignment and realignment of selected veterinary cordon fences, while simultaneously expanding access to regional and international markets for animals and animal-derived products via adoption of the above-described enlightened and practical disease control policies and practices.

The WCS-AHEAD programme, in conjunction with WWF, has also supported a study of land-use options in relation to FMD control in Namibia's Caprivi. The Caprivi Region of Namibia (recently renamed the Zambezi Region) lies at the heart of the 440,000+ km$^2$ KAZA TFCA and an experiment in producing exportable meat from within an FMD-infected zone is underway. The pilot effort tests the potential to release the TFCA from the need for geographically defined FMD-free zones based on veterinary cordon fences. Eastern Caprivi includes national parks, forest reserves and communal agro-pastoral small-scale farming areas, together with several communal land conservancies. Fences within the Caprivi Strip are largely absent and livestock and wildlife share the available range. The Caprivi shares boundaries with Angola, Botswana and Zambia. Game fences occur along parts of the Botswana border. In the past, livestock owners were able to market their livestock through an abattoir in Katimo Mulimo that exported beef to South Africa. More recently, frequent outbreaks of FMD in the area have severely curtailed exports and alternative 'non-geographic' options for disease control to allow beef exports are being explored (Penrith and Thomson, 2012; Barnes, 2013; Cassidy *et al.*, 2013). The studies by Barnes (2013) and Cassidy *et al.* (2013) explored various scenarios for wildlife, livestock and disease (FMD) management in the eastern Caprivi, namely: (i) community wildlife conservancies and the status quo in terms of geographical separation of cattle and wildlife; (ii) application of value-chain disease-risk management and commodity-based trade[4] in line with World Organisation for Animal Health (OIE) guidance allowing the export of appropriately processed de-boned beef; (iii) development of community wildlife conservancies as for scenarios (i) and (ii) but with the addition of cooking meat as part of processing; and (iv) the introduction of fenced FMD-free compartments within the Caprivi. The results of a thorough economic analysis of the four options indicated that commodity-based trade was the most efficient at both national and local levels (Fig. 21.3) and offers the greatest potential to optimize economic and environmental trade-offs, maximize economic returns and effectively integrate livestock- and wildlife-based enterprises.

As Barnes (2013) concluded:

> initiatives aimed at introduction of CBT [commodity-based trade] as part of a value chain approach to sanitary risk management offers significant economic potential. At the same time, this approach can assist in meeting other TFCA objectives such as maintenance of diverse ecosystems with greater biodiversity across large, connected landscapes – reducing risk to natural systems and providing greater resilience in the face of, for example, natural catastrophes, disease outbreaks and climatic challenges.

Cassidy *et al.* (2013), using a comprehensive multi-criteria decision analysis (MCDA) framework, examined an essentially similar set of development options and scenarios for the Caprivi. Their analysis, using 18 criteria, was

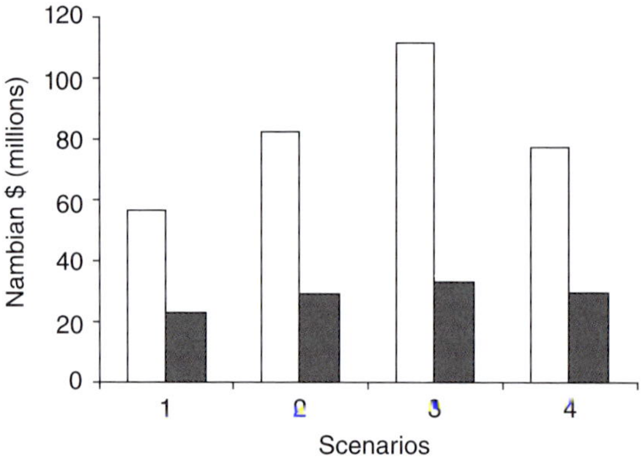


**Fig. 21.3.** Annual contributions to net national income (open columns) and to private incomes (filled columns) for four policy option scenarios (Namibian dollars, 2012). Scenarios: 1, status quo; 2, commodity-based trade of deboned steak; 3, commodity-based trade of deboned steak and cooked meat; 4, fenced foot and mouth disease-free areas (data from Barnes, 2013).

able to include an additional range of social and environmental factors. They reached similar conclusions to the analysis by Barnes (2013). Overall, the analysis yielded positive net flows for scenarios based on commodity-based trade (scenarios 2 and 3) and negative net flows for the status quo and fenced FMD-free compartments (scenarios 1 and 4).

## Open Landscapes, Health and Multispecies Systems

The nascent moves in southern Africa towards a return to open landscapes raise several ecological, social and economic questions. In the context of One Health, a key question is whether open landscapes and multispecies systems in arid and semi-arid rangelands are likely to result in improved livelihoods and healthier people, healthier wild and domestic animals and healthier ecosystems. An equally important question is: how feasible is it to establish multispecies systems given present land tenure and land-use systems? Clearly, areas with high and reliable rainfall and rich soils that can sustainably support intensive agriculture will be excluded from consideration. It is within the drier savannahs and arid rangelands that cover some 60% of southern Africa (and include most of the region's TFCAs) that the development of open systems may be most appropriate.

The ecological basis for maintaining open, multispecies systems in African savannahs is well established. African savannahs support a higher diversity of ungulate species than any other biome or continent. This diversity is functionally linked to the characteristically high spatial heterogeneity and plant species diversity of African savannah ecosystems (du Toit and Cumming, 1999). In turn, the range in body size and feeding strategies within intact ungulate communities (usually 20 or more species) has strong feedbacks on rangeland structure and function. Replacing this tightly coupled system, which evolved over millions of years, with one or two species of livestock at high densities has been responsible for the loss of plant species diversity and rangeland degradation over extensive areas (e.g. Dean and Macdonald, 1994; Milton *et al.*, 1994). Associated with reduced diversity and heterogeneity is declining resilience in the face of highly variable spatial and temporal patterns of rainfall, frequent droughts, and increasing aridity as a result of climate change.

Many wild ungulates move seasonally to take advantage of widely distributed key resources. Seasonal variability in access to water is a key driver of movement, resulting in dry-season concentrations at water points but with dispersal during the wet season. Spatial and seasonal changes in the availability of food and key nutrients, such as phosphorus required by pregnant and lactating animals, may also drive migrations such as those of the wildebeest in the Serengeti. Access to spatially dispersed key nutrients, such as sodium, calcium and phosphorus, may play an important role in the seasonal movement and migration of ungulates (Murray, 1995). Migratory species tend to occur in numbers that are an order of magnitude greater than sedentary species (Fryxell *et al.*, 1988) as a result of their ability to take advantage of key resources, move to fresh pastures, and escape predators that are not able to follow them.

In southern Africa both wild and domestic animal seasonal dispersal patterns and migrations have been greatly curtailed by fences and changes in land use. However, it is possible for migrations to be re-established, as the recent removal of cordon fences separating the Makgadikgadi and Chobe components of the KAZA TFCA in Botswana has shown (Bartlam-Brooks *et al.*, 2011). Zebra have re-established an annual migration that preceded the living memory of the current zebra population, involving a round trip of approximately 500 km between the Nxai Pan and Chobe National Parks. Some consideration is now being given to the potential advantages of re-establishing herding in the management of livestock on communal rangeland in South Africa (Salomon *et al.*, 2013) and northern Namibia (Namibian Economist, 2011). The ecological, socio-economic and system health ramifications of restoring animal migrations and seasonal movements over larger landscapes have still to be more fully researched – as does the question of where in the region they may be re-established to best advantage.

The social and cultural features relating to multispecies systems have not, to our knowledge, been specifically investigated. On private land in southern Africa landowners control the management of livestock and wildlife within the constraints of national policy and legislation. On communal land stockowners manage their herds but the legal use of wildlife is generally controlled by the state. However, in this case, both grazing and wildlife are common property resources. As such both resources may be subject to the 'tragedy of the commons' (Hardin, 1968) or instead be managed under adaptive co-management regimes that sustain resources and achieve an equitable distribution of benefits through community-based natural resource management programmes (Suich *et al.*, 2009). Few, if any, of these programmes cover large landscapes. In addition, appropriate institutions to manage multispecies systems in landscapes covering a diversity of tenure (and national) systems, such as occur in TFCAs, are yet to emerge.

The financial and economic viability of wildlife-based land use on private ranches in southern Africa is well established and is evidenced by the rapid increase in game ranching in the region over the last 50 years (e.g. Jansen *et al.*, 1992; Van Schalkwyk *et al.*, 2010). Community-based natural resource management focused on benefits from wildlife-based tourism has experienced varying levels of success (Cumming *et al.*, 2013a). Arguably the most successful programme has been in Namibia, where 71 community wildlife conservancies (that include wild and domestic ungulates) have been registered. Wildlife populations and associated returns to both local and national economies from conservancies have shown continuing growth over a period of 15 years (e.g. Suich *et al.*, 2009; Van Schalkwyk *et al.*, 2010). However, in Namibia and elsewhere in the region, many key issues related to resource management and equitable distribution of returns from common property resources to individuals and households remain to be resolved. Cumming *et al.* (2013b) review many of the constraints and issues being faced in realizing both conservation and improved livelihoods for rural people in the development of TFCAs in southern Africa (see also Suich *et al.*, 2009 and Torquebiau and Taylor, 2009). Despite the difficulties facing the development and extension of wildlife and multispecies systems as recognized, productive forms of land use in the region, their economic contribution is significant.

Zoonotic and non-zoonotic diseases and their influence on health in southern African rangelands, in the sense of improved human, animal and ecosystem health, is a central issue in moving beyond fences and towards open landscapes in TFCAs and elsewhere (Osofsky *et al.*, 2005, 2008). The interactions between disease management at the human–animal interface and the livelihoods of rural people are complex (Fig. 21.4). They are greatly influenced by cross-scale dynamics of export markets, global pricing structures and subsidies for commodities such as beef, and by global economic trends that affect the ability of tourists to visit wildlife areas.

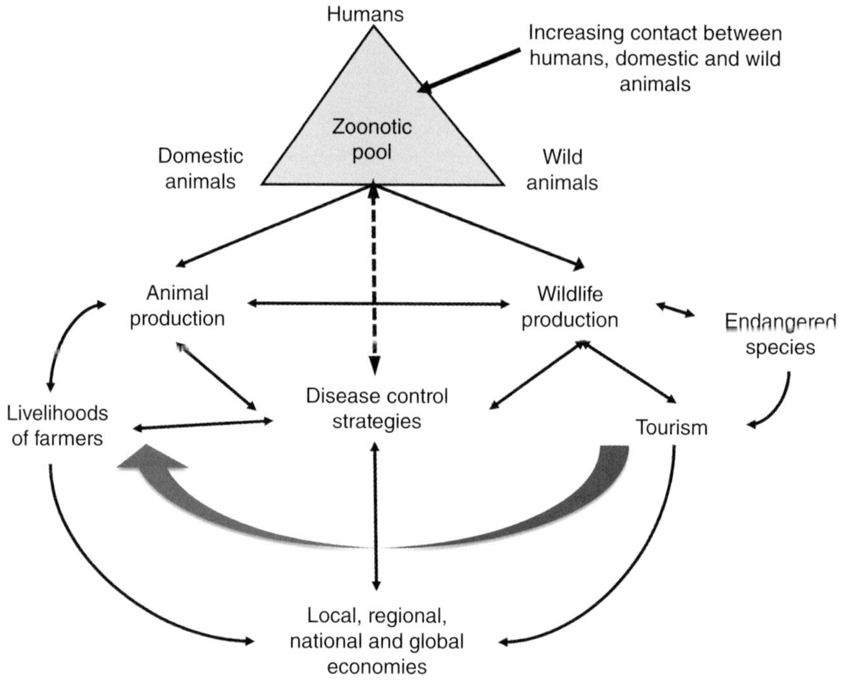


**Fig. 21.4.** Diagram showing the linkages between wild and domestic animals and humans and the central role of disease management strategies in influencing land use, livelihoods and economies at different scales (modified after Cumming *et al.*, 2007).

## Concluding Comment

Perhaps the greatest contribution that a One Health approach has brought to the debate about land use, fences and disease management in southern Africa is the importance of interdisciplinary and cross-sectoral approaches to resolving critical issues of development, system health and sustainability. In part, key debate and dialogue has been fostered by the AHEAD initiative in its involvement in the Great Limpopo and Kavango Zambezi TFCAs and is reflected in the following key questions that need to be addressed at the scale of large landscapes (revised from Cumming *et al.*, 2007).

**1.** What types and patterns of land tenure will enhance system health, productivity and resilience (sustainability) of the social-ecological system (SES) of the landscape or TFCA in question?
**2.** What is the state and trend of the five capitals (natural, human, social, financial and physical) in each land-use/land tenure component of the landscape/TFCA and how might these change and influence system health under differing development scenarios?
**3.** How will the biodiversity, environmental, social and economic trade-offs and opportunity costs of alternative patterns of land use influence adaptability and resilience of the SES?
**4.** What cross-subsidies exist within the system and how vulnerable are they to disturbance or shocks?
**5.** What are the levels of external subsidy to the landscape/TFCA system and how dependent is the system on, or vulnerable to, external subsidies?
**6.** How do external subsidies support or hinder the development of self-organization, adaptability, transformability and resilience of the SES?

There is little doubt that large, open landscapes that simulate or restore the functional integrity of southern Africa's rangelands are greatly undervalued. A recent comprehensive study of land use in the UK, in which the full value of ecosystem services was included, revealed the bias (and thus weakness) that is inherent in valuing rural land only in terms of its agricultural value (Bateman *et al.*, 2013).

While southern Africa does not have at its disposal the depth of detailed information that is available in the UK, the region would do well to move towards a much more in-depth analysis of the value of alternative (and potentially complementary) land-use options.

## Notes

[1] In the context of this chapter southern Africa refers to the area south of the Kunene–Zambezi rivers and includes Botswana, Lesotho, part of Mozambique, Namibia, South Africa, Swaziland and Zimbabwe.
[2] Formerly Bechuanaland, a British Protectorate until independence in 1966.
[3] The collaborative effort of multiple disciplines – working locally, nationally and globally – to attain optimal health for people, animals and the environment (AVMA, 2008).
[4] While there is no single accepted definition of commodity-based trade (CBT), it is considered to represent an array of alternatives that can be used to ensure that the production and processing of a particular commodity or product are managed so that identified food safety and animal health hazards are reduced to appropriate risk levels. OIE Terrestrial Animal Health Code guidelines now recognize a disease management scenario under which commodity-based trade, a non-geographic approach to disease management, could be effectively implemented.
[5] In this context 'health' refers to animal, human and ecosystem health – the One Health concept.

## References

American Veterinary Medical Association (AVMA) (2008) One Health: a new professional imperative. One Health Initiative Task Force final report, AVMA, Washington, DC.

Andersson, J.A. and Cumming, D.H.M. (2013) Defining the edge: boundary formation and TFCAs in southern Africa. In: Anderson J.A., de Garine-Wichatitsky, M., Cumming, D.H.M., Dzingirai, V. and Giller, K.E. (eds) *Transfrontier Conservation Areas: People Living on the Edge*. Routledge, London, pp. 25–61.

Andersson, J.A., de Garine-Wichatitsky, M., Cumming, D.H.M., Dzingirai, V. and Giller, K.E. (eds) (2013) *Transfrontier Conservation Areas: People Living on the Edge*. Routledge, London.

Barnes, J.I. (2013) Economic analysis of land use policies for livestock, wildlife and disease management in Caprivi, Namibia, with potential wider implications for regional transfrontier conservation areas. Technical Report to the Wildlife Conservation Society's AHEAD Program and the World Wildlife Fund. Available at: http://www.wcs-ahead.org/kaza/kaza_additional_resources.html (accessed 20 August 2013).

Barrett, M.A. and Osofsky, S.A. (2013) One Health: interdependence of people, other species, and the planet. In: Katz, D.L., Elmore, J.G., Wild, D.M.G. and Lucan, S.C. (eds) *Jekel's Epidemiology, Biostatistics, Preventive Medicine, and Public Health*, 4th edn. Elsevier/Saunders, Philadelphia, pp. 364–377 (and online supplement pp. 407(e1)–416(e10) at studentconsult.com).

Bartlam-Brooks, H.L.A., Bonyongo, M.C. and Harris, S. (2011) Will reconnecting ecosystems allow long-distance mammal migrations to resume? A case study of a zebra *Equus burchelli* migration in Botswana. *Oryx* 45, 210–216.

Bateman, I.J., Harwood, A.R., Mace, G.M., Watson, R.T., Abson, D.J., Andrews, B., Binner, A., Crowe, A., Day, B.H., Dugdale, S., Fezzi, C., Foden, J., Hadley, D., Haines-Young, R., Hulme, M., Kontoleon, A., Lovett, A.A., Munday, P., Pascual, U., Paterson, J., Perino, G., Sen, A., Siriwardena, G., van Soest, D. and Termansen, M. (2013) Bringing ecosystem services into decision-making: land use in the United Kingdom. *Science* 341, 45–50.

Caron, A., Cross, P.C. and du Toit, J.T. (2003) Ecological implications of bovine tuberculosis in African buffalo herds. *Ecological Applications* 13, 1338–1345.

Cassidy, D., Thomson, G. and Barnes, J. (2013) Establishing priorities through the use of multi-criteria decision analysis for a commodity based trade approach to beef exports from the East Caprivi Region of Namibia. Technical Report to the United States Agency for International Development (USAID)/Southern Africa Sanitary and Phytosanitary Support (SPS) Program for Regional Trade in Southern Africa. Available at: http://www.wcs-ahead.org/kaza/kaza_additional_resources.html (accessed 20 August 2013).

Child, G.F.T. and Riney, T. (1987) Tsetse control hunting in Zimbabwe, 1919–1958. *Zambezia* XIV, 11–71.

Child, G., Smith, P. and von Richter, W. (1970) Tsetse control hunting as a measure of large mammal population trends in the Okavango Delta, Botswana. *Mammalia* 34, 34–75.

Cumming, D.H.M. (2004) Performance of parks in a century of change. In: Child, B. (ed.) *Parks in Transition: Biodiversity, Development and the Bottom Line*. Earthscan, London, pp. 105–124.

Cumming, D.H.M. and Atkinson, M.W. (2012) Land-use paradigms, wildlife and livestock: Southern African challenges, choices and potential ways forward. In: Karesh, W. (ed.) *Animal Health and Biodiversity – Preparing for the Future*, Compendium of the OIE Global Conference on Wildlife, 23–25 February 2011, Paris. OIE (World Organisation for Animal Health), Paris, France, pp. 101–112.

Cumming, D.H.M. and Lynam, T.J.P. (1997) Land use changes, wildlife conservation and utilisation, and the sustainability of agro-ecosystems in the Zambezi Valley: final technical report. European Union Contract B7-5040/93/06. WWF Programme Office, Harare.

Cumming, D., Biggs, H., Kock, M., Shongwe, N. and Osofsky, S. (2007) The AHEAD (Animal Health for the Environment And Development) - Great Limpopo Transfrontier Conservation Area (GLTFCA) Programme: key questions and conceptual framework revisited. Available at: http://wcs-ahead.org/workinggrps_limpopo.html (accessed 15 August 2013).

Cumming, D.H.M., Dzingirai, V. and de Garine-Wichatitsky, M. (2013a) Land and natural resource-based livelihood opportunities in TFCAs. In: Andersson, J., de Garine-Wichatitsky, M., Cumming D.H.M., Dzingirai, V. and Giller, K. (eds) *Transfrontier Conservation Areas: People Living on the Edge*. Routledge, London, pp. 163–191.

Cumming, D.H.M., Andersson, J., de Garine-Wichatitsky, M., Dzingirai, V. and Giller, K. (2013b) Whither TFCAs and people on the edge in southern Africa? In: Andersson, J., de Garine-Wichatitsky, M., Cumming, D.H.M., Dzingirai, V. and Giller, K. (eds) *Transfrontier Conservation Areas: People Living on the Edge*. Routledge, London, pp. 192–203.

D'Amico Hales, J., Osofsky, S.A. and Cumming, D.H.M. (2004) Wildlife health in Africa: implications for conservation in the decades ahead. In: Burgess, N., D'Amico Hales, J., Underwood, E., Dinerstein, E., Olson, D., Itoua, I., Schipper, J., Ricketts, T. and Newman, K. (eds) *The Terrestrial Ecoregions of Africa and Madagascar: A Conservation Assessment*. Island Press, Washington, DC, pp. 129–130.

Dean, W.R.J. and Macdonald, I.A.W. (1994) Historical changes in stocking rates of domestic livestock as a measure of semi-arid and arid rangeland degradation in the Cape Province, South Africa. *Journal of Arid Environments* 26, 281–298.

De Garine-Wichatitsky, M., Caron, A., Gomo, C., Foggin, C., Dutlow, K., Pfukenyi, D., Lane, E., Le Bel, S., Hlokwe, T. and Michel, A. (2010) Bovine tuberculosis in buffaloes, southern Africa. *Emerging Infectious Diseases* 16, 884–885.

Denbow, J.R. and Wilmsen, E.N. (1986) Advent and course of pastoralism in the Kalahari. *Science* 234, 1509–1510.

du Toit, J.T. and Cumming, D.H.M. (1999) Functional significance of ungulate diversity in African savannas and the ecological implications of the spread of pastoralism. *Biodiversity and Conservation* 8, 1643–1661.

Eldridge, D.J., Bowker, M.A., Maestre, F.T., Roger, E., Reynolds, J.F. and Whitford, W.G. (2011) Impacts of shrub encroachment on ecosystem structure and functioning: towards a global synthesis. *Ecology Letters* 14, 709–722.

Fryxell, J.M., Greever, J. and Sinclair, A.R.E. (1988) Why are migratory ungulates so abundant? *American Naturalist* 131, 781–798.

Gadd, M.E. (2012) Barriers, the beef industry and unnatural selection: a review of the impacts of veterinary fencing on mammals in southern Africa. In: Somers, M. and Hayward, M. (eds) *Fencing for Conservation: Restriction of Evolutionary Potential or a Riposte to Threatening Processes?* Springer, New York, pp. 153–186.

Hamandawana, H. (2012) The impacts of herbivory on vegetation in Moremi Game Reserve, Botswana: 1967–2001. *Regional Environmental Change* 12, 1–15.

Hardin, G. (1968) The tragedy of the commons. *Science* 162, 1243–1248.

Jack, R.W. (1914) Tsetse fly and big game in Southern Rhodesia. *Bulletin of Entomological Research* 5, 97–110.

Jack, R.W. (1923) Tsetse fly: a four-year experiment in game elimination. *Rhodesia Agriculture Journal*, Bulletin, No. 460.

Jansen, D.J., Child, B. and Bond, I. (1992) Cattle, wildlife, both or neither: results of a financial and economic survey of commercial cattle ranches in southern Zimbabwe. WWF Multispecies Animal Production Systems Project, *Project Paper Number 27*. World Wildlife Fund, Harare, Zimbabwe.

Knight, A.T., Driver, A., Cowling, R.M., Maze, K., Desmet, P.G., Lombard, A.T., Rouget, M., Botha, M.A., Boshoff, A.F., Castley, J.G., Goodman, P.S., Mackinnon, K., Pierce, S.M., Sims-Castley, R., Stewart, W.I. and Von Hase, A. (2006) Designing systematic conservation assessments that promote effective implementation: best practice from South Africa. *Conservation Biology* 20, 739–750.

Lindsey, P., du Toit, R., Pole, A. and Romañach, S. (2009) Savé Valley Conservancy: a large-scale African experiment in cooperative wildlife management. In: Suich, H., Child, B. and Spenceley, A. (eds) *Evolution and Innovation in Wildlife Conservation: Parks and Game Ranches to Transfrontier Conservation Areas*. Earthscan, London, pp. 163–184.

Mack, R. (1970) The great African cattle plague epidemic of the 1890's. *Tropical Animal Health and Production* 2, 210–219.

Margules, C.R. and Pressey, R.L. (2000) Systematic conservation planning. *Nature* 405, 243–253.

Mbaiwa, J.E. and Mbaiwa, O.I. (2006) The effects of veterinary fences on wildlife populations in Okavango Delta, Botswana. *International Journal of Wilderness* 12, 17–23.

Milton, S.J., Dean, W.R.J., du Plessis, M.A. and Siegfried, W.R. (1994) A conceptual model of rangeland degradation: the escalating cost of declining productivity. *Bioscience* 44, 70–76.

Murphree, M.W. and Cumming, D.H.M. (1993) Savanna land use: policy and practice in Zimbabwe. In: Young, M.D. and Solbrig, O.T. (eds) *The World's Savannas: Economic Driving Forces, Ecological Constraints and Policy Options for Sustainable Land Use*. Man and the Biosphere Series Vol. 12. UNESCO and Parthenon Publishing Group, Paris, pp. 139–178.

Murray, M.G. (1995) Specific nutrient requirements and migration of wildebeest. In: Sinclair, A.R.E. and Arcese, P. (eds) *Serengeti II: Dynamics, Management, and Conservation of an Ecosystem*. University of Chicago Press, Chicago, Illinois, pp. 231–256.

Namibian Economist (2011) Teaching Africans how to tend cattle. Available at: http://www.economist.com.na/2011-12-07-11-05-31/agriculture/2967-teaching-africans-how-to-tend-cattle (accessed 10 August 2013).

Osofsky, S.A., Cleaveland, S., Karesh, W.B., Kock, M.D., Nyhus, P.J., Starr, L. and Yang, A. (eds) (2005) *Conservation and Development Interventions at the Wildlife/Livestock Interface: Implications for Wildlife, Livestock and Human Health*. IUCN, Gland, Switzerland and Cambridge, UK. Available at: http://www.wcs-ahead.org/wpc_launch.html (accessed 15 December 2014).

Osofsky, S.A., Cumming, D.H.M. and Kock, M.D. (2008) Transboundary management of natural resources and the importance of a 'One Health' approach: perspectives on southern Africa. In: Fern, E. and Redford, K.H. (eds) *State of the Wild 2008–2009: A Global Portrait of Wildlife, Wildlands, and Oceans*. Island Press, Washington, DC, pp. 89–98. Available at: http://www.wcs-ahead.org/documents/transbound_sotw.pdf (accessed 15 December 2014).

Penrith, M.-L. and Thomson, G.R. (2012) Analysis of the status of transboundary animal diseases and their control in the SADC region during the period 2005–2011, focusing on the five countries that contribute land to the Kavango Zambezi (KAZA) Transfrontier Conservation Area (TFCA). Technical Report to the Wildlife Conservation Society's AHEAD Programme, Wildlife Conservation Society, New York, 74 pp. Available at: http://www.wcs-ahead.org/kaza/rpt_tads_status&control_tad_sci_ltr_final.pdf (accessed 15 December 2014).

Perkins, J. (2010) Fences and landscape scale degradation. In: Ferguson, K. and Hanks, J. (eds) *Fencing impacts: A review of the environmental, social and economic impacts of game and veterinary fencing in Africa with particular reference to the Great Limpopo and Kavango-Zambezi Transfrontier Conservation Areas*. Mammal Research Institute, University of Pretoria, pp. 83–95. Available at: http://www.wcs-ahead.org/gltfca_grants/pdfs/ferguson_final_2010.pdf (accessed 15 December 2014).

Pilson, R.D. and Pilson, B.M. (1967) Behaviour studies of *Glossina morsitans* Westw. in the field. *Bulletin of Entomological Research* 57, 227–257.

Robertson, A.G., Kluge, E.B., Kritzinger, D.A. and De Sousa, A.E. (1972) The use of residual insecticides in the reclamation of the Rhodesia-Mozambique border region, the Sabi/Save and Limpopo Rivers from *Glossina morsitans* Westwood. *Proceedings and Transactions of the Rhodesia Scientific Association* 55, 34–62.

Rouget, M., Cowling, R.M., Lombard, A.T., Knight, A.T. and Kerley, G.I.H. (2006) Designing large scale corridors for pattern and process. *Conservation Biology* 20, 549–561.

Salomon, M., Cupido, C. and Samuels, I. (2013) The good shepherd: remedying the fencing syndrome. *African Journal of Range and Forage Science* 30, 71–75.

Scholes, R.J. (2009) Syndromes of dryland degradation in southern Africa. *African Journal of Range and Forage Science* 26(3), 113.

Suich, H., Child, B. and Spenceley, A. (2009) *Evolution and Innovation in Wildlife Conservation: Parks and Game Ranches to Transfrontier Conservation Areas*. Earthscan, London.

Torquebiau, E. and Taylor, R.D. (2009) Natural resource management by rural citizens in developing countries: innovations still required. *Biodiversity and Conservation* 18(10), 2537–2550.

Vale, G.A., Lovemore, D.F., Flint, S. and Cockbill, G.F. (1988) Odour-baited targets to control tsetse flies, *Glossina* sp., in Zimbabwe. *Bulletin of Entomological Research* 78, 31–49.

Van Schalkwyk, D.L., McMillin, K.W., Witthun, R.C. and Hoffman, L.C. (2010) The contribution of wildlife to sustainable natural resource utilization in Namibia: a review. *Sustainability* 2(11), 3479–3499.

Weitz, B. (1963) The feeding habits of *Glossina*. *Bulletin of the World Health Organization* 28, 711–729.

# 22 Better Together: Identifying the Benefits of a Closer Integration Between Plant Health, Agriculture and One Health

**Eric Boa,[1]* Solveig Danielsen[2] and Sophie Haesen[3]**
*[1]Independent Consultant, New Malden, UK; [2]CABI, Leusden, the Netherlands; [3]Swiss Tropical and Public Health Institute, Basel and University of Basel, Switzerland*

## Introduction

There is a long association between human and animal health. After all, humans and livestock, horses, cats and dogs – to name a few in regular contact with people – are all mammals, linked by biology and behaviours and affected by the same diseases. Medical and veterinary procedures and processes have naturally evolved to deal with these shared threats, but there has also been further reflection and sharing of lessons learned on how best to organize services and train health professionals.

The increasing confluence of human and animal health has been prompted by a surge in the importance of zoonotic diseases and is reflected in terms such as 'one medicine' and now One Health. One Health has stimulated new ideas about a wider vision of health that encompasses society at large, livelihoods and the natural world, as in the ecohealth movement. Broader integrated thinking has encouraged transdisciplinary research that examines the complexity of interactions between people, animals and their surroundings.

Despite the burgeoning movements and initiatives on 'health' in its widest sense, plant health is frequently missing or only briefly mentioned. The purpose of this chapter is to redress this imbalance and discuss the reasons why more attention should be given to plant health. We hope that a broad definition and exploration of plant health will suggest and stimulate new links and joint actions across the different health sectors, which will improve human lives and help sustain the natural environment.

The launch of the One Health Initiative, which 'seeks to promote, improve and defend the health and well-being of all species',[1] is an important recognition of how linking human and animal health has prompted new ideas and actions. Surprisingly, plant health is not explicitly addressed by the initiative, although lack of food and malnutrition make people ill and more prone to infections (Rice *et al.*, 2000). There are an estimated 400 million small (less than 2 ha) farms worldwide, more than 90% of which are in Asia and Africa (Nagayets, 2005). Despite the importance of crop production and agriculture to poor people, plant health is a marginal, if not invisible, topic within the wider debate about One Health. This needs to change.

*E-mail: eric_boa@hotmail.com

We review past and recent work in plant health, to show examples of how new approaches and ideas from plant health clinics (Boa, 2009a) could strengthen One Health and improve health outcomes for all. We consider the strategic and practical role of plant health in One Health through three areas: joint service delivery, cross-sectoral coordination and cross-sectoral learning. Our target audience includes the broad community of actors brought together through the One Health movement, as well as the people and organizations active in plant health and related aspects of agriculture. We also hope this chapter will be of general interest to people working in development and human and animal health.

Service delivery in plant, human and animal health has many common features. Joint service delivery for human and animal health saves money (Zinsstag *et al.*, 2005). What works in one sector could work in another; opportunities exist for combining plant health services with human or animal health. Good coordination between human health and agriculture has identified solutions to malnutrition (Stern *et al.*, 2007) and could be used to manage the threat of mycotoxins more effectively. Research on human health systems has provided new ideas and tools for plant health systems (Danielsen *et al.*, 2012). It is additionally true that lessons from running plant clinics are relevant to other health sectors.

We compare the current view of plants as part of One Health and related movements and the meaning of plant health more generally: it is more than crop protection or Integrated Pest Management (IPM). Recent developments in service delivery and health systems are reviewed for plants, people and animals. Last, we propose a tripartite approach to plant, human and animal health and show how this could help stimulate and shape cross-sectoral actions.

This is a timely moment to consider plant health. The Millennium Development Goals (MDGs) will be superseded by new sustainable development goals[2] in 2015, including goals that specifically address agriculture. The strong emphasis on human health remains. The importance of including plant health in broader movements such as One Health and ecohealth has never been greater.

## An Overview of Three Major Health Movements and Their Relation to Plant Health

Human and animal health are closely connected to plants for at least four reasons: (i) food and feed security – enough food and feed at the right time to sustain people and animals; (ii) food and feed safety – plant products free from mycotoxins, pesticide residues, and human and animal disease contaminants; (iii) livelihoods – agriculture is the world's most important enterprise, fundamental to economic growth in developing countries; and (iv) medicinal plants – the origin of pharmaceutical sciences and a continuing source of novel compounds for drugs used in human and animal health.

Three strong movements have emerged over the last decade or so: One Health, agriculture and health (AH) and ecosystem approaches to health (ecohealth). All stress the importance of multidisciplinary approaches and wide collaborations to improve health outcomes. One Health and AH have substantial overlap in content and rhetoric, yet have different origins and emphases. One Health has a long history rooted in 'one medicine' (Zinsstag *et al.*, 2011) and zoonotic diseases. One Health has largely been driven by the scientific community in the developed world, with its agenda influenced by pandemics such as avian flu and SARS, and perceived bio-terrorism threats. Ecohealth strives for sustainable health of people, animals and ecosystems, using knowledge drawn from natural, social and health sciences and the humanities (Charron, 2012; Zinsstag, 2012).

Zoonotic diseases remain a strong focus of One Health, though its aims have broadened to address improvements to the health and well-being of people, animals and the environment. The aims may have broadened, yet change is slow to arrive. Although the United States Department of Agriculture (USDA) is part of the One Health initiative, there is little mention of agriculture or integrated responses to hunger, inadequate diet and poor quality food and feed.

Enthusiasm for and interest in One Health is growing, particularly in developed countries where public concern about zoonoses is most clearly articulated. The One Health Global Network[3] says that One Health began as 'a concept that became an approach and then a movement'. The network's aim is to 'improve health and well-being through the prevention of risks and the mitigation of effects of crises that originate at the interface between humans, animals and their various environments'.

The One Health movement has gained wide official approval through the joint endorsement by the World Health Organization (WHO), Food and Agriculture Organization of the United Nations (FAO) and the World Organisation for Animal Health (OIE) and a 'tripartite global framework to address health risks at the human–animal–ecosystems interface' (FAO-OIE-WHO, 2010). One Health has spawned many new ideas, yet few include suggestions for linking to plant health. One possible exception is the potential for joint service delivery (Schelling *et al.*, 2007) to include plant health, which is considered later in this chapter.

The AH movement is more diffuse, though nutrition is a large part of its agenda. AH is driven by a 'South agenda' defined around the MDGs, with the International Food and Policy Research Institute (IFPRI) taking a leading role since 2005. The World Bank 2008 annual report on agriculture for development was a significant milestone in revitalizing donor and government interest in agriculture (World Bank, 2007). AH was further bolstered by an international assessment of agricultural knowledge, science and technology and its role in development (McIntyre *et al.*, 2009).

The close links between agriculture and human health are clearly illustrated by HIV/AIDS, a disease which has had disastrous effects on agricultural production. The failure chain is simple and direct: if you get sick, you are unable to farm; if you are unable to farm, families suffer. An increase in widow-and-orphan-headed households in Uganda led to a 'downward spiral of livelihood degradation for vulnerable households' (Parker *et al.*, 2009). Good nutrition, also part of AH, is essential for managing the long-term health outcomes of HIV-positive people and improving their quality of life.

Two programmes under the AH movement stress the importance of cross-sectoral approaches. The CGIAR collaborative research programme on Agriculture for Nutrition and Health (A4NH)[4] includes partner centres active in agriculture, agroforestry, development policy, livestock and fish. The Leverhulme Centre for Integrative Research on Agriculture and Health (LCIRAH)[5] is a coalition of researchers from diverse disciplines, including human health, sociology, anthropology and economics, among others.

These programmes have overlapping research themes that range from diet and non-communicable diseases in development and biofortification, to 'agrihealth' and 'enhanced nutrition'. There is, however, little mention of plant health. One reason may be the limited contact between scientific researchers studying plant pests and diseases and their medical and veterinary counterparts, perhaps because, with rare exceptions, plant pathogens do not infect humans or animals. Few professional societies foster interdisciplinary engagement that might build bridges between the different health sectors.

A stronger connection between nutrition and agriculture offers new ways to link plants to people (see von Braun *et al.*, 2012). The United Nations Standing Committee on Nutrition produced ten key recommendations for improving nutrition through agriculture, which included incorporating 'explicit nutrition objectives' into programmes. The Tata-Cornell Agriculture and Nutrition Initiative promotes links through a 'research, development and education program'. These are steps in the right direction, but there are still more policy briefs and recommendations than direct actions.

Disciplinary isolation is a major obstacle to bringing human and veterinary medicine, agriculture, livestock and nutrition closer together. Weak ties within and between ministries, local governments, service providers, regulatory agencies and education further limit cross-sectoral coordination, integrated actions and coordinated responses (Schelling *et al.*, 2007; von Braun *et al.*, 2012).

Human, animal and plant diseases are all covered by ProMed-mail,[6] an internet-based reporting system for 'rapid global dissemination of information on outbreaks of infectious diseases and acute exposures to toxins that affect human health, including those in animals and in plants grown for food or animal feed'. Run by the Society for Infectious Diseases, alerts are issued on diseases affecting people, animals and plants. The UK Foresight Programme reviewed threats to human, animal and plant health for both the UK and sub-Saharan Africa (Foresight, 2007) and attempted to place plant health in a wider context, an encouraging sign of cross-sectoral thinking.

The Emerging Pathogens Institute (EPI)[7] at the University of Florida studies human, animal and plant diseases. EPI draws on scientific expertise in medicine, veterinary medicine and agricultural and life sciences. In 2011 the Southern African Centre for Infectious Disease Surveillance (SACIDS) initially included plants in their One Health framework, however they are missing from a 2013 mission statement.[8] The reason is unclear, but it may have been difficult to define concrete actions that addressed broader health outcomes.

Fletcher *et al.* (2009) argued for broadening One Health to include plant health. The authors highlighted the importance of plant health to nutrition, food security and food safety. They proposed improvements in scientific cooperation and technology development but did not discuss delivery mechanisms or extension and advisory services. These topics will be considered in detail later in this chapter.

## Understanding Plant Health

Plant health in practice has a limited scope, usually restricted to pests and diseases and their management. A broader definition is needed to consider all the possible links to human and animal health, one that would consider the overall vigour and health of plants. Expanding the scope of plant health will not be easy given the weak visibility of services. The 'plant health workforce' consists mainly of general extension workers who have a broad range of responsibilities. Plant health specialists such as plant pathologists are more visible, but most are based in research, with often ill-defined roles in extension.

In the context of One Health, the scope of plant health should be consistent with achieving improved health outcomes for people, animals and the environment. J.A. Browning, a leading US plant pathologist, proposed a national plant health system comprising research, training, education and extension (Browning, 1998). His definition of plant health included biotic and abiotic stresses and therefore covered soil fertility as well as pests and diseases, and crop protection.

Browning worked in IPM for many years before developing his vision of 'holistic plant health'. IPM promotes non-chemical methods, including biological control, and has many definitions (Pinstrup-Andersen, 2001), making it difficult to agree on its scope. The System-wide Program for IPM (SP-IPM) talks of 'improving established methods and developing new practices of pest and disease control' (Anon, 2010). Integrated Soil Fertility Management (ISFM) also embraces plant health (Vanlauwe and Zingore, 2011).

The SP-IPM has little advice to offer on how to improve service delivery, beyond encouraging others: 'Policymakers need to provide incentives to encourage the adoption and adaptation of IPM to local conditions through a strengthening of knowledge transfer to upgraded extension services' (Anon, 2010). An independent review of the impact of IPM extension confirmed the need to pay more attention to delivery mechanisms (Bentley, 2009), a recognized priority in human health: 'Biomedical discoveries cannot improve people's health without research to find out how to apply them specifically within different health systems, population groups, and diverse political and social contexts' (WHO, 2004).

Plant health services are only one part of general extension efforts. Diagnostic laboratories are more visible, but difficult for farmers to access (Smith *et al.*, 2008). Extension has subject matter specialists in crop protection, but they are few and too thinly spread.

Support from plant health specialists, such as plant pathologists and entomologists, is often dependent on project funding for specific problems. Plant health service delivery does not receive the attention it clearly needs.

Browning's proposal of a national plant health system was never consciously adopted, though the creation of a National Plant Diagnostic Network (Stack *et al.*, 2006) and the continuation of joint research–extension appointments at land grant universities are positive signs. The political commitment to agriculture at all levels goes back to the creation of the USDA in 1862 (Campbell *et al.*, 1999). Continuing support has done much to sustain a strong and effective plant health delivery system with more than a passing resemblance to a national plant health system.

A less encouraging picture emerges from developing countries, where extension–agriculture links are generally weak (Davis, 2007). When emerging diseases cause major damage or pose major threats (Anderson *et al.*, 2004), plant health gains a temporary boost, but this may not be sustained. Diagnostic services continue to suffer from weak technical capacity and uncertain funding, even in places where major plant diseases cause widespread damage, such as Uganda (Miller *et al.*, 2009).

Browning's ideas have helped to establish a post-graduate qualification for Doctor of Plant Medicine (Agrios, 2001). The idea of plant doctors is not new (Large, 1940) and has gained wider attention through courses begun by the Global Plant Clinic (GPC) in 2003 (Boa, 2009a). The Plantwise programme of CABI[9] has expanded this training since 2011 to over 30 countries. Numbers trained are still small, however, when compared to community-based animal health workers in Africa and Asia (Scoones and Wolmer, 2006).

Plant health is closely associated with phytosanitary regulations and the International Plant Protection Committee (IPPC). Each Ministry of Agriculture nominates a national plant protection organization (NPPOs), usually the government body responsible for crop protection, whose main responsibility is to monitor pests and diseases and work closely with extension services. The IPPC is much smaller than the WHO or the OIE and has a narrower mandate: 'to protect the world's cultivated and natural plant resources from the spread and introduction of pests of plants'.

Extension and research in plant health often struggle to work together. In Uganda, government agencies have overlapping mandates and sometimes competing interests in food safety, nutrition and agriculture, with poor coordination between nationally organized research and locally delivered extension (Danielsen *et al.*, 2012). Internationally, opportunities for consolidating activities in plant health could be better exploited. The IPPC is hosted by the FAO, with wide interests in crop protection and extension, and overlapping interests with the WHO in nutrition and food safety.

Wider agreement is needed on the importance of plant health. The most widely quoted source estimated up to 40% crop losses due to pests and diseases (Oerke, 2006), but individual instances can be much higher (e.g. cassava mosaic disease: see Anon, 1997). Up-to-date and comprehensive data are, however, hard to obtain and difficult to assess. More accurate data are available on losses due to mycotoxins, an important actor in plant health, with lost export earnings from Africa of around US$400 million each year (Anon, 2012). The well-documented consequences of plant pests and diseases on livelihoods, human welfare and natural resources have often failed to translate into support for research (Lenné, 2000).

The Global Forum for Rural Advisory Services (GFRAS) offers new opportunities for encouraging a move towards 'robust rural services' rather than ad hoc, crop-specific, technology-driven projects (Tripp *et al.*, 2005). Projects on crop pests and diseases are an unreliable way to sustain service delivery, the key to improving plant health and providing consistent help to farmers.

## Improving Health Outcomes Through Joint Responses

This section explores the basis and outcomes of cross-sectoral actions and the scope for stronger involvement of plant health, where joint responses to health issues have been weakest.

In Chad, combined health interventions ensured that vaccination of the children of nomadic pastoralists, which was optional, took place at the same time as compulsory vaccination of cattle. Delivery of human health services, organized around static health centres, piggy-backed on the animal health campaigns designed for mobile populations (Schelling *et al.*, 2005; Schelling *et al.*, Chapter 20, this volume). Prior to this approach, studies had failed to find one fully immunized nomadic child. The joint efforts not only improved child vaccination coverage, but also incurred savings of 15% when compared to separate campaigns to vaccinate animals and people. Pastoralists understood the concept of vaccination for their animals but not for themselves or their families. Researchers used this knowledge to encourage vaccination of 'the most neglected populations in remote rural areas'.

The potential for improved health outcomes from closer cooperation between animal and human sectors is already recognized (Zinsstag *et al.*, 2005). Managing zoonotic diseases is a constant incentive for joint actions. There are also compelling reasons for including plant health in joint actions but for different reasons: for example, reducing contamination of food and feed. Results so far have been uneven. A comprehensive review by GFRAS on the integration of nutrition into extension and advisory services noted the restricted ability of extension agents in Nigeria to improve agricultural practices and reduce mycotoxins in crops (Franzo *et al.*, 2013). The extension agents 'lack(ed) a clear agenda on mycotoxins, limiting their ability to provide good messages that improve food safety'.

Nutrition is already part of agricultural extension in some countries, through efforts to change what people grow and eat. World Neighbors, an international non-governmental organization (NGO), has led efforts to 'bring agriculture and health workers together' in the Philippines, Indonesia and Ecuador (Stern *et al.*, 2007). They found that many women had significant practical knowledge of food, but were unaware which crops were most nutritious. The project team included people with backgrounds in nutrition, agriculture and the social sciences, and it took some time to design a multidisciplinary approach on how to encourage women to plant nutrient-rich crops and address changes in diets. As the scope of projects widens, disciplinary biases need to be recognized and managed.

Joint actions on the diagnosis of plant, human and animal diseases would appear to be more straightforward. Similar methods are used to identify human, animal and plant pathogens (see Fletcher *et al.*, 2009 for in-depth review). Diagnostic techniques and tools are often developed first by medical scientists before being adapted to plant and animal pathogens. Rapid diagnostic testing of human, animal and plant pathogens often uses similar technologies, such as lateral flow devices.

Yet there is little contact between plant diagnostic services and other health sectors. Human and animal pathology services already collaborate in confirming zoonotic diseases, although there is further scope for sharing facilities (Zinsstag *et al.*, 2005). Molecular and immunological diagnostic tools are being increasingly used to identify fungi, bacteria and viruses, for example, but few plant diagnostic laboratories are able to perform such tests (Smith *et al.*, 2008). It is unclear how many human and animal laboratories might accept samples from plants, although to our knowledge, few efforts have been made to explore such possibilities.

The OIE and the WHO have designated reference laboratories for specific diseases, which help to coordinate responses to new diseases. International cooperation in diagnosing new and emerging plant diseases is much weaker, despite calls to improve networking and coordination (Smith *et al.*, 2008; Miller *et al.*, 2009). CABI is unusual, in that it provides specialist diagnostic services for plant diseases to developing countries (Aitchinson and Hawksworth, 1993). More than 50 new plant disease records were published by the CABI-related Global Plant Clinic from 2002 to 2011 (Boa and Reeder, 2009). Although the Plantwise Diagnostic and Advisory Service continues to receive samples from around the world, there is still considerable scope for strengthening international cooperation in plant diagnostics, while more could be done to link plant diagnostic services in developed countries. The USDA-supported National Plant Diagnostic Network (NPDN) coordinates US laboratories, but has only done so since 2002 (Stack *et al.*, 2006). The NPDN is a potential focal point for expanding links to human and animal health, given the international reach of the US Centers for Disease Control and Prevention (CDC).

A multidisciplinary research strategy to address contamination of food with human pathogens has recently been proposed (Fletcher *et al.*, 2013). But there are few signs that cross-sectoral approaches are being used in developing countries, where the use of 'night soil' to fertilize crops and unsanitary conditions pose considerable public health threats (Nguyen-Viet *et al.*, 2009; Pham-Duc *et al.*, 2013; Nguyen-Viet *et al.*, Chapter 9, this volume).

Plant and human health closely intersect where pesticides are widely used. The effects of pesticides on human health was comprehensively studied in Carchi province, Ecuador, a major potato-producing area with highly damaging plant health problems such as the Andean weevil and late blight (Yanggen *et al.*, 2004). Carchi has the highest incidence of pesticide poisoning in the world, and researchers used an eco-health approach to limit pesticide use (see Zinsstag *et al.*, 2011). The researchers were disappointed in their ability to bring about 'substantial changes in current practices'. Yet even though the health outcomes were less than expected, the study confirmed the validity of cross-sectoral approaches. The study also provided important lessons for others attempting similar approaches concerning other aspects of plant and human health.

Two FAO studies in Africa looked at emerging and re-emerging diseases of agricultural importance in all three health sectors in two locations, one on the border of Tanzania and Uganda (Rugalema and Mathieson, 2009), the other between Malawi and Mozambique (Bentley *et al.*, 2012). They considered the combined impact of plant, human and animal diseases from a broad livelihoods perspective. A separate paper from the larger Tanzania/Uganda study looked at local perceptions of diseases and why recommended control measures and strategies were often ignored (Rugalema *et al.*, 2009).

One of the overall conclusions was that a lack of professional collaboration between health professionals undermined attempts to limit the knock-on effect of diseases in other sectors. Most residents in the border region between Malawi and Mozambique crossed frequently and were 'rarely empty-handed, often taking plants and animals'. The studies said that it was better to share information about diseases occurring on both sides of the border, rather than attempt to limit travel and hinder trade that depended on plants and animals (Bentley *et al.*, 2012). These initial insights confirm the need to continue using a cross-sectoral approach to understand and minimize the human, animal and plant health risks associated with movement of people across borders.

Many NGOs already use cross-sectoral approaches to work with rural communities. They are less restricted by the disciplinary silos of formal approaches. The Village Vocations Program, a Kenyan NGO, works in all three health sectors, though only recently in plant health. One reason for this addition was the recognition that efforts to help families affected by HIV/AIDS should also include support for agriculture.

In summary, there are encouraging examples of joint responses and cross-sectoral coordination involving plant health, but they are still small scale. Further thought is needed on designing interventions and testing their effectiveness.

## A Unified Approach to Plant Health-care

Attempts to broaden the focus of plant health beyond specific interventions on particular crops and pests and diseases include a proliferation of 'integrated' approaches, such as IPM and IFSM. Their separate achievements stop some way short, however, of a unified approach to plant health-care. Taking inspiration from broad-based approaches to human and animal health, and their emphasis on service delivery and health systems (see Catley *et al.*, 2001 and Tollman *et al.*, 2006), this section discusses a plant health system approach and a model for analysing links, dependencies and interactions between human, animal and plant health.

Plant clinics began with the intention of providing regular support to farmers, filling major gaps in service delivery for plant health (Boa, 2009a). The aim was to work with organizations already active in extension, building on local knowledge to streamline advisory services. Plant health clinics began in Bolivia in 2003 (Bentley *et al.*, 2009) but made their biggest steps forward in Nicaragua from 2005 onwards (Danielsen and Fernandez, 2008).

Plant clinics are run mainly by extension workers, often known as 'plant doctors'. By 2009 there were eight countries running 80 clinics with the support of the Global Plant Clinic (Boa, 2009a), now a part of the expanded Plantwise programme of CABI (Romney *et al.*, 2013). Training modules for plant doctors were developed in Nicaragua (Danielsen and Fernandez, 2008) and have been an important tool in establishing networks of plant clinics and creating new partnerships (Boa, 2009b).

Local innovations in plant clinics and service delivery flourished as more countries and new partners took part. In Bangladesh, plant clinics promoted safe use of pesticides; plant doctors requested training in diagnosing pesticide poisoning (Kelly *et al.*, 2008). Some plant clinics in Nicaragua included qualified veterinarians hired by local co-operatives, who accepted queries about animal health. Many of the early innovations were in location and timing of plant clinics, as local staff found what worked best. In the Democratic Republic of the Congo and Kenya, mobile plant clinics alternated between sites to increase coverage and improve access. At Southern Horticultural Research Institute (SOFRI), a fruit research institute in Vietnam, workers stayed overnight at more remote locations in order to run several plant clinics in quick succession. They visited different areas two or three times a year in response to local requests.

A university diagnostic laboratory in Butembo, North Kivu, analyses plant specimens and human samples (though safety procedures are lax). Plant clinics in Nepal organized by the Society for Environment Conservation and Agricultural Research and Development (SECARD), an agricultural NGO (Adhikari *et al.*, 2013), mobilized female farmers linked to a partner NGO working with livestock. The Nepali clinics carried out simple soil tests while SECARD integrated plant clinics into its programmes on organic farming.

Concerns have been raised about the knowledge and qualification of extension workers to deal with 'any crop, any problem'. Similar concerns are expressed about primary health-care in rural locations (Tollman *et al.*, 2006). In Nicaragua, the plant doctors – local extension officers – asked for more diagnostic support. Discussions led to ideas about a plant health system, where extension, diagnostic services, research and input supply were better connected and worked more closely together (Danielsen *et al.*, 2013). The Plantwise programme of CABI is now taking forward the plant health system approach by strengthening service delivery, plant health information systems (Leach and Hobbs, 2013) and linkages between key actors in developing countries (Romney *et al.*, 2013).

The shift from services to system thinking was a natural consequence of thinking about plant health from a wider perspective. With the expansion in numbers of organizations and countries running plant clinics,[10] it became increasingly necessary to consider the wider policy and the institutional and organizational implications of providing primary plant health services and to identify tools and methods to measure outcomes and provide guidance on future interventions.

The WHO health systems framework from 2007 was adapted to plant health (Fig. 22.1) and used in Uganda for measuring performance of plant clinics (Danielsen *et al.*, 2012). The resulting Plant Health Systems (PHS) framework is a work in progress and needs wider testing and validation as well as agreement on ultimate (plant health) outcomes.

The PHS framework is a good example of cross-sectoral learning, sharing ideas and insights gained from human health. The framework emphasizes the importance of service delivery, as well as policies, governance and financing – three topics that would normally receive little attention in crop protection.

The PHS framework has been used to develop a three health model (3H) for plants, people and animals, shown in Fig. 22.2

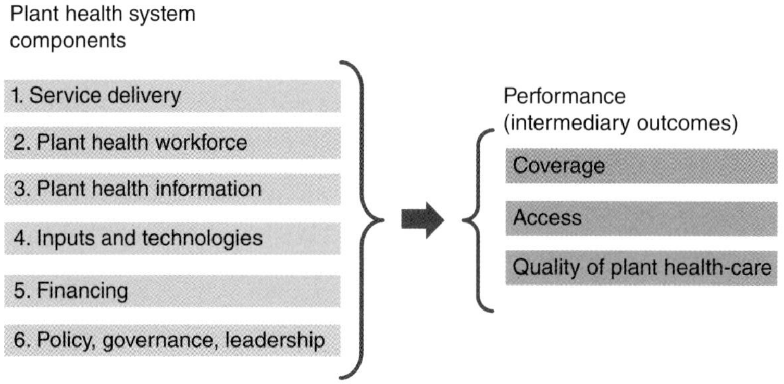


**Fig. 22.1.** Plant health system framework (Danielsen *et al.*, 2012).

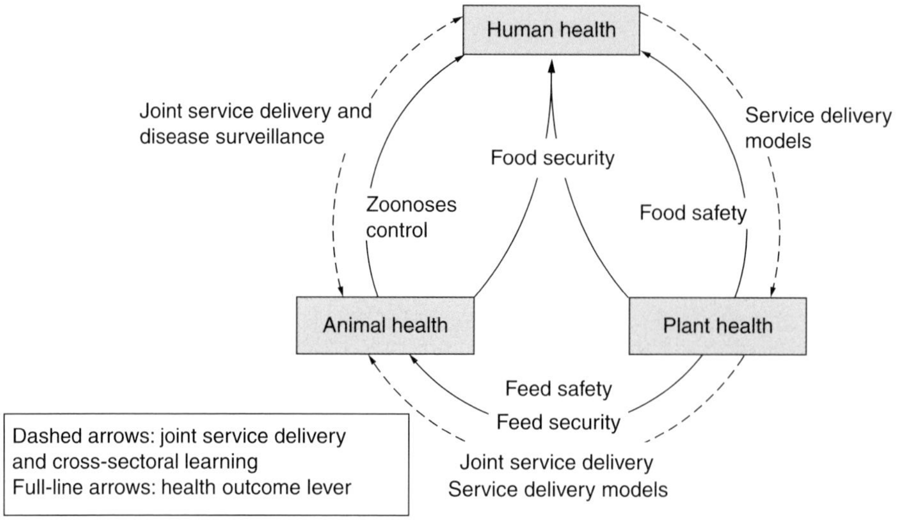


**Fig. 22.2.** Three health model (Danielsen, 2013).

(Danielsen, 2013). In its simplest reading, the 3H model is a way of showing links, dependencies and interactions between the different health sectors. It highlights important influences on food security (animal and plant health), for example, and the overall role of plant health in determining human health. The model has other potential uses, for example highlighting the need to coordinate disease surveillance across all health sectors, as well as the potential benefits of joint service delivery.

The 3H model emphasizes service delivery and exposes gaps in thinking about how to manage plant diseases at field level and organize extension services. Two of the most important conclusions, however, are to show the inter-relatedness of different health sectors and to emphasize the need to expand cross-sectoral actions.

## A Tripartite Approach to Plant, Human and Animal Health

Plant health is already part of the general debate on human health, animal health, agriculture, nutrition and ecosystem health, but there is little evidence of active engagement with other sectors. Practical suggestions on how to implement a tripartite approach that includes plant health are scarce, and new ideas need testing.

A decade's work on plant clinics in more than 30 countries is helping to strengthen links and widen partnerships through a plant health system approach. A better understanding of how extension is organized and how institutions function has identified opportunities to link different groups of people who have shared interests but who often struggle to work together. This helps to pave the way for tripartite approaches to health.

The MDGs have raised aspirations to alleviate poverty, and increased the importance of cross-sectoral actions. Complex problems demand complex responses and, as this chapter has shown, plant health has an important contribution to make in addressing such big issues. But first there must be better integration within plant health, with closer working ties between pre- and postharvest control of pests and diseases, and soil fertility and crop protection, for example. This is an essential precondition for embedding plant health more clearly in One Health and in preparation for new development goals for agriculture and human health (Independent Research Forum, 2013).

Plant clinics have articulated farmer and extension demand and stimulated new actions and partnerships, giving greater coherence to plant health. Human health systems thinking has helped develop a framework for measuring performance of plant clinics and understanding better how to strengthen plant health systems. Plant clinics have an important contribution to make in catalysing actions, stimulating partnerships, understanding the weaknesses and strengths of extension, improving surveillance, and linking to diagnostic services and input supply.

The PHS framework noted in the previous section still lacks long-term outcomes and indicators of success. These are important to assess the high expectations of the Plantwise programme (Romney *et al.*, 2013), for accountability as well as learning and improvement. Learning from human health systems has been critical in the transition from services (plant clinics) to systems, paying more attention to the delivery of primary plant health-care. Ideas from agricultural extension on seeking 'best fit' rather than 'best practice' (Birner *et al.*, 2005) also need to be considered. All of this is a long way from IPM and crop protection, but without a wider focus and perspective on plant health, little will change in how extension operates or impacts farmers and beyond.

Plant clinics have a wider role to play in general agriculture and human health, as noted previously: examples include diagnosis of pesticide poisoning and giving advice on safe use of pesticides, as well as planting nutritious crops. Advice on plant and animal health could be given at the same location. More plant samples could be diagnosed by medical and veterinary services. Adding new services and features to plant clinics will, however, require careful planning, additional training and better backstopping (Franzo *et al.*, 2013).

Sidai Africa[11] is a donor-funded attempt to improve the quality of advice on animal health through an agro-dealer franchise operation in Kenya. The same agro-dealers sell fertilizers and pesticides, which constitute 40% of their business. Although there is concern that agro-dealers give biased advice on plant health problems to promote sale of pesticides, work in Bangladesh has shown it is possible to create effective partnerships with plant clinics (Kelly *et al.*, 2008).

Another suggestion is to run plant clinics in parallel with other organized activities. Women who attend maternity clinics are often important producers and would benefit from crop advice that would improve nutrition (von Braun *et al.*, 2012). Village meetings or training events are opportunities to hold plant clinics, for delivery of advice on postharvest problems to reduce accumulation of mycotoxins. All these ideas need to be tested to see if they work and how they are best adapted to different locations and contexts.

Unpublished research in Uganda compares service delivery provided by village health teams and plant clinics. Both have similar challenges in paying staff and ensuring that the most serious illnesses and unknown problems are referred on to a reliable source. They also illustrate clear opportunities for human health and plant health to work more closely together.

A concise summary of (human) health systems (Mills, 2007) illustrates the challenges, opportunities and, above all, contributions made by effective primary health-care. The opening paragraph could just as easily apply to plant health:

> The term 'health system' is a shorthand way of referring to all the organizations, institutions and resources that are primarily concerned with improving health in a particular country. They ensure the provision of preventive, rehabilitative, curative, and other public health services, as well as the generation of the financial, physical, and human resources needed for service provision. Most importantly, health systems also encompass the management and governance arrangements that help ensure efficiency and equity in provision of service, responsiveness to patient needs, and accountability to communities and the broader society.

There are other opportunities for joint service delivery involving plant clinics, reducing costs, and increasing coverage and access to advice on crop protection, as well as other topics. The farmer demand for advice on mycotoxins is weak – to the best of our knowledge no queries have been received by plant clinics – yet the fundamental solutions to this human health liability lie in agricultural practice. A doctor will treat the symptoms of mycotoxin and other plant-related poisonings, but will not give advice on how to treat the root cause.

There have been other suggestions to promote tripartite approaches (Fletcher *et al.*, 2009) and links do exist between the health sectors. But much more could and should be done to establish a stronger role for plant health in One Health and to exploit new opportunities to improve health outcomes for all.

A unified vision of health and health-care is a powerful concept for tackling the complex challenges implicit in the MDGs and the new sustainable development goals. The 3H model is an important starting point for integrating plant health into One Health. However, it will require careful testing of assumptions about creating cross-sectoral collaborations, as well as new methods for assessing jointly agreed outcomes, if the model is to bring about demonstrable and measurable change.

## Acknowledgement

The preparation of this chapter was supported by the Plantwise programme of CABI.

## Notes

[1] http://www.onehealthinitiative.org
[2] http://www.sustainabledevelopment.un.org
[3] http://www.onehealthglobal.net
[4] http://www.a4nh.cgiar.org
[5] http://www.lcirah.ac.uk
[6] http://www.promedmail.org
[7] http://www.epi.ufl.edu
[8] http://www.sacids.org
[9] http://www.plantwise.org
[10] Plantwise budget about US$60 million in 2013
[11] http://www.sidai.com

## References

Adhikari, R.K., Regmi, P.P., Boa, E., Dhoj, Y. and Thapa, R.B. (2013) Innovation in plant health extension services: the case of plant clinics in Nepal. *Economia agro-alimentaire* 15, 235–245.

Agrios, G. (2001) The Doctor of Plant Medicine program at the University of Florida: growers, agricultural agencies, industries need plant doctors. *Plant Health Progress* DOI:10.1094/PHP-2001-0724-01-PS.

Aitchinson, E.M. and Hawksworth, D. (1993) *IMI: Retrospect and Prospect. A Celebration of the Achievements of the International Mycological Institute 1920–92.* International Mycological Institute, Egham, UK.

Anderson, P.K., Cunningham, A.A., Patel, N.G., Morales, F.J., Epstein, P.R. and Daszak, P. (2004) Emerging infectious diseases of plants: pathogen pollution, climate change and agrotechnology drivers. *Trends in Ecology and Evolution* 19, 535–544.

Anon. (1997) Mastering mosaic: the fight for cassava production in Uganda. *Gatsby Occasional Paper*. Gatsby Foundation, London, 28 pp.

Anon. (2010) *Integrated Pest Management and Crop Health – bringing together sustainable agroecosystems and people's health*. White Paper. SP-IPM Secretariat, International Institute of Tropical Agriculture (IITA), Ibadan, Nigeria, 17 pp.

Anon. (2012) Aflatoxin: a synthesis of the research in health, agriculture and trade. Feed the Future, USAID East Africa Regional Mission, Nairobi, Kenya. Available at: http://www.aflatoxinpartnership.org/~/media/Files/Projects/Aflatoxin%20microsite/PACA%20general%20documents/Aflatoxin%20Desk%20Study%20Final%20Report%202012.pdf (accessed 25 April 2014).

Bentley, J. (2009) Impact of IPM extension for smallholder farmers in the tropics. In: Peshin, R. and Dhawan, A.K. (eds) *Integrated Pest Management: dissemination and impact*. Springer, New York, pp. 333–346.

Bentley, J.W., Boa, E., Danielsen, S., Franco, P., Antezana, O., Villarroel, B., Rodríguez, H., Ferrrufino, J., Franco, J., Pereira, R., Herbas, J., Díaz, O., Lino, V., Villarroel, J., Almendras, F. and Colque, S. (2009) Plant health clinics in Bolivia 2000 – 2009: operations and preliminary results. *Food Security* 1, 371–386.

Bentley, J.W., Robson, M., Sibale, B.B., Nkhulungo, E., Tembo, Y. and Munthali, F. (2012) Travelling companions: emerging diseases of people, animals and plants along the Malawi-Mozambique border. *Human Ecology* 40, 557–569.

Birner, R., Davis, K., John Pender, J., Nkonya, E., Anandajayasekeram, P., Ekboir, J., Mbabu, A., Spielman, D., Horna, D., Benin, S. and Kisamba-Mugerwa, W. (2005) *From 'Best Practice' to 'Best Fit'. A Framework for Designing and Analyzing Pluralistic Agricultural Advisory Services*. IFPRI Policy Brief, Washington, DC.

Boa, E. (2009a) How the Global Plant Clinic began. *Outlooks on Pest Management* 20, 112–116.

Boa, E. (2009b) Plant Healthcare for poor farmers around the world: gathering demand and innovative responses. In: Hardwick, N.V. and Guillano, M. (eds) *Knowledge and Technology Transfer for Plant Pathology*. Springer, the Netherlands.

Boa, E.R. and Reeder, R. (2009) *New Disease Records from the Global Plant Clinic*. CABI, Egham, UK.

Browning, J.A. (1998) One phytopathologist's growth through IPM to holistic plant health: the key to approaching genetic yield potential. *Annual Review of Phytopathology* 36, 1–24.

Campbell, C.L., Peterson, P.D. and Griffith, C.S. (1999) *The Formative Years of Plant Pathology in the United States*. American Phytopathological Society, St Paul, Minnesota.

Catley, A., Blakeway, S. and Leyland, T. (2001) *Community-based Approaches to Animal Healthcare: a practical guide to improving primary veterinary services*. Practical Action, UK, 368 pp.

Charron, D.F. (2012) Ecosystem approaches to health for a global sustainability agenda. *EcoHealth* 9, 256–266.

Danielsen, S. (2013) Including plant health in the 'one health' concept - in theory and in Uganda. In: Olson, A., Ørnbjerg, N. and Winkel. K. (eds) *A Success Story in Danish Development Aid (1964–2012)*. University of Copenhagen, Denmark.

Danielsen, S. and Fernandez, M. (2008) *Public Plant Health Services for All*. FUNICA, Managua.

Danielsen, S., Matsiko, F., Mutebi, E. and Karubanga, G. (2012) *Second Generation Plant Clinics in Uganda: measuring clinic performance from a plant health systems perspective 2010–2011*. University of Copenhagen, Makerere University, Kampala and CABI, UK.

Danielsen, S., Centeno, J., López, J., Lezama, L., Varela, G., Castillo, P., Narváez, C., Zeledón, I., Pavon, F. and Boa, E. (2013) Innovations in plant health services in Nicaragua: from grassroots experiment to a systems approach. *Journal of International Development* 25(7), 968–986.

Davis, K. (2007) Extension in sub-Saharan Africa: overview and assessment of past and current models, future prospects. *Journal of International Agricultural and Extension Education* 15, 15–28.

FAO-OIE-WHO (2010) Sharing responsibilities and coordinating global activities to address health risks at the animal-human-ecosystems interfaces: a tripartite concept note. Available at: http://www.who.int/influenza/resources/documents/tripartite_concept_note_hanoi_042011_en.pdf (accessed 25 April 2014).

Fletcher, J., Franza, D. and LeClerc, J.E. (2009) Healthy plants: necessary for a balanced 'One Health' concept. *Veterinaria Italiana* 45(1), 79–95.

Fletcher, J., Leach, J.E., Eversole, K. and Tauxe, R. (2013) Human pathogens on plants: designing a multidisciplinary strategy for research. *Phytopathology* 103, 306–315.

Foresight (2007) Detection and Identification of Infectious Diseases Project. One year review: April 2006 - May 2007. Available at: http://webarchive.nationalarchives.gov.uk/20121212135622/http://www.bis.gov.uk/assets/foresight/docs/infectious-diseases/one-year_review_-_report_-_may_2007 (accessed 29 April 2014).

Franzo, J., Marshall, Q., Wong, J., Merchan, R.I., Jaber, M.I., Souza, A. and Verjee, N. (2013) The integration of nutrition into extension and advisory services: A synthesis of experiences, lessons and recommendations. Global Forum for Rural Advisory Services, Lindau, Switzerland. Available at: http://www.fsnnetwork.org/sites/default/files/gfras_nutrition_report.pdf (accessed 25 April 2014).

Independent Research Forum (2013) Post-2015: framing a new approach to sustainable development. Available at: http://sustainabledevelopment.un.org/content/documents/1690IRF%20Framework%20Paper.pdf (accessed 25 April 2014).

Kelly, P., Bentley, J., Harun-ar-Rashid and Zakaria, A. (2008) Plant health clinics help curb pesticide use in Bangladesh. *Pesticide News* 81, 16–17.

Large, E.C. (1940) *The Advance of the Fungi*. Jonathan Cape, London.

Leach, M. and Hobbs, S. (2013) Plantwise knowledge bank: delivering plant health information to developing country users. *Learned Publishing* 26, 180–185.

Lenné, J. (2000) Pests and poverty: the continuing need for crop protection research. *Outlook on Agriculture* 29(4), 235–250.

McIntyre, B.D., Herren, H.R., Wakhungu, J. and Watson, R.T. (eds) (2009) *Agriculture at a Crossroads. International Assessment of Agricultural Knowledge, Science and Technology for Development, synthesis report*. Island Press, Washington, DC, 97 pp.

Miller, S., Beed, F.D. and Harmon, C.L. (2009) Plant disease diagnostic capabilities and networks. *Annual Review of Phytopathology* 47, 15–38.

Mills, A. (2007) Strengthening health systems. In: Commonwealth Secretariat (ed.) *Commonwealth Health Ministers Book 2007*. Henley Media Group Ltd, London.

Nagayets, O. (2005) Small farms: current status and key trends. Information Brief. Paper presented at Future of Small Farms, Research Workshop. UK, Wye College, June 26–29, 2005.

Nguyen-Viet, H., Zinsstag, J., Schertenleib, R., Zurbrügg, C., Obrist, B., Montangero, A., Surkinkul, N., Doulaye, K., Morel, A., Cisse, G., Koottatep, T., Wangsuphachart, V., Bonfoh, B. and Tanner, M. (2009) Improving environmental sanitation, health and well-being – a conceptual framework for integral interventions. *EcoHealth* 6(2), 180–191.

Oerke, E.-C. (2006) Crop losses to pests. *Journal of Agricultural Science* 144, 31–43.

Parker, D.C., Jacobsen, K.H. and Komwa, M.K. (2009) A qualitative study of the impact of HIV/AIDS on agricultural households in southeastern Uganda. *International Journal of Environmental Research and Public Health* 6, 2113–2138.

Pham-Duc, P., Nguyen-Viet, H., Hattendorf, J., Zinsstag, J., Phung-Dac, C., Zurbrügg, C. and Odermatt, P. (2013) *Ascaris lumbricoides* and *Trichuris trichiura* infections associated with wastewater and human excreta use in agriculture in Vietnam. *Parasitology International* 62, 172–180.

Pinstrup-Andersen, P. (2001) The future world food situation and the role of plant diseases. *The Plant Health Instructor* DOI: 10.1094/PHI-I-2001-0425-01.

Rice, A.L., Sacco, L., Hyder, A. and Black, R.E. (2000) Malnutrition as an underlying cause of childhood deaths associated with infectious diseases in developing countries. *Bulletin of the World Health Organization* 78, 1207–1221.

Romney, D., Day, R., Faheem, M., Finegold, C., LaMontagne-Godwin, J. and Negussie, E. (2013) Plantwise: putting innovation systems principles into practice. *Tropical Agriculturist* 18, 27–31.

Rugalema, G. and Mathieson, K. (2009) *Disease, Vulnerability and Livelihoods on the Tanzania-Uganda Interface Ecosystem to the West of Lake Victoria*. FAO, Rome.

Rugalema, G., Muir, G., Mathieson, K., Measures, E., Oehler, F. and Stloukal, L. (2009) Emerging and re-emerging diseases of agricultural importance: why local perspectives matter. *Food Security* 1, 441–455.

Schelling, E., Wyss, K., Béchir, M., Moto, D.D. and Zinsstag, J. (2005) Synergy between public health and veterinary services to deliver human and animal health interventions in rural low income settings. *British Medical Journal* 331(7527), 1264–1267.

Schelling, E., Béchir, M., Ahmed, M.A., Wyss, K., Randolph, T.F. and Zinsstag, J. (2007) Human and animal vaccination delivery to remote nomadic families, Chad. *Emerging Infectious Diseases* 13, 373–378.

Scoones, I. and Wolmer, W. (2006) Livestock, Disease, Trade and Markets: Policy Choices for the Livestock Sector in Africa. *IDS Working Paper 269*. Institute of Development Studies, UK.

Smith, J., Waage, J., Woodhall, J.W., Bishop, S.J. and Spence, N.J. (2008) The challenge of providing plant pest diagnostic services for Africa. *European Journal of Plant Pathology* 121, 365–375.

Stack, J., Cardwell, K., Hammerschmidt, R., Byrne, J., Loria, R., Snover-Clift, K., Baldwin, W., Wisler, G., Beck, H., Bostock, R., Thomas, C. and Luke, E. (2006) The National Plant Diagnostic Network. *Plant Disease* 90, 128–136.

Stern, L.J., Killough, S., Borja, R., Sherwood, S., Hernidiah, N., Joicey, P. and Berti, P.R. (2007) Bringing agriculture and health workers together. *LEISA Magazine* 23, 6–8.

Tollman, S., Doherty, J. and Mulligan, J.-A. (2006) General primary care. In: Jamison, D.T., Breman, J.G., Measham, A.R., Alleyne, G., Claeson, M., Evans, D.B., Jha, P., Mills, A. and Musgrove, P. (eds) *Disease Control Priorities in Developing Countries*, 2nd edn. WHO, Geneva, pp. 1193–1209.
Tripp, R., Wijeratne, M. and Piyadasa, V.H. (2005) What should we expect from Farmer Field Schools: a Sri Lanka case study. *World Development* 33, 1705–1720.
Vanlauwe, B. and Zingore, S. (2011) Integrated soil fertility management: an operational definition and consequences for implementation and dissemination. *Better Crops* 95, 4–7.
von Braun, J., Ruel, M.T. and Gillespie, S. (2012) Bridging the gap between the agriculture and health sectors. In: Fan, S. and Pandya-Lorch, R. (eds) *Reshaping Agriculture for Nutrition and Health*. IFPRI, Washington, DC, pp. 183–190.
WHO (2004) *World Report on Knowledge for Better Health*. WHO, Geneva, Switzerland.
WHO (2007) *Everybody's Business, Strengthening Health Systems to Improve Health Outcomes: WHO's framework for action*. WHO, Geneva, Switzerland.
World Bank (2007) *World Bank Development Report 2008: Agriculture for Development*. World Bank, Washington, DC.
Yanggen, D., Cole, D.C., Crissman, C. and Sherwood, S. (2004) Pesticide use in commercial potato production: reflections on research and intervention efforts towards greater ecosystems health in northern Ecuador. *EcoHealth* 1, 72–83.
Zinsstag, J. (2012) Convergence of EcoHealth and One Health. *EcoHealth* 9, 371–373.
Zinsstag, J., Schelling, E., Wyss, K. and Mahamat, M.B. (2005) Potential of cooperation between human and animal health to strengthen health systems. *Lancet* 366, 2142–2145.
Zinsstag, J., Schelling, E., Waltner-Toews, D. and Tanner, M. (2011) From 'one medicine' to 'one health' and systemic approaches to health and well-being. *Preventive Veterinary Medicine* 101, 148–156.

# 23 Food Security, Nutrition and the One Health Nexus

**Mahamat Béchir Mahamat,[1]* Lisa Crump,[2,3] Abdessalam Tidjani,[4] Fabienne Jaeger,[2,5] Abderahim Ibrahim[4] and Bassirou Bonfoh[5]**

*[1]Centre National de Nutrition et de Technologie Alimentaire du Ministère de la Santé Publique au Tchad, N'Djaména and Centre de Support en Santé Internationale, N'Djaména, Chad; [2]Swiss Tropical and Public Health Institute, Basel, Switzerland; [3]University of Basel, Basel, Switzerland; [4]Université de N'Djaména, Faculté des Sciences et de la Santé, N'Djaména, Chad; [5]Centre Suisse de Recherches Scientifiques en Côte d'Ivoire, Abidjan, Côte d'Ivoire*

## Introduction

This chapter describes interdependent linkages between animal health and human health by considering connections through food availability and quality as well as nutrition. Plant health is clearly also an integral aspect (Boa *et al.*, Chapter 22, this volume). A recent case study and continuing research are presented to illustrate the added value of a closer cooperation between veterinary and public health.

Periodic food insecurity and hunger, along with numerous associated diseases, are common in many parts of the world, especially in low and middle-income countries. Worldwide, one in eight people suffered from chronic hunger in 2011–13, and the prevalence of undernourishment in sub-Saharan Africa was estimated to be nearly 25%, affecting over 200 million people (FAO *et al.*, 2013). In 2012, a food crisis devastated the Sahel region, affecting 18 million people and putting an estimated 1 million children at risk of death from acute malnutrition (UN, 2012). The factors affecting food security and nutrition are many and complex. Natural disasters, conflicts and climate shocks have major impacts, as do limited access to resources and markets and weak government structure (Ford, 2013).

It is possible to prevent human diseases and micronutrient deficiencies through interventions both in the environment and in animals. The global burden of disease attributable to different risk factors has shifted substantially in the last three decades. Childhood underweight was the leading risk factor for loss of health in 1990, but the rank fell to eighth globally among risk factors evaluated in 2010 (Murray and Lopez, 2013). However, the extent to which the epidemiological shifts occurred varied greatly across regions, with childhood underweight and inadequate breastfeeding remaining as leading risks in most of sub-Saharan Africa (Lim *et al.*, 2012). While the drivers of these global transitions are broad, including demographic change and change in causes of death and disability (Murray and Lopez, 2013), it must be noted

*E-mail: mahamatbechir@yahoo.fr

that, in the case of under-nutrition, the causes are associated with poverty (Lim *et al.*, 2012) and are largely preventable. Development is most vulnerable in the youngest age groups, therefore focusing interventions on early life, such as the 'first 1000 days', helps to minimize the consequences of malnutrition, even in adults (Horton, 2008).

Livestock plays a central role in the Sahel, contributing to 44% of the agricultural gross domestic product (GDP) and 34% of household income (Zoundi and Hitimana, 2008). In pastoral communities, animal products provide the majority of the essential proteins and micronutrients, as the diet is based on milk and cereals, with fruits and vegetables rarely consumed (Holter, 1988; Zinsstag *et al.*, 2002).

Despite an important economic value, animal source food production is not robust and is insufficient to cover the demands of local populations in most of Africa. The most current figures available (2009) show that total African annual production was equivalent to 43 kg of milk and 18 kg of meat per person, which is only a fraction of that available in developed countries. Switzerland, for instance, produced the equivalent of 312 kg of milk and 74 kg of meat per person in the same year (FAOSTAT, 2013).

In addition to the quantity, the quality of food is an extremely important aspect of food security. The nutrition provided by animal source food, and thus the contribution toward a balanced diet, is highly dependent upon environmental factors where the animals are raised. For example, serum retinol levels in nomadic women and children depend on livestock milk consumption and milk retinol levels, which in turn depend on the quality of the grazed pastures (Zinsstag *et al.*, 2002; Béchir *et al.*, 2012a). Increases in total production as well as production efficiency of animal source food are necessary to cover the needs of populations, particularly where milk is an essential food. Increased milk production would also improve protein intake, which has been estimated to be low in malnourished children in Chad (Bechir *et al.*, 2012b). Food hygiene is an important factor for increasing quality (Bonfoh *et al.*, 2003; Hetzel *et al.*, 2004; Racloz *et al.*, Chapter 8, this volume, on foodborne risk assessment and Nguyen-Viet *et al.*, Chapter 9, this volume, on sanitation).

## Global Framework on Food Security

In 1996, the World Food Summit described food security as 'when all people, at all times, have physical, social and economic access to sufficient, safe and nutritious food to meet their dietary needs and food preferences for an active and healthy life' (FAO, 1996). The Declaration of the World Summit of Food Security in 2009 extended the concept by describing four pillars of food security: 'availability, access, utilization and stability' (FAO, 2009). This framework has recently been further integrated in a systems approach, which considers overlapping paradigms and the complex interactions between and among sectors (Ecker and Breisinger, 2012). Food security is linked to nutrition security, with a consideration of the macro- and micro-dimensions. The factors have linkages across sectors and levels.

International factors, such as global crop prices or widespread trade issues, in addition to various national factors, influence food security in different populations. On a country level, this encompasses policy orientation on agriculture and livestock, education and economy, while on the individual level, the factors include nutritional status, health and well-being, all of which contribute to nutritional outcomes. Figure 23.1 illustrates the multiple bridges that link different levels.

## Interaction Between Animal Source Food and Crops

Animals can have a substantial impact on human well-being and health through improving livelihoods and food diversification and providing high quality proteins and micronutrients through animal-sourced products. These contribute a particularly important role in pastoral areas and in cold climates where there is a short growing season.

It has been argued that production of animal source food is resource intensive, while

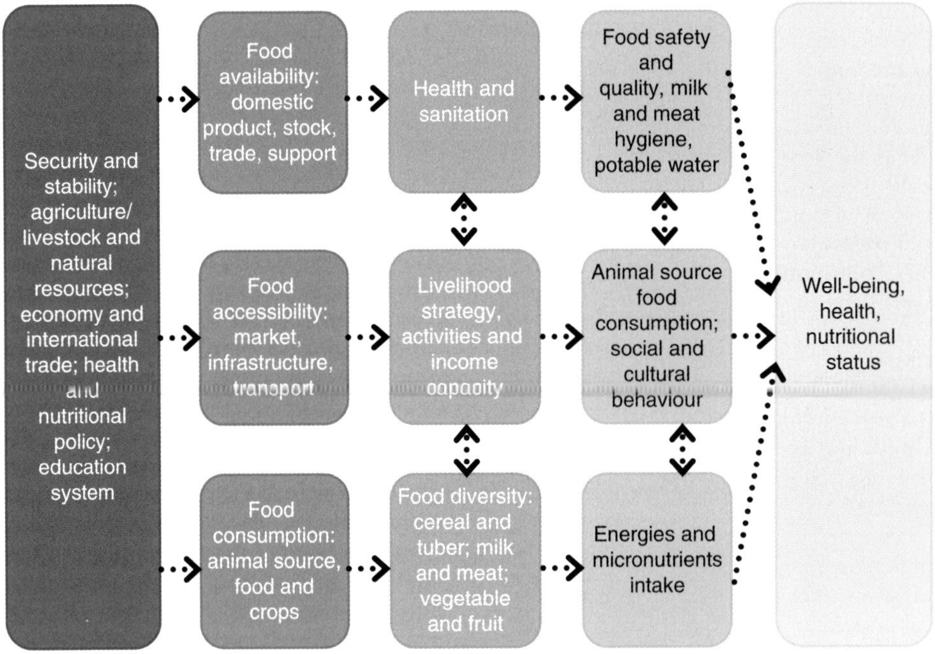


**Fig. 23.1.** A framework for linking food security and health (adapted from Guidelines for National Food Insecurity and Vulnerability Information and Mapping Systems, Background and Principles: Linkage between the overall development context, the food economy, household and individual measure of wellbeing; FAO, 2000).

producing a large share of greenhouse gas emissions (Steinfeld *et al.*, 2006), so expanding the use of animal-derived foods to feed increasingly large populations is not advisable. In most developing countries, however, food availability and accessibility is seasonal, with food storage often being problematic (Gubbels, 2011). In many areas, a dichotomy exists between animal source food and cereal production. For example, in the Sahel there is a supply shortfall from June to September, which is the rainy season, when cereal is not yet harvested but grass pastures are widely available. This causes an increased availability of milk and butter during the pre-harvest period, so prices for animal source food decrease while cereal prices increase. Milk and dairy products are used together with cereals and play an important role to mitigate the burden of food insecurity in pastoral areas. The settled communities also have access to dairy products with affordable prices at the village markets. This interaction is illustrated by a case-study from Chad (Box 23.1 and Fig. 23.2).

The case study from rural Chad illustrates important seasonal variations in price and shows clearly how access to valuable animal and non-animal products may vary according to season. During the pre-harvest period, settled communities also have better access to dairy products, which are more widely available in markets as prices decrease. The complementary use of dairy products with cereals provides an excellent source of proteins and vitamins, which are particularly important for children. It is important to note that land use for crops and livestock must be balanced and equitably regulated to prevent over-use of the fragile environment and reduce conflicts.

Animal source food also plays an important role for ensuring food security in other areas such as cold climates, where crop farming is limited or impossible due to the short growing season (e.g. Alaskan Inuit). In Kyrgyzstan and Mongolia, pastoral communities migrate during the winter for protection against bitterly cold temperatures and food scarcity. In these communities, meat, animal fat and milk products are

**Box 23.1.** A Chadian case study (adapted from Béchir *et al.*, 2013).

**2008 local commodity prices, Lake Chad region**
(average yearly price in 48 weekly village markets)

Maize: 19,313 FCFA (95% IC 17,777–20,848) for 100 kg = US$10.92 per bushel (US$1 = 447 FCFA):

- Lowest price (10,000 FCFA) observed in December;
- Highest price (29,000 FCFA) observed in August;
- World market prices varied around US$8.00 per bushel;
- Notably less than market price in the study area.

Milk: 121 FCFA (95% IC 108–134) for 1 l:

- Lowest price (25 FCFA) observed in August;
- Highest price (225 FCFA) observed in February.

Butter: 2597 FCFA (95% IC 2492–2701) for 1 l:

- Lowest price (1950 FCFA) observed in August;
- Highest price (3330 FCFA) observed in May.

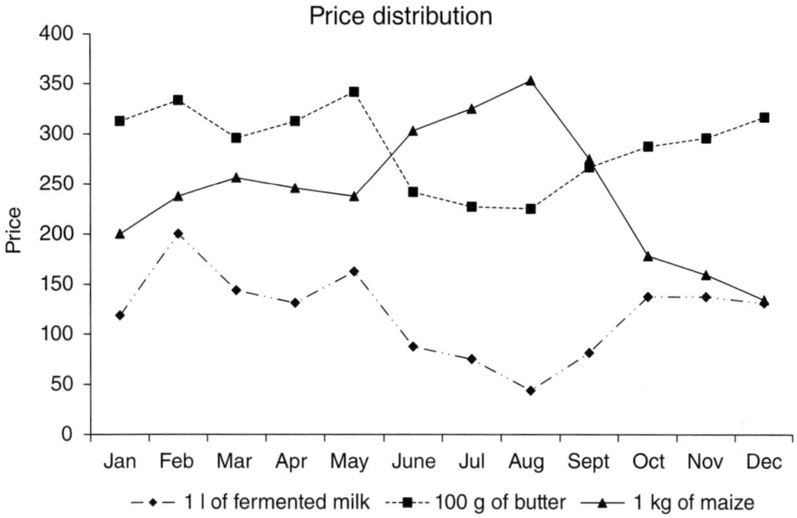


**Fig. 23.2.** Annual variation in food prices (FCFA) at the Gredaya, Chad village market (Béchir *et al.*, 2013).

crucial for survival. Extreme weather conditions can also have a sporadic impact, such as when heavy snowfall, or dzud, causes a total decimation of livestock herds (Zinsstag *et al.*, 2005), which subsequently leads to human famine.

## Micronutrient Deficiencies

Micronutrient deficiencies, also known as hidden hunger, are widespread in developing countries, particularly in remote communities (Muthayya *et al.*, 2013). The most important risk factors in terms of effect on total child mortality are deficiencies of vitamin A and zinc (Black *et al.*, 2008). Iodine and iron deficiencies result in small disease burdens; however, iron-deficiency anaemia is an important contributor to maternal mortality (Stoltzfus *et al.*, 2004). Vitamin A deficiency (VAD) continues to be a central health issue and an underlying cause of disease (Ramakrishnan and Martorell, 1998; Gogia and Sachdev,

2010). Low serum retinol concentration (<0.70 μmol/l) affects an estimated 190 million pre-school-age children and 19.1 million pregnant women worldwide, corresponding to 33.3% of the pre-school-age population and 15.3% of pregnant women in populations at risk for VAD, globally. Africa and South-east Asia are most affected by vitamin A deficiency (WHO and UNICEF, 1995).

Pastoralist populations, which practise transhumance (moving livestock from one grazing area to another in a seasonal cycle) in response to the needs of their animals, are nutritionally unique. Due to the seasonal mobility necessitated by variable resources, their diet is primarily based on milk and cereals, with fruits and vegetables being rarely consumed (Holter, 1988; Schelling *et al.*, 2005). The micronutrient status of these populations is largely unknown. We investigated vitamin A status in mobile pastoral and settled communities in the south-eastern Lake Chad region, finding a high prevalence of moderate to severe retinol deficiency (Zinsstag *et al.*, 2002), which was dependent on lifestyle (Béchir *et al.*, 2012a), with a direct dependence of human serum retinol to (consumed) cows' milk retinol (Fig. 23.3). This supported the idea that, in these populations, human vitamin A status was directly dependent on livestock vitamin A status. In turn, this indicator for animal nutrition and health should be dependent on the available ß-carotene in the grazed fodder (Calderón *et al.*, 2007). It was therefore expected that seasonal variation would be seen in vitamin A status as a result of the cyclic availability of green grass. Animals were expected to graze solely on standing hay during the dry season. Paradoxically, the milk of Fulani cattle contained especially high levels of vitamin A during the dry months. However, it was observed that these herds remained at the shore of Lake Chad, even grazing on the islands within the lake, thereby ensuring constant access to green grass as a result of the nomadic lifestyle (Zinsstag *et al.*, 2002). There is yet another nutritional aspect brought into play through this practice. Although the herds grazing at the lake have access to better fodder, they are at the same time highly exposed to *Fasciola* spp. (Jean-Richard, 2013). *Fasciola* trematodes use snails in the lake as an intermediate host. The consequences of these flukes are highly significant in cattle, causing severe reductions in milk and meat yield, as well as lower replacement stock numbers due

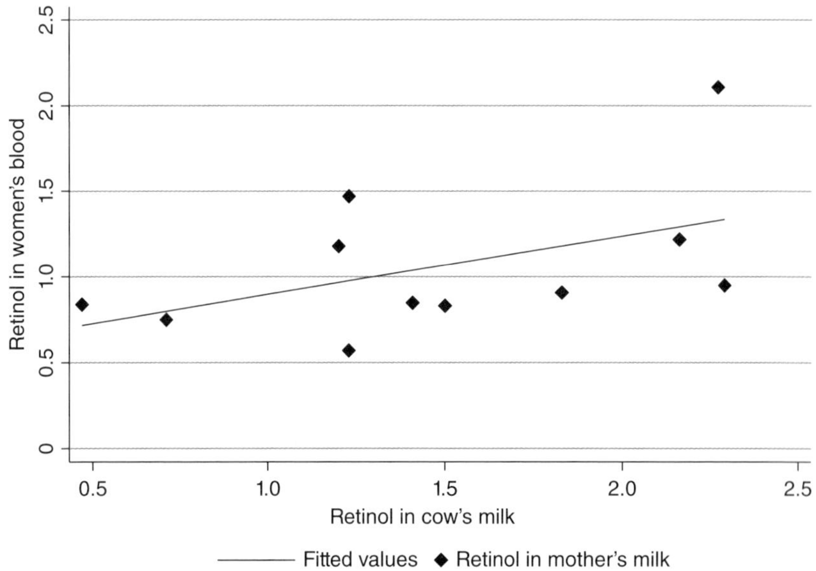


**Fig. 23.3.** Regression of pastoralist women's blood retinol and cows' milk retinol (Béchir *et al.*, 2012a).

to the decreased fertility in the herds (Abunna *et al.*, 2010; Sariozkan and YalCin, 2011).

Ongoing work is examining ecological linkages and environmental determinants, postulating that data on the availability and quality of pastures in remote areas of Chad are good indicators of the nutritional and health status of Sahelian livestock and people. We are investigating seasonal variation in ß-carotene in pasture grass, retinol levels in livestock milk and ß-carotene and retinol levels in human blood to further quantify the prevalence of VAD and identify the critical time period(s) for human nutritional interventions. This information will facilitate evidence-based recommendations on intervention timing for authorities making policy decisions. Additionally, we are using remote sensing to map pasture quality and availability. By correlating vegetative indices with local information in a transdisciplinary manner, we aim to develop a broadly useful predictive tool, as remote livestock-keeping communities are living in the most fragile areas of the ecosystem and could serve as sentinels for the entire rural population.

These investigations are only possible in such populations where dietary retinol sources are limited, primarily to milk, through lifestyle adaptation. The added value of a One Health approach is that human health benefits are realized through investigation into animal health. Knowledge about animal nutritional status becomes an essential part of planning effective, cost-efficient human food security interventions.

## Malnutrition

More than one-third of child deaths and more than 10% of the total global disease burden have been attributed to maternal and child under-nutrition. Inadequate infant feeding practices are responsible for two-thirds of child mortality due to malnutrition (WHO and UNICEF, 2003). Stunting, severe wasting and intra-uterine growth restriction, along with vitamin A and zinc deficiency, are important public health problems (Black *et al.*, 2008). In developing countries, malnutrition linked to a lack of adequate food intake can manifest as either acute or chronic malnutrition.

Wasting, defined as low weight-for-height, indicates acute weight loss. Worldwide, 52 million (9%) children under the age of 5 suffer from acute malnutrition, with 29 million (5%) being affected by the severe form. Most of these children live in developing countries with high periodic food insecurity, which further exacerbates their vulnerability (UNICEF, 2013).

The prevalence of acute malnutrition in regions of the Sahel recurrently reaches the threshold of 15%, defined by the World Health Organization as an emergency situation (WHO, 2000). The highest risk of mortality, particularly among children under 5 years, is in those affected by the severe forms of malnutrition, marasmus and kwashiorkor. The standard treatment of severe forms of malnutrition is based on fortified therapeutic milk, F100 and F75 (Golden and Grellety, 2012), and ready-made therapeutic foods.

Chronic malnutrition results in stunting caused by continuous inadequate nutrient intake, which restricts growth and manifests as a low height-for-age. Stunting affected at least 165 million children younger than 5 years of age in 2011 (Black *et al.*, 2013). The lack of adequate food has severe consequences, particularly during the first years of life. Growth and cognitive development also share this period of peak vulnerability (Black *et al.*, 2013), with the result that good nutrition and healthy growth in early life have lasting benefits through adulthood. A review of published work and analysis of data from longstanding prospective cohorts in Brazil, Guatemala, India, the Philippines and South Africa found a strong association between under-nutrition and shorter adult height, less schooling and reduced economic productivity. The authors concluded that under-nutrition has the long-term effect of lowering human capital, with height-for-age at 2 years of age being the best predictor (Victora *et al.*, 2008).

Underweight impacts 101 million children under the age of 5 worldwide, with 59 million in Asia and 30 million in Africa. It describes children with a low weight-for-age and is one indicator used to monitor progress towards the first Millennium Development Goal: 'to halve between 1990 and 2015 the proportion of people who suffer from hunger' (UN, 2000; Black *et al.*, 2013).

The key to prevention of all of these types of malnutrition is the provision of adequate food rich in micronutrients, energy and protein. A survey in a rural, settled district in Chad indicated that acutely malnourished children under 5 years of age often had diets that were relatively low in protein (Jaeger, Chad, 2011, personal communication). Animal source food, especially when locally available, offers highly bio-digestible nutrients and essential amino acids and may contribute to nourishment in an essential way. In addition to meat, fish and poultry may also help improve diets although they are often locally less available. While some cultural differences exist, such as eggs being considered as inadequate for children or heads of families being given priority when food is in scarce supply, the availability of animals also influences the level of protein consumption in developing countries (Speedy, 2003; Steinfeld, 2003).

## Over-nutrition and Disease

Another form of malnutrition is over-nutrition, which is defined as the excessive intake of food, particularly in unbalanced proportions. For many years, over-nutrition was primarily a problem in developed countries. However, now it is also prominent in developing countries, affecting 40 million people worldwide, with 10 million in Africa and 7 million in Asia. In 1990, 18 million people in developing countries were estimated to be overweight, and the number has increased dramatically to 43 million in 2011.

Studies have shown an association between food insecurity and overweight, but questions still remain about causal relationships. A limited number of studies have been carried out in developing countries, and results have been inconsistent. Variations in setting and complex interactions between factors, such as physical activity level and food support from relief efforts, must be adequately considered. In Iran, among women in moderately food insecure households, the possibility of overweight was lower than those of food secure households (OR 0.41, CI 95% 0.17–0.99), while the risk of abdominal obesity was 2.82 (CI 95% 1.12–7.08) times higher for women in severely food insecure compared to food secure households (Mohammadi *et al.*, 2013). Similar results were found in Malaysia (Shariff and Khor, 2005). In a study in rural Uganda, after adjustment for confounding effects, the association of food insecurity with overweight was diminished (Chaput *et al.*, 2007). In Morocco and Tunisia, the views of key stakeholders towards a range of policies designed to prevent obesity were investigated. In this context, obesity was not clearly recognized as a major public health priority, so raising awareness amongst decision makers is a crucial aspect (Holdsworth *et al.*, 2012).

According to WHO (WHO and PHAC, 2005), chronic diseases are the leading cause of deaths, at over 60% worldwide, with four out of five chronic disease deaths occurring in low- or middle-income countries. The largest increase in deaths from chronic diseases is predicted for sub-Saharan Africa and other developing countries (Alwan, 2011). Among chronic diseases, diabetes and cardiovascular diseases are rapidly increasing in sub-Saharan Africa (Dalal *et al.*, 2011) and together cause over 50% of deaths in developing countries (Abegunde *et al.*, 2007).

Relationships between food insecurity and metabolic control in adults have also been investigated. Even after adjustment for socio-economic and health factors, food insecurity was still significantly associated with poor glycaemic control (OR 1.53, 95% CI 1.07–2.19). There was also an association between food security and poor low density lipoprotein (LDL) control (68.8 mg/dl versus 49.8 mg/dl) before and after adjustment (OR 1.86, 95% CI 1.01–3.44) (Berkowitz *et al.*, 2013).

Clearly, the context is important, and finding the right dietary balance is imperative. Animal source products can be essential in some communities to meet dietary needs, but overconsumption of particular animal products can exacerbate disease. For instance, increased consumption of animal fat is associated with increased LDL and an increased risk of cardiovascular disease

(Stradling *et al.*, 2013). Another example is gout, which is caused by high levels of uric acid in the blood and associated with purine-rich foods, especially meat and seafood (Choi *et al.*, 2004; see also Turner, Chapter 19, this volume).

## Infectious Disease and Food Security

The relation between infectious disease and food security is bi-directional. Animal disease influences livestock production and thus availability of animal sourced food. Infectious bronchitis, for example, is a common poultry disease, which causes decreased egg laying and poor quality eggshells, resulting in a loss of productivity (Cavanagh and Gelb, 2008). The disease can easily be prevented through use of an oral vaccine mixed into the drinking water. Zoonotic diseases, such as brucellosis (Zinsstag *et al.*, Chapter 14, this volume) and bovine tuberculosis (Tschopp, Chapter 15, this volume), remain a significant public health problem in many regions, impacting food security and economies through reduced fertility and limited milk production (Zinsstag *et al.*, 2008; Bonfoh *et al.*, 2011). Fasciolosis, as described above in the section on micronutrients, is also endemic in many areas, with a significant adverse effect on livestock production (Malone *et al.*, 1998; Jean-Richard, 2013). Wise investing into animal health is an integral investment toward improved human health (Zinsstag *et al.*, Chapter 12, this volume).

Additionally, food insecurity and malnutrition are aggravating factors for opportunistic infections. A Canadian study (Anema *et al.*, 2013) observed that food insecurity remains significantly associated with mortality despite adjusting for multiple confounders in people living with HIV/AIDS (adjusted hazard ratio =1.95, 95% CI 1.07–3.53). HIV/AIDS also impacts the livestock sector, particularly in rural areas, although the full extent and complex factors are not well described (Goe, 2005). There is surprisingly little peer-reviewed research published on the economic impact of HIV/AIDS (Feulefack *et al.*, 2013); however, adaptations in affected households can include reorganization of labour responsibilities and sale of animals to meet expenses (Sauerborn *et al.*, 1996; Bollinger and Stover, 1999). In Zimbabwe, cattle products were found to be 29% lower in affected families (Kwaramba, 1997).

Malnutrition is a major risk factor for disease (Horton, 2008), directly and indirectly responsible for more than half of all child deaths globally, including mortality due to pneumonia, diarrhoea, malaria, measles and HIV/AIDS (Lopez *et al.*, 2006).

## Conclusion

Health, at both the individual and the population level, depends on nutrition, and food quality is dependent on good health of animals and crops produced in healthy environments (Boa *et al.*, Chapter 22, this volume). Animal source food plays an important role, particularly in pastoral areas where it provides an essential source of protein and micronutrients. This is especially important before the harvest season when plant products are not yet available and during food shortages in order to prevent and combat malnutrition.

Micronutrient deficiencies are widespread in developing countries. Vitamin A deficiency continues to be an important issue, particularly for women of child-bearing age, and an underlying contributor to disease, especially in children. Milk production is an essential source of vitamin A in pastoral areas.

In developing countries, malnutrition due to a lack of adequate food intake affects the health and development of many children, contributing to the high mortality rates. Increased animal source food production, particularly in semi-arid areas, could be a significant part of the solution. In juxtaposition with under-nutrition, there is the problem of over-consumption of animal source food. While causal relationships are not clearly established, diet, metabolic control and non-communicable disease in humans have complex associations which must be further considered.

Animal source food, with use of livestock in a moderate manner, is important for human life and livelihood. The holistic approach with a One Health concept remains one of the main avenues to tackle the direct and underlying causes of food insecurity, malnutrition and poor health and maximize human, animal and environmental well-being. The added value of a One Health approach is that human health benefits are realized through simultaneous investigations into human and animal health. Knowledge about animal nutritional status becomes an essential part of planning effective, cost-efficient human food security interventions. In addition to economic and human health benefits derived from investing into animal health, land use policies are also important. In fragile areas where there is insufficient pasture, overstocking and high grazing pressures, it is a waste of resources to neglect animal health, resulting in decreased productivity and increased mortality. Valuable pasture is consumed, but relatively little milk or meat is produced. The same amount of pasture allocated to a healthy animal maximizes production. These complex intersectoral linkages must be carefully considered for optimal resource utilization and sustainability.

## Acknowledgement

The preparation of this chapter was supported by National Centre of Competence in Research North-South (NCCR North-South) SKP Food Security.

## References

Abegunde, D., Mathers, C., Adam, T., Ortegon, M. and Strong, K. (2007) The burden and costs of chronic diseases in low-income and middle-income countries. *Lancet* 370(9603), 1929–1938.

Abunna, F., Asfaw, L., Megersa, B. and Regassa, A. (2010) Bovine fasciolosis: coprological, abattoir survey and its economic impact due to liver condemnation at Soddo municipal abattoir, Southern Ethiopia. *Tropical Animal Health and Production* 42(2), 289–292.

Alwan, A. (2011) *Global Status Report on Noncommunicable Diseases 2010*. World Health Organization, Geneva, Switzerland.

Anema, A., Chan, K., Chen, Y., Weiser, S., Montaner, J. and Hogg, R. (2013) Relationship between food insecurity and mortality among HIV-positive injection drug users receiving antiretroviral therapy in British Columbia, Canada. *PLoS ONE* 8(5), e61277.

Béchir, M., Schelling, E., Kraemer, K., Schweigert, F., Bonfoh, B., Crump, L., Tanner, M. and Zinsstag, J. (2012a) Retinol assessment among women and children in Sahelian mobile pastoralists. *EcoHealth* 9(2), 113–121.

Béchir, M., Schelling, E., Hamit, M.A., Tanner, M. and Zinsstag, J. (2012b) Parasitic infections, anemia and malnutrition among rural settled and mobile pastoralist mothers and their children in Chad. *EcoHealth* 9(2), 122–131.

Béchir, M., Zinsstag, J., Tidjani, A., Schelling, E., Ibrahim, A., Bonfoh, B. and Tanner, M. (2013) Food security and resilience among mobile pastoral and settled community around Lake Chad in Sahel. In: Srivastava, Y. (ed.) *Advances in Food Science and Nutrition*. Queen's College of Food Technology & Research Foundation, Aurangabad, India, pp. 90–106.

Berkowitz, S., Adam, T., Abegunde, D., Huskey, K. and Wee, C. (2013) Food insecurity and metabolic control among US adults with diabetes. *Diabetes Care* 36(10), 3093–3099.

Black, R.E., Allen, L.H., Bhutta, Z.A., Caulfield, L.E., de Onis, M., Ezzati, M., Mathers, C. and Rivera, J. (2008) Maternal and child undernutrition: global and regional exposures and health consequences. *Lancet* 371(9608), 243–260.

Black, R.E., Victora, C.G., Walker, S.P., Bhutta, Z.A., Christian, P., de Onis, M., Ezzati, M., Grantham-McGregor, S., Katz, J., Martorell, R., Uauy, R. and Maternal and Child Nutrition Study Group (2013) Maternal and child undernutrition and overweight in low-income and middle-income countries. *Lancet* 382(9890), 427–451.

Bollinger, L. and Stover, J. (1999) *The economic impact of AIDS in South Africa*. The Futures Group International in collaboration with Research Triangle Institute (RTI), The Centre for Development and Population Activities (CEDPA).

Bonfoh, B., Wasem, A., Traoré, A., Fané, A., Spillmann, H., Simbé, C., Alfaroukh, I., Nicolet, J., Farah, Z. and Zinsstag, J. (2003) Microbiological quality of cows' milk taken at different intervals from the udder to the selling point in Bamako (Mali). *Food Control* 14(7), 495–500.

Bonfoh, B., Zinsstag, J., Fokou, G., Weibel, D., Ould Taleb, M., Inam-ur-Rahim, Maselli, D., Kasymbekov, J. and Tanner, M. (2011) Pastoralism at the crossroads: new avenues for sustainable livelihoods in semi-arid regions. In: Wiesmann, U. and Hurni, H. (eds) *Research for Sustainable Development: foundations, experiences, and perspectives*. NCCR North-South, Centre for Development and Environment (CDE) and Institute of Geography, University of Bern, pp. 549–570.

Calderón, F., Chauveau-Duriot, B., Pradel, P., Martin, B., Graulet, B., Doreau, M. and Nozière, P. (2007) Variations in carotenoids, Vitamins A and E, and color in cow's plasma and milk following a shift from hay diet to diets containing increasing levels of carotenoids and Vitamin E. *Journal of Dairy Science* 90(12), 5651–5664.

Cavanagh, D. and Gelb, J. (2008) Infectious bronchitis. In: Saif, Y.M., Fadly, A.M., Glisson, J.R., McDougald, L.R., Nolan, L.K. and Swayne, D.E. (eds) *Diseases of Poultry*. Wiley-Blackwell, Ames, Iowa.

Chaput, J.-P., Gilbert, J.-A. and Tremblay, A. (2007) Relationship between food insecurity and body composition in Ugandans living in urban Kampala. *Journal of the American Dietetic Association* 107(11), 1978–1982.

Choi, H.K., Atkinson, K., Karlson, E.W., Willett, W. and Curhan, G. (2004) Purine-rich foods, dairy and protein intake, and the risk of gout in men. *New England Journal of Medicine* 350(11), 1093–1103.

Dalal, S., Beunza, J.J., Volmink, J., Adebamowo, C., Bajunirwe, F., Njelekela, M., Mozaffarian, D., Fawzi, W., Willett, W., Adami, H.-O. and Holmes, M.D. (2011) Non-communicable diseases in sub-Saharan Africa: what we know now. *International Journal of Epidemiology* 40(4), 885–901.

Ecker, O. and Breisinger, C. (2012) *The Food Security System: A New Conceptual Framework*. International Food Policy Research Institute, Washington, DC.

FAO (1996) Rome Declaration on World Food Security and World Food Summit Plan of Action. Available at: http://www.fao.org/docrep/003/W3613E/W3613E00.htm (accessed 13 February 2014).

FAO (2000) *Guidelines for National FIVIMS, Background and principles*. FAO, Rome.

FAO (2009) *Declaration of the World Summit on Food Security*. FAO, Rome.

FAO, IFAD and WFP (2013) *The State of Food Insecurity in the World 2013: The multiple dimensions of food security*. FAO, Rome.

FAOSTAT (2013) FAOSTAT. Available at: http://faostat3.fao.org/faostat-gateway/go/to/browse/C/CL/E (accessed 9 December 2013).

Feulefack, J.F., Luckert, M.K., Mohapatra, S., Cash, S.B., Alibhai, A. and Kipp, W. (2013) Impact of community-based HIV/AIDS treatment on household incomes in Uganda. *PLoS ONE* 8(6), e65625.

Ford, E. (2013) *Learning the Lessons in the Sahel*. Oxfam International.

Goe, M.R. (2005) *Linkages Between Livestock Production and HIV/AIDS in Countries in Eastern and Southern Africa*. Food and Agriculture Organization of the United Nations, Rome.

Gogia, S. and Sachdev, H.S. (2010) Maternal postpartum vitamin A supplementation for the prevention of mortality and morbidity in infancy: a systematic review of randomized controlled trials. *International Journal of Epidemiology* 39(5), 1217–1226.

Golden, M. and Grellety, Y. (2012) *For the Integrated Management of Severe Acute Malnutrition: in- and out-patient treatment*. ACF International, Jamaica.

Gubbels, P. (2011) *Escaping the Hunger Cycle: Pathways to resilience in the Sahel*. Sahel Working Group, UK.

Hetzel, M., Bonfoh, B., Farah, Z., Traoré, M., Simbé, C.F., Alfaroukh, I.O., Schelling, E., Tanner, M. and Zinsstag, J. (2004) Diarrhoea, vomiting and the role of milk consumption: perceived and identified risk in Bamako (Mali). *Tropical Medicine & International Health* 9(10), 1132–1138.

Holdsworth, M., El Ati, J., Bour, A., Kameli, Y., Derouiche, A., Millstone, E. and Delpeuch, F. (2012) Developing national obesity policy in middle-income countries: a case study from North Africa. *Health Policy and Planning* DOI: 10.1093/heapol/czs125.

Holter, U. (1988) Food habits of camel nomads in the north west Sudan: food habits and foodstuffs. *Ecology of Food and Nutrition* 21(1), 1–15.

Horton, R. (2008) Maternal and child undernutrition: an urgent opportunity. *Lancet* 371(9608), 179.

Jean-Richard, V. (2013) *Crowding at Lake Chad: An Integrated Approach to Demographic and Health Surveillance of Mobile Pastoralists and Their Animals*. University of Basel, Basel.

Kwaramba, P. (1997) *The Socio-Economic Impact of AIDS on Commercial Agricultural Production Systems in Zimbabwe*. Zimbabwe Farmer's Union and Friedrich Ebert Stiftung, Harare.

Lim, S.S., Vos, T., Flaxman, A.D., Danaei, G., Shibuya, K., Adair-Rohani, H., Amann, M., Anderson, H.R., Andrews, K.G., Aryee, M., Atkinson, C., Bacchus, L.J., *et al*. (2012) A comparative risk assessment of burden of disease and injury attributable to 67 risk factors and risk factor clusters in 21 regions, 1990–2010: a systematic analysis for the Global Burden of Disease Study 2010. *Lancet* 380(9859), 2224–2260.

Lopez, A.D., Mathers, C.D., Ezzati, M., Jamison, D.T. and Murray, C.J. (2006) Global and regional burden of disease and risk factors, 2001: systematic analysis of population health data. *Lancet* 367(9524), 1747–1757.

Malone, J.B., Gommes, R., Hansen, J., Yilma, J.M., Slingenberg, J., Snijders, F., Nachtergaele, F. and Ataman, E. (1998) A geographic information system on the potential distribution and abundance of *Fasciola hepatica*

and *F. gigantica* in east Africa based on Food and Agriculture Organization databases. *Veterinary Parasitology* 78(2), 87–101.
Mohammadi, F., Omidvar, N., Harrison, G.G., Ghazi-Tabatabaei, M., Abdollahi, M., Houshiar-Rad, A., Mehrabi, Y. and Dorosty, A.R. (2013) Is household food insecurity associated with overweight/obesity in women? *Iranian Journal of Public Health* 42(4), 380–390.
Murray, C.J.L. and Lopez, A.D. (2013) Measuring the global burden of disease. *New England Journal of Medicine* 369(5), 448–457.
Muthayya, S., Rah, J.H., Sugimoto, J.D., Roos, F.F., Kraemer, K. and Black, R.E. (2013) The global hidden hunger indices and maps: an advocacy tool for action. *PLoS ONE* 8(6), e67860.
Ramakrishnan, U. and Martorell, R. (1998) The role of vitamin A in reducing child mortality and morbidity and improving growth. *Salud Publica de Mexico* 40(2), 189–198.
Sariozkan, S. and YalCin, C. (2011) Estimating the total cost of bovine fasciolosis in Turkey. *Annals of Tropical Medicine and Parasitology* 105(6), 439–444.
Sauerborn, R., Adams, A. and Hien, M. (1996) Household strategies to cope with the economic costs of illness. *Social Science & Medicine* 43(3), 291–301.
Schelling, E., Daoud, S., Daugla, D., Diallo, P., Tanner, M. and Zinsstag, J. (2005) Morbidity and nutrition patterns of three nomadic pastoralist communities of Chad. *Acta Tropica* 95(1), 16–25.
Shariff, Z.M. and Khor, G.L. (2005) Obesity and household food insecurity: evidence from a sample of rural households in Malaysia. *European Journal of Clinical Nutrition* 59(9), 1049–1058.
Speedy, A. (2003) Animal source foods to improve micronutrient nutrition in developing countries. *Journal of Nutrition* 133, 4048S–4053S.
Steinfeld, H. (2003) Economic constraints on production and consumption of animal source foods for nutrition in developing countries. *Journal of Nutrition* 133, 3875S–3878S.
Steinfeld, H., Gerber, P., Wassenaar, T., Castel, V., Rosales, M. and de Haan, C. (2006) *Livestock's Long Shadow*. Food and Agriculture Organization of the United Nations, Rome.
Stoltzfus, R., Mullany, L. and Black, R. (2004) Iron deficiency anaemia. In: Ezzati, M., Lopez, A., Rodgers, A. and Murray, C. (eds) *Comparative Quantification of Health Risks: global and regional burden of disease attributable to selected major risk factors*. World Health Organization, Geneva, pp. 163–209.
Stradling, C., Hamid, M., Fisher, K., Taheri, S. and Thomas, G.N. (2013) A review of dietary influences on cardiovascular health: Part 1: the role of dietary nutrients. *Cardiovascular & hematological disorders-Drug Targets* 13(3), 208–230.
UN (2000) United Nations Millennium Development Goals. Available at: http://www.un.org/millenniumgoals/poverty.shtml (accessed 22 November 2013).
UN (2012) *Sahel Regional Strategy 2013*. United Nations, New York.
UNICEF (2013) *Improving Child Nutrition: the achievable imperative for global progress*. UNICEF.
Victora, C.G., Adair, L., Fall, C., Hallal, P.C., Martorell, R., Richter, L., Sachdev, H.S. and the Maternal and Child Undernutrition Study Group (2008) Maternal and child undernutrition: consequences for adult health and human capital. *Lancet* 371(9609), 340–357.
WHO (2000) *The Management of Nutrition in Major Emergencies*. World Health Organization, Geneva.
WHO and PHAC (2005) *Preventing Chronic Diseases: a vital investment*. World Health Organization, Geneva; Public Health Agency of Canada, Ottawa.
WHO and UNICEF (1995) *Global Prevalence of Vitamin A Deficiency*. World Health Organization, Geneva.
WHO and UNICEF (2003) *Global Strategy for Infant and Young Child Feeding*. World Health Organization, Geneva.
Zinsstag, J., Schelling, E., Daoud, S., Schierle, J., Hofmann, P., Diguimbaye, C., Daugla, D.M., Ndoutamia, G., Knopf, L., Vounatsou, P. and Tanner, M. (2002) Serum retinol of Chadian nomadic pastoralist women in relation to their livestocks' milk retinol and beta-carotene content. *International Journal for Vitamin and Nutrition Research* 72(4), 221–228.
Zinsstag, J., Roth, F., Orkhon, D., Chimed-Ochir, G., Nansalmaa, M., Kolar, J. and Vounatsou, P. (2005) A model of animal-human brucellosis transmission in Mongolia. *Preventive Veterinary Medicine* 69(1–2), 77–95.
Zinsstag, J., Schelling, E., Roth, F. and Kazwala, R. (2008) Economics of bovine tuberculosis. In: Thoen, C.O., Steele, J.H. and Gilsdorf, M.J. (eds) *Mycobacterium Bovis Infection in Animals and Humans*. Blackwell Publishing Ltd, Oxford, UK, pp. 68–83.
Zoundi, J.S. and Hitimana, L. (2008) *Élevage et marché régional au Sahel et en Afrique de l'Ouest: Potentialités et défis*. Club du Sahel et de l'Afrique de l'Ouest, Paris.

# 24 One Health Into Action: Integrating Global Health Governance with National Priorities in a Globalized World

Anna Okello,[1*] Alain Vandersmissen[2] and Susan C. Welburn[1]
[1]Division of Infection and Pathway Medicine, The University of Edinburgh, UK;
[2]European Union, European External Action Service, Brussels, Belgium

## Introduction

In this chapter we review the evolution of Global Health Governance (GHG), from the early years of International Health Diplomacy in the 19th century, to a discussion of the systems, actors and networks that currently hold a stake in GHG today. Through describing the changing relationships between health policy and practice, the authors explore and provide an analysis of the various options, considerations and challenges that may be required to sustainably operationalize One Health on a global scale in the future.

## Challenges of health governance in a globalized world

Global Health Governance (GHG) in the 'Global Health Decade' (Hotez and Fenwick, 2009) acknowledges the rising stake of 'non-traditional health actors' (Clark *et al.*, 2010) in a sphere previously dominated by a limited number of key actors including the World Health Organization (WHO), the World Organisation for Animal Health (OIE), some bilateral partnerships and several key research institutes. Globalization, re-emerging disease threats, the rise in philanthropic initiatives by private companies and individuals, international pressure to achieve the Millennium Development Goals (MDGs) and the Sustainable Development Goals (SDGs), have all been credited with generating increased visibility and funding for global health issues within the political sphere in recent years. Moving into the second decade of the 21st century, the need to understand and communicate the potential benefits of One Health practices within a wide range of governance contexts is growing.

Mapping the pathways of International Health Diplomacy from the 19th century illustrates several similarities and challenges faced by previous international health actors, many of which remain pertinent to global health today. By examining the evolution of health policy and governance into – and beyond – the 20th century, valuable lessons can be drawn regarding how to navigate the current 'explosion' of often-competing donors, systems and policy narratives that define contemporary GHG networks. Examining the trajectory of WHO since 1948, for example, in light of its

*E-mail: Anna.Okello@ed.ac.uk

'global political legitimacy' (Clark *et al.*, 2010) provides insight into the interconnections, alliances and priorities that have formed within and between the major health actors over time, and within which One Health must become embedded.

The rise of a global public goods (GPG) perspective as a means to 'solve' world health problems is also pertinent in light of the 'broad consensus' that One Health is a public good (CDC and EU, 2011). Addressing global health concerns through health securitization and/or trade policy narratives may not be key priorities in developing countries that provide limited access to trade, and where pressure to prioritize the 'big three' of MDG 6 (HIV/AIDs, malaria and tuberculosis), overwhelm national health budgets. An analysis of options that may serve to motivate and encourage developing countries to invest in alternative One Health approaches is essential.

## Globalization and global health governance

Globalization is defined as the process of increasing social, economic and political interdependence; recognizing that events in one part of the world have an ever-growing effect on people and places in another (Fidler, 2001). Globalization evolves as people, goods, concepts, capital, ideas and values diffuse across national borders, with 'critical implications for public health and global health governance' that affects sustainability of health systems worldwide (Taylor, 2002). However, for many sectors globalization is a double-edged sword, as mass flows of people, animals, goods and services across borders ensure that health determinants, status and outcomes can no longer be guaranteed solely by the actions of individual national governments. This realization drives the current discourse around international collective action that urges health actors to look beyond government sectors to include various private and third-party actors in order better to manage the growing health risks associated with globalization. It has been argued that the effects of globalization may ultimately undermine sovereignty, resulting in changes to traditional health governance whereby nation states are forced to adopt innovative transnational strategies that engage both state and non-state actors, in order to ensure the health of their own country (Ng and Ruger, 2011). External non-health influences can also impact on human, animal and environmental health determinants within a country or region, such as transportation systems, trade, migration (legal and illegal), illicit activities, communication technologies and environmental destruction. Globalization is perceived to amplify such issues, further depleting the extent to which individual nations can fairly, responsibly and sustainably tackle health issues alone (Lee and Pang, 2014). Indeed, the term Global Health Governance has evolved from questions surrounding the ways in which human populations can better meet their increasing collective health needs; loosely defined as 'the agreed rules, processes and institutional arrangements for achieving collective health needs across populations and geographies' (Lee and Pang, 2014).

## The first 100 years of international health governance: 1851–1951

International platforms for public health diplomacy have been in place, in some form, since the 19th century and examining the history of international health governance can provide important lessons that may guide 21st-century decisions (Fidler, 2001). For example, although quarantine practices in Europe can be traced back to the 14th century (Bell *et al.*, 2010), *international* cooperation for control of global risks to human health did not emerge until the mid-19th century. Original shifts from national to international governance evolved largely as a response to increasing public health threats from infectious disease, opium and alcohol, trans-boundary pollution and occupational hazards at the time.

The first International Sanitary Conference occurred in 1851, when European states gathered to discuss cholera, yellow fever and plague. National quarantine policies had become compromised, largely due to technological advances in transportation such as improved rail networks and faster ships, with cholera in particular becoming an important 'emerging' infectious disease of the 19th century (Fidler, 2001).

Following the first International Sanitary Conference, a number of 'global' public health initiatives were established; nation states adopted treaties, staged conferences and created international health organizations with various mandates to facilitate cooperation on infectious disease control (Table 24.1). Science took a lead role in informing policy and treaty development; for example advances in germ theory established by Koch and Pasteur (Fidler, 2001). There followed a rapid expansion of initiatives and actors in international health cooperation, particularly for infectious disease, with the private sector playing a major role in exerting pressure on states to cooperate on laws and policies for control. Several non-governmental organizations including the Rockefeller Foundation and the International Union against Tuberculosis became instrumental in supporting and developing international treaties and laws. By 1951, this movement had resulted in the creation of five international health organizations,[1] the International Sanitary Regulations (a precursor to the International Health Regulations, Box 24.1) and the OIE Codes for animal health (Box 24.2).

Notably, veterinary physicians became early pioneers of transnational response mechanisms for highly contagious and deadly infectious diseases in animals that ultimately led to a similar concept of cross-national coordination

**Table 24.1.** International treaties for human infectious diseases 1892–1951 (adapted from Fidler, 2001).

| Year | Treaty |
|---|---|
| 1892–1912 | Series of seven International Sanitary Conventions (including one Pan-American Sanitary Convention) |
| 1924 | Pan American Sanitary Code |
| | Agreement Respecting Facilities to be Given to Merchant Seaman for the Treatment of Venereal Disease |
| 1926 | International Sanitary Convention, modifying the 1892–1912 International Sanitary Conventions |
| 1927 | Additional protocol added to the Pan American Sanitary Convention |
| 1928 | Pan American Sanitary Convention for Aerial Navigation |
| 1930 | Convention Concerning Anti-Diphtheritic Serum |
| | Agreement regarding measures to be taken against Dengue |
| 1933 | International Sanitary Convention for Aerial Navigation |
| 1934 | International Convention for Mutual Protection Against Dengue Fever |
| 1938 | International Sanitary Convention, amending the 1926 International Sanitary Convention |
| 1944 | International Sanitary Convention, modifying the 1926 International Sanitary Convention |
| 1944 | International Sanitary Convention for Aerial Navigation, modifying the 1933 International Sanitary Convention for Aerial Navigation |
| 1946 | Protocols to Prolong the 1944 International Sanitary Conventions |
| 1951 | International Sanitary Regulations (precursor to the current International Health Regulations, IHR – see Box 24.1). |

**Box 24.1.** International Health Regulations of the WHO.

'To prevent, protect against, control and provide a public health response to the international spread of disease in ways that are commensurate with and restricted to public health risks, and which avoid unnecessary interference with international traffic and trade.' (WHO, 2005)

Consolidation of the numerous sanitary conventions of the 19th and 20th centuries resulted in a single set of rules; officially named the International Health Regulations 1969. The IHR are updated to reflect major changes in the world health picture, for example smallpox eradication in 1981. The only *legally binding* set of international rules on infectious disease control for all 194 WHO member states, the current IHR was endorsed in 2007 to reflect 21st-century threats such as emerging infectious diseases and other public health emergencies such as nuclear meltdowns.

**Box 24.2.** The Codes of the OIE (WTO, 2014).

The World Organisation for Animal Health, recognized by the SPS Agreement, is implementing its mission with various instruments. The most prominent ones are the Animal Health Codes.

The two OIE Codes are the International Animal Health Code (for terrestrial animals: mammals, birds and bees) and the International Aquatic Animal Health Code (for fish, molluscs and crustaceans). The Codes as well as their associated Manuals are designed as reference documents to be used by the veterinary administrations or the competent authorities of the member countries, to assist them in establishing the health regulations that their countries should apply to the import and export of live animals and animal products, so that the spreading of pathogens responsible for diseases to other animals or to human beings is avoided.

In addition to recommendations specific to diseases, the OIE has also developed general principles relating to risk analysis methodology, comprised of four components, namely import risk assessment, assessment of veterinary services, zoning/regionalization, and surveillance and monitoring.

As scientific knowledge on disease agents and their ways of diffusion increases every day, new diagnostic techniques become available, and control methods become more refined, the OIE Codes and Manuals are revised. For the development of OIE recommendations, the procedures within the OIE encourage the active participation of countries in drawing up the rules that will apply both to others and to themselves. These recommendations are established by consensus by members' chief veterinary officers.

The standards of OIE have also proved an important reference point for the dispute settlement mechanisms of the WTO.

of human health services. There are two drivers for this: (i) animal health actors must often consider the needs of a population over the needs of an individual; and (ii) the economic impact of animal diseases is a potentially huge, and often a highly visible, threat. Rinderpest for example, has been of global economic importance since its emergence in Egypt in 3000 BC, with efforts for control beginning in earnest in the 18th century. The unexpected emergence of rinderpest in Belgium in 1920, from a shipment of Zebu cattle transiting in Antwerp en route from India to Brazil, was the motivation for 28 pioneer states to sign an international agreement creating the Office International des Epizooties (OIE), known today as the World Organisation for Animal Health; 27 years before the creation of the United Nations (Table 24.2). Within the European Union (EU), animal health has been a full community competence for a considerable period of time, with attempts to harmonize animal health legislation starting as early as 1957. In contrast human health, even after the Maastricht and Lisbon Treaties, remains mostly a national competence.

The global health situation a century ago 'exhibited the same paradox as has been identified by contemporary analysis of the globalization of public health' (Fidler, 2001). States, non-state actors and international health organizations need to be realistic as to what may be accomplished through international law and other policy templates alone as a means for tackling global health issues.

## Through the eyes of the World Health Organization: the transition from 1950s 'International Health Diplomacy' to the Global Health Governance of the 21st century

Since the inception of the WHO in 1948, tensions between socio-economic and technical approaches to health-care, and the systems for its delivery, have been defined by shifting global politics and dominant international actors (Brown *et al.*, 2006). The role of WHO as 'unquestionable leader' in international health was severely challenged towards the end of the 20th century (Godlee, 1994; Brown *et al.*, 2006; Lidén, 2014). Understanding the changing role of WHO since its formation in 1948 serves to provide a background to the current global health contexts within which One Health finds itself today.

### *Early years of the World Health Organization (1940s and 1950s)*

The concept of permanent institutions for world health trace back to 1902 with the Pan

**Table 24.2.** Agreements made by the World Organisation for Animal Health (OIE) (1924–2014).

| Year | Treaty |
|---|---|
| 1924 | International agreement – 28 states – creating the Office International des Epizooties |
| 1928 | Geneva conference establishing the basis for an international sanitary police |
| 1952 | Agreement with the Food and Agriculture Organization of the United Nations – created in 1951 |
| 1960 | Agreement with the World Health Organization (WHO) |
| 1993 | Agreement with the Inter-American Institute for Cooperation on Agriculture (IICA) |
| 1998 | Agreement with the World Trade Organization (WTO) |
| 1999 | Agreements with the Organismo Internacional de Sanidad Agropecuaria (OIRSA) and the Secretariat of the Pacific Community (SPC) |
| 2000 | Agreement with the Pan-American Health Organization/World Health Organization (PAHO/WHO) |
| 2001 | Agreement with the World Bank |
| 2002 | Agreements with the Organization of African Unity – Inter-African Bureau for Animal Resources (OAU-IBAR), the World Veterinary Association (WVA), the International Federation for Animal Health (IFAH) and various others |
| | New agreement with WHO |
| 2004 | New agreement with FAO. Exchange of letters with the European Commission. Agreements with the Andean Community and various others |
| 2005 | Agreement with the General Secretariat of the South Asian Association for Regional Cooperation (SAARC) and various others |
| | At the Geneva conference of 7–9 November, National Veterinary Services are recognized as a Public Good |
| 2006 | Agreement with the Arab Organization for Agriculture Development (AOAD) |
| 2007 | Agreement with the Economic Community of West African States and five others |
| 2008 | Agreement with the International Council for the Exploration of the Sea (ICES), the International Air Transport Association (IATA), the Inter-American Development Bank (IDN), the West African Economic and Monetary Union (WAEMU), the International Poultry Council (IPC) and the International Council for Laboratory Animal Science (ICLAS) |
| 2009 | Cooperation agreement with the WAEMU |
| 2011 | Agreement with the International Council for Game and Wildlife Conservation (CIC), the Arab Maghreb Union (AMU), the International Organization for Standardization (ISO) and the World Small Animal Veterinary Association (WSAVA) |
| 2012 | Agreement with the United Nations Office for Disarmament Affairs (UNODA), the International Union for Conservation of Nature and Natural Resources (IUCN), the Caribbean Community (CARICOM) and the Commonwealth Veterinary Association (CVA) |

American Sanitary Bureau, which eventually became the Pan American Health Organization (PAHO). In 1907, the Office International d'Hygiène Publique (OIHP) was mandated with the overall administration of the international sanitary agreements (Table 24.1). In 1923, the Health Organization of the League of Nations established its offices in Geneva, extending the work of the OIHP through supporting international disease commissions via epidemiological intelligence and technical reports. The formal establishment of the WHO constitution occurred on 7 April 1948, incorporating the OIHP, the League of Nations Health Organization and the Health division of the UN Relief and Rehabilitation Administration (UNRRA). Early indications of possible tensions between the European health actors and the USA were evident however, when the Pan American Health Organization (PAHO) opted to remain autonomous in the Americas in the interest of 'national security' (Brown *et al.*, 2006).

### *African independence and shifting world power relations (1960s and 1970s)*

The 1960s and 1970s saw emphasis on socio-economic reforms, attributed to independence from former colonial powers and the spread of socialist movements such as the civil rights movement in the USA. Unlike the World

Bank and other large agencies where national votes are weighted according to financial contribution, all member states of the WHO share an equal vote in the World Health Assembly (WHA). The broadening WHO agenda during this period is largely attributed to this increase in WHO member-states – by the late 1960s, Latin American, Asian and African states held over two-thirds majority in the WHA (Walt, 1993). WHO's technical mandate had largely spared it the 'political conflicts wracking the rest of the United Nations', but the new demands of health systems in developing nations was the beginning of WHO's 'key role' in international health policy (Godlee, 1994; Brown *et al.*, 2006).

### *World Health Organization in crisis (1980s and 1990s)*

The 1990s saw a rise in publications in prominent journals that both questioned and affirmed the role at the time of the WHO, reflecting the wider dialogue (Walt, 1993; Godlee, 1994; Lee *et al.*, 1996; Vaughan *et al.*, 1996; Silver, 1998; Yach and Bettcher, 1998). Extra budgetary funding overtook that from WHO member states for the first time in 1991 (Table 24.3) resulting in the World Bank, United Nations Development Programme (UNDP) and wealthier nation states 'largely calling the shots' through a series of vertical programmes (Walt, 1993). Demands for the international health agenda to align with donor interests led to 'a cycle of decline, with donors expressing their lack of faith in its central management by placing funds outside the management's control' (Walt and Gilson, 1994).

**Table 24.3.** Shifting trends in WHO extra budgetary funding 1950–2011.

| Year | WHO budget Member States (US$ million) | Extra budgetary funding (US$ million) |
|---|---|---|
| 1950 | 6 | 0 |
| 1971 | 75 | <25 |
| 1986–1987 | 543 | 437 |
| 1990–1991 | 654 | 770 |
| 1998–1999 | 842 | 956 |
| 2002–2003 | 830 | 1.5 bn |
| 2010–2011 | 945 | 2.9 bn |

### *Increased 'growth and complexity' of the World Health Organization (1998–2003)*

Former Norwegian Prime Minister Dr Gro Harlem Brundtland was appointed in 1998 to revitalize and reposition WHO as a key actor in global health (Kickbusch, 2000; Lidén, 2014). Brundtland's leadership saw the emergence of the 'Global Health Decade' (Hotez and Fenwick, 2009). Stakeholders from the private and non-governmental sectors were brought together with governments and other agencies to strengthen WHO's financial position, expanding extra-budgetary funding and leading to an explosion of public–private partnerships (later termed Global Health Initiatives or GHIs). Brundtland oversaw the creation of new initiatives where gaps were perceived in the health architecture, or where actors required greater coordination or dialogue (Lidén, 2014). These new initiatives included Roll Back Malaria (1998), the Global Alliance for Vaccines and Immunisation (GAVI) (1999), the Medicines for Malaria Venture (MMV, 1999), Stop TB (2001), the Global Programme to Eliminate Lymphatic Filariasis (GPELF, 2000) and the Global Fund (2002). With a 'general consensus' that its leadership had improved, WHO again became 'a credible and highly visible contributor' to the global health agenda (Brown *et al.*, 2006; Lidén, 2014).

### *Further loss of the World Health Organization's traction in global health matters (2003 onwards)*

Between 1998 and 2003 health become a 'central theme' on the international political agenda, with a myriad of externally funded health partnerships and alliances and philanthropic organizations such as The Bill & Melinda Gates Foundation rising in prominence; by 2005 over 70 international partnerships had been created. However, the technical mandate of the WHO, historically its strongest advantage, was slipping away as Global Health Actors (GHAs) gained traction and confidence in their expertise on health matters, for example, the US President's Emergency Plan for AIDS Relief (PEPFAR) sought expertise from American academic institutes and non-governmental organizations rather than from the WHO (Lidén, 2014). Moreover, the perceived disconnect between the national health ministries that govern the WHA, and those responsible for financing health issues, appeared to be growing, challenging the organization's ability to reform and provide the much-needed direction and leadership of the global health agenda (Lidén, 2014).

In conclusion, fundamental events in the history of WHO have been heavily influenced and shaped by overarching global political events and a rapidly changing health landscape since the end of World War II. The independence from former colonial powers in the 1960s, followed by shifting financial leadership in the 1980s and the rising fear of 'global health threats' towards the end of the 20th century (driven largely by the HIV/AIDS epidemic and political and economic turbulence following the collapse of the Soviet Union) all illustrate the close linkages between global health indicators and political events.

## The Drivers for One Health's Increasing Political Traction in the First Decade of the 21st Century

### From HIV to SARS: health securitization as an early driver for One Health

The emergence of high-profile emerging disease threats such as SARS and H5N1 highly pathogenic avian influenza (HPAI) in the early 2000s helped propel a new concept, One Health, into the centre of global health policy dialogue. Securitization describes the politicization (in relation to security concerns) of an issue that was previously not a major issue for the public, or at least not a reason to fear; a 'model that explains the transition by which an issue such as influenza can be moved from the non-political sphere to the political sphere, and ultimately into the realm of security' (Collins, 2007). Securitization of a topic demands a combination of two key elements; (i) the voice of a credible authority; and (ii) the belief of the listeners. Once an issue is perceived as negative to a country's or region's well-being, for example, in terms of human deaths, high costs of control, or long-term detriment to financial and natural resources, it becomes increasingly important to utilize part of a nation's resources to protect against the threat in question (Leboeuf and Broughton, 2008).

The 'Health as Securitization' narrative has emerged frequently in recent years – particularly in the context of emerging infectious diseases and One Health. However, the notion of controlling disease in another country for the benefit of one's own has existed for much longer. A speaker at the third session of a joint WHO/FAO meeting on malaria in 1948 claimed: 'Africa cannot be fully exploited, because of the danger of flies and mosquitoes; if we can control them the prosperity of Europe will be enhanced' (Packard, 1997). Similar views were expressed during the 1950s and 1960s, with the belief that health improvements in developing countries would expand markets for US goods (Packard, 1997). Malaria control was used as a political tool for 'winning hearts and minds' of underdeveloped nations in the war against communism (Brown *et al.*, 2006). Towards the end of the 20th century, health became increasingly conceptualized as 'a limited resource to be defended'; US President Bill Clinton famously stated that infectious diseases such as HIV posed 'a threat to US national security because of its catastrophic social consequences, particularly in the developing world' (Leboeuf and Broughton, 2008).

Health securitization can have both positive and negative impacts on how a health issue is managed, both by politicians and the implementers of health policy. The high-profile securitization of HIV/AIDS undoubtedly resulted in a huge amount of advocacy and resources; including the creation of a specific UN agency (UNAIDS), explicit reference in the MDGs and debate at the UN Security Council (Leboeuf and Broughton, 2008). However, those working at the community level to 'normalize social perceptions' of HIV/AIDS in many countries viewed this approach to disease control through the 'narrow framework of security' as detrimental to HIV-positive individuals, 'wrongly identified as the risk rather than the referent object' (Elbe, 2006; Collins, 2007). The same could be said for any high-profile disease including

SARS, HPAI and tuberculosis, highlighting the fine line between the health rights of the nation versus the health rights of its individual citizens in the era of globalization.

*Health securitization case study 1: severe acute respiratory syndrome in 2003: the 'nail in the coffin' for conventional international health governance*

Severe acute respiratory syndrome (SARS), the 'first severe infectious disease to emerge in the globalized society of the 21st century', is considered to have permanently changed the way in which global health is governed. SARS was a new disease and therefore not subject to the IHR (Fidler, 2004) and the international response to SARS led to a permanent 'change in attitude' by the traditional gatekeepers of disease control, culminating in a renewed version of the IHR being approved in 2005 (Lidén, 2014). The SARS response demonstrated how epidemiological information in a globalized world does not respect sovereignty. When the Chinese government showed reluctance to report openly on the magnitude of the problem in China, WHO had to rely on innovative approaches to gain epidemiological information, including the media, the Internet and individual case reports. Previous restrictions on external international agencies to 'dictate' outbreak control measures in the name of sovereignty were overruled, with the WHO demonstrating an unprecedented power over nation states at the time (Fidler, 2004; Lidén, 2014). Ethical issues also arose during management of the SARS outbreak; for example the balance of professional duty with fears for personal safety, economic losses against containment of disease and other balancing acts required to ensure public health while simultaneously protecting human rights (Singer *et al.*, 2003; Fidler, 2004).

*Health securitization case study 2: the unprecedented global response to avian influenza*

The Global Response to Avian Influenza (GRAI) is based on a political initiative launched at the first International Ministerial Conference on Avian and Pandemic Influenza (IMCAPI) in Beijing, January 2006, triggered by the EU. The GRAI was founded on strong ad hoc collaboration and joint leadership of the EU, the USA and the United Nations System Influenza Coordination (UNSIC) office, who, in collaboration with the World Bank, the OIE and relevant UN agencies, developed policies and set up mechanisms for the crisis response. A major outcome of the GRAI has been the successful coordination at the international level between political stakeholders, development partners, UN agencies and the OIE. Control of HPAI continues to attract considerable investment, primarily driven by policy narratives around global health security and pandemic preparedness (EU, 2010).

The GRAI benefited from two closely related drivers. The first was the process of securitization of previous sanitary crises, largely due to SARS but also from weaknesses in responses to several natural catastrophes (e.g. the heat wave in France in summer 2003 and Hurricane Katrina in the USA in August 2005). The second was the rapid setup of partnerships directed against H5N1, including strong leadership from the EU and the USA that together contributed the political driving force for broader networking from individual countries, the UN, the OIE and the World Bank.

Partnerships established through the GRAI provided a firm foundation for the development and application of One Health approaches globally, further translated into strategies and policies at sub-national levels (Okello *et al.*, 2011). The One Health approach was put forward on the international scene at the 3rd IMCAPI in New Delhi in December 2007 and a joint strategic framework developed by FAO, OIE, WHO, UNSIC, UNICEF and the World Bank (FAO *et al.*, 2008) was presented at the 4th IMCAPI in 2008 in Sharm-el-Sheikh.

In 2010 the tripartite (FAO, OIE, WHO) published a concept note on sharing responsibilities, collaboration and coordination of global activities and integration of control systems for disease control. This concept note acknowledges that while integration has been attempted in some countries, there remains limited collaborative work in the control systems of many countries (FAO *et al.*, 2010). This led to the tripartite High-Level Technical Meeting (HLTM) of 2011 in Mexico providing a platform for stakeholders to discuss priorities at the human–animal–ecosystem interface within the One Health vision (USAID *et al.*, 2011). The HLTM highlighted rabies as an important topic along with zoonotic influenza and antimicrobial resistance; a positive sign that advocacy for these diseases may be increasing. This interaction between stakeholders from these three sectors encouraged by the tripartite and the collaboration in control efforts may serve to pave the way for zoonotic diseases to move higher on the agenda of disease control and international health (Vandersmissen and Welburn, 2014).

## Expanding the securitization narrative – One Health as a global public good?

Global Public Good (GPG) theory offers a second political narrative for global health approaches that builds on health securitization. A public good is that which is non-excludable and non-rival: one person's consumption does not restrict its availability to another, and everyone in a particular community can simultaneously benefit from its provision. This is in contrast to private goods, which demonstrate high excludability and high rivalry; those who do not or cannot afford to pay will not benefit, and once the good is 'consumed', it cannot be consumed again. In the economic context, GPGs can be thought of as 'public goods with significant cross border benefits on a global level' (Smith *et al.*, 2004). An expanded definition of GPG pertaining to health is 'a good which it is rational, from the perspective of a group of nations collectively, to produce for universal consumption and for which it is irrational to exclude an individual nation from consuming' (Smith and MacKellar, 2007).

In terms of infectious disease control, One Health principles align well with a key component of GPG theory: the promotion of *international collective action*, a political process that ensures the benefits of controlling a disease within one's country are maintained in the absence of 'free-riding' by other nations (Smith, 2003; Smith *et al.*, 2004). However, interventions for the control of diseases that only occur within a specific socio-economic or geographic domain – for example the suite of neglected tropical diseases – cannot be promoted as a true GPG. Some have also argued that GPG theory has 'fuelled the proliferation of specific infectious disease-targeted programmes' (Smith and MacKellar, 2007). Promoting One Health as a GPG could therefore inadvertently encourage the recent explosion of vertical approaches to health challenges, such as seen with the international response to HPAI and numerous GHIs, conflicting with wider philosophies surrounding horizontal and more holistic approaches to health outside a crisis situation.

## One Health as a means to refocus attention on strengthening health systems and integrated approaches to disease control

Concerns about the large investments that have been directed into vertical disease approaches for HPAI and the 'big three' (HIV/AIDS, tuberculosis and malaria) have been raised in recent years (England, 2007; Leboeuf and Broughton, 2008; Molyneux, 2008; Maudlin *et al.*, 2009). Opponents argue that the tendency for GHIs to concentrate resources on single disease interventions can result in the creation of parallel systems outside of existing health systems, leading to criticism that GHIs are ignoring the state of health *systems* in many countries (Marchal *et al.*, 2009). The entire 2005, Uganda Ministry of Health budget (US$112 million) was swamped by US$167 million in HIV/AIDS funding from PEPFAR, the World Bank and the Global Fund (Marchal *et al.*, 2009).

Rhetoric surrounding integrated approaches to disease control and strengthening of the wider health systems in developing countries is often in stark contrast with the reality of the 'top down efforts to control particular diseases, one at a time' that has emerged in recent years (de Savigny *et al.*, 2004). Increased funding from a number of GHIs has also resulted in concern that pressure to demonstrate 'impact' has created a bias against a longer term, more systemic approach to health care (de Savigny *et al.*, 2004). This is compounded by the fact that the 'systems thinking' mechanism evolved relatively late in global health discourse; even now our understanding of how to improve health systems, and the available frameworks for doing so, remain limited (de Savigny *et al.*, 2004; de Savigny and Adam, 2009). The result is that despite the huge increases in spending on global health, many global health systems do not have the processes in place to accurately measure their weaknesses and constraints, leaving policy makers 'unsure of what should actually be strengthened' (de Savigny *et al.*, 2004).

It is this third narrative, promoting integrated approaches and a more participatory, problem-focused approach to disease control and health system management at the district level, that has afforded One Health further traction in recent years away from the pandemic to endemic narrative (Bechir *et al.*, 2004; Schelling *et al.*, 2005; Zinsstag *et al.*, 2007; Okello *et al.*, 2011; Godfroid *et al.*, 2013; Leach and Scoones, 2013; Vandersmissen and Welburn, 2014). The realization that packaged, integrated solutions to human and animal health are vital to avoid overburdening district health units has led to several projects promoting integrated interventions and effective approaches to coexisting health issues, as opposed to 'stand alone interventions' (de Savigny *et al.*, 2004; de Savigny and Adam, 2009; ICONZ, 2014).

Political support for a transdisciplinary One Health approach to endemic disease control is growing. Many One Health networks are emerging across Asia and Africa that are applying a One Health approach for both epidemic and endemic zoonoses (Saarnak *et al.*, 2014; Vandersmissen and Welburn, 2014). There is greater recognition that 'packaged' interventions simultaneously addressing a variety of health conditions for both humans and animals may reduce the risk of disease emergence and re-emergence if delivered via a sustainable livelihoods approach (WHO *et al.*, 2006, 2009, 2011). For example, the joint human and animal vaccine services for pastoralists in Chad demonstrates some of the earliest evidence of One Health in the 21st century; the focus on the district health offices remained central to the intervention (Bechir *et al.*, 2004; Schelling *et al.*, 2005; Schelling *et al.*, Chapter 20, this volume).

The growing evidence for the advantages of joint human–animal health systems in the diagnosis, prevention and control of the neglected zoonotic diseases (NZDs) has led to an overarching recommendation to 'work towards the concept of One Health' (WHO *et al.*, 2006; Maudlin *et al.*, 2009). A One Health approach for the NZDs in Africa is now firmly acknowledged, targeting eight endemic diseases: anthrax, bovine tuberculosis, brucellosis, cysticercosis, cystic echinococcosis, leishmaniasis, rabies and zoonotic trypanosomiasis (WHO *et al.*, 2006; Maudlin *et al.*, 2009; Gibbs, 2014).

## One Health Policy into Practice: Actors, Networks and Partnerships

### Examining the interrelationships between prominent global health actors and their role in One Health

The realization that diseases such as SARS, HIV/AIDS and HPAI could affect nations regardless of their geographic location, resulted in a 'new urgency to address health on a global scale' (Ng and Ruger, 2011). Today within the global health sector alone, there are estimated to be over 40 bilateral donors, 26 UN agencies, 20 global and regional funds and 90 global health initiatives (Sridhar, 2010). Despite criticisms that there is 'no architecture to global health', a review of recent literature implies a vaguely defined structure does indeed exist, captured in Fig. 24.1 (Ng and Ruger, 2011).

#### *Nation states*

Individual nation states maintain an ongoing responsibility for GHG, with bilateral funding still comprising most international health assistance (Ng and Ruger, 2011). Disease surveillance and control depends on the capacity and cooperation of nation states as implementers of international decisions, pertinently seen with China's response to requests

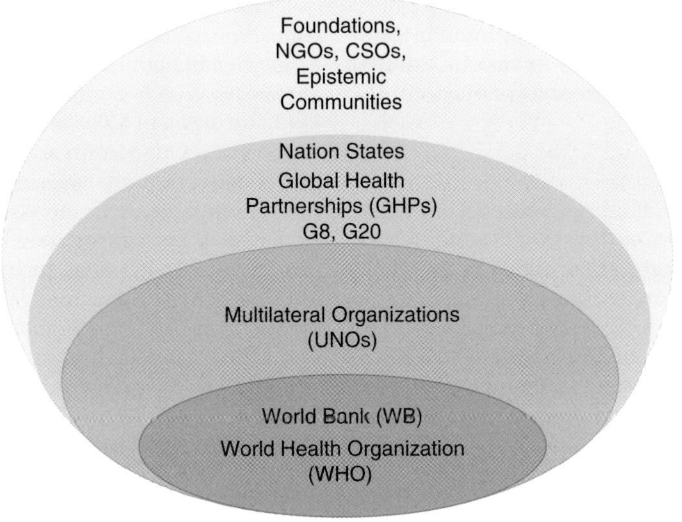


**Fig. 24.1.** Prominent global health governance actors in the 21st century (Ng and Ruger, 2011).

for information during the SARS outbreak. Individual nations, particularly the rich and powerful, can affect health outcomes through trade agreements and agenda setting within the WHO, for example through the provision of extra-budgetary funding.

In terms of One Health, several nation states have promoted the approach within various national or regional frameworks. For example in the Asia Pacific region, national-level platforms have become key for building surveillance capacity, supporting implementation of the International Health Regulations and frameworks such as APSED. These platforms are also essential for the bi-regional strategy of WHO South and East Asia Regional Office (SEARO) and Western Pacific Regional Office (WPRO). At the district level in some countries, participatory One Health platforms further build local leadership, ownership, together enabling a transdisciplinary culture to tackle health and ecosystem challenges.

In Africa, the national response to sleeping sickness and animal trypanosomiasis in Uganda is a good example of a One Health working platform (Welburn and Coleman, Chapter 18, this volume). The Co-ordinating Office for the Control of Trypanosomiasis in Uganda (COCTU) is the formal Secretariat of the Ugandan Trypanosomiasis Control Council (UTCC) formed by a parliamentary act in 1992. This permanently funded inter-ministerial platform coordinates policy for all stakeholders involved in tsetse and trypanosomiasis control in Uganda. Both forms of human sleeping sickness, and all forms of nagana, are managed in coordination by COCTU to deliver a cross-sectoral response to human and animal disease. Sleeping sickness is normally endemic but can rapidly become epidemic due to a range of human, animal and ecological factors. It is perhaps not surprising that lessons learned from over 100 years of human and animal disease control resulted in a One Health platform for disease management and risk mitigation for this particular disease.

One Health approaches have also been implemented at the national level in several developed countries; examples include the key role of the Canadian Public Health Agency in launching the process of 'operationalizing One Health' (Public Health Agency of Canada, 2009; CDC, 2010). The US Department of State has been crucial to the GRAI, along with the creation of One Health structures in the US Department of Agriculture and the US Centers for Disease Control (CDC). In Europe, the EU has also made One Health the flagship of its veterinary public health policy at domestic level, aside from promoting and integrating the approach in various external actions (Vandersmissen and Welburn, 2014).

### *United Nations organizations*

Outside the WHO, broad-based UN development agencies such as UNDP and UNICEF have increasingly been accused of 'taking the initiative' on health, resulting in some degree of animosity between the agencies. The 1993 launch of UNAIDS effectively removed WHO's largest budget from its control (Godlee, 1994), while the 1990 Children's Vaccine Initiative proposed by UNICEF, UNDP, Rockefeller and several others was seen by the WHO as nothing less than an 'attempted coup' on WHO (Muraskin, 1998; Brown *et al.*, 2006). Despite these shortcomings, and in the absence of any real alternative, the WHO remains for now the authoritative voice on GHG, with its perceived neutrality on health issues offering combined 'institutional mandate, legal authority and public health expertise' (Ng and Ruger, 2011). Whilst WHO's relationship with the Food and Agriculture Organization of the United Nations (FAO) has been at times strained, particularly regarding the priority given to veterinary public health in the organization, the GRAI was instrumental in building alliances between these UN agencies, resulting in the unprecedented WHO/FAO/OIE tripartite partnership that promoted integration of foodborne, neglected zoonotic and tropical diseases within the One Health movement.

### *The World Organisation for Animal Health*

The OIE Codes (for Terrestrial and Aquatic Animals) adopted and applied by the 178 OIE member states have constantly been ahead of similar mechanisms in human health; over 50 agreements with political and technical organizations have been made since 1952. The highly centralized normative power of the OIE and its link to international trade may explain this profound influence of the OIE on its members (more so than those of WHO or the FAO).

OIE, as the 'guardian of the Codes', took some time to consider whether embarking on a One Health path was realistic and appropriate (as did WHO). Once OIE became committed to the concept (2008 onwards), the amplification of a One Health approach across the global network of the veterinary services has been impressive, with the veterinary profession widely promoting the One Health approach to address issues such as food safety, food security, antimicrobial resistance, climate change and the human–animal bond. The GRAI promoted alliances between the OIE and UN agencies to develop the Global Early Warning System (GLEWS) that builds on the added value of combining and coordinating alert mechanisms for WHO, FAO and OIE. The 2009 H1N1 influenza pandemic, quickly and successfully controlled largely as a result of the coordination mechanisms developed for H5N1, served to further strengthen the relationship between the WHO and OIE. If One Health is going to survive, it is axiomatic that the veterinary profession remains a strong advocate of multidisciplinary approaches to solving the complex challenges of global health and is in a position to provide decisive leadership. The sustained response of the veterinary profession in meeting the precepts and being a champion of One Health is a litmus test for the future of the profession (Gibbs and Gibbs, 2013; Gibbs, 2014).

### *The World Trade Organization, World Bank, G8, G20*

The World Bank is considered by some to have the ultimate power in setting the global health agenda, with its increasing recognition of the linkages between human health and development and ability to mobilize huge amounts of funds – often exceeding the WHO's total annual budget – affording them a large stake in GHG (Ng and Ruger, 2011). From the first loan for family planning in 1970 to the establishment of the Department of Population, Health and Nutrition in 1979, it is argued that World Bank assistance to governments could help overcome developing-country health problems while simultaneously promoting economic growth (Brown *et al.*, 2006). In terms of One Health, the World Bank has maintained a presence in the international dialogue, being an important stakeholder for the GRAI and a contributing member to the aforementioned 2008 Strategic Framework.

The World Trade Organization (WTO) is also becoming an increasingly important 21st-century stakeholder in global health. Trade regimes controlled by the WTO can have a significant impact on access to medicines and other health system inputs, as well as influencing the distribution of non-communicable disease risks such as tobacco and food safety. For animal health, the Marrakech Agreement in April 1994 that established the WTO and the agreement of May 2008 between the OIE and WTO have considerably reinforced the role and the powers of OIE, with OIE standards becoming an important reference point in trade relations (in particular in the dispute settlement mechanisms) of the WTO.

The G8 has been flagged as a potential 21st-century leader in global health, with examples such as the Global Fund emerging out of this informal and therefore relatively flexible network (Ng and Ruger, 2011). Concerns have nevertheless been raised as to the extent to which the G8 can make objective decisions about global health, given its access to significant human and financial resources, or conversely, feel forced to act given their status; a phenomenon described as the 'great global guilt trip' (Garrett and Alavian, 2010). Alternatively, the G20, of which most member states are developing or recently emerging economies such as Brazil, China, Indonesia and Egypt, have been suggested as potentially powerful stakeholders in future health governance, particularly since they are 'not vulnerable to such pleas to share their wealth' (Garrett and Alavian, 2010). Whereas the G8 has traditionally used health within a security or development narrative, the G20 appears to be using health to pursue some quite different policy issues, for example Indonesia's recent challenge to the WHO's long-standing influenza virus sharing agreements (Fidler, 2004). Despite this, there is hope the G20 countries will 'voice' the concerns of the developing world in the global health agenda, particularly against trade and intellectual property rules that for example hinder access to medicines. However, there are growing economic concerns of several G8 countries as to the future role of the G20 within global health power.

### *Non-government organizations and civil society organizations*

Non-government organizations (NGOs) and civil society organizations (CSOs) are considered by some to have the greatest potential to override national state efforts in health service delivery in many low-income countries (Ng and Ruger, 2011). NGOs now wield a considerably larger influence on GHG than they did previously, partly through their access to communities and resulting flexibility towards health issues that may lie outside existing government agendas, and partly through their admission as formal stakeholders on the Global Fund, GAVI, UNITAID and UNAIDS boards (Lidén, 2014). However, competition for donor funds, territorialization and underlying religious mandates can all affect the design and delivery of health programmes to beneficiaries. Questions of NGO accountability are often raised, with accusations that the highly inflated salaries and benefits paid to NGO staff in developing countries result in 'brain drain' from national administrations, research institutes and government departments (Ng and Ruger, 2011). (See also Stephen and Waltner-Toews, Chapter 32, this volume.)

### *The private sector, public–private partnerships and philanthropic foundations*

The explosion of private sector and philanthropic authority into the arena of global health into the 21st century has been highly visible. Some have attributed this to the 'longer standing trend towards the private' as a result of World Bank structural adjustment programmes, whilst others credit it to the new direction taken by WHO under Brundtland (Williams and Rushton, 2011). Historically, philanthropy and health have always held close interconnections; for example the Rockefeller Foundation played a lead role in attempts at global malaria eradication in the 1960s (Brown *et al.*, 2006). The current weight of private philanthropic foundations, of which the Bill & Melinda Gates Foundation is probably the most influential at present, is unprecedented: 'When Bill speaks, they listen. And as long as the Gates Foundation has the ability to deploy such huge resources, these organizations will continue to listen' (Williams and Rushton, 2011).

Despite the positives, reports of 'unease and some tension' at the decreasing financial importance, and thus influence, of traditional health actors are beginning to surface. For example consider claims that spending on global health by the Bill & Melinda Gates Foundation in 2007 was almost equal to WHO's annual budget for the same year (Clark *et al.*, 2010). There are reservations about the long-term sustainability of public–private partnerships (PPPs), with fears that private sector actors, particularly the smaller or less publicized, could be tempted to use development projects as a public relations manoeuvre, promoting short-term corporate social responsibility (CSR) strategies to the detriment of any long-term investment into actual change. Others maintain that 'the private sector reaps the benefits whilst the public sector carries the risk', thus jeopardizing long-term, sustainable approaches to improvement of health systems in developing countries (Ollila, 2005; Ng and Rugen, 2011).

Despite some advances in recent years, most notably in the veterinary sector, the engagement of NGOs, the private sector and PPPs in the One Health movement is still limited. There appears to be little mention of One Health in the numerous Global Health Initiatives focused on human health and livelihoods; for example despite the GAVI Alliance describing the 'added value' of vaccination programmes (http://www.gavialliance.org/About/Value/Added-value), there is as yet no specific reference to working in a One Health space. Conversely, similar global health approaches driven by the veterinary sector are strong supporters of One Health; for example the Global Alliance for Rabies Control[2] (GARC) (Léchenne *et al.*, Chapter 16, this volume) and the Global Alliance for Livestock Veterinary Medicines[3] (GALVmed). Similarly for the private sector, relatively few acknowledgements of One Health exist, again the exceptions being mainly from the veterinary sector, for example the veterinary pharmaceutical company CEVA Santé Animale.[4] Opportunities for greater inclusion of One Health approaches to be utilized by these agencies, alliances and companies, for example the promotion of joint human and animal vaccination programmes, should be identified and acted upon in order to improve the efficacy of existing efforts.

The overwhelming message arising from this analysis of the multitude of actors, networks and alliances that govern global health today is the requirement for *balance*: to balance the needs of individuals with that of populations, of donors with their beneficiaries, of agenda-setting from powerful GHIs with the traditional technical and research actors with the ability to adequately address systemic issues in health service delivery. It is within this complex maze of interactions that One Health could potentially play a role of 'overseer'. Through exerting a non-biased authority over cooperation and collaboration between differing GHAs, One Health could help ensure the underlying philosophies of a holistic approach to health – incorporating transdisciplinarity and a *whole of systems* approach – remains prominent.

## One movement, many interpretations: is governing One Health 'mission impossible'?

Operationalizing One Health is founded on strong linkages between human and animal health, environment and policies. Advocacy, political support, governance and networks are crucial building blocks for One Health sustainability. The acceleration of institutional and individual effort to promote One Health led to a concern that obtaining a complete picture of what was going on was almost impossible, resulting in an urgent need for 'a global network of networks to optimize information sharing globally and to keep information up to date' (quote by Alain Vandersmissen, cited in CDC and EU, 2011). Whilst conceding that One Health should not be 'owned' by any single organization or institution, a requirement for some form of coordinating body to keep all the 'puzzle pieces' of One Health current and relevant has been acknowledged (CDC and EU, 2011).

The concept of a One Health Global Network[5] (OHGN) and the web portal attached to it emerged from a 'How to Make It Happen' expert-based process that began in 2009 in Winnipeg, Canada, that was further refined in 2010 at Stone Mountain, USA and in 2011 in Atlanta, USA (Okello *et al.*, 2011; Vandersmissen and Welburn, 2014). The OHGN Working Group was given two specific objectives: (i) to advocate and garner international support for One Health; and (ii) to promote One Health and enable connectivity through a centralized area (CDC, 2010). As a first step towards development of the OHGN, test phase questionnaires were sent to 29 'key One Health respondents' in June 2011, to gain their insights as to what One Health was perceived to be and what a 'network of networks' could look like. All respondents were familiar with the One Health approach; but their understanding of it varied, usually in accordance to their professional background or representative institution. There was consensus that One Health involved 'to some extent' the integration of disciplines across human and animal health; but responses were largely biased towards epidemic and zoonotic diseases, with little reference to the wildlife/ecosystem aspects and the endemic or non-communicable diseases. One respondent mentioned the economic benefits of interdisciplinary collaboration: '(One Health) is any added value in terms of health gains in all species, or economic savings from closer cooperation ... if we cannot show such an added value in any way it is not really "One Health"' (Key informant, 2011) (Zinsstag *et al.*, Chapter 5, this volume). Two respondents mentioned the need for One Health to be 'sustainable and locally relevant', broadening the definition from Scoones' 'outbreak narrative' (Scoones, 2010). A valuable concluding remark captured what many One Health advocates feel to be a weakness for One health to date, highlighting the 'unfinished agenda' of interdisciplinary collaboration: 'One Health is mainly supported and known by animal health specialists ... a strong outreach effort towards human health, wildlife and environment specialists, development specialists and economists should be supported by the network, and all of its members who all have connections in fields other than animal health' (Key Informant, 2011).

The first Expert Meeting on One Health Governance and the Global Network was held in November 2011 in Atlanta, USA. The meeting convened 20 One Health experts to develop a proposal for the governance of One Health, while recognizing it is not necessary for any one organization to 'own' or 'lead' the approach and to consolidate the nascent OHGN. Many were not comfortable with the word 'governance' and consensus was to form of a 'One Health Global Guidance Group' – the '3G' (emphasizing 'governance with a small g') with a mandate that includes advocacy, championing of One Health approaches, provision of input into a biannual One Health conference, and facilitating and enabling collaboration, connection and synergies, including funding opportunities.

The question today is not 'how to set up and sustain a One Health movement' but how to monitor its rapid growth and establish a model of governance that is acceptable to all One Health stakeholders. The emerging OHGN does not aim to replace any existing One Health initiative or structure (e.g. http://www.onehealthinitiative.com), but rather proposes a 'network of networks' with the website serving as a portal to One Health websites, case studies and resources. The group of experts providing voluntary contributions to the development of the network supports a soft governance structure for the One Health movement. The choice of soft governance for the emerging One Health movement is both unique and challenging, the complexities of One Health governance appear similar to the challenges surrounding any global health approach in the fast moving, multi-actor 21st century. The emergence of One Health as a discipline at professional and academic level together with the growing references to a One Health culture undoubtedly offers new opportunities (Gibbs, 2014).

## Maintaining and Building One Health Momentum – How Can Existing Global Health Actors, Networks and Alliances Promote a Global Approach in the Future?

### Demonstrate the added value of One Health

Universally it is accepted that One Health expertise is required to tackle the human, animal and environmental challenges of the 21st century – to identify, control and manage human and animal diseases in complex ecosystems and mitigate risk (Zinsstag *et al.*, 2007; Okello *et al.*, 2011; Welburn, 2011). Prevention of disease outbreaks is economically preferable to addressing a global pandemic. However, preventative measures require long-term financial commitments, difficult to justify if the total health impact is not calculated in national, regional or even global terms. Validated evidence demonstrating the added value of One Health in socio-economic terms is therefore the key to the sustainability of the approach. Estimations of total societal burden of emerging and endemic zoonoses (the combined human, animal and environmental costs of disease for the public and private sectors including indirect impacts on food security of smallholder farmers and micro- and macroeconomic impacts of disease on livestock productivity losses and health) can provide compelling evidence for the value of operationalizing One Health (Narrod *et al.*, 2012).

Determination of the combined human, animal and environmental costs of disease to both the public and private sectors should therefore be prioritized by One Health practitioners, incorporating indirect impacts on food security of smallholder farmers with the economic effect of disease on livestock productivity and health. Operationalizing One Health in this way requires an appreciation and validation of the multi-disciplinary linkages between human and animal health, ecosystems, livelihoods and policy processes, demanding support and consultation from all sectors or industries with a stake in health governance (Public Health Agency of Canada, 2009; CDC, 2010; USAID *et al.*, 2011; FAO *et al.*, 2012).

### Build on existing regional and sub-national platforms for One Health

To date, the threat of emerging pandemics has been a major driver for the proliferation of One Health projects and platforms that attempt to link animal, human and ecosystem health at both national and transnational levels, for example the Asia Pacific Strategy for Emerging Diseases (APSED) (Association of Southeast Asian Nations, 2010; UNSIC and World Bank, 2010; European Commission, 2011a,b; European Union, 2011).

The challenge across all regions is to support, build upon and broaden the existing One Health platforms that were established for detection of emerging threats to encompass the endemic infectious disease burden of communities. Long-term institutional approaches to zoonoses management that sustainably strengthen the regional and national institutional base for One Health will require a rigorous assessment of governance structures, policy processes and actor-networks, to better understand and inform decision-makers on ways to optimize existing structures that promote One Health (Okello *et al.*, 2014). Engaging key sub-national actors has been shown to build understanding and shared learning between community members, local organizations and public services. Moreover, interventions that translate gender, knowledge, cultural practices and risk perception into disease control programmes, particularly those deemed 'community-led', are invaluable to improve acceptance and understanding (European Commission, 2008; Scoones, 2010).

Notwithstanding the significant political will and financial commitment required, building on established national and regional platforms originally developed for emerging infectious diseases can facilitate a One Health culture, strengthening existing ties between key stakeholders from the environmental, private and local community sectors. One Health working practices benefit regional organizations such as the Association of South East Asian Nations (ASEAN) and other biosecurity and bilateral trade agreements that contribute to regional integration and to development.

Across Asia, several transnational networks have been 'operationalizing One Health', with the successes and challenges of these networks well documented (European Union, 2011; Vandersmissen and Welburn, 2014). It would be timely to build upon these networks. Regional networks, for example the Mekong Basin Disease Surveillance (MBDS) network established in 1999 that monitors 25 cross-border surveillance sites in Cambodia, China, Lao PDR, Myanmar, Vietnam and Thailand for 18 infectious diseases (including avian influenza, dengue, typhoid, cholera, influenza and SARS) could include surveillance for endemic zoonoses within these border communities. MBDS had been effective in promoting regional cooperation and information exchange between local actors and policy makers via inter-ministerial collaboration in border communities where political, environmental and human and animal health issues are key for effective disease management.

In January 2014 the EU launched its INNOVATE One Health programme, an on-the-ground continuation of EU One Health engagement in Asia (since 2005), focusing on the collaboration between NGOs, civil society and academia to develop the One Health movement and aiming at better addressing the environmental dimension of One Health.

In Africa, several successful surveillance networks and partnerships have been operationalizing One Health, for example the Coordinating Office for Control of Trypanosomiasis (COCTU) Uganda and the Stamp Out Sleeping Sickness programme (http://stampoutsleepingsickness.org); the Southern African Centre for Infectious Disease Surveillance (SACIDS) and Animal and Human Health for the Environment and Development (AHEAD). However, evidence of One Health working practice outside of the Asia Pacific region remains limited and platforms and service providers for One Health remain patchy in many areas of high zoonotic disease risk (European Union, 2011). While it is acknowledged that prevention of disease outbreaks and management of endemic infection is preferable and less costly, long-term financial commitments are difficult to obtain when the health impact, or consequences of emerging or endemic zoonoses are not realized in global terms as is the case with the endemic neglected zoonoses. However, estimations of *total societal burden* of emerging and endemic zoonoses can provide compelling evidence for the value of operationalizing One Health (the combined human and animal +/– environmental costs of disease for the public and private sectors including indirect impacts on food security of smallholder farmers and micro- and macroeconomic impacts of disease on livestock productivity losses and health) (Narrod *et al.*, 2012) and can provide compelling evidence for investment in One Health (Centre for Global Development and Social Finance, 2013).

## Considering the needs of all nations – both developed and developing

Constraints in many developing countries for infectious disease control include limited human resources, finances, and discrepancies within government structures such as decentralization that prevent 'national' disease control programmes from operating smoothly (Okello *et al.*, 2014). Moreover, many biomedical programmes to date have lacked a true cross-disciplinary angle incorporating environmental, sociocultural and socio-political research investigations, which mar the successful uptake of infectious disease control even more (Allotey *et al.*, 2010; Bardosh *et al.*, 2014). As a result, national or regional surveillance and control programmes are often difficult to execute. Government and research institutions, and animal and human health systems, will require strengthening if disease control under a One Health approach is to be realized without long-term subsidies from international donors. Enhancement of biosecurity and surveillance mechanisms is required for long-term sustainable control of infectious disease in poor communities but at the same time the endemic diseases affecting local communities could also be addressed under One Health, increasing the motivation for a wide number of countries to embrace the approach. Cost, tradition, lack of income diversity and lack of alternatives to current practices are often given as reasons as to why effective surveillance does not take place.

In developing countries in particular, the available human and financial resources to undertake in-depth participatory approaches to policy development and execution remain thin on the ground. Training, educational and professional networks can play a key role in filling this gap, with various donors responding with investments that target the next generation for delivery of One Health training at undergraduate, post-graduate and continuous professional development levels (http://www.onehealthinitiative.com; Marcotty et al., 2013; Gibbs, 2014). Closer working practices for the next generation are expected to optimize the development and uptake of successful One Health models by district, national and regional policy makers, thereby avoiding future duplication of effort.

## Conclusion

With the right drivers, it has been possible to mobilize considerable political and financial support to achieve national, sub-regional and regional integrated approaches for the control of emerging or re-emerging zoonotic disease. The rapid evolution from the 'simple' response to H5N1 towards an international coordinated response to the AI/H1N1 pandemic and the emergence of a longer-term One Health movement have been unprecedented and timely in terms of global public health (Buzan et al., 1998; European Union, 2010; Scoones, 2010).

Addressing new and recurring global health challenges requires a long-term, strategic approach to GHG. Management of the disease risks arising from interactions between animals, humans and the environment demands integrated action from both human and animal health sectors, with support from other sectors or industries with a stake in health governance. The capacity for detection of emerging zoonoses and control of existing disease can be further increased with committed advocacy strategies, both at the higher policy levels and via engagement with affected communities to improve local disease surveillance networks. Institutional and private support for One Health is growing; a series of high-profile meetings initiated and supported by the EU, FAO, WHO and OIE, amongst others, has helped to foster political consensus and increase advocacy within the international community, highlighting the intersectoral action required for the 'new' approach to health.

There is presently wide consensus that 'One Health is a public good, that it cannot be owned, and that it should remain flexible, based on a broad pool of multiple expertises that cross disciplines and countries' (CDC and EU, 2011). While consensus acknowledges and attempts to include the wide variety of contexts and countries involved in any global approach, there is a need to look deeper into the emerging narratives of global health to see how best One Health may fit.

In conclusion, innovative solutions towards GHG will need to be found in order to overcome the challenges of global One Health coordination – given the wide variety of actors and agendas that now hold a stake. The global response to avian influenza was fundamental to the establishment of a longer term One Health movement and the promotion of innovative partnerships at political, institutional and technical levels; however, this now requires expansion and ownership within regional and national policy frameworks.

While One Health offers a rational choice where cumulative effects of disease on food and economic security are considered, rolling out the approach requires a fundamental change in institutional operations, accompanied by long-term financial solutions, for which demonstrating the added value of One Health in socio-economic terms will be key.

## Notes

[1] The Pan American Sanitary Bureau (1902), the Office International d'Hygiène Publique (1907), the Health Organization of the League of Nations (1923), the Office International des Epizooties – now the World Organisation for Animal Health (1924) and the World Health Organization (1951).

[2] http://www.rabiesalliance.org/what-we-do/asia/one-health-challenge
[3] http://www.galvmed.org/2012/03/galvmed-shares-one-health-message
[4] http://www.ceva.com.au/News-Media/News/One-World-One-Health-One-Ceva-March-2011
[5] http://www.onehealthglobal.net

## References


Allotey, P., Reidpath, D.D. and Pokhrel, S. (2010) Social sciences research in neglected tropical diseases 1: the ongoing neglect in the neglected tropical diseases. *Health Research Policy and Systems* 8, 32.

Association of Southeast Asian Nations (2010) ASEAN Ministerial Statement on ASEAN Cooperation on Animal Health and Zoonoses: Avian Influenza and Beyond. 32nd Meeting of ASEAN Ministers on Agriculture and Forestry (32nd AMAF), Phnom Penh, 23 October 2010.

Bardosh, K., Inthavong, P., Xayaheuang, S. and Okello, A.L. (2014) Controlling parasites, understanding practices: the biosocial complexity of a One Health intervention for neglected zoonotic helminths in northern Lao PDR. *Social Science and Medicine* 120, 215–223.

Bechir, M., Schelling, E., Wyss, K., Daugla, D.M., Daoud, S., Tanner, M. and Zinsstag, J. (2004) An innovative approach combining human and animal vaccination campaigns in nomadic settings of Chad: experiences and costs. *Revue de la Médecine Tropicale* 64, 497–502.

Bell, R., Taylor, S. and Marmot, M. (2010) Global health governance: Commission on Social Determinants of Health and the imperative for change. *Journal of Law, Medicine and Ethics* 470–485.

Brown, T.M., Cueto, M. and Fee, E. (2006) The World Health Organization and the transition from international to global public health. *American Journal of Public Health* 96(1), 62–72.

Buzan, B., Waever, O. and de Wilde, J. (1998) *Security: A New Framework for Analysis*. Lynne Rienner Publishers, Boulder, Colorado, p. 25.

Centers for Disease Control and Prevention (CDC) (2010) Operationalizing 'One Health': A policy perspective – taking stock and shaping an implementation roadmap. Meeting Overview 4–6 May 2010, Stone Mountain, Georgia.

Centers for Disease Control and Prevention (CDC) and European Union (EU) (2011) Atlanta Report 2011: Expert Meeting on One Health Governance and Global Network, 31 October 31–1 November 2011, Atlanta, Georgia. Available at: http://eeas.europa.eu/health/docs/2011_report-experts-atlanta_en.pdf (accessed 11 January 2014).

Centre for Global Development and Social Finance (2013) Investing in Social Outcomes: Development Impact Bonds. Report of the Development Impact Bond Working Group Consultation. Available at: http://www.socialfinance.org.uk/work/developmentimpactbonds (accessed 28 April 2014).

Clark, W.C., Szlezak, N.A., Moon, S., Bloom, B.R., Keusch, G.T., Michaud, C.M., Jamison, D.T., Frenk, J. and Kilama, W.L. (2010) The Global Health System: Institutions in a Time of Transition. *CID Working Paper No. 193*. Center for International Development, Harvard University.

Collins, A. (ed.) (2007) *Contemporary Security Studies*, 2nd edn. Oxford University Press, New York.

de Savigny, D. and Adam, T. (eds) (2009) Systems thinking for health systems strengthening. Alliance for Health Policy. World Health Organization.

de Savigny, D., Kasale, H., Mbuya, C. and Reidde, G. (2004) Fixing Health Systems. International Research Development Centre. Available at: http://dspace.cigilibrary.org/jspui/bitstream/123456789/11434/1/Fixing%20Health%20Systems.pdf?1 (accessed 28 April 2014).

Elbe, S. (2006) Should HIV/AIDS be securitized? The ethical dilemma of linking HIV/AIDS and security. *International Studies Quarterly* 50(1), 119–144.

England (2007) Are we spending too much on HIV? *British Medical Journal* 334, 344.

European Commission (2008) *Study on the Gender Aspects of the Avian Influenza Crisis in Southeast Asia*. Directorate-General External Relations Avian Influenza External Response Coordination, Brussels.

European Commission (2011a) *HPED Networking Event. Linking the Actors of the EU Asia Regional One Health Programme*, Bangkok, 18–19 January 2011. Directorate General for Development and Cooperation, EuropeAid, Brussels.

European Commission (2011b) *Cross Border Cooperation in Animal and Human Health – EU Regional HPED Programme*. Directorate General for Development and Cooperation, EuropeAid, Brussels.

European Union (2010) *Outcome and Impact Assesment of the Global Response to the Avian Influenza Crisis 2005–2010*. Publications Office of the European Union, Luxembourg.

European Union (2011) Implementation of the One Health approach in Asia and Europe – How to set-up a common basis for action and exchange of experience – Preparatory Study.
FAO, OIE, UNSIC, UNICEF, WHO and World Bank (2008) Contributing to OWOH – A strategic framework for reducing risks at the Animal-Human-Ecosystems Interface. Consultation Document. UNSIC, FAO,WHO, UNICEF, OIE, WBG 14 October 2008.
FAO, OIE and WHO (2010) The FAO-OIE-WHO Collaboration: Sharing responsibilities and coordinating global activities to address health risks at the animal-human-ecosystems interfaces. Tripartite concept note.
FAO, OIE and WHO (2012) High-Level Technical Meeting to Address Health Risks at the Human-Animal-Ecosystems Interfaces. Mexico City, Mexico.
Fidler, D. (2001) The globalization of public health: the first 100 years of international health diplomacy. *Bulletin of the World Health Organization* 79, 842–849.
Fidler, D. (2004) Germs, governance and global public health in the wake of SARS. *Journal of Clinical Investigation* 113(6), 799–804.
Garrett, L. and Alavian, E. (2010) Global health governance in a G20 world. Global Health Governance, Vol. IV, No. 1 (FALL 2010). Available at: http://www.ghgj.org (accessed 11 January 2014).
Gibbs, E.P.J. (2014) The evolution of One Health: a decade of progress and challenges for the future. *Veterinary Record* doi: 10,1136/vr.g143.
Gibbs, S.E.J. and Gibbs, E.P.J. (2013) The historical, present, and future role of veterinarians in One Health. *Current Topics in Microbiology and Immunology* 365, 31–47.
Godfroid, J., Dahouk, S., Pappas, G., Roth, F., Matope, G., *et al.* (2013) A 'One Health' surveillance and control of brucellosis in developing countries: moving away from improvisation. *Comparative Immunology, Microbiology and Infectious Diseases* 36(3), 241–248.
Godlee, F. (1994) WHO in retreat; is it losing its influence? *British Medical Journal* 309, 1491–1495.
Hotez, P.J. and Fenwick, A. (2009) Schistosomiasis in Africa: An Emerging Tragedy in Our New Global Health Decade. *PLoS Neglected Tropical Diseases* 3(9): e485. doi:10.1371/journal.pntd.0000485
ICONZ (2014) Integrated Control for Neglected Zoonoses in Africa. European Commission. Available at: http://www.iconzafrica.org (accessed 28 April 2014).
Kickbusch, I. (2000) The development of international health priorities - accountability intact? *Social Science and Medicine* 51, 979–989.
Leach, M. and Scoones, I. (2013) The social and political lives of zoonotic disease models: narratives, science and policy. *Social Science and Medicine* 88, 10–17.
Leboeuf, A. and Broughton, E. (2008) *Securitization of Health and Environmental Issues: Process and Effects. A research outline*. Health and Environment Working Document, Institut Français des Relations Internationales (Ifri), ISBN: 978-2-86592-305-2.
Lee, K. and Pang, T. (2014) WHO: retirement or reinvention? *Public Health* 128, 119–123.
Lee, K., Collinson, S., Walt, G. and Gilson, L. (1996) Who should be doing what in the international health: a confusion of mandates in the United Nations? *British Medical Journal* 312, 302–307.
Lidén, J. (2014) The World Health Organization and global health governance: post-1990. *Public Health* 128, 141–147.
Marchal, B., Cavalli, A. and Kegels, G. (2009) Global health actors claim to support health system strengthening. Is this reality or rhetoric? *PLoS Medicine* 6(4): e1000059. doi:10.1371/journal.pmed.1000059.
Marcotty, T., Thys, E., Conrad, P., Godfroid, J., Craig, P., Zinsstag, J., Meheus, P., Boukary, A.R., Abdou Badé, M., Sahibi, H., Filali, H., Hendrickx, S., *et al.* (2013) Intersectoral collaboration between the medical and veterinary professions in low-resource societies: the role of research and training institutions. *Comparative Immunology, Microbiology and Infectious Diseases* 36(3), 233–239.
Maudlin, I., Eisler, M.C. and Welburn, S.C. (2009) Neglected and endemic zoonoses. *Philosophical Transactions of the Royal Society B* 364, 2777–2787.
Molyneux, D.H. (2008) Combatting the other diseases of MDG 6: changing the paradigm to achieve equity and poverty reduction? *Transactions of the Royal Society of Tropical Medicine and Hygiene* 102, 509–519.
Muraskin, W. (1998) *The Politics of International Health: the children's vaccine initiative and the struggle to develop vaccines for the third world.* SUNY Press, Albany, New York.
Narrod, C., Zinsstag, J. and Tiongco, M. (2012) A one health framework for estimating the economic costs of zoonotic diseases on society. *EcoHealth* 9(2), 150–162.
Ng, N. and Ruger, J.P. (2011) Global Health Governance at a Crossroads. Global Health Governance, Vol. III, No.2 (Spring 2011). Available at: http://www.ghgj.org (accessed 11 January 2014).

Okello, A.L., Gibbs, E.P.J., Vandersmissen, A. and Welburn, S.C. (2011) One Health and the neglected zoonoses: turning rhetoric into reality. *Veterinary Record* 169, 281–285.
Okello, A.L., Welburn, S.C. and Smith, J. (2014) Crossing institutional boundaries: mapping the policy process for the control of neglected zoonotic disease in sub-Saharan Africa. *Health Policy and Planning* 1–9. doi:10.1093/heapol/czu059.
Ollila, E. (2005) Global health priorities - priorities of the wealthy? *Global Health* 1, 6
Packard, R.M. (1997) Malaria dreams: postwar visions of health and development in the third world. *Medical Anthropology: Cross-Cultural Studies in Health and Illness* 17(3), 279–296.
Public Health Agency of Canada (2009) One World One Health™ : from ideas to action. Report of the Expert Consultation, March 16–19, Winnipeg, Manitoba, Canada.
Saarnak, C., Johansen, M.V. and Mukaratirwa, S. (2014) ADVANZ: establishing a Pan-African platform for neglected zoonotic disease control through a One Health approach. *Onderstepoort Journal of Veterinary Research* 81(2), E1–3.
Schelling, E., Wyss, K., Béchir, M., Daugla, D. and Zinsstag, J. (2005) Synergy between public health and veterinary services to deliver human and animal health interventions in rural low income settings. *British Medical Journal* 331(7527), 1264–1267.
Scoones, I. (2010) *Avian Influenza: Science, Policy and Politics*. Routledge Earthscan, London.
Silver, G.A. (1998) Editorial: international health services need an interorganizational policy. *American Journal of Public Health* 88(5), 727–729.
Singer, P.A., Benatar, S.R., Bernstein, M., Daar, A.S. *et al.* (2003) Ethics and SARS: lessons from Toronto. *British Medical Journal* 327, 1342–1344.
Smith, R. (2003) Global public goods and health. *Bulletin of the World Health Organization* 81(7), 475.
Smith, R.D. and MacKellar, L. (2007) Global public goods and the global health agenda: problems, priorities and potential. *Globalization and Health* 3(9) doi:10.1186/1744-8603-3-9.
Smith, R., Woodward, D., Acharya, A., Beaglehole, R. and Drager, N. (2004) Communicable disease control: a 'Global Public Good' perspective. *Health Policy and Planning* 19(5), 271–278.
Sridhar, D. (2010) Seven Challenges in International Development Assistance for Health and Ways Forward. Global Health Governance Vol. II, No.2 (Fall 2010). Available at: http://www.ghgj.org (accessed 11 January 2014).
Taylor, A.L. (2002) Global governance, international health law and WHO: looking towards the future. *Bulletin of the World Health Organization* 80, 975–980.
UNSIC and World Bank (2010) Animal and Pandemic Inflenza: A framework for sustaining momentum. 5th Global Progress Report, July 2010. UN System Influenza Coordination (UNSIC) and World Bank, 2010.
USAID, United Nations System and World Food Programme (2011) Beyond Pandemics: a whole of society approach to disaster preparedness.
Vandersmissen, A. and Welburn, S.C. (2014) Current initiatives in 'One Health' consolidating the One Health global network. In: *OIE Scientific and Technical Review* 33(2), August.
Vaughan, J.P., Mogedalb, S., Kruseb, S., Kelley, L., Walt, G. and Wilde, K. (1996) Financing the World Health Organization: global importance of extrabudgetary funds. *Health Policy* 35, 229–245.
Walt, G. (1993) WHO under stress: implications for health policy. *Health Policy* 24, 125–144.
Walt, G. and Gilson, L. (1994) Reforming the health sector in developing countries: the central role of policy analysis. *Health Policy and Planning* 9(4), 353–370.
Welburn, S.C. (2011) One Health the 21st Century challenge. *Veterinary Record* 168, 614–615.
WHO, FAO, DFID and OIE (2006) *The control of neglected zoonotic diseases: a route to poverty alleviation.* WHO, Geneva, Switzerland.
WHO, EU, ILRI, DBL, FAO, OIE and AU (2009) Integrated Control of Neglected Zoonotic Diseases in Africa: Applying the 'One Health' Concept. WHO, Geneva, Switzerland.
WHO, ICONZ, DFIF-RIU, SOS, EU, TDR, FAO, ILRI and OIE (2011) *The control of Neglected Zoonotic Diseases: community based interventions for prevention and control.* WHO, Geneva, Switzerland.
Williams, O.D. and Rushton, S. (2011) Are the 'Good Times' Over? Looking to the Future of Global Health Governance. *Global Health Governance* V(1). Available at: http://www.ghgj.org (accessed 11 January 2014).
World Trade Organization (2014) Available at: http://www.wto.org/english/thewto_e/coher_e/wto_oie_e.htm (accessed 25 January 2014).
Yach, D. and Bettcher, D. (1998) The globalization of public health, I: Threats and opportunities. *American Journal of Public Health* 88(5), 735–738.
Zinsstag, J., Schelling, E., Roth, F., Bonfoh, B., de Savigny, D. and Tanner, M. (2007) Human benefits of animal interventions for zoonosis control. *Emerging Infectious Diseases* 13, 527–531.

# 25 One Health in Policy Development: an Integrated Approach to Translating Science into Policy


**Susan C. Cork,[1]* Dorothy W. Geale[2] and David C. Hall[1]**

*[1]Department of Ecosystem & Public Health, Faculty of Veterinary Medicine, University of Calgary; [2]Canadian Food Inspection Agency, Port Hope, Ontario*


## Introduction

The application of the One Health concept to the development and delivery of science-based policy is not new, but it has been revived in the past decade with a growing awareness of the need to engage transdisciplinary teams to solve complex problems. The composition of these teams depends very much on the issue(s) to be addressed, but for emerging diseases of significance to human and animal health the team might include animal and human health professionals, wildlife experts, biologists, ecologists, disease specialists, agricultural economists, epidemiologists and social scientists. As well as fostering an enlightened approach to problem solving, the engagement of a broader range of expertise has also resulted in a more integrated approach to translating science into policy. Taking a more integrated approach, as well as engaging a One Health team when developing policy, ensures that the policies developed are more relevant and likely to be accepted and implemented by relevant stakeholders. Developing good partnerships between scientists, communities, industry stakeholders and policy makers also helps to improve communication, which is a key component of successful policy acceptance. Another important factor that should be considered when taking a One Health approach is the need for good governance. In this chapter we will use case studies from New Zealand and South-east Asia to illustrate the added value of using a One Health approach in policy development and the benefits of taking an integrated transdisciplinary approach when translating science into policy.

## Biosecurity Science and One Health – a New Zealand Perspective on Avian Influenza

New Zealand has developed some of the most respected biosecurity systems in the world. These systems were originally developed to protect the primary production industries such as livestock agriculture, horticulture and forestry, which are the cornerstone of New Zealand's economic stability. Now, these systems also seek to protect New Zealand's unique natural environment including several rare and endangered species of birds. With the rapid growth in tourism and trade, the number


*E-mail: sccork@ucalgary.ca

of ways that pests and diseases can enter the country continues to grow. At the same time, economic, environmental, social and cultural considerations, particularly *Tikanga Maori*,[1] have required changes to the way that pests and diseases are managed. New Zealand's biosecurity systems have evolved to meet these challenges. In the following text we use the example of avian influenza, a potentially significant zoonotic pathogen, to illustrate how disease prevention and control policies have been developed in New Zealand using a transdisciplinary One Health approach.

## Introduction to avian influenza – a constantly evolving threat

Several times in recorded history avian influenza viruses have evolved to cause significant morbidity and mortality in human populations (Alexander and Brown, 2000). Avian influenza, or influenza A viruses are zoonotic pathogens with multiple animal reservoirs including domestic poultry and pigs (Webby *et al.*, 2007). Although these viruses can infect numerous vertebrate host species including swine and many avian species, the aquatic bird population, especially the anseriformes (i.e. ducks and geese), are considered to be the main natural reservoir (Hinshaw *et al.*, 1980; Stanislawek *et al.*, 2002). Influenza A viruses are known to adapt rapidly within a population and can readily cross from one species to another when selection pressure is high. These viruses are typically described according to their surface glycoproteins, haemagglutinin (HA) and neuraminidase (NA), which have been found in combinations of 16 HA and 9 NA serologic subtypes (Webby *et al.*, 2007). There are two key mechanisms by which influenza A viruses change antigenically. These are referred to as: (i) antigenic drift; and (ii) antigenic shift. Antigenic drift occurs as a result of substitution of amino acids at the antigenic sites of the HA molecule and subsequent selection within the host for variants able to evade the immune system. This continual selection for antigenically novel variants allows influenza A virus to reappear seasonally within populations. Antigenic shift occurs less frequently and refers to the emergence of a novel HA subtype within a population. This can occur as a result of interspecies transfer of a whole virus or through the process of genetic re-assortment events associated with interhost transmission (Alexander *et al.*, 1987; Brown, 2000; Lei and Shi, 2011). The resultant progeny viruses can have an unpredictable antigenicity due to the mixture of genomic segments inherited. Although any influenza A virus has the potential to cause disease, most of the significant outbreaks of avian influenza in poultry have been caused by H5 and H7 subtypes (Alexander *et al.*, 1987). Other subtypes have been associated with disease outbreaks in turkeys, horses, dogs and marine mammals (Webby *et al.*, 2007; Capua and Alexander, 2009). Human influenza is more frequently associated with subtypes H1, H2 and H3, but strains of other subtypes e.g. H5, H7 and H9 have the capability to become zoonotic (Capua and Alexander, 2009). The complex evolution of avian influenza viruses was recently elucidated for the emergence of the zoonotic H7N9 avian influenza in China (March 2013). The authors suggest that the continuing prevalence of H7 viruses in poultry could lead to the generation of highly pathogenic variants and further sporadic human infections with a risk of acquiring human-to-human transmissibility (Lam *et al.*, 2013).

Given the natural ecology of influenza in wild bird populations and the interaction between wildlife, domestic animals and humans, it is important to understand the factors that drive emergence of new strains of influenza A. The complexity of the natural system, and the constantly changing situation as new influenza A viruses emerge, requires regulatory authorities to take a One Health approach to the development of disease control and prevention policies.

## Pandemic planning, biosecurity science and disease response in New Zealand

In 2007 a Biosecurity Science Strategy for New Zealand/*Mahere Rautaki Putaiao Whakamaru* was released. This strategy built on the recommendations of *Tiakina Aotearoa, Protect New Zealand: The Biosecurity Strategy for New*

*Zealand* (MPI, 2003, 2007), which identified the need for adaptation and change in response to new threats, and emphasized the critical role that science plays in underpinning the biosecurity system. The strategy recognized that achieving good biosecurity outcomes is dependent on multidisciplinary and multi-sectoral approaches and cooperation across the different government agencies responsible for biosecurity outcomes.

New Zealand has never had a case of highly pathogenic avian influenza (HPAI) in domestic poultry. Surveillance for avian influenza has included active and passive surveillance programmes for both wild birds and commercial poultry (Tana *et al.*, 2007; Frazer *et al.*, 2008; Rawdon *et al.*, 2008, 2010, 2012a,b; Stanislawek *et al.*, 2011). The Ministry of Agriculture and Forestry (MAF), now the Ministry for Primary Industries (MPI), has conducted avian influenza surveillance in migratory birds and in wild mallard ducks (*Anas platyrhynchos*) in conjunction with the Ornithological Society of New Zealand (OSNZ) migrating bird banding programme, regional and local councils, the Department of Conservation (DOC) and other stakeholders. To date, avian influenza viruses have been reported in healthy mallard ducks (Austin and Hinshaw, 1984; Stanislawek, 1990, 1992; Stanislawek *et al.*, 2002) but not in samples from migratory shorebirds (Langstaff *et al.*, 2009). The MPI has also worked with the New Zealand poultry industry to ensure that strict import health standards are in place to prevent the entry of avian influenza and other diseases in imported commodities. However, another reason that domestic poultry have remained free of HPAI viruses may be the absence of migratory waterfowl in New Zealand. The latter are thought to play a key role in transferring new strains of influenza from one region to another and can be important with regard to transmitting virus to free-range outdoor poultry.

The migratory shore birds sampled in the New Zealand surveillance programme include the bar-tailed godwit (*Limosa lapponica*) and the red (lesser) knot (*Calidras canutus*). These species are caught soon after their arrival at Miranda, their main North Island arrival site, in late September to November (Stanislawek *et al.*, 2011). Shore birds are targeted because their migration pathway extends from the Arctic regions of Asia and North America, in the case of the godwit, and from the Arctic via the Pacific coast of Asia for the knot (Williams *et al.*, 2004). Resident waterfowl, predominantly mallard ducks, are tested over the summer months throughout New Zealand with a particular focus on coastal areas where they may have contact with migratory shore birds or where large numbers of juvenile mallards mix (Stanislawek *et al.*, 2011). Enhanced active and passive surveillance was put in place in 2004 in response to the spread of H5N1 across Asia and concern about its arrival to New Zealand via the flyways from East Asia. In addition to surveillance programmes, MPI operates a 24-h toll-free exotic pest and disease emergency hotline, which receives calls from the public, veterinarians, regional laboratory pathologists and others relating to suspected exotic pests and diseases including calls about sick and dead wild and domestic birds. Investigators follow up on cases of interest in order to rule in, or rule out, suspected cases of avian influenza and other exotic diseases (Rawdon *et al.*, 2007a,b).

Due to the potential for a new influenza pandemic in humans, the New Zealand Government also updated its pandemic preparedness plan. It was agreed that the MPI would take the lead in implementing the plan if the first cases occurred in poultry or wild birds but that the Ministry of Health (MOH) would take over if human cases occurred with subsequent human–human transmission. A number of public education campaigns were also launched through these lead agencies as well as through the DOC for issues associated with wild birds.

### *Pandemic planning and the need for good governance*

Pandemic planning requires coordinated global actions as well as actions at the national level. Good governance is essential and New Zealand has developed good relationships with other countries and international organizations operating in the Asia-Pacific region. Internationally, to enhance global efforts to detect and deal with potential disease threats, the Food and Agriculture Organization (FAO), the World Organisation for Animal Health (OIE) and the World Health Organization (WHO) developed a framework for countries to engage in dialogue and negotiations to address health risks at the human–animal–ecosystem interface (FAO, 2010). To avoid duplication and ensure coordination, the three organizations have combined their alert and response mechanisms to form the Global Early Warning and Response System for Major Animal Disease (GLEWS). In addition, the OIE and FAO, the two principal agencies dealing with transboundary animal health issues, launched the Global Framework for the progressive control of Transboundary Animal Diseases (GF TADs) to address endemic and emerging infectious diseases including zoonoses. Under this framework, FAO/OIE Regional Animal Health Centres provide member countries with technical support and evaluate national and regional projects. Such joint regional and national efforts generally lead to stronger and sustainable political support for integrated disease prevention and promote trust, transparency and cooperation. It is well recognized that the prevention of emergence and cross-border spread of human and animal infectious diseases, such as avian influenza, is a global public good with benefits that extend to all countries, people and generations.

### *A 'whole of government' approach and disease response policies*

In New Zealand, a suite of documents have been developed to outline the roles and responsibilities of the multitude of players that would be engaged in an avian influenza response (MAF, 2008, 2011). To ensure an integrated approach, a 'whole-of-government' response[2] would need to be adopted for avian influenza virus strains affecting animals that could affect humans, while for non-zoonotic strains, the response would be managed within the MAF's (now MPI) *Memorandum of Understanding (MOU) on biosecurity activities between MAF and the DOC, Ministry of Fisheries (Min Fish, now within MPI) and the MOH*, 31 October 2006 and an operational guideline between DOC and MAF, December 2008. The 'whole-of-government' approach to an influenza A 'response' is founded on the Domestic and External Security Coordination (DESC) system, which outlines expectations for the information and resources each agency would provide (MAF, 2011). The importance of information sharing was specified between key agencies, i.e. the MPI, MOH, DOC, Ministry of Foreign Affairs and Trade (MFAT), Reserve Bank, Treasury, Ministry of Civil Defence and Emergency Management (MCDEM), New Zealand Police, New Zealand Defence Force (NZDF), Ministry of Transport (MOT), Ministry of Social Development (MSD), Ministry of Economic Development (MED), Ministry for the Environment (MfE) and Te Puni Kokiri (Ministry of Maori Development).

Within MAF (MPI) a generic *Policy for MAF's Response to Risk Organisms* was developed to outline responses to organisms that could harm people, the environment and/or the economy (MAF, 2008). This was to be used in conjunction with MAF's more detailed internal biosecurity response management processes including *Technical Response Policies for Avian Influenza Viruses of Regulatory Concern*, which provided an overview of approved policies following inter-departmental and industry consultation (Geale and Rawdon, 2005; MAF, 2006) and *Technical Response Plans*, which described in detail the application of policies and generic procedures to a particular circumstance. The basis for all biosecurity response plans in New Zealand is the Biosecurity Act 1993. A series of standards (formerly termed 153 standards) set out the CTO's operational requirements with respect to the investigation, control and eradication of exotic organisms that are suspected to be present in New Zealand.[3]

### *Evolving regulations and international reporting requirements*

In 2004 all isolations of H5 and H7 avian influenza subtypes in poultry were made notifiable to the OIE and were classified as either highly pathogenic notifiable avian influenza (HPNAI) or low pathogenicity notifiable avian influenza (LPNAI) (OIE, 2004). Previous to 2004, only highly pathogenic avian influenza was required to be reported by the OIE. The change was implemented because it had been recognized that LPNAI strains had the potential to become highly pathogenic (HPNAI) when circulating in poultry. Other subtypes are not notifiable in poultry but can become pathogenic under some circumstances (Capua and Alexander, 2009). The reporting of human influenza strains in New Zealand is handled through the public health laboratory system in collaboration with the MOH and WHO (Jennings, 2005; Huang *et al.*, 2008).

In 2013, the OIE dropped the term 'notifiable', with HPNAI referred to as high pathogenicity avian influenza (HPAI) and LPNAI as low pathogenicity avian influenza (LPAI) (OIE, 2013). The definition of HPAI includes not only H5 and H7 subtypes, but also any influenza A virus meeting the criteria for highly pathogenic, which can be measured by laboratory protocols *in vivo* or by using molecular techniques that can identify multiple basic amino acids at the cleavage site which are similar to those of previous HPAI isolates.[4]

In 2005 when the initial MPI policies were developed, the OIE definition of poultry excluded the adjective, 'domesticated', referring simply to 'all birds' or 'for the breeding of these categories of birds' (OIE, 2005). Due to the importance of New Zealand's unique avifauna, birds other than poultry are specifically incorporated and, unlike most other developed countries, New Zealand's *Technical Response Policies* also covered the H9N2 subtype which is endemic in the Middle East and Asia and intermittently associated with high mortality in poultry.[5] Thus the New Zealand *Technical Response Policies* for avian influenza remain broader in scope than currently required by the OIE guidelines.

### *Surveillance for avian influenza and research*

In New Zealand, a cross-sectional serological survey stratified by production sector (broiler, caged/barn layer, free-range layer, pullet rearer and turkey broiler) found no evidence of active infection with H5 or H7 AI viruses in commercial turkeys and chickens and only historic exposure to H5 subtypes in free-range layer flocks (Rawdon *et al.*, 2010). Further surveillance, and a research study to examine the natural disease ecology and transmission of non-pathogenic influenza A viruses, was conducted on a subset of backyard poultry operations adjacent to wetlands where waterfowl had been tested. Only 3.6% of the poultry samples (309) showed evidence of exposure to influenza A while 30% (54) of duck sera were positive, confirming exposure of backyard flocks to non-notifiable low pathogenic avian influenza viruses (Zheng *et al.*, 2010).

Since 1984, surveillance of wild waterfowl (healthy mallard ducks) has resulted in the isolation of a number of low pathogenic avian influenza viruses, including two H5 LPAI isolates in 1997 and one H7 isolate in 2005 (Tana *et al.*, 2007). As all avian influenza virus isolations have been from wild waterfowl, New Zealand's avian influenza freedom status is not affected.

### *New Zealand's technical response policies for avian influenza viruses of regulatory concern*

MPI's suite of response documents typically include: (i) a technical analysis (disease monograph); (ii) technical response policies (high-level statements and response objectives); (iii) an operational plan (detailed procedures); (iv) resource requirements (specific human and physical resources for likely scenarios); and (v) a communication plan. Due to the complex disease ecology of avian influenza and the range of susceptible species (including humans), a matrix of response actions was created. Categories of what the OIE then defined as poultry included: (i) commercial galliformes; (ii) commercial anseriformes; (iii) commercial other (game birds, quail, ratites etc.); (iv) backyard poultry; (v) captive birds (pigeons, aviaries, public sanctuaries, etc.); and (vi) wild birds in sanctuaries including threatened indigenous birds protected under the Wildlife Act (1953) in private DOC sanctuaries. Response actions for HPAI, LPAI and other exotic emerging avian influenza subtypes were determined for each category. These ranged from 'stamping out' to a 'measured response' such as phased eradication for low pathogenic H5 and H7 in commercial galliformes, or only monitor (low pathogenic in captive birds such as some zoo/cage birds) or no action (endangered birds except for HPNAI). Measured responses are determined at the time and developed by the Technical Advisory Group (TAG) and Stakeholder Advisory Group (SAG), and endorsed by CTO generally for the presence of LPAI in other than commercial galliformes where phased eradication or vaccination may be indicated. These graduated responses recognize that the natural reservoir of LPAI and other avian influenza viruses is in aquatic avian species where they are enteric rather than systemic and generally cause minimal or no clinical disease. By stipulating a response decision process for LPAI response, inherent flexibility exists contingent on a risk assessment based on current scientific knowledge, the epidemiology of the virus isolated and in which of six designated compartments the virus is detected. The potential conversion of LPAI to HPAI and the subsequent risk to animal and human health and well-being associated with continued passage of virus in chickens, turkeys, quail or other species must be assessed by the TAG and SAG. Due to the changing risk profile of avian influenza viruses, and the range of different situations that might be presented, a prescribed response is often not realistic but agreement on the process to define appropriate and transparent response actions is critical.

A key to the success of New Zealand's response actions are the multi-sectoral and multi-disciplinary TAG and SAG. The TAG may comprise technical experts such as virologists, epidemiologists, biologists, ornithologists and veterinarians who review the scientific context and assess the associated risks and recommend appropriate technical response management option(s) to the response manager (previously the CTO or CVO). The need to increase the inter-disciplinary co-operation between these professional groups in the management of avian influenza is recognized internationally. TAG members are paid by MPI and sign a conflict of interest document for confidentiality and scientific impartiality. The SAG normally reviews TAG-proposed response management option(s) in light of primary production/commerce, environment, social (including human health) and cultural values. It is comprised of individuals with skills and experience in these matters, including policy advisers from the MOH and DOC and industry advisers from the Poultry Industry Association of New Zealand (PIANZ), Egg Producers Federation of New Zealand (EPFNZ), Ostrich and Emu Standards Council (OESC), Australasian Regional Association of Zoological Parks and Aquaria (ARAZPA), Game Preserves and the MAF Maori Strategic Unit with knowledge of Tikanga Maori. Both the TAG and SAG contributed to the current version of the *Technical Response Policies*. In the event of a response, the situation circumstances could dictate a change in the terms of reference and membership of the TAG and SAG by the CTO.

## The One Health team and biosecurity – a New Zealand perspective

There is no magic formula for the success of a One Health approach but good governance and a clear set of agreed goals and objectives should be an integral component. MPI's TAG and SAG in New Zealand represent a two-tiered approach to a One Health team separating technical/scientific aspects, which are then reviewed from the socio-economic perspective. The acronym STEEPLE, i.e. considering a proposal from a range of angles – Social, Technological, Environmental, Economic, Political, Legal and Ethical (Robert Burke, Mt Eliza Business School, 2012, personal communication) may be aptly applied to consideration of a One Health team.

The application of the One Health concept is especially important with regard to the development and delivery of disease prevention and control policies to address influenza A viruses. Taking a more integrated approach, as well as engaging a One Health team, has ensured that the policies developed are acceptable to the public and to relevant industry stakeholders and are therefore more readily implemented (Geale *et al.*, 2006). Developing good partnerships between scientists, communities, industry stakeholders and policy makers has also helped to improve communication, which is a key component of successful policy acceptance and implementation.

## Policy at the Local, National and Regional Level – Examples from South-east Asia

With two examples from South-east Asia, this section will illustrate that where health policy is to be effective in preventing zoonotic disease transmission in a highly populated region with multiple political borders, policy must be developed and implemented at local, national and regional levels. Such policy depends on the successful integration of transdisciplinary teamwork that includes social scientists and community members in decision making and recognition of the complexity of the ecology of diseases such as avian influenza.

### Highly pathogenic avian influenza in South-east Asia

Outbreaks of HPAI H5N1 have occurred in poultry in almost every country in South-east Asia. Although the incidence of human cases is far lower than that for poultry, the high rate of hospitalization and mortality of humans known to be clinically infected with HPAI H5N1 (WHO, 2013) means that HPAI H5N1 remains a disease of serious concern in South-east Asia. The threat of pandemic emergence remains a concern in the region and globally due to several factors related to the biology of avian influenza and the lack of biosecurity and effective disease control policy to deal with the disease. The ability of the avian influenza virus to re-assort and cross species barriers has been noted earlier. This is all the more worrying where biosecurity is weak or compromised due to management factors that permit mixing of species including anseriformes, galliformes and swine, especially at live animal markets where biosecurity standards are not enforced. In many South-east Asian countries there are also few practices in place to prevent entry of wildlife to farmsteads and there is often low compliance with other biosecurity features such as vaccination or one-way travel of species from farm to market. The lack of biosecurity is typically most problematic at the level of the small scale (i.e. 'backyard') producer who tends to rely on livestock production for income supplementation as well as food security. Mid- to large-scale facilities in South-east Asia have been improving biosecurity for many years in response to consumer demand, and many operate with high standards of disease prevention. Thus, a policy problem has presented itself to South-east Asian governments with respect to HPAI H5N1: how to formulate strict and enforceable biosecurity standards for all actors – including small-scale producers – while minimizing the need for costly development of alternative forms of livelihood at the village level. The latter has been a legitimate concern of producers in all sectors of the poultry industry in South-east Asia.

#### *Policy responses to H5N1 in South-east Asia*

Policy responses to HPAI H5N1 in South-east Asia began at the national and regional level. From 2003 to 2005, as Vietnam, Thailand, Indonesia and China came to grips with the rapid spread of the H5N1 virus, provincial and national authorities were challenged to revise biosecurity measures and implement new human and veterinary health policy measures to contain and possibly eradicate the virus (Sims *et al.*, 2005). In the early years of the epidemic (2003–2007) there was considerable reliance on expert advice and technical assistance from international organizations, including FAO and the OIE. Country-level policies with clear and consistent strategies for controlling H5N1 were slow to emerge for a number of reasons, including debate over federal versus local authority, right to vaccinate poultry and lines of reporting. As a result, without a strong voice to guide policy, valuable response time was not used most effectively to respond to outbreaks or to develop a regionally harmonized prevention strategy.

Notably absent from input to guiding regional policy support directed at containment of spread of the disease across Asia was the only regional political representation in Asia, the Association of South-east Asian Nations (ASEAN). Much of the effort for developing a strategy for regional containment was led by FAO, OIE and WHO, in consultation with member states in South-east Asia. This initiated a criticism of ASEAN that remains a point of contention today (Pitsuwan, 2011; Duc, 2012; Tay, 2012). The ten-nation institution failed to develop a regional statement, a first step in regional policy formulation, that could have been effective to guide development of a consistent regional control strategy, leverage distribution of needed resources, implement essential trade restrictions and sanction compensation and recovery measures in member countries where needed. The importance of this is to note that a regional institution charged with policy formulation did not act, for whatever admittedly complicated reasons, in a tangled political and social context. From a strategic point of view, ASEAN missed an opportunity that was not only lost to FAO, OIE and WHO to influence regional health policy, but also to be recognized as an effective formulator of policy important to South-east Asian economic and biologic health.

### *The response to HPAI H5N1 in Vietnam*

In Asia, Vietnam has experienced the second highest number of human fatalities due to HPAI H5N1 after Indonesia, and by far the largest number of reported outbreaks causing extensive economic impact exceeding half a billion dollars (Jonas, 2008; Herington, 2010; Government of Vietnam, 2011). The development of Vietnam's response to HPAI H5N1 is interesting in terms of the role of the government and farmers in addressing the disease locally and nationally and their contribution to a more regional effort. Initially, the policy response from Vietnam was led by the national government, which sought to eliminate a key precipitating factor in the spread of the disease, i.e. eliminate or control movement of roaming ducks in rice paddies. With input from provincial authorities, commune leaders and rural development advisors, a solution was developed to simply allow netting of the ducks in a fairly large, but confined, space. The inelegant solution overshadows a far more important development in HPAI policy formulation that addressed an element absent at the OIE-FAO-WHO June 2007 technical meeting in Rome (Scoones and Forster, 2010) and absent in general prior to that point. The Government of Vietnam was including social and cultural perspectives (livelihoods, rural economics and public choice) in national policy formulation coupled with science-based decision making. A key One Health pillar was now being addressed. This was noted in an interim evaluation of the Government of Vietnam policy to control HPAI H5N1 (Hall and Le, 2009) with the recommendation, subsequently adopted, that an ecohealth/One Health approach be integrated into zoonotic disease control policy in the future.

The more general approach of the Government of Vietnam was to build on the level of rapport that existed between specific government health ministries and their United Nations (UN) counterparts, other international agencies and provincial authorities. Lines of communication across government ministries were less open, although a concerted effort to improve communication developed within the first 2 years of the HPAI H5N1 outbreaks. From this history, it was a natural extension for Vietnam to agree to be a pilot country for the One-UN Plan for UN reform in 2005 (UN, 2013), affording it the opportunity to engage with domestic and international policy makers in a transdisciplinary framework addressing health policy in terms of communication, participatory development, epidemiology, finance and economics, change management and education.

Vu (2009) identified five characteristics of the country's policy-making context, listed here with commentary on relevance: (i) party state dominance over civil society, which may appear heavy-handed but does result in rapid mobilization of disease control measures when needed; (ii) differentiation from central to local policy intent and results, which allows for local adaptation but potentially reduces effectiveness of centrally designed policy; (iii) marginalization of farmers in policy making, which risks alienating key stakeholders in decision making and implementation; (iv) dependence on foreign aid, a feature particularly true of the response to HPAI H5N1, making the coordinated response highly vulnerable to donor fatigue and international politics; and (v) general lack of an appropriate scale of attention to agriculture, both in terms of fiscal planning and degree of extension activities.

These key factors drove avian influenza policy development in Vietnam in the context of a political issue, a technical problem, a social concern, a matter of high economic impact, an issue of institutional capacity and governance and a topic of sensitive socio-cultural context. Numerous institutional leaders emerged both domestically and internationally including: the Government of Vietnam Ministries of Agriculture and Rural Development (MARD), Health (MOH) and Finance (MF); the UN agencies FAO, WHO, UNICEF and UNDP; OIE; the World Bank and countless donors; non-governmental organizations (NGOs); and farmers, traders and consumers. While philosophical differences were bound to emerge and competing institutional interests complicated strategy, in general the co-operation between MARD and FAO, MOH and WHO, donors and NGOs and local organizations and commune leaders has been exemplary. The cornerstone policies of mass culling and vaccination coupled with communication and behaviour change programmes have resulted in a complicated multi-faceted approach to disease control but one that aligns well the interests of Vietnam, regional partners and international agencies.

Despite issues yet to be resolved, including a compensation programme inconsistently implemented, limited adoption of change by farmers despite high-level understanding of the cause of H5N1 and uneven technical responses to outbreaks, Vietnam's technical capacity to prevent and respond to an emerging infectious disease domestically and to contribute to regional biosecurity has improved significantly.

### Food safety and small-scale poultry in northern Thailand

Food safety has become increasingly important to Asian consumers, and this has played an important role in government policy making in South-east Asia (Hall *et al.*, 2013). Response is developing to demand for training in interdisciplinary approaches to zoonotic disease prevention, particularly within higher academic institutions in Indonesia, Thailand and Vietnam. Ministerial agencies responsible for food safety show clear organizational overlap between human and veterinary authorities, although this is not always reflected in communication and cooperation in policy development, partly because of limited training in One Health concepts and rigid institutional frameworks for problem solving.

An example of a One Health approach to food safety policy formulation is small-scale slaughterhouse food safety policy in northern Thailand, developed jointly by local and national governments, academics and small-scale industry (Chotinun *et al.*, 2013). High levels of foodborne pathogens including *Salmonella* and *Campylobacter* in poultry meat from small-scale slaughterhouses in peri-urban and rural areas of Chiang Mai, Thailand prompted local public health authorities to discuss possible interventions with their veterinary counterparts. Recent training in One Health approaches received by several of the actors and the newly established Ecohealth/One Health Resource Center at Chiang Mai University, Faculty of Veterinary Medicine, influenced discussion of a One Health development of policy solutions. This included examination of the problem from five key perspectives including public health, policy support, veterinary and human health, socio-economics and community engagement.

Policy development for food safety in Thailand included a review of laws and regulations for poultry slaughterhouses, in-depth interviews and focus-group discussions with key stakeholders, and participatory engagement with 41 small-scale slaughterhouses to examine epidemiologic and socio-cultural aspects of the factors relating to zoonotic disease. However, none of the slaughterhouses were able to meet current food safety regulations and obtain proper licensing. As a result, revised standards, reflecting locally appropriate standards, were generated. This allowed consumers access to locally produced affordable food, which was not intended for export. This One Health approach to policy formulation was interesting in that it modified nationally mandated food hygiene regulations using locally driven demands while incorporating socio-cultural norms with science-based decision making.

## Conclusion

In the examples provided above we have used case studies to illustrate some of the successes and challenges of developing science-based policies for the prevention and control of infectious diseases such as avian influenza and foodborne pathogens. In New Zealand, we found that taking a more integrated approach and engaging a One Health team facilitated the development of policies that were generally acceptable to the public and to relevant industry stakeholders. In South-east Asia the application of the One Health concept to the development and delivery of science-based policy is not new but challenges remain with regard to engaging communities and stakeholders in the development of policy. This is especially true where there are political and economic constraints and a lack of a cohesive policy framework across the different countries in the regions which share borders. New Zealand has been able to implement a sound policy framework to deal with many potential pathogens. This is partly because it is surrounded by ocean, and therefore has the potential to implement strict biosecurity to reduce the risk of disease entry, but also because it has a strong economic base, good governance for both the primary industry sector and public health authorities and an active public education programme. The latter is especially important with regard to ensuring public compliance with biosecurity guidelines and disease control policy. The policy examples provided in this chapter also illustrate the importance of disease reporting, transparency and good cooperation between countries especially for diseases that rapidly spread within and between countries. Whereas not everything fell into place during the H5N1 pandemic in South-east Asia, there were many lessons learned, which have helped governments and international organizations such as the FAO, WHO and OIE develop improved guidelines for responding to disease outbreaks. If done well, taking a One Health approach can promote the development of good partnerships between government agencies as well as engage the public and industry stakeholders in the development and delivery of policy. At the same time, using a One Health approach effectively should also ensure that community engagement and public education are core to the policy process (Zinsstag *et al.*, 2005).

## Acknowledgements

The authors would like to thank Dr Wlodek Stanislawek, Toni Tana and Richard Norman from the Ministry of Primary Industries, New Zealand for their comments on an earlier draft of this chapter and Brenda Moore for proofreading the final draft.

## Notes

[1] Tikanga can be described as general behaviour guidelines for daily life and interaction in Māori culture. Tikanga is commonly based on experience and learning that has been handed down through generations. It is based on logic and common sense associated with a Māori world view.

[2] Current policy outlined in http://www.dpmc.govt.nz/sites/all/files/publications/national-security-system.pdf

[3] The role of the CTO in a response has changed more recently and some of the responsibilities during an outbreak have been transferred to a designated response manager and the response is managed, coordinated and led using a response strategic leadership team, http://brkb.biosecurity.govt.nz

[4] Occurrence is restricted to infection of poultry or a product derived from poultry, where poultry is currently defined by the OIE as:

all domesticated birds, including backyard poultry, used for the production of meat or eggs for consumption, for the production of other commercial products, for restocking supplies of game, or for breeding these categories of birds, as well as fighting cocks used for any purpose. Birds that are kept in captivity for any reason other than those reasons referred to in the preceding paragraph, including those that are kept for shows, races, exhibitions, competitions or for breeding or selling these categories of birds as well as pet birds, are not considered to be poultry. (Available at: http://www.oie.int/international-standard-setting/terrestrial-manual/access-online/)

[5] Human cases of H9N2 were documented in China in the late 1990s and recent research shows transmissibility to, and between, other mammals including dogs (Amirsalehy *et al.*, 2012). H9N2 is not notifiable to the OIE unless associated with high mortality, and experts conjecture under-reporting of animal (and human) cases. In addition, co-circulation of H9N2 and H5N1 in Egypt raises a public health concern (Capua, 2013). New Zealand has also made provision for emerging pathogenic influenza A (exotic strains) along with the notifiable H5 and H7 subtypes in legislation (unwanted organism designation) in 2005.

## References

Alexander, D.J. and Brown, I.H. (2000) Recent zoonoses caused by influenza A viruses. OIE *Revue Scientifique et Technique* 19(1), 197–225.
Alexander, D.J., Allan, W.H., Parsons, D.G. and Parsons, G. (1987) The pathogenicity of four avian influenza viruses for fowls, turkeys and ducks. *Research in Veterinary Science* 24, 242–247.
Amirsalehy, H.H., Nili, H. and Mohammadi, A. (2012) Can dogs carry the global pandemic candidate avian influenza virus H9N2? *Australian Veterinary Journal* 90(9), 341–345.
Austin, F.J. and Hinshaw, V.S. (1984) The isolation of influenza A viruses and paramyxoviruses from feral ducks in New Zealand. *Australian Journal of Experimental Biology and Medical Science* 62, 355–360.
Brown, J.H. (2000) The epidemiology and evolution of influenza viruses in pigs. *Veterinary Microbiology* 74, 29–46.
Capua, I. (2013) Three open issues on Avian Influenza – H5, H7, H9 against all odds. *British Poultry Science* 54, 1–4.
Capua, I. and Alexander, D.J. (2009) Ecology, epidemiology and human health implications of avian influenza virus infections. In: Capua, I. and Alexander, D.J. (eds) *Avian Influenza and Newcastle Disease*. Springer, Berlin, pp. 1–18.
Chotinun, S., Rojanasthien, S., Unger, F. and Suwan, M. (2013) Achieving food safety, the improvement of small-scale slaughterhouses through policy engagement. *Proceedings of the Veterinary Public Health Centre for Asia Pacific*, 2–6 July 2013. Veterinary Public Health Centre for Asia Pacific, Chiang Mai, Thailand, 235 pp.
Duc, K.V. (2012) Time for a new Asian way. *Asian Times*. Available at: http://www.atimes.com/atimes/South-east_Asia/NI11Ae01.html (accessed 21 August 2013).
FAO (2010) FAO-OIE-WHO Collaboration: A Tripartite Concept Note. Available at: http://www.fao.org/docrep/012/ak736e/ak736e00.pdf (accessed 27 June 2013).
Frazer, J., Rawdon, T. and Stanislawek, W. (2008) Avian influenza surveillance programme. *Surveillance* 36(2), 14–16.
Geale, D. and Rawdon, T. (2005) Response Planning for Avian Influenza in New Zealand. *Proceedings of the Food Safety and Biosecurity, and Epidemiology and Animal Health Management Branches of the NZVA*. FCE Publication 245(Jan 2005), pp. 113–122.
Geale, D.W., Gerber, N.D., Marks, D.A., Tana, T.A., Rawdon, T.G. and Murray, A. (2006) Biosecurity risk profile - a foundation for poultry sector exotic disease contingency planning. International Symposia on Veterinary Epidemiology and Economics proceedings, ISVEE 11: *Proceedings of the 11th Symposium of the International Society for Veterinary Epidemiology and Economics, Cairns, Australia*, Theme 3 - Animal health delivery and response: Emergency response session, Aug 2006, p. 778.
Government of Vietnam (2011) The Vietnam Integrated National Operational Program on Avian Influenza, Pandemic Preparedness and Emerging Infectious Diseases (Aiped), 2011–2015. *Strengthening responses and improving prevention through a One Health approach*. Ministry of Agriculture and Rural Development (MARD) and Ministry of Health (MOH), Hanoi.
Hall, D.C. and Le, Q.B. (2009) Evaluation of the Government of Viet Nam–UN Joint Programme on Avian Influenza. *Report and Policy Recommendations*. Government of Vietnam and FAO-UN.
Hall, D.C., Nguyen-Viet, H., Willyanto, I., Tung, D. and Chotinun, S. (2013) Improving food safety in Asia through increased capacity in ecohealth. *Journal of Epidemiology and Public Health* 5(8), 336–340.

Herington, J. (2010) Securitization of infectious diseases in Vietnam: the cases of HIV and avian influenza. *Health Policy and Planning* 25, 467–475.
Hinshaw, V., Webster, R. and Turner, B. (1980) The perpetuation of orthomyxoviruses and paramyxoviruses in Canadian waterfowl. *Canadian Journal of Microbiology* 26, 622–629.
Huang, Q.S., Lopez, L.D., McCallum, L. and Adlam, B. (2008) Influenza surveillance and immunization in New Zealand, 1997–2006. *Influenza and Other Respiratory Viruses* 2(4), 139–145.
Jennings, L.C. (2005) New Zealand's preparedness for the next influenza pandemic. *New Zealand Medical Journal* 118, 1–3.
Jonas, O. (2008) Update on coordinated international assistance. *Sixth International Ministerial Conference on Avian and Pandemic Influenza, Sharm El-Sheikh* 24–26 October 2008.
Lam, T.T.-Y., Wang, J., Shen, Y., Zhou, B., Duan, L., Cheung, C.-L., Ma, C., Lycett, S.J., Leung, C.Y.-H. Chen, X., Li, L., Hong, W., Chai, Y., Zhou, L., Liang, H., Ou, Z., Liu, Y., Farooqui, A., Kelvin, D.J., Poon, L.L.M., Smith, D.K., Pybus, O.G., Leung, G.M., Shu, Y., Webster, R.G., Webby, R.J., Peiris, J.S.M., Rambaut, A., Zhu, H. and Guan, Y. (2013) The genesis and source of the H7N9 influenza viruses causing human infections in China. *Nature*, advance online publication. DOI: 10.1038/nature12515.
Langstaff, I.G., McKenzie, J.S., Stanislawek, W.L., Reed, C.E.M., Poland, R. and Cork, S.C. (2009) Surveillance for highly pathogenic avian influenza in migratory shorebirds at the terminus of the East Asian–Australian flyway. *New Zealand Veterinary Journal* 57(3), 160–165.
Lei, F. and Shi, W. (2011) Prospective of genomics in revealing transmission reassortment and evolution of wildlife-borne avian influenza A (H5N1) viruses. *Current Genomics* 1297, 466–474.
Ministry for Primary Industries (MPI) (2003) Tiakina Aotearoa Protect New Zealand: The Biosecurity Strategy for New Zealand. Available at: http://www.biosecurity.govt.nz/biosec/sys/strategy/biostrategy/biostrategynz (accessed 10 August 2013).
Ministry for Primary Industries (MPI) (2007) Biosecurity Science Strategy for New Zealand/Mahere Rautaki Putaiao Whakamaru. Available at: http://ww.biosecurity.govt.nz/biosec/research (accessed 10 August 2013).
Ministry of Agriculture and Forestry (MAF) (2006) Technical Response Policies for Avian Influenza Viruses of Regulatory Concern (Version 2.4). Available at: http://www.biosecurity.govt.nz/pests/bird-flu/response-policies (accessed 27 June 2013).
Ministry of Agriculture and Forestry (MAF) (2008) MAF's Response to Risk Organisms. Available at: http://www.biosecurity.govt.nz/bio-strategy/library/policy-incursion.htm (accessed 27 June 2013).
Ministry of Agriculture and Forestry (MAF) (2011) Whole-of-Government BIOSECURITY Response Guide August 2011. Available at: http://brkb.biosecurity.govt.nz/reference/whole-of-govt-bs-response-guide.pdf (accessed 27 June 2013).
OIE (World Organisation for Animal Health) (2004) Terrestrial Animal Health Code, 13th edn. Chapter 2.7.12 Avian Influenza. Available at: http://www.oie.int/doc/ged/D6450.pdf (accessed 28 August 2013).
OIE (World Organisation for Animal Health) (2005) Terrestrial Animal Health Code, 145th edn. Chapter 2.7.12 Avian Influenza. Available at: http://www.oie.int/doc/ged/D6428.PDF (accessed 18 July 2013).
OIE (World Organisation for Animal Health) (2013) Infection with Avian Influenza Viruses. Available at: http://www.oie.int/index.php?id=169andL=0andhtmfile=chapitre_1.10.4.htm (accessed 6 September 2013).
Pitsuwan, S. (2011) Challenges in infection in ASEAN. *Lancet* 377, 619–621.
Rawdon, T., McFadden, A., Stanislawek, W.L. and Bingham, P. (2007a) Public reports of avian mortality. Part 1: Risk profiling and investigation. *Surveillance* 34(3), 10–13.
Rawdon, T., Thornton, R., McKenzie, J. and Gerber, N. (2007b) Biosecurity risk pathways in New Zealand's commercial poultry industry. *Surveillance* 34(3), 4–9.
Rawdon, T., Tana, T., Frazer, J., Thornton, R. and Chrystal, N. (2008) Biosecurity risk pathways in the commercial poultry industry: free-range layers, pullet-rearers and turkey broilers. *Surveillance* 35(4), 4–9.
Rawdon, T.G., Tana, T., Thornton, R.N., McKenzie, J.S., Stanislawek, W.L., Kittelberger, R., Geale, D., Stevenson, M.A., Gerber, N. and Cork, S.C. (2010) Surveillance for avian influenza virus subtypes H5 and H7 in chickens and turkeys farmed commercially in New Zealand. *New Zealand Veterinary Journal* 58(6), 292–298.
Rawdon, T., Zheng, T., Adlam, B., Williman, J. and Huang, S. (2012a) Disease risk pathways associated with backyard poultry-keeping in New Zealand – Part 1: Animal health implications. *Surveillance* 38(2), 12–19.
Rawdon, T., Zheng, T., Stanislawek, W., Adlam, B., Williman, J. and Huang, S. (2012b) Disease risk pathways associated with backyard poultry keeping in New Zealand – Part 2: Human health implications. *Surveillance* 39(1), 7–11.
Scoones, I. and Forster, P. (2010) Unpacking the international response to avian influenza: actors, networks and narratives. In: Scoones, I. (ed.) *Avian Influenza: Science, Policy and Politics*. Routledge, London, pp. 19–64.

Sims, L., Domenech, J., Benigno, C., Kahn, S., Kamata, A., Lubroth, J., Martin, V. and Roeder, P. (2005) Origin and evolution of highly pathogenic H5N1 avian influenza in Asia. *Veterinary Record* 157, 159–164.
Stanislawek, W.L. (1990) Avian influenza of New Zealand wild ducks. *Surveillance* 17(2), 13–14.
Stanislawek, W.L. (1992) Survey of wild ducks for avian influenza, 1988–90. *Surveillance* 19(1), 21–22.
Stanislawek, W.L., Wilks, C.R., Meers, J., Horner, G.W., Alexander, D.J., Manvell, R.J., Kattenbelt, J.A. and Gould, A.R. (2002) Avian paramyxoviruses and influenza viruses isolated from mallard ducks (*Anas platyrhynchos*) in New Zealand. *Archives of Virology* 147, 1287–1302.
Stanislawek, W.L., Frazer, J., Rawdon, T., McFadden, A. and Lee, E. (2011) Avian influenza surveillance programme. *Surveillance* 38(3), 19–21.
Tana, T., Rawdon, T. and Stanislawek, W.L. (2007) Avian influenza surveillance programme. *Surveillance* 34(2), 11–13.
Tay, S. (2012) ASEAN risks being ineffective and neutered. Din Merican. Available at: http://dinmerican.wordpress.com/2012/07/27/asean-risks-being-ineffective-and-neutered (accessed 25 August 2013).
United Nations (2013) Available at: http://unvietnam.wordpress.com/category/one-un-in-viet-nam (accessed 2 September 2013).
Vu, T. (2009) The Political Economy of Avian Influenza. Response and Control in Vietnam. *STEPS working paper* 19. Brighton, UK.
Webby, R.J., Webster, R.G. and Richt, J.A. (2007) Influenza viruses in animal wildlife populations. In: Childs, J.E., Mackenzie, J.S. and Richt, J.A. (eds) *Wildlife and Emerging Zoonotic Diseases: The Biology, Circumstances and Consequences of Cross-Species Transmission*. Current Topics in Microbiology and Immunology 315. Springer, Berlin, pp. 67–83.
Williams, M., Gummer, H., Powlesland, R. and Taylor, G. (2004) Migrations and movements of birds to New Zealand and surrounding seas. *Department of Conservation Science and Research Unit Publication* 12(13), 111–112.
WHO (2013) Cumulative number of confirmed human cases for avian influenza A(H5N1) reported to WHO, 2003–2013. August 9, 2013. WHO, Geneva.
Zheng, T., Adlam, B., Rawdon, T.G., Stanislawek, W.L., Cork, S.C., Hope, V., Buddle, B.M., Grimwood, K., Baker, M.G., O'Keefe, J.S. and Huang, Q.S. (2010) A cross-sectional survey of influenza A infection, and management practices in small rural backyard poultry flocks in two regions of New Zealand. *New Zealand Veterinary Journal* 58(2), 74–80.
Zinsstag, J., Schelling, J.E., Wyss, K. and Bechir, M. (2005) Potential of cooperation between human and animal health to strengthen health systems. *Lancet* 366, 2142–2145.

## Appendix: List of Abbreviations

Association of South-east Asian Nations (ASEAN)
Australasian Regional Association of Zoological Parks and Aquaria (ARAZPA)
Chief Technical Officer (CTO)
Chief Veterinary Officer (CVO)
Department of Conservation (DOC)
Domestic and External Security Coordination (DESC)
Egg Producers Federation of New Zealand (EPFNZ)
Food and Agriculture Organization (FAO)
Global Early Warning and Response System for Major Animal Disease (GLEWS)
Global Framework for the progressive control of Transboundary Animal Diseases (GF TADs)
Government of Vietnam Ministries of Agriculture and Rural Development (MARD)
Government of Vietnam Ministry of Finance (MF)
Government of Vietnam Ministry of Health (MOH)
gross domestic product (GDP)
high pathogenicity avian influenza (HPAI)
highly pathogenic avian influenza (HPAI)
highly pathogenic notifiable avian influenza (HPNAI)
low pathogenicity notifiable avian influenza (LPNAI)

low pathogenicity avian influenza (LPAI)
Memorandum of Understanding (MOU)
Ministry of Agriculture and Forestry (MAF)
Ministry of Civil Defence and Emergency Management (MCDEM)
Ministry of Economic Development (MED)
Ministry for the Environment (MfE)
Ministry of Fisheries (Min Fish)
Ministry of Foreign Affairs and Trade (MFAT)
Ministry of Health (MOH)
Ministry for Primary Industries (MPI)
Ministry of Social Development (MSD)
Ministry of Transport (MOT)
New Zealand Defence Force (NFDF)
non-governmental organization (NGO)
notifiable avian influenza (NAI)
Ostrich and Emu Standards Council (OESC)
Poultry Industry Association of New Zealand (PIANZ)
Stakeholder Advisory Group (SAG)
Technical Advisory Group (TAG)
United Nations (UN)
United Nations Children's Fund (UNICEF)
United Nations Development Programme (UNDP)
World Health Organization (WHO)
World Organisation for Animal Health (OIE)

# 26 Evolution of the One Health Movement in the USA

**Carol S. Rubin,[1]* Rebekah Kunkel,[1] Cheri Grigg[1] and Lonnie King[2]**
*[1]One Health Office, National Center for Emerging and Zoonotic Infectious Diseases, Centers for Disease Control and Prevention, Atlanta, Georgia;*
*[2]College of Veterinary Medicine, Ohio State University, Columbus, Ohio*

## Introduction

Throughout the history of the USA, collaboration among human, animal and environment sectors has waxed and waned according to situational demand for working across disciplines. Several events in the early 21st century renewed interest in the One Health concept, broadly defined as the inter-connectedness of human, animal and environmental health sectors.

In 1992, the Institute of Medicine (IOM) published a report entitled 'Emerging Infections: Microbial Threats to Health in the United States' highlighting the importance of recognizing and preventing emerging infectious diseases. In response to the report, the US Centers for Disease Control and Prevention (CDC) and the National Institutes of Allergy and Infectious Diseases requested that IOM convene the Forum on Emerging Diseases, later renamed the Forum on Microbial Threats (National Academy of Sciences, 2013a). Under the leadership of Nobel laureate Dr Joshua Lederberg, the Forum provided a structured opportunity to discuss emerging communicable diseases in humans, plants and animals.

In 2004, the Wildlife Conservation Society (WCS) and Columbia University convened a meeting in New York City that called for a renewal of transdisciplinary collaboration to 'protect human health' (Wildlife Conservation Society, 2004). During that meeting physician William Foege delivered an address that outlined the necessity for collaboration (Foege, 2004), and the conveners released a list of 12 fundamental reasons for taking a One Health approach. This list has come to be known as the Manhattan Principles (Wildlife Conservation Society, 2004). (See also Cumming and Cumming, Chapter 4, this volume.)

Leadership by subject matter experts involved in the IOM and WCS meetings provided the basis for a series of concurrent activities among scientific and service communities, including US government agencies, non-governmental organizations (NGOs), academic institutions and professional membership groups. Situational demand for this One Health resurgence included recognition that: emerging and re-emerging zoonotic infectious diseases (EIDs) pose a new and substantial threat to human health; climate change nationally and globally impacts food safety and security; and the demonstrated importance of biosecurity preparedness necessitates working with non-traditional partners.

We are now in a period of opportunity in which we can use the One Health approach to institutionalize and operationalize problem

*E-mail: carolrubin.dvm@gmail.com

solving that crosses professional boundaries of expertise. This chapter highlights the work that has been accomplished or at least initiated in a variety of sectors. We describe the current status of One Health in the USA, and the challenges that we face in sustaining communication and collaboration across sectors and disciplines.

## Recognition of the Need for One Health by the US Scientific Community

Progression of One Health in the USA has been championed by a series of visionaries within the scientific community (Box 26.1). The majority of these individuals came from the animal health sector, probably because several tenants of One Health, including the emphasis on population rather than individual health, the fundamental association between health and food safety and the necessity to take a systems approach to problem solving, have historically been more integral to veterinary rather than human medical training. One Health visionaries articulated this concept and provided a foundation for others to integrate One Health approaches into a variety of scientific disciplines. This process can be traced by reviewing IOM publications produced during the past several decades.

The National Academies, which functions independently and is not directly funded by the US federal government (USG), includes the IOM and the National Research Council (NRC) (National Academy of Sciences, 2013b). These two bodies conduct targeted reviews of specific scientific questions, with the intention of providing unbiased expert advice to policy makers and the general public. The end-products include rigorously reviewed IOM/NRC consensus reports as well as IOM workshop summaries that are the opinions of subject matter experts rather than consensus conclusions and recommendations. A recent paper reviewing all IOM and NRC reports between 1991 and 2013 found multiple reports and recommendations that address One Health concepts, activities and approaches even when the term 'One Health' was not specifically used (Rubin *et al.*, 2013). The recommendations can be grouped into seven topical categories: Surveillance and Response (16 recommendations); Governance and Policy (ten recommendations); Laboratory Networks (four recommendations); Training Needs (six recommendations); Research Needs (11 recommendations); Communication Needs (three recommendations); and Partnerships (five recommendations). These categories offer some insight into the areas that scientists in the USA recognize as likely to benefit from inclusion of a One Health approach.

## Sentinel Examples of How a One Health Approach Has Enhanced Public Health Response in the USA

### Example – public health response to foodborne disease

The PulseNet and FoodNet surveillance systems exemplify how the most basic One Health principle of cross-sectoral communication can increase public health effectiveness. Traditionally, foodborne disease investigations in the USA were conducted locally and relied upon epidemiological investigation tools to implicate a potentially contaminated product. Multiple outbreaks caused by a single animal or common source of contamination were rarely connected, especially if the product was distributed across several state jurisdictions (Woteki and Kineman, 2003). Human health and animal health agencies at both state and national levels fell under different governmental jurisdictions. The lack of cross-agency communication and collaboration made it less likely that multiple human foodborne outbreaks with a single source of contamination would be identified and thus mitigated in a time frame likely to decrease morbidity and mortality.

A multi-state foodborne outbreak of *E. coli* 0157:H7, spanning 1992–1993, brought attention to the need for a nationally integrated system for detecting and responding to food contamination before widespread human illness occurred. In response to the illness and death caused by this outbreak, congressional

**Box 26.1.** Quotes from selected One Health visionaries.

1807 – Benjamin Rush, MD

By extending our knowledge of the causes and the cure of the diseases of domestic animals, we may add greatly to the certainty and usefulness of the profession of medicine as far as it relates to the human species.

1964 – Calvin W. Schwabe, DVM, MPHD, ScD

Veterinary Medicine is the field of study concerned with the diseases and health of non-human animals. The practice of veterinary medicine is directly related to man's well-being in a number of ways.

2000 – Joshua Lederberg, PhD

An axiomatic starting point for progress is the simple recognition that humans, animals, plants and microbes are cohabitants of this planet. That leads to refined questions that focus on the origin and dynamics of instabilities within this context of cohabitation. These instabilities rise from two main sources loosely definable as ecological and evolutionary.

2004 – Rita R. Colwell, PhD, MS

Health issues are no longer just a matter between patient and physician – if they ever were – but now encompass an individual's complex relationship with the global environment.

2007 – Ronald M. Davis, MD

I'm delighted that the AMA House of Delegates has approved a resolution calling for increased collaboration between the human and veterinary medical communities and I look forward to seeing a stronger partnership between physicians and veterinarians. Emerging infectious diseases, with the threats of cross-species transmission and pandemics, represent one of many reasons why the human and veterinary medical professions must work more closely together.

2007 – Roger K. Mahr, DVM

It is my fervent hope and vision that we as health science professionals, and as professional associations, will assume our collaborative responsibility … to protect and promote our immeasurable value, to utilize that value to its fullest, and to make sure that our future is a promising future … a future of even greater value.

2008 – James H. Steele, DVM, MPH

You cannot have good public health unless you have good animal health. And you can't have good animal health unless you have good public health.

2009 – Ronald M. Atlas, PhD

Given that 75% of newly emerging human infectious diseases originate within wildlife and domesticated animals, and that global warming and other environmental changes are likely to have significant health impacts, it is essential that the medical, veterinary, and public health sectors join forces.

2011 – William H. Foege, MD, MPH

…you cannot deal with the health of people without dealing with the health of animals – the two are inseparable.

2013 – James M. Hughes, MD, FDSA

The veterinary medical community deserves credit for generating interest in the importance of a One Health approach involving transdisciplinary collaboration and opening communication channels across professional categories. Physicians who are interested in or involved with influenza, antimicrobial resistance, healthcare-associated infections, foodborne diseases, blood, organ, and tissues safety, pathogen discovery, biosafety or biosecurity programs, or bioterrorism preparedness should be supportive and willing to reach out to veterinary medical colleagues.

2013 – Lonnie J. King, DVM, MS, MPA

The convergence of people, animals and our environment has created a new dynamic characterized by a profound and unprecedented interdependence of these domains that are now inextricably linked and elaborately connected and has also resulted in new threats to the health of each of these 3 domains. We can no longer focus on these threats separately.

legislation allocated funding to establish the enhanced sentinel surveillance systems PulseNet and FoodNet, for detecting outbreaks across state and agency jurisdictions (Swaminathan *et al.*, 2001; Allos *et al.*, 2004). Although this event pre-dates the term One Health, the USG actions taken in response to this outbreak can be viewed as one of the first One Health successes in the USA.

The effectiveness of these integrated surveillance and response systems has led to development of additional nationally coordinated systems, including ArboNET, which integrates human, animal and vector surveillance (Lindsey *et al.*, 2012), and MicrobeNet, which links CDC laboratory expertise with state and local laboratories to rapidly identify infectious pathogens (Centers for Disease Control and Prevention, 2013a).

### Example – Zoonoses Education Coalition

In response to the increasing number of large, multistate zoonotic outbreaks, CDC proposed partnering with the pet industry in order to more effectively address human illness associated with pet exposure. In 2013, the Zoonoses Education Coalition (ZEC) was formed to develop a set of evidence-based, plain language recommendations which can be used consistently across the pet industry. The ZEC is a multi-sectoral collaboration with representatives from the American Veterinary Medical Association, the Food and Drug Administration, the National Association of State Public Health Veterinarians, the Pet Industry Joint Advisory Council, the pet industry and CDC. This partnership between the public and private sector will result in scientifically accurate information which can more effectively reach consumers.

The ZEC is currently embarking on a pilot project to help consumers understand how to prevent *Salmonella* infections resulting from direct and indirect contact with reptiles and amphibians. In addition to the core members listed above, representatives from the pet reptile and amphibian industry will also be involved in the pilot project. The group has developed a series of messages that can be adapted by partners for use in any of their communication products, such as print materials, newsletters and websites. Based on evaluation of the pilot, the project may be expanded to include additional partners and to develop targeted messages to prevent other zoonotic issues.

### Example – human and animal health agency responses to novel influenza viruses

The 2009 emergence of novel influenza A H1N1 and the subsequent pandemic highlighted both challenges and successes of implementing a One Health response to EIDs in the USA. When the novel virus emerged, scientists in the USA were able quickly to determine the origin and begin tracking cases. Antigenic and genetic characteristics of the identified virus indicated that it was most closely related to North American swine-lineage H1N1 and Eurasian lineage swine-origin H1N1 influenza viruses (Garten *et al.*, 2009). Unfortunately, this rapid determination of the genetic makeup of the virus resulted in public health authorities initially referring to the virus as 'swine flu' (Centers for Disease Control and Prevention, 2009; World Health Organization, 2009). The subsequent public misconceptions about risk factors for contracting the virus from swine and pork products resulted in substantial loss in revenue for the US swine industry, even before official detection of the virus in pigs in the USA (Butler, 2009). In order to mitigate further losses, the United States Department of Agriculture (USDA) organized calls with a wide variety of key stakeholders, including human health and industry, to agree upon speaking points for when the inevitable first case of 2009 pH1N1 would be diagnosed in swine in the USA (Gostin and Hanfling, 2009). This forward-thinking One Health communication campaign was instrumental in preventing further trade restrictions and avoiding what could have been a US$456 million revenue loss (Zering, 2009).

Lessons learned from the 2009 H1N1 pandemic were effectively applied to the 2011 emergence of swine origin influenza A H3N2 variant virus (H3N2v). From the initial detection of the virus, the public health, animal health and animal industries worked together to assess the situation and produce recommendations to protect both people and swine.

## US Government Acknowledgement of One Health

USG agencies at the federal, state and local levels are responsible for human, animal and environmental health. These agencies have different mandates and regulatory authority, which may impede collaboration. The lack of integrated federal funding that cuts across sectors is also a major impediment to the development of One Health partnerships. This long-standing separation sometimes manifests as distrust towards other agencies, further preventing the formation of interagency partnerships (Rabinowitz and Conti, 2013).

Despite these challenges, government entities have found ways to overcome traditional barriers. Several federal agencies have created One Health-dedicated units, which promote both internal and external collaboration. In addition to internal structural changes at some agencies, a Federal Interagency One Health Working Group has been created to improve interagency communication and cooperation.

### United States Department of Agriculture

USDA is a regulatory organization analogous to a ministry of agriculture and is formally led by a Secretary of Agriculture who is appointed by the President of the USA. USDA recently established a One Health Joint Working Group that includes members from USDA agencies with interests in One Health. The Working Group supports the USDA implementation of One Health principles and improves the outcomes of USDA programmes for global public health, animal and plant health and environmental health. USDA's Animal and Plant Health Inspection Service (APHIS), Veterinary Service (VS) has also broadened the scope of its mission to address the animal component of One Health issues. The commitment of APHIS VS to One Health is reaffirmed in their mission statement: 'As the recognized animal health leader and trusted partner, Veterinary Services safeguards the health of animals, people and the environment' (United States Animal and Plant Health Inspection Service, 2011).

The APHIS VS has developed a strategic plan for implementing One Health activities within VS which outlines a set of goals to increase the credibility of USDA within the One Health community and includes: aligning policy, programmes and infrastructure with the VS One Health vision; building and sustaining partnerships, particularly with other US government agencies; spearheading outreach and communication; and building new skill sets within the VS workforce (VS 2015 One Health Working Group, 2010). To help achieve those One Health goals, APHIS VS formed a One Health Coordination Office in 2012 (Animal and Plant Health Inspection Service, 2012). The Office has employees working throughout USDA and with other USG agencies to promote and improve collaboration and communication among federal, state, local and tribal governments and private industry.

### Centers for Disease Control and Prevention

CDC is an agency within the US Department of Health and Human Services (HHS), which is led by a presidentially appointed Secretary of Health; HHS is loosely equivalent to a ministry of health. Other HHS agencies include the National Institutes of Health and the Food and Drug Administration.

CDC's National Center for Emerging Zoonotic and Infectious Diseases (NCEZID) is home to most of the scientists who work on pathogens that can be passed from animals to humans. NCEZID (Centers for Disease Control and Prevention, 2013b) focuses on:

> diseases that have been around for many years, emerging diseases (those that are new or just recently identified) and zoonotic diseases (those spread from animals to people). [The Center's] work is guided in part by a holistic One Health strategy, which recognizes the vital interconnectedness of

> microbes and the environment. Through a comprehensive approach involving many scientific disciplines, we can attain better health for humans and animals and improve our environment.

The One Health Office was established in 2009 to promote One Health both within and outside of CDC. Currently located within NCEZID, the office serves as the CDC programmatic home for many of the One Health activities that involve collaboration of subject matter experts in different internal units. For example, the office organizes an internal Zoonoses Working Group that builds collaboration among CDC scientists working on different pathogens. The office also serves as a point of contact for external animal health and agriculture organizations. The One Health Office recently designed a comprehensive website to provide greater insight into One Health and highlight public health activities that use a One Health approach (http://www.cdc.gov/onehealth).

The One Health Office at CDC has also stationed Animal-Human Interface (AHI) Officers in strategic international locations to work collaboratively with in-country partners on public health issues related to zoonotic diseases at the AHI. The CDC Global Detection (GDD) Regional Centers have recognized the value of the AHI Officers and have established the One Health/Zoonoses capacity as one of six GDD core capacities (Centers for Disease Control and Prevention, 2011).

## National Park Service

The National Park Service (NPS), established in 1916, is a bureau in the Department of the Interior. The National Park Service preserves more than 84 million acres of natural and cultural resources in US states and territories. With over 275 million visitors annually, national parks offer a unique opportunity to practise One Health. The Wildlife Health Branch and Office of Public Health within NPS have partnered to promote One Health through the development of a One Health Network which serves to 'promote and protect the health of all species and the parks that we share' (National Park Service, 2013).

The NPS One Health Network uses a management approach that provides guidance and recommendations which consider the impacts on humans, animals and the environment. The Network also promotes research and education on the health benefits of biodiversity, with NPS resources as 'living laboratories' for health promotion and research. The network emphasizes interdisciplinary response; a disease outbreak investigation team, consisting of a medical epidemiologist, wildlife veterinarian, veterinary epidemiologist and public health consultant, is available to provide technical assistance to park units regarding human and wildlife disease outbreaks. NPS is also exploring combining human and wildlife surveillance systems to better detect disease outbreaks and clusters, and using a One Health paradigm to study disease transmission.

NPS recently created a position for a One Health Coordinator. The One Health Coordinator provides rapid assistance in disease response and communications with other departments within the National Park Service, the media and the public. The coordinator also promotes One Health through research, education and programmes that explore the interconnectedness of all species.

## Federal Interagency One Health Working Group

In 2011, individual members of several federal agencies came together to discuss ways to increase collaboration and communication among One Health focal points within each agency. The result of these discussions was the formation, in 2012, of a Federal Interagency One Health Working Group (FIOHWG). The primary purpose of the FIOHWG is to enhance exchange of information and foster USG implementation of One Health principles. The Working Group focuses on four key functions to improve human, animal, plant and environmental health: (i) increasing awareness throughout the government of One Health principles and practices; (ii) improving communication regarding One Health activities to improve cooperation and efficiency of government resources; (iii) providing a forum for government programme managers and subject matter experts to communicate; and (iv) facilitating coordination of personnel to support government initiatives.

Participation in the Working Group is voluntary and open to programme managers and subject matter experts at any government agency. The group currently has participants from 14 federal agencies whose primary mission areas represent all three sectors of One Health. Participating agencies include CDC, the Department of State, the USDA, the US Geological Survey and the Department of the Interior. The group is not led by any single department or agency; rather, leadership is shared across agencies with rotating meeting chairs. The group meets quarterly via conference call to exchange information and keep abreast of topics of interest.

## One Health Activities in the US Non-governmental Sector

NGOs have been instrumental in the USA in drawing attention to One Health both as a term and also in demonstrating the utility of One Health as an approach to working across traditional boundaries. Two of the more well-known entities, the One Health Initiative and the One Health Commission, were early leaders in garnering supporters among the scientific community. These organizations were formed around the same time but had distinctly separate missions, activities and leadership. Several other non-profit organizations, such as the Marine Mammal Foundation, have officially established One Health components and incorporated a One Health approach into their research agenda. Similarly, several internationally focused NGOs (e.g. Wildlife Conservation Society, EcoHealth Alliance) are based in the USA but function globally to prevent emerging infectious diseases in developing countries by using a One Health approach.

### Examples of NGOs that have championed One Health

#### *One Health Initiative (OHI)*

After the introduction of the Manhattan Principles, in 2008 the terms 'One Health' and 'One World–One Health'™ began to be used more frequently but there was no organized point of contact for information exchange. Several well-known leaders in the One Health community recognized the need to provide a platform for networking scientists and activists, as well as educating the lay public about the activities that were included under the One Health umbrella. To meet this need, the OHI website (http://onehealthinitiative.com) was created in 2008 to increase communication and collaboration among human, animal and ecosystem health professionals. In 2010 the OHI formed an honorary Advisory Board consisting of 30 professionals drawn from the human medical, animal health, public health and environmental sector, including members from academia, state and federal government agencies and international organizations.

Several aspects of the OHI are of note and have contributed to its longevity and success. Perhaps most importantly, the founding members include two physicians and a veterinarian. This combination of professionals is of importance because it marks one of the few One Health efforts in the USA that have emerged primarily from the human health community. Its descriptive name, along with its professional logo that promotes both human and animal health, has also contributed to the success of the OHI. It is also of note that the OHI formally includes the importance of 'mental health via the human–animal bond phenomenon' in its mission statement. This wording is reflective of the overall inclusivity of the OHI.

#### *American Veterinary Medical Association*

The American Veterinary Medical Association (AVMA), a not-for-profit association founded in 1863, is a professional organization that represents over 84,000 US veterinarians (American Veterinary Medical Association, 2013b). AVMA functions to improve animal and human health through advancing its relationship to public health, biological science and agriculture (American Veterinary Medical Association, 2013a). In accordance with this mission, AVMA has displayed a commitment to supporting the integration of One Health in approaches to address global challenges to human, animal and environmental health. In 2007, a One Health Initiative Task Force (OHITF) was formed to study the feasibility of a campaign to 'facilitate collaboration and cooperation among health science professions, academic institutions, governmental agencies and industries to help with the assessment, treatment and prevention of cross-species disease transmission and mutually prevalent, but non-transmitted, human and animal diseases and medical conditions' (King *et al.*, 2008). The OHITF examined current challenges to global health, and identified specific areas that would benefit from a more integrated approach to facing these challenges. Potential barriers and solutions were described in the OHITF final report, *One Health: A New Professional Imperative* (American Veterinary Medical Association, 2008).

### *One Health Commission*

The One Health Commission (OHC) was officially chartered in Washington, DC on 29 June 2009 as a 501 (c) (3) corporation and designated as a public charity (One Health Commission, 2013b). The Commission was created to improve the health of 'people, domestic animals, wildlife, plants and our environment' by promoting the establishment of closer professional interactions, collaborations and educational and research opportunities across the health science professions together with their related disciplines (One Health Commission, 2013a).

In 2012, OHC established a new membership model with a tiered contribution structure, including membership categories for organizational institutions, industry and individuals. The management of the Commission is under a Board of Directors drawn from a variety of animal, human and ecosystem health sectors. A Council of Advisors is appointed by the Board to serve in an advisory capacity with respect to policy matters and pursuing activities in support of the educational and scientific purposes of the Commission.

### *National Marine Mammal Foundation*

The National Marine Mammal Foundation (NMMF) is a non-profit organization with a mission to protect and improve life for marine mammals and humans through medicine, research and education (National Marine Mammal Foundation, n.d.,a). The NMMF was founded in San Diego, California in 2007 to expand on the research initiatives of the US Navy Marine Mammal Program.

NMMF features a One Health Medicine & Research Program that expands on the basic definition of One Health to include comparative medicine. Activities are broad-ranging but currently focus on the human health implications of research into marine mammal ageing, diabetes and infectious diseases (National Marine Mammal Foundation, 2012). Notable NMMF accomplishments include the discovery by Foundation scientists that bottlenose dolphins can serve as a natural animal model for type 2 diabetes and the ongoing study of elephant seal metabolic adaptations to fasting for clues to human metabolic disorders (National Marine Mammal Foundation, n.d.,b).

## Academic Institutions

In the late 19th century, as scientific knowledge increased and the professions became more specialized, human and veterinary medical training diverged (American Veterinary Medical Association, 2008; Chaddock, 2012). Additionally, veterinary medicine in the USA has long been associated with agriculture and production animals. Consequently, most of the veterinary colleges in the USA are located at land grant institutions in rural areas, while the majority of medical schools are located in urban population centres. The geographic discontinuity and separate training curricula for these professional programmes have resulted in compartmentalization, further impeding the development of interdisciplinary programmes.

Although changing this deep-rooted separation is difficult, One Health leaders in the USA have begun to revise existing training programmes to prepare a One Health-ready workforce. Several universities in the USA have adopted an inter-professional education model to bring together professionals from multiple disciplines, including human and veterinary medicine, for collaborative learning. Other universities have created unique DVM/MPH programmes and academic programmes specifically focused on One Health. The following universities, all of which have co-located schools of human medicine and veterinary medicine, demonstrate that traditionally separate departments can come together to create training programmes that prepare students to face the interdisciplinary challenges of the 21st century (see also Buntain *et al.*, Chapter 28, this volume).

### Western University of Health Sciences

In January 2010, Western University of Health Sciences (WesternU) implemented an innovative education curriculum at the university's campuses in California and Oregon (Western University of Health Sciences, 2013). The programme brings together groups of seven to nine students from different professional programmes, including medical and veterinary students, for collaborative learning experiences. Each year more than 900 students participate. The multi-disciplinary education curriculum focuses on several core competencies, one of which is One Health.

During the programme, students solve case studies using a cross-disciplinary collaborative approach under the guidance of a skilled facilitator. Through this process, students build communication and interpersonal skills and gain an understanding of the roles of other professions. Moreover, the programme helps the students build lasting networks with professionals from other disciplines, encouraging future integration of these professions in the workforce.

### University of Minnesota

The University of Minnesota (UMN) has several training programmes to prepare professionals for the One Health workforce. One of these programmes is the DVM/MPH veterinary public health programme, which is the largest dual DVM/MPH programme in the country (University of Minnesota School of Public Health, 2013). The programme is unique among DVM/MPH programmes because it combines distance and traditional courses, which allows students from any accredited veterinary school to attend. Although the programme began as a joint effort between the College of Veterinary Medicine and the School of Public Health, it has now expanded to include the School of Dentistry, Medical School, School of Nursing, College of Pharmacy and College of Food, Agricultural and Natural Resource Sciences (University of Minnesota College of Veterinary Medicine, 2012).

UMN continues to explore novel training opportunities. The university recently piloted an inter-professional education programme called the 1Health Initiative (Brandt *et al.*, 2010; University of Minnesota Academic Health Center Office of Education, 2013). The programme provides students from a variety of professional programmes, including medicine, nursing, public health and veterinary medicine, with the opportunity to build skills for professional collaborative practice (University of Minnesota Academic Health Center Office of Education, 2013). Additionally, faculty from the Colleges of Veterinary Medicine, Public Health, Nursing and Medicine are currently using newly identified One Health core competencies to build partnerships within academic health centres across UMN and with other institutions.

### The Ohio State University

In 2005, The Ohio State University (OSU) created a Veterinary Public Health specialization within the Masters of Public Health degree programme. This programme, developed by the College of Veterinary Medicine in collaboration with the College of Public Health, provides training in veterinary public health for veterinarians and students intending to earn an advanced degree (DVM, MPH, PhD). The programme provides students with the skills, knowledge and resources to protect human health using a One Medicine approach

(Hoet *et al.*, 2008). Students receive a broad-based public health education with special emphasis on infectious disease epidemiology, zoonotic diseases and biostatistics. Students are also required to complete at least 120 h of field experience in veterinary public health. The degree usually takes 1.5–2 years to complete. The Veterinary Public Health specialization at OSU is also recognized by the American College of Veterinary Medicine.

### University of Florida

The University of Florida (UF) is the first university in the USA to provide formal academic training for One Health. The Department of Environmental and Global Health at UF has partnered with professionals from seven UF colleges to develop two new graduate programmes for One Health training. One is a 40 credit programme for a Masters of Health Science with a concentration in One Health (University of Florida Department of Environmental & Global Health College of Public Health and Health Professions, 2013b). The second programme is a 90 credit PhD programme in Public Health with a One Health concentration (University of Florida Department of Environmental & Global Health College of Public Health and Health Professions, 2013c). The first cohort of PhD students began in the summer of 2012 (Special Wildlife Health Issue, 2012).

UF has also created a Certificate in One Health to provide One Health training to veterinary, environmental and public health professionals and students (University of Florida Department of Environmental & Global Health College of Public Health and Health Professions, 2013a). The programme enrols around 50 professionals each year who participate in 18–20 days of intensive training at UF and one term of distance learning.

## One Health Progress, Challenges and Future Direction

One Health is gaining momentum in the USA and globally, and the progress that has been made nationally has occurred in synchronization with international partners, including the World Health Organization (WHO), the World Organisation for Animal Health (OIE) and the Food and Agriculture Organization of the United Nations (FAO).

### Progress

The preceding sections and cited examples elucidate the many aspects of progress toward a One Health approach in the USA. Each step toward enhanced collaboration has been somewhat situation-specific and varied from congressionally mandated and funded integration of surveillance and response to outbreaks to independently initiated formation of the federal interagency working group focused on One Health activities.

During the past decade a great many meetings have been convened at both the state and national level that included the term One Health in the title of the meeting or at least designated a substantial section of the meeting to a One Health topic area. These meetings served the important function of bringing professionals from different areas together to actively debate the utility of a One Health approach. Often, meetings thematically devoted to One Health brought together scientists and other professionals who had not previously met to discuss formally subject matter areas where their interests and activities overlapped. An example of tangible progress from such a meeting was demonstrated by outcomes from the 2010 Stone Mountain meeting, 'Operationalizing "One Health": A Policy Perspective – Taking Stock and Shaping an Implementation Roadmap' (Rubin, 2013). CDC led the organization of this conference and worked collaboratively with the WHO, OIE, FAO, the World Bank and the European Union Commission to convene the meeting. Six Work Groups that were formed during this meeting continue to function more than 3 years later, producing carefully defined outputs that were identified during the meeting as essential components to demonstrating the utility of a One Health approach. For example, the Work Group tasked with identifying proof of concept for One Health published an extensive literature search (Rabinowitz *et al.*, 2013) and assembled concept papers for field studies to demonstrate added benefit. The Work Group focused on One Health training has made course listings available (http://www.onehealthglobal.net) and collaborated with others to formalize core competencies for One Health practitioners. With the assistance of World Bank funding, the Country-Level Needs Assessment Work Group has designed tools for state and national governments to assess their capacity for using a One Health approach; these are currently being piloted within the USA and internationally.

The extent to which a One Health approach has been embraced by the academic community is perhaps the most significant milestone toward institutionalizing One Health in the USA. Adding new course areas to established professional curriculums, integrating course requirements among professional schools and founding new advanced degree programmes are daunting tasks. None the less, these tasks have been accomplished at several academic institutions in the USA. These changes will produce a workforce uniquely qualified to function across historically defined divisions between human, animal and environmental disciplines. Optimally, it will be the success of this workforce that institutionalizes the One Health approach.

## Challenges and opportunities to further implementation of One Health nationally

Despite the great deal of progress that has been made during the past decade in integrating surveillance and response among animal and human health sectors and increasing training in the One Health concept, several barriers and challenges to implementation remain. At the most basic level, these challenges can be summarized under the headings of inertia, lack of trust and funding discrepancies. It is difficult to move beyond the status quo and work with non-traditional partners. Most public health, animal health and academic professionals are busy; the pressure of completing required time-sensitive tasks takes precedence over bringing in new collaborators and potentially delaying, and even complicating, completion of deliverables. We are at a point in the One Health movement in which the collaborative approach is likely to be more time consuming as we build new relationships with new partners. The act of collaboration, based upon a deliberate decision to reach across traditional disciplinary divisions, must be a goal in and of itself.

Institutionalization of One Health is also challenged by a lack of trust among agencies that have well-defined, albeit different, mandates. Open communication is necessary to overcome entrenched misconceptions that can prevent the level of trust that is essential to true collaboration. Cross-training, exchange of embedded liaisons among agencies with different mandates and successful collaborative experiences will slowly chip away at even long-standing divides. Examples of overcoming this barrier in the USA include: the WesternU requirement that professional students have at least one class with peers from other professional schools to focus on cross-discipline problem-solving; embedding USDA/APHIS, USDA/FSIS and FDA staff within CDC; and joint human and animal surveillance and outbreak response to diseases caused by novel influenza viruses.

An additional challenge to the successful adaptation of One Health is the differences in funding streams and funding levels and the restrictions imposed upon discretionary use of funds. Funding is frequently pathogen-specific and organizations have limited flexibility in using budgetary funds allocated by Congress. This is a multi-faceted situation without an easy solution. However, it is of note that when funding is directly allocated toward a One Health approach to addressing a defined problem, as was done with the creation of PulseNet and FoodNet in response to foodborne pathogens, then both efficiency and effectiveness are enhanced. Drawing attention to successful efforts and more formal evaluation of One Health approaches may lead to further integration of funding.

## Future direction of One Health in the USA

Overall, movement toward a One Health approach in the USA has made substantial headway, especially during the past 15 years, and it continues to evolve and demonstrate added value. The global realities that underscore the need for this cross-sector collaboration in the USA and elsewhere include rapid movement of people and products nationally and internationally, increasing demand for protein sources, encroachment of humans into animal habitats, climate changes that alter vector distribution and increasing antimicrobial resistance to pathogens. These realities will only intensify with time, and the need for cross-sector and cross-disciplinary collaboration will also escalate.

The vision of national intersectoral and transdisciplinary collaboration has been well-articulated, and the necessity for such a One Health approach is becoming more accepted. Challenges are being recognized and addressed; scientists in the USA from both the public and private sector are reaching out to colleagues in other disciplines. A One Health community is gaining foothold in the USA, and future leaders from the human, animal and environmental health sectors are stepping forward.

## Note

The findings and conclusions in this chapter are those of the authors and do not necessarily represent the official position of the US Centers for Disease Control and Prevention.

## References

Allos, B.M., Moore, M.R., Griffin, P.M. and Tauxe, R.V. (2004) Surveillance for sporadic foodborne disease in the 21st century: the FoodNet perspective. *Clinical Infectious Diseases* 38(Suppl. 3), S115–120.

American Veterinary Medical Association (2008) One Health: A New Professional Imperative. One Health Initiative Task Force: Final Report. Available at: https://www.avma.org/KB/Resources/Reports/Pages/One-Health.aspx (accessed 7 October 2014).

American Veterinary Medical Association (2013a) AVMA Mission and Objective. Available at: https://www.avma.org/About/WhoWeAre/Pages/mission.aspx (accessed 7 October 2014).

American Veterinary Medical Association (2013b) Who We Are. Available at: https://www.avma.org/About/WhoWeAre/Pages/default.aspx (accessed 7 October 2014).

Animal and Plant Health Inspection Service (2012) One Health. Available at: http://www.aphis.usda.gov (accessed 7 October 2014).

Brandt, B., Buchanan, J. and Kostka, S. (2010) 1Health, the Center for Interprofessional Education, The University of Minnesota. *Journal of Allied Health* 39(3), e-143–144.

Butler, D. (2009) Testimony of the National Pork Producers Council on the US Pork Industry Economic Crisis before the US House Committee on Agriculture Subcommittee on Livestock, Dairy, and Poultry, October 22. Available at: http://agriculture.house.gov/testimony/111/h102209/Butler.pdf (accessed 7 October 2014).

Centers for Disease Control and Prevention (2009) Swine influenza A (H1N1) infection in two children – Southern California. *Morbidity and Mortality Weekly Report* 58, 400–402.

Centers for Disease Control and Prevention (2011) Global Disease Detection (GDD). Available at: http://www.cdc.gov/globalhealth/gdder/gdd (accessed 7 October 2014).

Centers for Disease Control and Prevention (2013a) National Antimicrobial Resistance Monitoring System for Enteric Bacteria (NARMS). Available at: at: http://www.cdc.gov/narms/index.html (accessed 7 October 2014).

Centers for Disease Control and Prevention (2013b) National Center for Emerging and Zoonotic Infectious Diseaes (NCEZID). Available at: http://www.cdc.gov/ncezid (accessed 7 October 2014).

Chaddock, M. (2012) Academic veterinary medicine and One Health education: it is more than clinical applications. *Journal of Veterinary Medical Education* 39(3), 241–246.

Foege, W.H. (2004) One World, One Health, Could We Muddle Through? One World, One Health: Building Interdisciplinary Bridges. Available at: http://www.oneworldonehealth.org/sept2004/presentations/eve_foege.html (accessed 9 September 2013).

Garten, R.J., Davis, C.T., Russell, C.A., Shu, B., Lindstrom, S., Balish, A., Sessions, W.M., Xu, X., Skepner, E., Deyde, V., Okomo-Adhiambo, M., Gubareva, L., Barnes, J., *et al.* (2009) Antigenic and genetic characteristics of swine-origin 2009 A (H1N1) influenza viruses circulating in humans. *Science* 325(5937), 197–201.

Gostin, L.O. and Hanfling, D. (2009) National preparedness for a catastrophic emergency: crisis standards of care. *Journal of the American Medical Association* 302(21), 2365–2366.

Hoet, A.E., Caswell, R.J., DeGraves, F.J., Rajala-Schultz, J., Gebreyes, W.A., Saville, J.A.W. and Wittum, T.E. (2008) A new approach to teaching veterinary public health at the Ohio State University. *Journal of Veterinary Medical Education* 35(2), 106–165.

King, L.J., Anderson, L.R., Blackmore, C.G., Blackwell, M.J., Lautner, E.A., Marcus, L.C., Meyer, T.E., Monath, T.P., Nave, J.E., Ohle, J., Pappaioanou, M., Sobota, J., *et al.* (2008) Executive summary of the AVMA One Health Initiative Task Force report. *Journal of the American Veterinary Medical Association* 233(2), 259–261.

Lindsey, N.P., Brown, J.A., Kightlinger, L., Rosenberg, L. and Fischer, M. (2012) State health department perceived utility of and satisfaction with ArboNET, the US National Arboviral Surveillance System. *Public Health Reports* 127(4), 383–390.

National Academy of Sciences (2013a) Forum on Microbial Threats - Institute of Medicine. Available at: http://www.iom.edu/Activities/PublicHealth/MicrobialThreats.aspx (accessed 7 October 2014).

National Academy of Sciences (2013b) The National Academies, Advisors to the Nation on Science, Engineering and Medicine. Available at: http://www.nationalacademies.org (accessed 7 October 2014).

National Marine Mammal Foundation (n.d.a) Mission. Available at: http://nmmf.org/mission (accessed 7 October 2014).

National Marine Mammal Foundation (n.d.b) Research. Available at: http://nmmf.org/?type=scientific-research (accessed 7 October 2014).

National Marine Mammal Foundation (2012) *One Health Medicine & Research Program Overview and 5-Year Investment Strategy: FY12-FY16.*

National Park Service (2013) NPS One Health Network News. Available at: http://www.nps.gov/public_health/info/newsletters/2013/OneHealth_newsletter_Spring%202013.pdf (accessed 10 September 2013).

One Health Commission (2013a) About Us. Available at: https://www.onehealthcommission.org (accessed 7 October 2014).

One Health Commission (2013b) History. Available at: https://www.onehealthcommission.org/en/why_one_health/about_us/history (accessed 7 October 2014).

Rabinowitz, P. and Conti, L. (2013) Links among human health, animal health, and ecosystem health. *Annual Review of Public Health* 34, 189–204.

Rabinowitz, P., Kock, R.A., Kachani, M., Kunkel, R., Thomas, J., Gilbert, J., Wallace, R., Blackmore, C.G., Wong, D., Karesh, W., Natterson, B., Dugas, R. and Rubin, C. (2013) Towards proof of concept of a 'One Health' approach to disease prediction and control. *Emerging Infectious Diseases* DOI: 10.3201/eid1912.130265.

Rubin, C. (2013) Operationalizing One Health: Stone Mountain and beyond. *Current Topics in Microbiology and Immunology* 366, 173–183.

Rubin, C., Myers, T., Stokes, W., Dunham, B., Harris, S., Lautner, L. and Annelli, J. (2013) Review of Institute of Medicine and National Research Council Recommendations for One Health Initiative. *Emerging Infectious Diseases* 19(12), 1913–1917.

Special Wildlife Health Issue (2012) One Health Newsletter. Available at: http://www.doh.state.fl.us/environment/medicine/One_Health/FallOHNL2012.pdf (accessed 9 September 2013).

Swaminathan, B., Barrett, T.J., Hunter, S.B. and Tauxe, R.V. (2001) PulseNet: the molecular subtyping network for foodborne bacterial disease surveillance, United States. *Emerging Infectious Diseases* 7(3), 382–389.

United States Animal and Plant Health Inspection Service (2011) *VS 2015: A New Perspective*, no.91-05-007. US Dept of Agriculture, Animal and Plant Health Inspection Service, Hyattsville, Maryland.

University of Florida Department of Environmental and Global Health College of Public Health and Health Professions (2013a) Certificate in One Health. Available at: http://egh.phhp.ufl.edu/academic-programs/certificate-programs/certificate-in-one-health (accessed 7 October 2014).

University of Florida Department of Environmental and Global Health College of Public Health and Health Professions (2013b) Master of Health Science One Health. Available at: http://egh.phhp.ufl.edu/academic-programs/masters-programs/mhs-one-health (accessed 7 October 2014).

University of Florida Department of Environmental and Global Health College of Public Health and Health Professions (2013c) PhD in One Health. Available at: http://egh.phhp.ufl.edu/academic-programs/doctoral-programs/phd-in-one-health (accessed 7 October 2014).

University of Minnesota Academic Health Center Office of Education (2013) What is 1Health? Available at: http://www.ahceducation.umn.edu/1Health (accessed 7 October 2014).
University of Minnesota College of Veterinary Medicine (2012) Pioneers in One Health. College of Veterinary Medicine Profiles. Available at: http://www.cvm.umn.edu/prod/groups/cvm/@pub/@cvm/documents/asset/cvm_asset_420620.pdf (accessed 9 September 2013).
University of Minnesota School of Public Health (2013) Veterinary Public Health DVM/MPH. Available at: http://sph.umn.edu/programs/vph (accessed 7 October 2014).
VS 2015 One Health Working Group (2010) *Strategic Plan For Implementing One Health Activities Within USDA APHIS VS*. Hyattsville, Maryland.
Western University of Health Sciences (2013) Interprofessional Education (IPE): Overview: Planning Process. Available at: http://www.westernu.edu/interprofessional-planning (accessed 7 October 2014).
Wildlife Conservation Society (2004) Conference Summary. Available at: http://www.oneworldonehealth.org/sept2004/owoh_sept04.html (accessed 7 October 2014).
World Health Organization (2009) *Swine influenza- update 3; 27 April 2009*. WHO, Geneva.
Woteki, C.E. and Kineman, B.D. (2003) Challenges and approaches to reducing foodborne illness. *Annual Review of Nutrition* 23, 315–344.
Zering, K. (2009) Economic Disaster in the US Pork Industry and Implications for North Carolina. NC State Swine Extension Swine News 32(09). Available at: http://www.ncsu.edu/project/swine_extension/swine_news/2009/sn_v3209%20 (september).htm (accessed 9 September 2013).

# 27 Institutional Research Capacity Development for Integrated Approaches in Developing Countries: an Example from Vietnam

**Hung Nguyen-Viet,[1,2,3,4]* Vi Nguyen,[1] Phuc Pham-Duc,[1] Le Vu Anh,[1] Phung Dac Cam,[5] Marcel Tanner,[2,3] Della Grace,[1,7] Christian Zurbrügg,[6] Tran Thi Tuyet Hanh,[1] Tu Vu-Van,[1] Luu Quoc Toan,[1] Dang Xuan Sinh,[1] Pham Thi Huong Giang[1] and Jakob Zinsstag[2,3]**

*[1]Centre for Public Health and Ecosystem Research, Hanoi School of Public Health, Hanoi, Vietnam; [2]Swiss Tropical and Public Health Institute, Basel, Switzerland; [3]University of Basel, Basel, Switzerland; [4]International Livestock Research Institute, Hanoi, Vietnam; [5]National Institute of Hygiene and Epidemiology, Hanoi, Vietnam; [6]Eawag: Swiss Federal Institute of Aquatic Science and Technology, Department of Water and Sanitation in Developing Countries (Sandec), Dübendorf, Switzerland; [7]International Livestock Research Institute, Nairobi, Kenya*

## Introduction

Global health architecture, environmental change, rapid economic development and other unprecedented global changes complicate present and future development. This is demonstrated in the United Nation's World Water Day (UNW, 2014) 'water and energy nexus' theme and development policies, programmes and tools lagging behind these global changes (Moss, 2011; UNW, 2014). The former refers to the interdependence of water and energy resulting in challenges in attaining some of the Millennium Development Goals, which depend on progress in access to water, sanitation, power and energy sources (UNU-INWEH, 2014). Conversely, lack of access to these resources impedes sustainable economic development, which is a major consideration in combating global poverty. The latter means a greater focus on results-based innovation and aid, investment in solutions with impacts beyond single countries and the move towards non-aid tools for global interactions such as trade, investment and migration (Moss, 2011). Ultimately, a larger role for science, technology, innovation and partnerships requires research to contribute both the vision and space to test potential solutions to global challenges.

Research can be a driver of development within a nation. Universities typically host and conduct research and create innovative solutions for a society. In the developing world, universities tend to have more teaching than research activities; however, it is largely accepted that research-based universities are an important trend. This model is

*E-mail: h.nguyen@cgiar.org

being implemented in many developing countries with an expectation to bridge the gap between developing and developed country higher education programmes and create innovation capacity within developing countries (Whitworth *et al.*, 2008).

Vietnam is no exception in this discussion, as its universities are generally teaching-oriented institutions. Research is not always prioritized and is given limited resources. This leads to modest visibility in the international sphere, especially with regard to internationally recognized publications, research funding and impact on society when compared to the research from national research institutes in other, particularly developed, countries (Nguyen and Pham, 2011). In Vietnam, the concept of research centres at universities has been developed and has allowed the emergence and development of many research groups to strengthen research capacity at the university level. However, many research centres have been developed to implement specific projects that are usually supported by international donor and research funding. As a result, the sustainability of these centres beyond the lifespan of the funded research projects is questionable, as they cannot function without funding.

As it becomes increasingly clear that our health, ecosystems and economies are interdependent, the challenge of keeping up with the pace of development and its implications for different sectors brings us back to the issue of research capacity development. Current challenges facing our health and the environment require an innovative approach that integrates different types of knowledge and involves a larger range of stakeholders. One Health and ecosystem approaches to health (ecohealth) are among a family of integrated research approaches that recognize and attempt to address this interdependence (Charron, 2012).

This chapter presents one case of developing the institutional capacity for integrated research in developing countries. We will describe the emergence of a research group in environmental health, rooted from a North-South partnership research programme in Switzerland and how they developed and became integrated in a national institution and its work to address local needs and contribute to informed policy.

## From a Post-doctoral Research Project to a Research Group

The National Centre of Competence in Research North-South (NCCR North-South) was a research programme from Switzerland, from 2001 to 2013, working on sustainable development research with a North-South research partnership spirit (Wiesmann and Hurni, 2011). Its first phase focused on the training of many PhD students in North-South research partnership, as such training still remains an important focus of capacity development in the future. Recent programmes put a new emphasis on post-doctoral fellows (postdoc), because they operate within a unique space, as there is often no or very few mid-level staff between established professors and their PhD students. Postdocs have the potential to start new research groups, often bringing new fields of study to their institutions. The intermixing of disciplines could be an essential ingredient for integrated research. However, the concept of research group nuclei through postdocs is rather new to African and Asian academic institutions with limited resources.

The NCCR North-South research programme had a postdoc project on environmental sanitation and health in South-east Asia and West Africa beginning in 2007. The postdoc was hosted by the Swiss Tropical and Public Health Institute and the Swiss Federal Institute of Aquatic Science and Technology, Department of Water and Sanitation in Developing Countries (Sandec/Eawag). With the goal of undertaking research for development, our efforts initially grew by developing North-South research networks focused on building partnerships and capacities locally. The research activities were guided by a conceptual framework for improving health and environmental sanitation in peri-urban areas (Nguyen-Viet *et al.*, 2009; Nguyen-Viet *et al.*, Chapter 9, this volume). We worked on the premise that research on environmental sanitation and health often lacks an integrated approach and any intervention in this interdisciplinary field must consider a comprehensive assessment that guides the design of socially and culturally accepted, cost-effective interventions that are often context-specific.

The project began with institutional support from the National Institute of Hygiene and Epidemiology (NIHE) in 2007 and expanded to the Hanoi School of Public Health (HSPH) in 2009, both of which are Vietnamese institutions in Hanoi. At each of these institutions, we worked with the staff and recruited graduate students to form a research group. This started from a study site and sanitation problem in Ha Nam Province – about 60 km south of Hanoi – where most of the field research activities take place (Nguyen-Viet *et al.*, Chapter 9, this volume). This research project has been able to flourish because of the building of partnerships with academic as well as the local community institutions (the health stations in Hoang Tay and Nhat Tan communes). Relationship building required more than just gaining approval to do research. Part of these efforts focused on recruiting Vietnamese graduate students and providing them with both national and international opportunities, which offered training with new methods and a forum for knowledge exchange.

The different components of the conceptual framework thus brought several Vietnamese graduate students to work together in the same study site and on different aspects of the health and environmental sanitation issues. This was the case with a PhD that focused on the health risks and environmental impacts of wastewater and excreta reuse in northern Vietnam (Pham Duc, 2012; Pham Duc *et al.*, 2011, 2013). There were three MSc students involved in this research project, which opened up opportunities to further study in Japan and Switzerland while maintaining a network and collaboration in Vietnam (Nga *et al.*, 2011; Nguyen-Cong *et al.*, 2011; Tu *et al.*, 2011). The research efforts also focused on training health station staff and village health workers on collecting health data and interviewing community members. These interactions gave opportunities for Vietnamese researchers to engage in a dialogue with community leaders and farmers to gain a richer understanding of the local context. The outcomes of this process of developing partnerships and capacities locally were mainly empirical research results and learning new methods. This lays the foundation for doing integrated research, as the work started with the ambitious intentions of using integrated approaches, but this also required building up an evidence base that provides a rationale for changing the way research and decision-making is done. It also provides a rationale for addressing the problem of sanitation at different levels and training researchers for future leadership in integrated approaches.

## Emergence of a Research Group and its Institutionalization

Beyond individuals and groups of researchers, research for development requires developing institutional research capacities to ensure the sustainability of such efforts. Thus, infrastructure is important and this is where research centres can emerge. With the vision to foster South-South networks, mutual learning and more coordinated efforts (through pooling resources, for example), having an official platform to officially and easily build partnerships and interact with stakeholders, it was necessary to have an official status for the research group. Therefore, after 3 years of forming a research group at NIHE, and almost 3 years at HSPH, HSPH founded the Centre for Public Health and Ecosystem Research (CENPHER) on the basis of our research group.

CENPHER was founded on 1 June 2012 as a research centre of HSPH to conduct and strengthen interdisciplinary research within the university. The centre focuses on three main pillars to develop the research links between health and the environment at the national and regional levels: research, training and services. Our mission is to study the health impacts of environmental, cultural, socio-economic and demographic factors using the integrative approaches of ecohealth/One Health, with a special focus on South-east Asia and links to analogous issues in Africa.

Specifically, our focal issues include the links between health and agriculture, infectious and zoonotic diseases, chemical pollution, food safety and nutrition. Research is conducted at different levels of organization (molecular, individual and population) and ranges from the laboratory to the field. Our ultimate goal is to understand the health issues related to pressures on ecosystems and to use research outputs to inform policy for health improvements of vulnerable populations.

The support of HSPH leadership to embed CENPHER within the university shows their recognition of CENPHER's work and its relevance to the local context, as well as the importance of developing institutional research capacity. HSPH is a young university (founded in 2001) and has continually been open to opportunities and development. The establishment of CENPHER at HSPH has yielded the benefit of improved visibility of HSPH nationally and internationally; therefore, this is a win–win situation for both parent and child institutions, with CENPHER functioning as a self-funded unit. The partnership with HSPH has also allowed CENPHER to be recognized as a legal entity within the university. Presently, the group is involved with university teaching on environmental health topics, supervising undergraduate and post-graduate students doing these, and is developing more projects to grow as a research centre (Table 27.1). These projects cover research fields defined in the strategic plan of CENPHER 2012–2020.

Our research group started with five people at HSPH and CENPHER staff, and has varied between eight and ten people, comprising one head, one postdoc, three PhD and three MSc students, and two to three research assistants. All staff positions are completely funded by research projects. This is one of the challenges of CENPHER, as there are no permanent positions at CENPHER. Fortunately, CENPHER works with staff from different departments of HSPH, in particular the

**Table 27.1.** Past and currently acquired projects.

| | Timeline | | | | | | |
|---|---|---|---|---|---|---|---|
| Project/Programme | 2007–2012 | 2013 | 2014 | 2015 | 2016 | 2017 | Donors |
| EH: Sanitation and Health – NCCR North-South | ■ | ■ | | | | | SDC/SNSF, KFPE |
| EH: PAMS QMRA | ■ | | | | | | SDC/SNSF |
| EH: PAMS waste | ■ | ■ | | | | | SDC/SNSF |
| EH: RRR | | ■ | | | | | SDC |
| EH: FBLI Ecohealth | ■ | ■ | ■ | ■ | ■ | ■ | IDRC |
| EH: FBLI coordinating unit | ■ | ■ | ■ | ■ | ■ | ■ | IDRC |
| EH: Leptospirosis and Regional ecohealth course | | ■ | ■ | | | | CGIAR – CRP4 |
| EH: VOHUN–One Health | | ■ | ■ | | | | USAID |
| FS: Book QMRA | ■ | | | | | | WHO |
| FS: FOOD-RISK | | ■ | ■ | | | | SDC |
| FS: PigRISK | ■ | ■ | ■ | ■ | ■ | ■ | ACIAR/ILRI |
| FS: Risk assessment taskforce for Vietnam | | ■ | ■ | | | | CGIAR – CRP4 |
| FS: QMRA research | | ■ | | | | | MARD |
| FS: QMRA training | | ■ | | | | | MOH |

ACIAR , Australian Centre for International Agricultural Research; EH, Ecohealth and One Health; FBLI, Field Building Leadership Initiative; FOOD-RISK, Strengthening the capacity of risk assessment application for managing food safety within a Food production–Environment–Health interaction context in Vietnam; FS, Food Safety; IDRC, International Development Research Centre; ILRI, International Livestock Research Institute; MARD, Ministry of Agriculture and Rural Development; MOH, Ministry of Health; PAMS, Partnership Action for Mitigation of Syndromes (of NCCR North-South); FBLI, Field Building Leadership Initiative; PigRISK, reducing disease risks and improving food safety in smallholder pig value chains in Vietnam; QMRA, Quantitative Microbial Risk Assessment; RRR, Resource, Recovery and Reuse; TASKFORCE, Risk assessment taskforce for food safety management; VOHUN, Vietnam One Health University Network

Department of Environmental Health, and this joint force has resulted in productive research and training with novel research topics for post-graduates (Toan *et al.*, 2013; Tung *et al.*, 2013). Moreover, the Swiss Tropical and Public Health Institute has contributed to the core funding of CENPHER, covering some administrative and routine research expenses and capacity building, whereas HSPH has offered working spaces to CENPHER.

Building the capacity of staff and career orientation development are important activities at CENPHER. Several international and regional scholarships have been granted to CENPHER collaborators for graduate studies overseas (Belgium, Thailand and Switzerland) and attendance at short courses. While this is good for both individual and institutional development, the personnel flow presents a challenge for the work organization of a small group like CENPHER.

## Approaching Strategic Donors and International Partners, Research Portfolio and Outputs

As mentioned previously, CENPHER is a self-funded centre within HSPH; therefore, it is crucial for the centre to mobilize financial resources. The seed funding from NCCR North-South for the current Phase 3 has served as the backbone for a PhD study on productive sanitation. More significantly, it has given the group independence and flexibility to do research and helped build up the group. This link to the NCCR North-South in Switzerland has allowed CENPHER staff to have access to international networks and partnerships.

A first partnership was with the International Livestock Research Institute (ILRI) in Kenya to conduct a scoping study on ecohealth of zoonotic diseases in South-east Asia. This small project was an entry point for CENPHER to approach the International Development Research Centre (IDRC) in Canada, from which CENPHER acquired two competitive research and partnership projects (2012–2016), becoming part of their funded research projects in South-east Asia (Table 27.2). The latter has offered a large range of infectious diseases research networks in the region. Projects funded by IDRC helped CENPHER develop and conduct research and training activities on Ecohealth and One Health, promoting integrated approaches, as stated in the centre's strategic plan. Through the partnership with ILRI, CENPHER obtained funding from the Australian Centre for International Agricultural Research (ACIAR, 2012–2017) to work on food safety, a second research axis of CENPHER (Table 27.2). In addition, we have

**Table 27.2.** CENPHER's research, training and knowledge translation outputs (2009–2014).

| Type of publication/output | Number of outputs | Field | Capacity building |
|---|---|---|---|
| International peer-reviewed papers | 18 | Interdisciplinary | |
| National peer-reviewed papers | 15[a] | Interdisciplinary | |
| Text books | 3 | Environmental Sciences<br>Public Health | |
| Book chapters | 4 | Interdisciplinary | |
| Policy briefs | 3 | Food safety, Sanitation | |
| Practical guidelines | 1 | Sanitation | |
| Short courses | 6 | Risk assessment, Ecohealth, One Health | X |
| PhD training | 1 accomplished<br>3 ongoing | Interdisciplinary | X |
| MSc theses | 8 | Public Health | X |
| BSc final research projects | 7 | Public Health | X |

[a]Most of these papers were published in two special editions: (i) In June 2013, the *Vietnamese Journal of Preventive Medicine* published a special edition on 'Risk Assessment for Health Research in Vietnam'; and (ii) in November 2011, the *Vietnamese Journal of Public Health* published a special edition on 'Sanitation and Health'

acquired other short-term grants, from 6 to 24 months, from various donors, including the Swiss Agency for Development and Co-operation (SDC), World Health Organization (WHO), US Agency for International Development (USAID), Consultative Group on International Agricultural Research (CGIAR) – Agriculture for Nutrition and Health Research Program (A4NH) and national funding from the Ministry of Health, Ministry of Agriculture and Rural Development with partners. We have conducted consultancies upon request, which are related to core competencies of CENPHER. In short, CENPHER has diversified its research portfolio and regional partners and secured other international partners and funding. These collective research efforts led to the research outputs presented in Table 27.2.

## Knowledge Translation

One of CENPHER's principles is to translate research outputs (evidence) into practice and use it to inform policy. Therefore, the centre actively builds bridges for knowledge exchange between researchers, practitioners and policy makers. In just a short time frame, it has already leveraged scientific capacity and produced targeted policy briefs for issues that need to be tackled in the short term. For example, food safety is a pressing issue currently for Vietnam's informal (wet) markets, where most of the country's consumers buy and sell food products, but also as Vietnam develops its domestic and international markets for agricultural commodities. The major implication is to a shift in focus of food safety policy towards a basis on risks (probability of harm occurring) instead of hazards (presence of harmful substances). The National Law of Food Safety, in effect since July 2011, mandates application of risk assessment to high-risk food products intended both for domestic consumption and for export. However, there is a lack of local capacity in the practical application of risk assessment. The situation is especially urgent in Vietnam's informal markets, where risk assessment is rarely applied.

CENPHER undertook an initiative to strengthen risk assessment capacity through a Risk Assessment Task Force, focusing on food, water and environmental hazards. It brings together representatives from Vietnam's Ministry of Health, its Ministry of Agriculture and Rural Development and researchers involved in risk assessment and food safety from key universities and research institutes. The Task Force is developing guidelines for use of risk assessment on behalf of food safety management in informal markets catering to local consumers. These guidelines will be used to train a wide range of decision makers, including high-level policy makers. A technical course and case studies of food safety in informal markets were used, followed by mentoring and on-the-job support (Nguyen-Viet *et al.*, 2013). With our project partners, we developed a policy brief on risk assessment for food safety in Vietnam, targeting the national Ministry of Health (MOH) and Ministry of Agriculture and Rural Development (MARD) (Nguyen-Viet *et al.*, 2013). On the request of the Department of Animal Health, Ministry of Agriculture and Rural Development (MARD), the CENPHER team ran two workshops on Risk Assessment for Food Safety for over 120 veterinary staff in Hanoi and Ho Chi Minh City in 2013. This is the model that CENPHER uses to inform policy based on our areas of expertise, for instance, environmental sanitation and waste re-use (Nguyen-Viet *et al.*, 2011; Phuc *et al.*, 2013). Finally, aside from influencing policy makers, we have worked with farmers to implement a field intervention examining how the combination of human and animal excreta composting influences helminth egg die-off in excreta, while still maintaining its nutrient value. The intervention aimed to improve the current storage practices of human excreta and identify the best option for the safe use of excreta in agriculture.

## Reflection, Conclusion and Ways Forward

As a driver of the development in developing countries, research conducted using

North–South partnerships is a good starting point to develop research capacity in the south (Tanner *et al.*, 1994; Whitworth *et al.*, 2008). We described a case of founding and early development of a research centre, which originated from a postdoc research project from Switzerland, leading to the formation, development and institutionalization of a research unit in Vietnam. Although still in its early stages, some key messages on the institutional capacity development of an integrated research centre can be made based on the process of CENPHER's development. These include the following messages.

Post-doctoral partnerships have the potential to make southern partners highly autonomous, and they can start driving their own research and move from North-South networks to South-South networks. This kind of research space is not common, as there are usually two types of researchers: a very senior group or early-career researchers. Fortunately, the status of postdocs is increasingly recognized in the south and more donors are providing grants for postdocs to build up their own research group (Afrique One – 'African Research Consortium on Ecosystem and Population Health' and SACIDS – 'Southern African Center for Infectious Diseases Surveillance'). Challenges to this model are that only a small proportion of postdocs may have the desire or capacity to lead research groups, postdocs lack the reputation that facilitates funding and publication, and postdocs may be seen both as a threat by senior researchers and lacking credibility by graduate fellows. We suggest that, to be successful, postdocs must have financial autonomy, low administrative barriers, access to regional and international networks and a forum of open exchange with peers and senior experts to shape their research approaches. The constant support both from the north and the south is extremely important for new research groups. In addition, support from institutional host leaders will allow an enabling environment for work with financial flexibility and less time for administration, which reserves more time for research. The development of new centres requires key donors to invest and commit support with major funding for at least the first 5–10 years. This will allow the centre to clearly shape priorities and position itself in the research and training landscape. This is particularly significant for self-funded research units, when national funding is not available or rarely available for core funding and the centre has to rely primarily on international grants. This is at once a threat to the sustainability of the centre and a motivation for the centre to be pro-active in seeking funding. In our experience, the emergence of a research group within a national institution and the efforts to approach international donors and partners and develop research portfolios and outputs together have helped strengthen the identities of this particular research hub/institution. Efforts at CENPHER have broadened research topics beyond what classical degrees could address to global health, ecohealth and One Health issues. This broadens the competence of researchers to deal with complex issues by using interdisciplinary approaches and strengthens their capacities for knowledge synthesis and translation and, therefore, impact. The last few decades have seen many approaches to build research capacity through projects, networks, post-doctoral support, graduate fellow training, centres and outposts of northern universities. There is a missed opportunity of better evaluating these initiatives to compare their relative impacts, efficiency and costs.

## Moving towards a vision for One Health (or integrated research)

In closing, we return to the vision of southern researchers becoming leaders in development. From a regional perspective, the way forward must address capacities on three fronts: research excellence, capacity building and knowledge to policy translation. At the research level, there is a need for more integrated and practically oriented case studies on One Health/ecohealth that generate results which can be directly used by research clients. At the same time, research must meet international standards of excellence. In terms of capacity building, degree training and short courses on ecohealth would help expand the knowledge of mainstream practitioners and policy makers. This would make the approach more sustainable and relevant beyond the research realm. However, we question the current emphasis on short courses, led by northern universities, which do not lead to recognized qualifications and are not grounded in local contexts. On the policy side, the efforts on strengthening both research and training capacities in health policy and research translation will be crucial to move beyond advocacy for ecohealth approaches towards influence on decision making. Decision makers increasingly look for research which is published in high-impact-factor journals and is well marketed through media and communications material. We believe focus on research excellence, capacity building and research to policy translation will extend the impact of the current investments in academic capacity development for integrated approaches. It will build researchers' capacity to leverage the human resources and form the structures required to convince national governments in the region to increase investment in their own research for development.

## Acknowledgements

We would like to thank Dr Dinh Xuan Tung and Dr Hein Mallee for their help in developing the concept of CENPHER. We thank Ms Nguyen Hong Nhung, Ms Nguyen Thi Thao and colleagues at Hanoi School of Public Health for their contributions to CENPHER. We thank donors and partners, in particular SDC, SNSF, IDRC, ACIAR, KFPE, Swiss TPH, Sandec/Eawag, ILRI and IFPRI for their support. Both HNV and VN contributed to this chapter equally.

## References

Charron, D. (2012) Ecohealth: origins and approach. In: Charron, D. (ed.) *Ecohealth Research in Practice: Innovative Applications of an Ecosystem Approach to Health*. Springer, Ottawa.

Moss, T. (2011) Development policy of the future and why we aren't ready. Available at: http://devpolicy.org/development-policy-of-the-future20110220 (accessed 4 March 2014).

Nga, D.T., Morel, A., Hung, N.V., Phuc, P.D., Nishida, K. and Kootattep, T. (2011) Assessing nutrient fluxes in a Vietnamese rural area despite limited and highly uncertain data. *Resources Conservation and Recycling* 55(9–10), 849–856.

Nguyen, T.V. and Pham, L.T. (2011) Scientific output and its relationship to knowledge economy: an analysis of ASEAN countries. *Scientometrics* 89, 107–117.

Nguyen-Cong, K., Th, B., Pham-Duc, P. and Nguyen-Viet, H. (2011) Assessment of diarrhea risk by micro-organisms in wastewater and excreta used in agriculture in Hanam. *Vietnam Journal of Public Health* 22, 14–20.

Nguyen-Viet, H., Zinsstag, J., Schertenleib, R., Zurbrugg, C., Obrist, B., Montangero, A., Surkinkul, N., Kone, D., Morel, A., Cisse, G., Koottatep, T., Bonfoh, B. and Tanner, M. (2009) Improving environmental sanitation, health, and well-being: a conceptual framework for integral interventions. *EcoHealth* 6(2), 180–191.

Nguyen-Viet, H., Tuan-Anh, V., Pham-Duc, P. and Van-Tu, V. (2011) Safe use of wastewater in agriculture and aquaculture. In: Thammarat Koottatep (ed.) *Evidence for Policy Series, Regional edition Southeast Asia, No. 2*. NCCR North-South, Pathumthani, Thailand.

Nguyen-Viet, H., Grace, D., Tran, T.T.H., Pham, D.P. and Tanner, M. (2013) Risk assessment for food safety in Vietnam. In: *Evidence for Policy Series, Regional edition Southeast Asia*. NCCR North-South, Pathumthani, Thailand.

Pham Duc, P. (2012) Wastewater and excreta use in agriculture in northern Vietnam: health risks and environmental impacts. Unpublished PhD, University of Basel, Swiss Tropical and Public Health Institute, Basel.

Pham Duc, P., Nguyen-Viet, H., Hattendorf, J., Zinsstag, J., Cam, P.D. and Odermatt, P. (2011) Risk factors for *Entamoeba histolytica* infection in an agricultural community in Hanam province, Vietnam. *Parasites & Vectors* 4.

Pham Duc, P., Nguyen-Viet, H., Hattendorf, J., Zinsstag, J., Cam, P.D., Zurbrugg, C. and Odermatt, P. (2013) *Ascaris lumbricoides* and *Trichuris trichiura* infections associated with wastewater and human excreta use in agriculture in Vietnam. *Parasitology International* 62, 172–180.

Phuc, P.-D., Hung, N.-V., Tu, V.-V., Zurbrugg, C. and Zinsstag, S. (2013) The Vietnamese double-vault composting latrine: fertilizer source or health risk? In: *Evidence for Policy Series, Regional edition Southeast Asia*. NCCR North-South, Pathumthani, Thailand.

Tanner, M., Kitua, A. and Degremont, A.A. (1994) Developing health research capability in Tanzania: from a Swiss Tropical Institute Field Laboratory to the Ifakara Centre of the Tanzanian National Institute of Medical Research. *Acta Tropica* 57(2–3), 153–173.

Toan, L.Q., Hung, N.V. and Huong, B.M. (2013) Risk assessment of Salmonella in pork in Hanoi, Vietnam. *Journal of Preventive Medicine* 24(4), 10–17.

Tu, V.v., Huong, N., Phuc, P.D., Hung, N.V. and Zurbrugg, C. (2011) Developing a questionnaire to measure awareness and behaviours of people in relation to wastewater use in agriculture at Hoang Tay commune and Nhat Tan commune. *Vietnam Journal of Public Health* 22, 14–20.

Tung, B.H., Hanh, T.T.T. and Hung, N.V. (2013) Risk assessment of arsenic contamination in tube-well drinking water in Hanam province. *Journal of Preventive Medicine* 23(4), 10–17.

UNU-INWEH (2014) *World Water Day Advocacy Guide*. United Nations University Institute for Water, Environment, and Health (UNU-INWEH), Hamilton

UNW (2014) UN World Water Day 2014: Water and Energy. Available at: http://www.unwater.org/worldwaterday/about-world-water-day/world-water-day-2014-water-and-energy/en (accessed 4 March 2014).

Whitworth, J.A., Kokwaro, G., Kinyanjui, S., Snewin, V.A., Tanner, M., Walport, M. and Sewankambo, N. (2008) Strengthening capacity for health research in Africa. *Lancet* 372(9649), 1590–1593.

Wiesmann, U. and Hurni, H. (2011) *Research for Sustainable Development: Foundations, Experiences, and Perspectives*. Perspectives of the Swiss National Centre of Competence in Research (NCCR) North-South, University of Bern, Vol. 6. Geographica Bernensia, Bern, Switzerland, 640 pp.

# 28 Enabling Academic One Health Environments

**Bonnie Buntain,[1]* Lisa Allen-Scott,[2] Michelle North,[3] Melanie Rock[4] and Jennifer Hatfield[5]**
[1]*Department of Ecosystem and Public Health, Faculty of Veterinary Medicine, Department of Community Health Sciences, Faculty of Medicine, University of Calgary;* [2]*Population and Public Health, Community Health Sciences, Faculty of Medicine, University of Calgary;* [3]*Department of Ecosystem and Public Health, University of Calgary;* [4]*Department of Community Health Sciences, Faculty of Medicine, Department of Ecosystem and Public Health, University of Calgary;* [5]*Global Health and International Partnerships, Faculty of Medicine, University of Calgary, Canada*

## Introduction

Academic institutions can play critical roles in nurturing emerging researchers and leaders in One Health. In particular, these institutions can foster the creation, translation and development of knowledge, skills and organizational capacities, all of which are needed to address complex problems that implicate human beings, non-human animals and ecosystems. Within this chapter, we illustrate the importance of academic institutions for promoting One Health. We begin with an overview of how 'One Medicine' has evolved toward One Health in Canada. This overview sets the stage for an analysis of the foundation and growth of the Faculty of Veterinary Medicine at the University of Calgary (UCVM) in Calgary, Alberta, Canada as a case study.

UCVM is an unusual case in two respects. First, UCVM does not operate a veterinary hospital; rather, UCVM is based on community partnerships with privately owned clinics and non-profit organizations, including governmental and non-governmental organizations, where veterinary medicine is practised and the principles of One Health are applied. Second, UCVM is predominantly collocated with the Faculty of Medicine at the University of Calgary (UCFM), which is firmly founded in comparative medical and public health research. Unlike a growing number of universities, wherein schools specializing in public health operate separately from medical schools, UCFM and UCVM include research, education and stakeholder engagement in public health. This transformative environment for One Health is perhaps unique in the world. By way of illustration, we trace the 'added-value' of One Health at the University of Calgary through quantitative measures and case examples.

We conclude our analysis with reflections on specific aspects of both the enabling academic environment and barriers for collaboration in One Health at the University of Calgary.

*E-mail: bonnie.buntain@ucalgary.ca

## Evolution of One Health in Canada

The beginning of One Health collaboration between medical and veterinary schools in Canada started long before the foundation of the UCVM in 2005. In the 1800s, Canada's Montreal Veterinary College in Quebec embarked on a professional training programme, incorporating high standards into teaching veterinary science. It was noteworthy that veterinary and medical students from McGill University in Montreal studied together; this ensured that both groups achieved the same standards. Throughout that century, the veterinary profession strove to be on par with human medical education, and often physicians taught in veterinary colleges. In 1889 McGill University assumed control of the Montreal Veterinary College and renamed it the Faculty of Comparative Medicine and Veterinary Science. Veterinary students studied botany, chemistry, physiology and histology at McGill with students in the medical school, and they studied anatomy, therapeutics and obstetrics at McGill's veterinary school. Arguably, this arrangement contributed significantly to Canada's collaborative foundation of comparative biomedical research and its relevance for human health. In this way, as well as through the influence of luminaries, most notably William Osler, Canada's distinctive approach to integrating comparative medicine and veterinary science spread throughout the USA. Canada became the 'cradle of veterinary science in America', as the Ontario Veterinary College (founded in 1862) graduated more Americans than all US schools combined (American Veterinary Medical Association, 2012).

During the 1900s, Canadian and US veterinary and medical colleges evolved separate paths as veterinary teaching hospitals were built in more rural areas away from most medical schools, and both professions developed clinical specializations. The concept of separate facilities became the norm. Veterinarians in comparative and laboratory medicine were often collocated in research institutes, contributing enormously to the development of animal experimental models and new pharmaceuticals, medical devices and vaccines (Committee on the National Needs for Research in Veterinary Science, 2005).

In 1999, the Canadian government was concerned about the global threat of zoonotic and other infectious diseases and started developing a new laboratory to address them. In the early 2000s, Canada experienced outbreaks from the global spread of severe acute respiratory syndrome (Centers for Disease Control and Prevention, 2003). In order to best address zoonotic diseases, the Public Health Agency of Canada collocated animal and public health laboratories and experts under one facility, the National Microbiological Laboratory (NML). As stated on their website (Public Health Agency of Canada, 2012).

> The NML is located at the Canadian Science Centre for Human and Animal Health in Winnipeg, the first facility in the world to have high containment laboratories for human and animal health in one building. It is recognized as a leader in an elite group of centres around the world, equipped with laboratories ranging from biosafety level 2 to level 4 designed to accommodate the most basic to the most deadly infectious organisms.

## From 'One Medicine' to One Health – The Road to The University of Calgary's Faculty of Veterinary Medicine

In Alberta, Canada, despite years of budgetary cutbacks during the early 21st century, the concept of a veterinary faculty with a focus on the convergence of animal, human and ecosystem health emerged. In 2003, this movement gained significant momentum with emergence of zoonotic diseases threatening the agricultural industry, most importantly the discovery of bovine spongiform encephalopathy (BSE) in an Alberta dairy cow. The financial and social impact of the trade barriers on Alberta was staggering (Forge and Fréchette, 2005; Le Roy *et al.*, 2006). In addition, the public had concerns about food safety, ecological changes due to intensive livestock production and the emergence of West Nile virus, highly pathogenic zoonotic avian influenza H5N1, chronic wasting disease (CWD) in deer and elk and transmission of tuberculosis (TB) and brucellosis from wildlife to livestock. As a consequence, politicians became very receptive to the link between animal and human health (University of Calgary Veterinary Medicine, 2012).

Although many presumed that an agricultural college would make the best home for a new Alberta veterinary faculty, in 2004 leaders in UCFM, in collaboration with key veterinary experts in Alberta, were successful in advocating aligning the veterinary school with the medical faculty. They convinced the Alberta government that the University of Calgary could create an interdisciplinary research-intensive and translational environment linking human and animal health. From the onset, this One Health mandate and contextual framework was established.

The province of Alberta gave UCVM clear mandates that promoted the One Health evolution. The new veterinary faculty was instructed to share resources and enhance collaborative teaching and research with medicine; therefore, UCVM was collocated with the medical faculty within the Foothills Medical Complex. Additionally, UCVM developed a community-based distributed clinical teaching model in collaboration with veterinary practices and government, corporate and non-governmental organizations. UCVM's early focus was on intensive research within the areas of emphasis of production animal and equine health, ecosystem and public health and investigative comparative medicine. Another instruction from the province was that UCVM's graduates must be well prepared to serve rural Alberta's veterinary needs with a broad-based general veterinary practice education.

The original plan for basic and translational research followed UCFM's highly successful model started in the 1970s of clustering researchers with similar interests and expertise in collocated institutes, laboratories and office spaces. UCFM had a non-traditional model of structure based on researchers' interests (e.g. cancer or neuroscience); faculty members in these interest groups were situated across various departments, but clustered in physical proximity to each other irrespective of departmental affiliation. This clustering evolved into centres and institutes whose faculty enjoyed success in obtaining grants. Consequently, UCVM faculty were integrated into this model, grouping veterinary clinicians and basic scientists with medical researchers in the Foothills Medical Complex, in accordance with their shared interests and expertise.

Initially UCFM was tasked with planning the veterinary curriculum in conjunction with other faculties and Alberta veterinarians. The first class was expected to be admitted in 2 years (2007). To begin this process, a retreat was held to create 100 cases, the foundation of a problem-based curriculum modelled after the medical school. Soon after the inaugural Dean was hired, researchers from within the UCFM and elsewhere at the University of Calgary joined UCVM as founding faculty with joint academic appointments. Based on faculty interests and the provincial mandates, four unique multi-disciplinary departments were created: Production Animal Health; Ecosystem and Public Health; Veterinary Clinical and Diagnostic Services; and Comparative Biology and Experimental Medicine. An administrative and research-intensive faculty was housed in the Foothills Medical Complex, and a separate state-of-the-art facility for animal-based education, the Veterinary Clinical Skills Building (CSB), was constructed 10 km away to ensure students achieved a strong grounding in clinical and professional skills. The Distributed Veterinary Learning Community (DVLC) was created to provide the final fourth year veterinary students 'real world' experiences in veterinary, government, corporate and non-governmental organizations. Despite political, economic and accreditation challenges, the innovative and non-traditional UCVM admitted its first undergraduate Doctor of Veterinary Medicine (DVM) class in 2008, successfully graduating them and receiving accreditation in 2012. The strategy of collocation, shared institutes and laboratories, joint appointments and community-based mission of UCVM and UCFM provided a fertile ground for a One Health enabling environment.

### UCVM One Health curriculum

Alberta's economy is driven by export-intensive agrifood, oil, gas and tourism industries. Because of this, the Government of

Alberta wanted UCVM to produce veterinarians competent in animal, public and ecosystem health practice and research. This One Health focus represented a cultural shift and new challenges in veterinary education.

The faculty created a 3-year foundational core curriculum described as an integration of basic theoretical and applied sciences, clinical cases, professional skills (communication, economics and evidence-based research) and hands-on general veterinary practice skills learned at the CSB. There are four Areas of Emphasis (AoE) integrated throughout the curriculum; however, in the fourth and final year students selected an additional 10 weeks in one AoE: Production Animal Health; Equine Health; Ecosystem and Public Health; or Investigative Medicine. The principles of One Health are integrated throughout the first 3 years of the curriculum. For example, during the first year students take the course Animals, Health and Society, emphasizing ecological, biological and social determinants of health that influence, or are influenced by, humans, terrestrial and aquatic animals and the environment. In the Professional Skills Communication Courses, social scientists from UCFM contribute cases teaching veterinary students how the care people provide to pets may serve as a window into the determinants of human health, people's health-related preferences and values and dilemmas inherent to chronic disease, such as diabetes.

The fourth year became the undergraduates' 40-week practicum in the Distributed Veterinary Learning Community, exposing them to a broad range of multi-disciplinary professional partners. The curriculum emphasized preventive medicine and health protection and promotion. One Health is a practicum focus for students selecting the Ecosystem and Public Health AoE in the 4th year. In all AoEs, students are exposed to many career options, from urban to remote private practice, government and international service, corporate practice, research and graduate training, wildlife and aquatic animal management, opportunities to work with aboriginal and underserved communities, and more. These practicum rotations are crucial to meeting the One Health educational and research mandates (Cribb and Buntain, 2009).

## Collocation of UCVM with UCFM: enabling and adding value to One Health research

In regard to the past 8 years (2005–2013), a critical question has arisen in relationship to the One Health foundation and unique collocation of UCVM and UCFM in the Foothills Medical Complex: what has been the added value to advancing the One Health approach to research? In the following, we propose preliminary quantitative measures linked to demonstrating the added value of One Health research attributable to collocation of the two faculties.

Although there is a substantial body of knowledge on creating effective interdisciplinary and transdisciplinary collaborations, there has been an urgent call to demonstrate potential added value to what human and animal health working alone can achieve (GRF Davos, 2012; Zinsstag *et al.*, 2012b). At the first One Health Summit in Davos, Switzerland, participants described the following qualitative added value to One Health approaches to research: a better understanding of researchers' past, present and future roles in creating and responding to barriers between human and animal disease research; promoting a more holistic risk management strategy; encouraging systems thinking; engaging a broader spectrum of stakeholders resulting in greater investment and support; and applying multiple disciplines from human, animal and environmental health, food safety and security and agricultural components, thereby making progress towards solving complex problems (GRF Davos, 2012). However, there is a paucity of quantitative measures related to enabling academic environments to support One Health research and collaboration. What follows proposes measures of the added value of the collocation of UCFM and UCVM in relationship to One Health research and education outcomes.

### *Publications*

The Government of Alberta envisioned that collocating UCVM and UCFM in a shared space would create a unique environment for interdisciplinary and transdisciplinary research collaboration. While this objective is laudable, scholarship on interdisciplinarity and transdisciplinarity suggests that team science is ultimately productive, yet can take time to become established (Stokols, 2006).

Since the announcement of the Millennium Development Goals (MDGs) and publications on Ecosystems and Human Well-Being (Corvalan *et al.*, 2005; UN, 2013), researchers have become more aware of the need to focus on social-ecological models in an attempt to address complex, or 'wicked', problems (Zinsstag *et al.*, 2011). Granting agencies became likely to encourage and reward large inter- or multidisciplinary teams (Wuchty *et al.*, 2007). Additionally, the application of transdisciplinary approaches to health in socio-ecological systems was emerging (Rosenfield, 1992; Schelling *et al.*, 2008; Lang *et al.*, 2012). However, progress on using transdisciplinary teams to address these complex issues has been reported to be slow by Parkes *et al.* (2005), due to the difficulty and threat of overcoming scientific and academic institutional power arrangements. In a recent study on collocation and collaboration, Lee *et al.* (2010) reported that even in the current culture of the Internet and other communication technologies, physical proximity of the research team was a positive predictor of success in publication of biomedical research. In that regard, 'the level of intra-building collaboration is positively associated with the impact of publications originating in that building' (Lee *et al.*, 2010, p. 2).

In an attempt to quantify the effect that proximity or collocation may play on the degree to which medical and veterinary researchers collaborate, the number of co-authored papers were determined for the University of Calgary's medical and veterinary faculties for the years 2006–2012. Using 'University of Calgary' and 'Faculty of Veterinary Medicine' to search the addresses of published articles in the databases PubMed, Scopus and Web of Science, a comprehensive overview of all veterinary research was compiled. From these results all articles that were co-authored by a member of UCFM were then selected and combined, with duplicates deleted. The definition of co-authorship was strictly adhered to, with only members of the two faculties mentioned above being accepted. Any ambiguous results were searched in order to accurately represent the effect of collocation. The final 107 publications were ordered and the number of co-authored papers per year was calculated and illustrated graphically. The resulting list of co-authored publications per year was graphed from a Microsoft Excel spread sheet (Fig. 28.1).

No co-authored publications were found in 2006. However, there was an exponential increase (doubling each year from 2007 to 2010) of co-authored publications. Many of the UCVM authors were jointly appointed to medicine, collocated in UCFM institutes, and/or housed in clusters by research expertise and interest. We propose that this facilitated a relatively rapid development of research grants from 2005, when the university's Board of Governors founded UCVM and faculty were collocated in the Foothills Medical Complex.

### *Cost effectiveness*

Several exceptional attempts to describe the added value of animal and human health collaboration have been published (Schelling *et al.*, 2005, 2007; Zinsstag *et al.*, 2007). In developing a One Health framework for the economic added value of zoonotic disease control programmes, Narrod *et al.* (2012) created a model based on a modified risk analysis process with cost-sharing options identified by using a separable cost method considering multiple sectors (see Zinsstag *et al.*, Chapter 12, this volume). These efforts have significant potential to impact policies, programmes and peoples' lives when we can demonstrate that research of health in social-ecological systems is clearly economically beneficial.

It is difficult to quantify the cost-effectiveness value of collocation of faculties within the Foothills Medical Complex; unlike the National Microbiological Laboratory (NML) in Winnipeg, Canada, the Foothills area was not purpose built for such collocation. This has been one of the barriers obstructing more efficient collaboration between the faculties. Emigration of new veterinary faculty and students into the medical complex resulted in competition for space and administrative stress because it interfered with medicine's

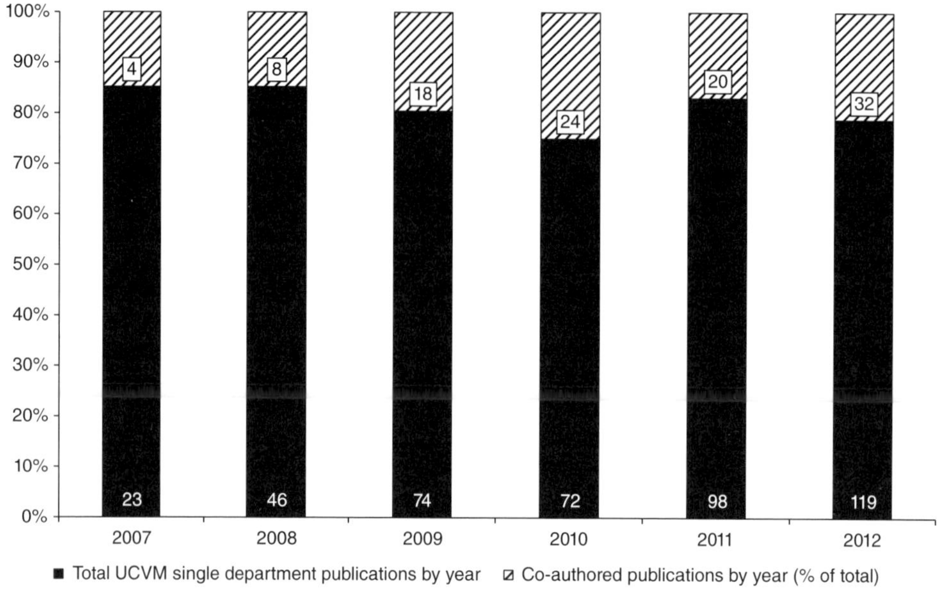


**Fig. 28.1.** UCVM and UCFM co-authored publications expressed as a percentage of total UCVM publications by year (2007–2012).

plans to expand laboratory, office, meeting areas and lecture halls. If a purpose-built facility, such as the NML, had coincided with UCVM's creation, a more efficient use of administrative time and space may have resulted. However, generalizations of collocation cost-effective savings within the Foothills Medical Complex include sharing resources, such as: information technology; teleconferencing; security; utilities; technical and administrative assistance; laboratory animal care, facilities and approval processes; expensive laboratory and diagnostic equipment; educational space; and other common infrastructure resources (e.g. dining, washrooms and public meeting areas).

Despite that the building complex was not purpose-built to house two faculties, we now provide further evidence that people are more likely to collaborate when collocated, contributing to creating the interdisciplinary culture needed for One Health research.

### *Added value of the research clustering model*

As proposed, the rapid early increase in co-authored publications (Fig. 28.1) could likely be due to early success in collaborative grant writing with subsequent joint publications. We were unable to find, within a similar timeframe, another collocated veterinary and medical research and education complex. Therefore, we hypothesize that based on collaboration theories, the publication proxy analysis is reasonable. We propose that key concepts of collaboration may be applied here to help provide context to our added-value conclusions.

One concept is that collaborators share the goal to solve common problems for the betterment of both parties that become a 'win–win' situation. Another is that they could also seek out those who can help provide additional power and resources, such as gaining grants and graduate students described as an 'opportunity-seeking venture' (Aniekwe *et al.*, 2012). During this growing research phase, an enabling research academic environment in the Foothills Medical Complex included clustering of researchers by interest areas, shared laboratory spaces and membership in institutes creating win–win and opportunity-seeking collaborations. UCVM faculty joined successful institutes and centres such as the Hotchkiss Brain Institute, Calvin, Phoebe and Joan Snyder Institute for Chronic

Diseases, McCaig Institute for Bone and Joint Health, Alberta Children's Hospital Research Institute for Child and Maternal Health, and later the Institute for Population and Public Health (IPH). These clustered early research leaders contributed to recruitment of new veterinary faculty, who were attracted to both the collocation and collaborative interdisciplinary One Health research environment developing within the Foothills Medical Complex. The early UCVM researchers became the *collaboration enablers* using their established networks and understanding of what disparate disciplines could bring to the research team (Patrick Whelan, 2013, personal communication). They engaged the established researchers with new veterinary faculty, assisting in overcoming communication problems and perceived power differentials. Therefore, these early collaboration enablers helped bring notably veterinary science, medical, kinesiology, biology, science and clinical veterinary and medical faculty together, building research capacity relatively rapidly and helping to reduce power differentials among well-established research programmes and the newer UCVM faculty. Over time, new collaborations expanded in new institutes, building the One Health theme into productive interdisciplinary research, including discovery in companion animal health in relationship to human population health, as exemplified in the Institute for Public Health.

### *Case example: Institute for Public Health*

The Institute for Public Health (IPH) evolved over the early 2000s and was officially established in 2009, as the seventh and newest institute supported by the Faculty of Medicine. Its more than 320 members represent faculties of Medicine, Nursing, Social Work, Arts, Kinesiology and Veterinary Medicine, along with officials from Alberta Health Services and City of Calgary. Clustered within IPH are researchers and practitioners committed to excellence in research and stakeholder engagement (University of Calgary, n.d.). With growing joint interests in animal and public health, UCFM and UCVM faculty joined the new Population Health and Inequities Research Centre established in 2013. This centre aims to bring together researchers in social sciences, humanities and health sciences (University of Calgary, Institute for Public Health, 2013). An example of collaboration with UCVM faculty is this centre's current funded research projects studying: the relationship of social injustice with pet ownership; people's pets and off-leash areas; analyses of population health promotion and exposure to zoonotic diseases; and animal–human bonds as windows into human health. Thus the IPH is a case study exemplifying ongoing collaboration between medical and veterinary medical-based faculty enhanced by collocation and joint institute membership.

### *Overcoming power differentials to enhance collaboration*

The more a partner is perceived to add value to a successful research grant programme, the more that partner is attractive as a collaborator (Adams *et al.*, 2007). However, an established research institution may not perceive a new faculty member as an added value co-researcher. As the veterinary faculty began to grow from 2005 to 2008, a key attraction for top-notch researchers to Calgary was the established and successful medical research programme at the Foothills Medical Complex. Like-minded comparative medicine researchers joined UCVM's Department of Comparative Biology and Experimental Medicine, creating an enabling environment to grow UCVM's capacity to attract major international, national and regional grants. UCVM was becoming a more attractive collaborator.

Funders became more supportive of integrative research teams that could potentially lead to collaboration across animal and human health disciplines (Natural Sciences and Engineering Research Council of Canada, 2012). Canada's major funding agencies are: Natural Sciences and Engineering Research Council of Canada (NSERC); Social Sciences and Humanities Research Council (SSHRC); Canadian Institutes of Health Research (CIHR); and the International Development Research Centre (IDRC). As UCVM faculty became more successful in leading team and other grants, the power differential between medicine and veterinary medicine began to lessen. At the same time, the efforts of the collaboration enablers were building more win–win teams, and medicine recognized the advantage of having veterinary applied clinical and basic comparative researchers on grants. UCVM's research focus on interdisciplinary biomedical, clinical, health policy and population and public health created common ground for One Health approaches, lessening perceived research power differentials and expanding the University of Calgary's research enterprise. An example of funders combining resources to address animal, public and ecosystem health was the 2007 Teasdale Corti Global Health Research Initiative (IDRC/CIDA/CIHR). The Teasdale-Corti Global Health Research Partnership Program supported teams of Canadian researchers collaborating with low- and middle-income countries to address health policy and system research, prevention and control of pandemics and chronic diseases, and interactions of health, environment and development. UCVM researchers were awarded more than CAN$1 million to improve veterinary public health as part of the global response to emerging diseases by building a sustainable model in Sri Lanka with extension to South and South-east Asia (Centre for Coastal Health, 2013). With this and other grant successes, UCVM gradually decreased the perceived power differential in relationship to research prowess. As a result, UCFM (as well as other faculties) engaged UCVM more in collaborative research (IDRC, 2013), as illustrated in growing co-authorship of publications (Fig. 28.1).

## Enabling academic One Health environments: joint professorships and interdisciplinary, integrative programmes

### *Bridging cultures: joint professorships*

Integrative academic teams have been proposed to add value to One Health research and programmes (Kahn *et al.*, 2008; Hall and Coghlan, 2011; Leung *et al.*, 2012). Integrative academic research teams have been challenged by reductionist thinking that rewarded veterinary and medical specializations (Gasparatos *et al.*, 2009). With the One Health approach focus and mission to advance health sciences, a culture of integrative research was rewarded. Within this spectrum, there are multi-, inter- and transdisciplinary team approaches to One Health. Multidisciplinary approaches are the least integrative and most sequential, limiting collaboration mostly to the individual's own discipline (Stock and Burton, 2011). Inter-disciplinarity (ID) crosses disciplinary boundaries, especially in shared decision-making, developing conceptual frameworks and establishing and achieving goals. At the University of Calgary, the concept of transdisciplinary (TD) teams to achieve integrative research was informed significantly by research from the Swiss Tropical and Public Health Institute (Swiss Tropical and Public Health Institute, 2013). TD teams engage non-academic participants actively in the research and solutions (Stokols, 2006). One Health research, by its definition, stimulates academia to build collaborative integrative research capacity by applying ID and TD approaches.

Several tools used by academic institutions to encourage collaborations include joint professorships, shared appointments, adjunct appointments, external sessional instructors, endowed chairs and distinguished scholars. A tool purposefully applied by leadership very early during the foundation of the UCVM was joint professorships in UCFM, bridging academic cultures, promoting collaborations, expanding network access and contributing to the diversity of culture between faculties and with external institutions. During the formative years of UCVM from 2005 to 2008 and in 2009, joint academic faculty appointments consisted of approximately 30% and 80%, respectively, of new faculty hires (Fig. 28.2). In the Foothills Medical Complex, they built trusting relationships critical to creating and maintaining multidisciplinary teams (Anholt *et al.*, 2012). Regardless of their official affiliation, they become the 'One Health faculty', integrating veterinary, medical and social sciences expertise into research opportunities. The resulting enabling environment rapidly promoted One Health research and teaching, as described in the following case examples.

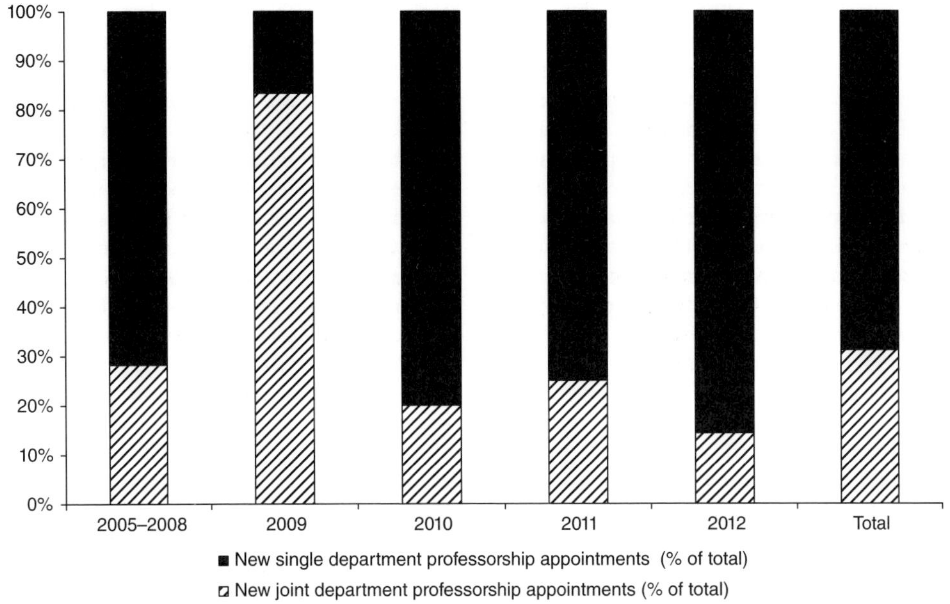


**Fig. 28.2.** University of Calgary percentage of total new joint and single departmental professorship appointments (2005–2012).

*Case example: joint professors in UCFM Department of Community Health Sciences and UCVM Department of Ecosystem and Public Health*

Perhaps the history of comparative medicine roots and the Department of Community Health Sciences (CHS) contributed to UCFM developing a welcoming environment and rapid evolution of collaboration in One Health. CHS' faculty include experts in biostatistics, epidemiology, medical education, health services and population and public health. In the UCVM, the Department of Ecosystem and Public Health (EPH) was founded to focus on the interconnectedness of animal, public and ecosystem health and to promote One Health initiatives. The department hired veterinary and non-veterinary faculty with expertise in public health, public service, wildlife biology, parasitology, parasitic genomics, disease ecology, agricultural economics, pathology, epidemiology, virology, bacteriology, prion disease and bioinformatics. Within a relatively concise period, the collocation environment of CHS and EPH developed into hubs for One Health research and learning.

A strategy used to build an enabling academic One Health environment was by purposefully appointing joint professors starting in the first year with two social anthropologists from CHS into EPH and two public health veterinarians into CHS. An early example of collaboration in One Health was a co-authored call to action to publication to 'create a space in which human health, veterinary, and social scientists may learn from one another, collaborate in research, and cooperate to clear the way for future generations of practitioners and researchers' (Rock *et al.*, 2009).

Another enabling tool promoting One Health was the Grant Gall One Health Research Student Award requiring UCFM and UCVM students to partner in projects building One Health research competencies. Joint professors from both faculties mentored and supervised these One Health students, some who entered graduate programmes in One Health, contributing ultimately to the university's priority to create interdisciplinary researchers (University of Calgary, 2012).

Human and financial resources were dedicated in deans' and departments' offices to encourage One Health interdisciplinary, integrative programmes as these CHS and EPH joint professors recognized win–win cross-disciplinary research and teaching opportunities. They applied transdisciplinary approaches and overcame barriers by: developing shared conceptual frameworks; creating a communication environment that promoted a common understanding of each other's professional language; recognizing and rewarding the time and effort involved in complex One Health research; and providing students with transdisciplinary One Health leadership training and community partnership experiences (Min *et al.*, 2013). The following examples demonstrate the added value of building One Health-enabling environments.

### *Case example: building One Health into Global Health*

Professors from CHS were significantly engaged in creating the Health and Society curriculum of medicine's Bachelor of Health Sciences (BHSc) programme. Formally started in 2005, the O'Brien Centre for the BHSc Health and Society programme focuses on providing a broad-based science foundation and opportunities to engage in global health issues. This programme aligned well with the mandate of UCVM, particularly with the Department of Ecosystem and Public Health (EPH) and the Office of the Assistant Dean of Government and International Relations, both founded in 2007.

UCVM had an established provincial mandate to create new One Health knowledge. There were pressing Global Health concerns and a call to action for academics to respond (Kaplan *et al.*, 2008) as well as international movements to improve collaboration (Oslo Ministerial Declaration, 2007). The UCFM faculty were building institutional capacity addressing these challenges locally and globally, and the early deans and department heads considered how the new veterinary faculty could contribute. In 2007, a new UCVM Office of Government and International Relations (OGIR) was created to represent the dean in partnership-building, especially to build common ground in applying the One Health approach to human health systems. One result was the merging of One Health and Global Health research and teaching through strategic education and research collaboration enabled by OGIR and medicine's Bachelor of Health Sciences (BHSc) programme. In 2007, the BHSc course 'One Health/Global Health' and the formation of the Tanzania Field School were initiated. What emerged was an enabling environment expanding the BHSc programme to include the complex interactions of animals, people and their shared ecosystems. Veterinary professors with research on arctic climate change impacts on caribou health and northern Canadian cultures, food security and safety and animal health were integrated into both initiatives, providing an instructional model of interdisciplinary collaboration needed for teams to solve complex health problems in social-ecological systems. Students learn to distinguish among the concepts of global public health, international health and globalization and challenges of creating and maintaining animal and human health systems in a culturally responsive way. Multidisciplinary instructors working in Tanzania and Canadian aboriginal underserved communities demonstrate how diverse disciplines contribute to equitable and sustainable health research partnerships. Ultimately the added value of this academic approach resulted in BHSc students pursuing mentors, honour supervisors, preceptorships and graduate research studies in One Health with UCVM faculty.

An institutional strategy emerged: building capacity in Global Health by purposefully integrating an interdisciplinary One Health approach. Successful characteristics of interdisciplinary collaboration supporting One Health have been described as: professional networks across disciplines; passionate leadership; a culture of trust and respect; and shared interests and vision (Anholt *et al.*, 2012). All of these characteristics evolved through the efforts of collocated faculty leaders, strategic joint appointments and visionary leadership to build institutional research and educational capacity in One Health approaches to Global Health.

### *Case example: Tanzania One Health/Global Health Field School*

The UCFM BHSc programme had developed relationships with a small hospital in the

Ngorongoro Conservation Area, serving approximately 80,000 Maasai pastoralists. In 2005, leadership in the BHSc Health and Society programme envisioned developing a community-based programme there. It is known that in the Maasai culture, health and food security was heavily dependent on livestock health, environmental changes and wildlife interactions. Therefore, in 2007, UCFM leadership approached UCVM and the Calgary Zoological Society to become engaged in the nascent field school. The Tanzania Field School began with the request of the local health clinic and the resident communities of Maasai to build their capacity in malaria diagnostics (Allen *et al.*, 2010, 2013), and subsequently in addressing zoonotic diseases, HIV-AIDS and food insecurity. In 2008, UCFM and UCVM faculty and undergraduate and graduate students worked together on projects and shared their disciplinary knowledge to advance One Health and Global Health approaches to community-based, transdisciplinary research. A ripple effect of cultural practices, social inequalities and worsening livestock income resulted in a significant reduction in people seeking medical attention at local rural clinics (University of Calgary, n.d.). These intersecting events contributed to complex animal and human health vulnerabilities, requiring social scientists, veterinarians and medical professionals to jointly work on community-based programmes. Building trusting relationships over the years with the affected communities has created a unique academic environment where One Health and Global Health competencies are learned and practised (Hatfield *et al.*, 2009). Leadership within the UCVM Office of Government and International Relations partnered and provided resources to the field school to foster integration of veterinary students and faculty into ongoing projects, contributing over time to bridging disciplinary and departmental cultures. More recently, the UCFM co-developed a Masters of Public Health with the Catholic University of Health and Allied Sciences (CUHAS) in Mwanza, to build Tanzanian research and education capacity that is integrating transdisciplinary One Health approaches into the MPH programme.

This case example exemplifies a far-reaching impact enabled by financial and human resources' support from UCFM and UCVM leadership enhanced by efforts of the collocated departments and joint professors. The leadership understood the importance of integrating One Health concepts into Global Health programmes, resulting in a unique educational transdisciplinary environment with community co-researchers. These two case examples of the Tanzanian Field School and the One Health/Global Health course also demonstrate how institutional support and resources created an enabling One Health/Global Health academic environment that flourished relatively quickly after UCVM was collocated within the Foothills Medical Complex. These cases emerged from UCFM strong Global Health leadership, allocation of resources and history of partnership building in low to middle income countries. These efforts were fundamentally enabled by the collocation of departments, allocation of shared institutional and financial resources, university strategic interdisciplinary support; all combined with the passionate dedication of the collaboration enablers to One Health's contributions to Global Health.

## Summary: Enabling Academic Environments for One Health Approaches to Research and Education

### Historic and political enablers

In the 1800s, Canada had a strong history of veterinary and medical education collaboration, especially in comparative biological medicine research. In the 1900–2000s, the global spread of zoonotic and foodborne emerging and re-emerging pathogens and the devastation in Alberta due to the BSE crisis created public pressure for Canada to be more proactive. This set the stage for the province of Alberta to build academic capacity to address the complex systems contributing to these threats. In 2004, the province supported the founding at the University of Calgary of a veterinary faculty to be collocated within the medical complex.

## Institutional enablers

### *One Health mandate and leadership vision*

The Alberta Province mandated UCVM to focus on animal, public and ecosystem health (One Health) in collocation and partnership with UCFM. The leaders of UCFM believed that health is a shared responsibility between medicine and veterinary medicine. The inaugural Dean of UCVM led the development of a community-based curriculum where One Health was embedded, established an Office of Government and International Relations and created a Department of Ecosystem and Public Health to institutionalize One Health internally and externally. UCFM leadership was committed to Global Health programmes and building institutional and individual capacity in them. The One Health mandate of UCVM with early leadership support of One Health approaches became fertile ground for adding value in One Health and Global Health research and education.

### *Collocation and clustering*

Collocation of a veterinary faculty within a unique medical complex opened opportunities for interdisciplinary integrative research among basic and applied researchers, social scientists and population and public health experts. UCFM's historical success of physically clustering researchers with similar expertise and interests within centres and institutes was applied to integrate the new veterinary researchers. We propose that a rapid increase in co-authorship of research publications (Fig. 28.1) is evidence of the added value of collocation of faculties and clustering of researchers. It also supports the finding by Lee *et al.* (2010) that physical proximity is positively associated with collaboration. We presented above a case where collaboration is enabled by collocation and is continuing to build UCFM-UCVM interdisciplinary work with formation of the new Institute of Public Health, where One Health research projects are emerging on pets and society and animal–human bonds as windows into human health.

### *Leadership and shared conceptual framework*

The university leadership institutionalized community-based programmes, especially in UCFM's Department of Community Health Sciences, Bachelor of Health Sciences programme and Global Health initiatives. This created a unique environment within a medical faculty where research, education and community stakeholder engagement in public health is practised. This shared conceptual framework of community-based programmes melded well with the newly collocated UCVM because it did not operate a veterinary hospital; rather, UCVM founding leaders relied on establishing community partnerships with privately owned clinics and non-profit organizations, including governmental and non-governmental organizations, where veterinary medicine is practised and the principles of One Health are applied. The leadership of UCFM and UCVM used this community-based conceptual framework upon which to build a transformative environment for One Health, perhaps unique in the world. The leadership encouraged the mutual integration of social, animal and ecosystem determinants of health to educate a new cadre of undergraduate and graduate students in One Health. Two case examples are described above, the BHSc Health and Society capstone courses, One Health/Global Health and the jointly led Tanzania Field School.

### *Joint professorships*

An effective institutional tool used to create added value in One Health collaboration was the application of strategically planned and early implementation of joint professorship appointments in medicine and veterinary medicine (Fig. 28.2). This tool bridged academic cultures, promoted collaborations and contributed to the diversity of culture between faculties and external institutions. UCFM and UCVM ensured the development of collaborative One Health research and education efforts resulting in an increase of co-authored publications among UCVM and UCFM faculty (Fig. 28.1). Regardless of their official affiliation, they become the One Health faculty *collaboration enablers*, integrating veterinary, medical, ecological and social sciences.

*Team grants enabling One Health integrative research and decreasing power differentials*

Major funding agencies became more supportive of integrative research teams that potentially led to collaboration across animal and human health disciplines (Natural Sciences and Engineering Research Council of Canada, 2012). The collocated faculties were able to quickly respond in a win–win approach, contributing to a decrease in power differentials between the well-established and new faculties.

*Internal support for One Health*

Internal funding from UCFM's Global Health and International Partnerships, UCVM's Government and International Relations and the University of Calgary's International Grant streams enabled One Health approaches to be integrated into undergraduate and graduate research programmes.

*University reward system*

The university's strategic plan promoted and rewarded interdisciplinary and global health initiatives. This enabled faculties to implement education, research and service that supported One Health. The reward system included central support to promote interdisciplinary collaboration enablers and improvements in valuing team work in faculty merit awards and promotion.

## Added Value of a One Health Academic Enabling Environment

In the final analysis, collocation of a medical and a veterinary faculty mandated to promote One Health demonstrates significant potential to shorten timelines to research productivity and ensures much-needed melding of interdisciplinary collaboration in both research and education.

Throughout this chapter we provided other examples of value added to this case study, including:

- cost-effective savings of medicine and veterinary medicine faculty collocation;
- creation of unique veterinary curriculum where One Health is taught and opportunities for research are integrated;
- creation of *collaboration enablers*, bridging academic cultures overcoming inherent academic power differentials, and encouraging win–win interdisciplinary and transdisciplinary collaborative One Health work; and
- institutional and individual capacity building in One Health/Global Health competencies required to address complex health systems' challenges, locally and globally.

## Recommendations

Although collocation of medical and veterinary medical faculties provided a unique enabling environment, academics must still overcome barriers inherent to One Health collaborations. From this University of Calgary case study, we can offer the following recommendations:

**1.** Plan from the beginning to build a centre to collocate veterinary and medical faculty administrators, educators and researchers, with a separate animal-based veterinary facility to teach veterinary clinical skills by instructors and community-based practitioners.
**2.** When conducting research and education under the One Health conceptual framework, from the beginning, plan an evaluation framework, including economic valuing, cost savings and qualitative criteria, such as: student and faculty satisfaction; faculty retention; performance evaluation and reward systems to value One Health approaches; new and productive One Health research partnerships; research awards for One Health work; and outcome evaluation of joint programmes encouraging inter- and transdisciplinary collaboration. Although operationalizing One Health is believed to have benefits, we must examine the processes that encourage institutions and their partners to communicate,

collaborate, share information, and partner in One Health initiatives (Hall and Coghlan, 2011). Evidence-based, quantitative and qualitative measures of added value are critically needed to positively influence funders of academia and policy makers who dictate resource allocation and mandates. Without such evidence, our efforts may devolve into separate silos, losing opportunities as academicians to make significant impacts to collaborate and solve complex health challenges throughout the world.

**3.** Additionally, our team proposes a 'call to action' for academic institutions to provide unique undergraduate and graduate career trajectories enabling a cadre of new One Health researchers. These students would develop specific competencies earlier in their research careers to overcome disciplinary barriers and potential power differentials among academics and communities and be able to negotiate between internal and external cultures. One Health-focused faculty has learned many of these competencies after years of experience in interdisciplinary and transdisciplinary research. However, we believe there is urgency for academia to create career trajectories and field experiences to quicken and stimulate individual capacity building for leaders in One Health research and education. Such academic degrees could span social, biomedical and health sciences and include bench and applied research, especially with significant experience in community-based research. The expert mentoring and supervision in interdisciplinary and transdisciplinary team work and leadership are essential. As time-consuming as this mentoring can be, the outcomes are equally rewarding. We believe that it is our responsibility to future generations to overcome real and perceived barriers to integrative research and education in socio-ecological One Health systems.

## Acknowledgements

First and foremost, we acknowledge our research assistant, Boh Min, for her dedicated work on references and data analysis. We are indebted to Dr John Kastelic, who provided expert editing advice and Lorraine Toews, who conducted a critically important SCOPUS literature search. Others who have contributed their time, encouragement, ideas and opinions are, in alphabetical order: Drs Susan Cork, Alistair Cribb, Ina Dobrinski, John Gilleard, Benedikt Hallgrimsson, Eugene Janzen, (Ms) Sarah Kempin, John Matyas and Patrick Whelan.

## References

Adams, J., Gurney, K. and Marshall, S. (2007) Patterns of international collaboration for the UK and leading partners (Summary report).

Allen, L.K., Hetherington, E., Manyama, M., Hatfield, J.M. and van Marle, G. (2010) Using the social entrepreneurship approach to generate innovative and sustainable malaria diagnosis interventions in Tanzania: a case study. *Malaria Journal* 9, 42.

Allen, L.K., Hatfield, J.M. and Manyama, M.J. (2013) Reducing microscopy-based malaria misdiagnosis in a low-resource area of Tanzania. *Tanzania Journal of Health Research* 15(1).

American Veterinary Medical Association (2012) *The AVMA: 150 Years of Education, Science, and Service.* American Veterinary Medical Association, Schaumburg, Illinois.

Anholt, R.M., Stephen, C. and Copes, R. (2012) Strategies for collaboration in the interdisciplinary field of emerging zoonotic diseases. *Zoonoses and Public Health* 59(4), 229–240.

Aniekwe, C.C., Hayman, R., Mdee, A., Akuni, J., Lall, P. and Stevens, D. (2012) Academic-NGO Collaboration in International Development Research: a reflection on the issues. Development Studies Association (UK and Ireland) and implemented by the International NGO Training and Research Centre (INTRAC), the University of Bradford and World Vision UK (September), 53 pp.

Centers for Disease Control and Prevention (2003) Update: Severe Acute Respiratory Syndrome – Toronto, Canada, 2003. *MMWR Weekly* 52(23), 547–550. Available at: http://www.cdc.gov/mmwr/preview/mmwrhtml/mm5223a4.htm (accessed 1 March 2014).

Centre for Coastal Health (2013) Integrating human, animal and environmental health since 1996. Available at: http://centreforcoastalhealth.ca (accessed 20 August 2013).

Committee on the National Needs for Research in Veterinary Science (2005) *Critical Needs for Research in Veterinary Science*. The National Academies Press, Washington, DC.

Corvalan, C., Hales, S. and McMichael, A. (2005) Ecosystems and human well-being. In: Sarukhan, J., Whyte A. and Weinstein, P. (eds) *Health Synthesis*. World Health Organization.

Cribb, A. and Buntain, B. (2009) Innovation in veterinary medical education: the concept of 'One World One Health' in the curriculum of the Faculty of Veterinary Medicine at the University of Calgary. *Revue scientifique et technique (International Office of Epizootics)* 28(2), 753–762.

Forge, F. and Fréchette, J.-D. (2005) Mad Cow Disease and Canada's Cattle Industry. Available at: http://www.parl.gc.ca/Content/LOP/researchpublications/prb0301-e.htm#consequencestxt (accessed 20 August 2013).

Gasparatos, A., El-Haram, M. and Horner, M. (2009) The argument against a reductionist approach for measuring sustainable development performance and the need for methodological pluralism. *Accounting Forum* 33(3), 245–256.

GRF Davos (2012) Global Risk Forum (GRF) One Health Summit 2012. Available at: http://www.grforum.org/pages_new.php/one-health/1013/1/938 (accessed 20 August 2013).

Hall, D. and Coghlan, B. (2011) Implementation of the One Health approach in Asia & Europe: How to set-up a common basis for action and exchange of experience. Available at: http://eeas.europa.eu/health/docs/2011_09_eeas_operationalizing_one_health_report_en.pdf (accessed 4 September 2013).

Hatfield, J.M., Hecker, K.G. and Jensen, A.E. (2009) Building global health research competencies at the undergraduate level. *Journal of Studies in International Education* 13(4), 509–521.

IDRC (2013) Global Health Research Initiative. In: Teasdale-Corti Global Health Research Partnership Program. Available at: http://www.idrc.ca/EN/Programs/Global_Health_Policy/Global_Health_Research_Initiative/Pages/Teasdale-Corti.aspx (accessed 4 September 2013).

Kahn, L.H., Kaplan, B., Monath, T.P. and Steele, J.H. (2008) Teaching 'One Medicine, One Health'. *The American Journal of Medicine* 121(3), 169–170.

Kaplan, J.P., Bond, T.C., Merson, M.H., Reddy, K.S., Rodriguez, M.H., Sewankambo, N.K. and Wasserheit, J.N. (2008) Towards a common definition of global health. *The Lancet* 373, 1993–1995.

Lang, D.J., Wiek, A., Bergmann, M., Stauffacher, M., Martens, P., Moll, P., Swilling, M. and Thomas, C.J. (2012) Transdisciplinary research in sustainability science: practice, principles, and challenges. *Sustainability Science* 7, 25–43.

Lee, K., Brownstein, J.S., Mills, R.G. and Kohane, I.S. (2010) Does collocation inform the impact of collaboration? *PloS ONE* 5(12), e14279.

Le Roy, D., Klein, K. and Klvacek, T. (2006) The Losses in the Beef Sector in Canada from BSE. Canadian Agricultural Trade Policy Research Network. Paper 2006-05. Available at: http://www.uoguelph.ca/catprn/publications_commissioned_papers.shtml (accessed 2 September 2013).

Leung, Z., Middleton, D. and Morrison, K. (2012) One Health and EcoHealth in Ontario: a qualitative study exploring how holistic and integrative approaches are shaping public health practice in Ontario. *BMC Public Health* 12(1), 1–15.

Min, B., Allen-Scott, L. and Buntain, B. (2013) Transdisciplinary research for complex One Health issues: a scoping review of key concepts. *Preventive Veterinary Medicine* 112, 222–229.

Narrod, C., Zinsstag, J. and Tiongco, M. (2012) A One Health framework for estimating the economic costs of zoonotic diseases on society. *EcoHealth* 9(2), 150–162.

Natural Sciences and Engineering Research Council of Canada (2012) Collaborative Health Research Projects. Available at: http://www.nserc-crsng.gc.ca/Professors-Professeurs/grants-subs/CHRP-PRCS_eng.asp (accessed 20 August 2013).

Oslo Ministerial Declaration (2007) Global health: a pressing foreign policy issue of our time. *Lancet* 369(9570), 1373–1378.

Parkes, M.W., Bienen, L., Breilh, J., Hsu, L., McDonald, M., Patz, J.A., Rosenthal, J.P., Sahani, M., Sleigh, A., Waltner-Toews, D. and Yassi, A. (2005) All hands on deck: transdisciplinary approaches to emerging infectious disease. *EcoHealth* 2, 258–272.

Public Health Agency of Canada (2012) National Microbiology Laboratory (NML) Overview. Available at: https://www.nml-lnm.gc.ca/overview-apercu-eng.htm (accessed 20 August 2013).

Rock, M., Buntain, B.J., Hatfield, J.M. and Hallgrímsson, B. (2009) Animal-human connections, 'One Health,' and the syndemic approach to prevention. *Social Science & Medicine* 68(6), 991–995.

Rosenfield, P.L (1992) The potential of transdisciplinary research for sustaining and extending linkages between the health and social sciences. *Social Science & Medicine* 35(11), 1343–1357.

Schelling, E., Wyss, K., Béchir, M., Moto, D.D. and Zinsstag, J. (2005) Synergy between public health and veterinary services to deliver human and animal health interventions in rural low income settings. *British Medical Journal (Clinical research edn)* 331(7527), 1264–1267.

Schelling, E., Bechir, M., Ahmed, M.A., Wyss, K., Randolph, T.F. and Zinsstag, J. (2007) Human and animal vaccination delivery to remote nomadic families, Chad. *Emerging Infectious Diseases* 13(3), 373–379.

Schelling, E., Wyss, K., Diguimbaye, C., Bechir, M., Taleb, M.O., Bonfoh, B., Tanner, M. and Zinsstag, J. (2008) Towards integrated and adapted health services for nomadic pastoralists and their animals: a north-south partnership. In: *Handbook of Transdisciplinary Research*. Springer-Verlag, New York, pp. 277–291.

Stock, P. and Burton, R.J. (2011) Defining terms for integrated (multi-inter-trans-disciplinary) sustainability research. *Sustainability* 3(8), 1090–1113.

Stokols, D. (2006) Toward a science of transdisciplinary action research. *American Journal of Community Psychology* 38(1–2), 63–77.

Swiss Tropical and Public Health Institute (2013) Home Page. Available at: http://www.swisstph.ch (accessed 2 September 2013).

United Nations (2013) The Millennium Development Goals Report. Available at: http://www.un.org/millenniumgoals/pdf/report-2013/2013 (accessed 2 September 2013).

University of Calgary (n.d.) Global Health and International Partnerships, Tanzanian Endulen Hospital Collaboration. Available at: http://www.ucalgary.ca/ghealth/projects/TZA_Endulen (accessed 20 August 2013).

University of Calgary (2012) University of Calgary 2012 Strategic Research Plan, 2012, 9 pp. Available at: http://www.ucalgary.ca/news/utoday/july12-2012/plan (accessed 16 October 2014).

University of Calgary, Institute for Public Health (2013) Research Groups. Available at: http://iph.ucalgary.ca/research_groups (accessed 4 September 2013).

University of Calgary Veterinary Medicine (2012) *University of Calgary Veterinary Medicine 2004–2008*. Faculty of Veterinary Medicine, Calgary.

Wuchty, S., Jones, B.F. and Uzzi, B. (2007) The increasing dominance of teams in production of knowledge. *Science* 316 (5827), 1036–1039.

Zinsstag, J., Schelling, E., Roth, F., Bonfoh, B., de Savigny, D. and Tanner, M. (2007) Human benefits of animal interventions for zoonosis control. *Emerging Infectious Diseases* 13(4), 527–531.

Zinsstag, J., Schelling, E., Waltner-Toews, D. and Tanner, M. (2011) From 'one medicine' to 'One Health' and systemic approaches to health and well-being. *Preventive Veterinary Medicine* 101(3–4), 148–156.

Zinsstag, J., Andrea, M., Schelling, E., Bonfoh, B. and Tanner, M. (2012a) From 'two medicines' to 'One Health' and beyond. *Onderstepoort Journal of Veterinary Research* 79(2), 1–5.

Zinsstag, J., Mackenzie, J.S., Jeggo, M., Heymann, D.L., Patz, J. and Daszak, P. (2012b) Mainstreaming One Health. *EcoHealth* 9(2), 107–110.

# 29 Individual and Institutional Capacity Building in Global Health Research in Africa

**Bassirou Bonfoh,[1,2]* Mahamat Béchir Mahamat,[3] Esther Schelling,[4,5] Karim Ouattara,[1,6] Aurélie Cailleau,[1,2] Daniel Haydon,[7] Sarah Cleaveland,[7] Jakob Zinsstag[4,5] and Marcel Tanner[4,5]**

*[1]Centre Suisse de Recherches Scientifiques en Côte d'Ivoire, Abidjan; [2]Consortium Afrique One, Ecosystem and Population Health: Expanding the Frontiers in Health, Abidjan, Côte d'Ivoire; [3]Centre de Support en Santé Internationale au Tchad, N'Djaména, Chad; [4]Swiss Tropical and Public Health Institute, Basel, Switzerland; [5]University of Basel, Basel, Switzerland; [6]Université Félix Houphouët-Boigny de Cocody, Abidjan, Côte d'Ivoire; [7]Boyd Orr Centre for Population and Ecosystem Health, Institute of Biodiversity, Animal Health and Comparative Medicine, University of Glasgow, UK*

## Introduction

Emerging and re-emerging diseases continue to pose a threat to human and animal health in Africa. At the same time, the intersecting demands of human population growth, economic development, food security and biodiversity conservation pose substantial challenges to human, animal and ecosystem health. These pressures are more intense in Africa than in most other parts of the world, but scientific capacities and knowledge are still limited in Africa. Public health systems are weak and fragmented and often unable to respond adequately in crisis and endemic disease situations (Bonfoh *et al.*, 2010). Subsequently, the prevailing, and often highly underreported, endemic diseases are rarely approached together with communities in equity-effective control programmes. Furthermore, African institutions are still poorly equipped to provide the interdisciplinary training needed to develop the next generation of professionals who can undertake research and formulate and implement policy across sectors to tackle these global health challenges.

In complex social and ecological systems, weak response capacities and lack of infrastructure increase the risk of diseases at the human–animal–environment interface (e.g. Ebola virus epidemic in Guinea, Sierra Leone and Liberia). Geographic and social barriers and disparities, as well as conflicts, limit the capacity of institutions to develop health services that are equity-effective, particularly in remote and rural zones. An equitable health service delivers quality services to all people. Approaches designed to increase coverage first among disadvantaged groups show most progress towards universal health coverage (Gwatkin and Ergo, 2011; Schelling *et al.*, Chapter 20, this volume). In terms of zoonotic diseases, preventive measures that are aimed at the animal source represent a potentially more equitable approach to disease prevention

*E-mail: bassirou.bonfoh@csrs.ci

than reliance on unreliable access to fragmented human health services.

In such contexts with a fragile health system, an overarching, comprehensive One Health framework offers good opportunities for operational research partnerships to work towards an adaptive health system. It provides evidence of how collaboration and communication between disciplines and sectors can reduce social and economic costs and add value in health services, community development, local economy and environmental services (Zinsstag *et al.*, Chapter 5, this volume).

The current chapter describes innovative concepts for raising the individual and institutional capacity across Africa. It covers our experiences in developing long-term, equitable and transparent international partnerships, research administration and management capacity, technical skills and capacity needed for One Health at individual and institutional levels, and finally, the chapter shows how these can contribute to global health improvement using the One Health concept.

We draw on two decades of experience in building inter- and transdisciplinary research partnerships involving northern institutions (Swiss TPH, University of Glasgow, Bergen University) and African partners in institutions across West and East Africa, with a hub at the Centre Suisse de Recherches Scientifiques in Côte d'Ivoire (CSRS) and, more recently, new partners in African and Asian countries. The research programmes have addressed issues relating to the health of pastoralists in the Sahel and Central Asia, focusing on control and prevention of zoonotic diseases (e.g. bovine tuberculosis, rabies, anthrax, brucellosis, Rift Valley fever, cysticercosis and toxoplasmosis) and supporting the design of health systems in developing countries with a basic interest in health delivery to mobile communities. We also build on the 12 years of the National Centre of Competence in Research North-South (NCCR North-South) including seven Swiss research institutes together with their partner institutes on four continents. This programme focused on natural resource management, conflict transformation, governance, livelihoods, health and urban planning. It was financed by the Swiss National Science Foundation (SNSF) and the Swiss Agency for Development and Cooperation (SDC). These research programmes facilitate interdisciplinary research on shared topics. In addition, mutual learning between scientists and communities are fostered, i.e. transdisciplinary research (Schelling and Zinsstag, Chapter 30, this volume).

## Long-term Commitments of Partners

The research landscape in Africa is weakly developed and complex. Laboratories and equipment are often inadequate. There are very few advanced training and mentoring programmes and few local research positions for post-graduates. Therefore, there is little incentive and support for the most academically gifted students to pursue a career in scientific research.

For those scientists who do embark on a research career, the most difficult transition is moving from graduate student to independent, internationally competitive researcher. Capacity-building initiatives and partnerships therefore need to address this challenge by providing facilities and career development opportunities for the most promising young scientists to become internationally competitive researchers in their home countries.

### Guidance in individual and institutional capacity in implementing innovative research

We experienced that supervision and mentorship were key for a promising young African scientist who implemented, throughout 7 years, the project titled 'Healthy Milk for the Sahel' from 2000 to 2007. This project, with the support of northern partners, brought together different disciplines, research institutions, non-governmental organizations (NGOs), governmental agencies, communities and funders in Mali to develop an innovative peri-urban dairy sector with higher yield and quality milk production system.

Local knowledge and expressed needs contributed to develop the approach 'High quality milk for technical and financial services'. For example, control of milk-borne zoonotic diseases, such as brucellosis and bovine tuberculosis, could be incentivized by payment of premiums paid on sale of uncontaminated milk through micro-finance and health assurance schemes that would also increase milk production (Bonfoh *et al.*, 2003, 2004).

A social science post-doctoral student was in charge of evaluating the social relevance of these activities, while having sufficient freedom to decide on the objectives and methods, but also the consistent opportunities to exchange with more senior researchers of the involved institutes. He could prepare publications and gain first experiences in teaching and own supervision of Masters' students.

## From North–South to South–South partnerships

The experiences on brucellosis from Mali and Chad within North–South research partnerships were used in Kyrgyzstan to support the design of estimation of representative seroprevalences of brucellosis in humans and livestock. Through the NCCR North-South, the South-South mutual learning and sharing of values in research capacity building was developed (Bonfoh *et al.*, 2012). The experience was further expanded to East Africa with a project entitled 'Enhancing the surveillance and control of bovine tuberculosis in Africa' funded by the Wellcome Trust initiative 'Livestock for Life'. The African bovine TB network with East and West African institutes was the starting point for moving from research teams to a broader consortium in 2009. Support was provided by the Wellcome Trust 'African Institutions Initiatives' at the Centre Suisse de Recherches Scientifiques, which currently has its second African director. The process of building a strong interdisciplinary scientific community of both individuals and institutions within the West African region and towards South–South collaborations took 15 years and several financial schemes to succeed. The strong North–South and South–South networks and strengthened institutions, in spite of the conflict crisis in Côte d'Ivoire, were the basis for seeking a new major programme. The CSRS with its partners had the capacity to lead the 6 year long, £6 million funded 'Afrique One' consortium (http: //www.afriqueone.net), which supports African researchers who are working on One Health at African private, national and university institutes.

Afrique One and the CSRS sustained the research that derives from a huge investment in infrastructure and the intercontinental building of research groups. In return, such a network can attract other grants to support their activities (Bonfoh *et al.*, 2011). However, the building up of successful research partnerships and networks depends on the long-term commitment of all partners and adhering to partnership principles such as mutual learning, setting the agenda together and enhancing capacities (KFPE, 1998). The CSRS has evolved through addressing local and regional priorities and, by so doing, engaging in equitable research partnerships with northern partners. These efforts led to a dynamic equilibrium between partners along the established networks as one of the KFPE partnership principles. European researchers then rethink their role in research in Africa and contribute to the spirit of 'mutual learning for change'.

As members of the community of practice of One Health, we believe that while research capacity requires strong institutions, institutional strength only comes through the contributions of talented and committed individuals. However, the commitments toward capacity building are not easy to judge when selecting new collaborators. We have witnessed how strong leaders can inspire collaborators in African institutions to lead and build up exciting, sustained and independent research programmes and groups. Once an African research group has developed the potential to continue competitive research over years, such a group should be recognized and supported by funding agencies since high-quality applications can lead to very exciting and relevant research.

## Research Governance and Sustainable Research Funding Schemes

The challenges in the African research landscape include good project design, individual capacity and career pathways and, finally, the access to funding. How to improve research capacity in Africa is one of the most demanding issues in designing, costing, monitoring and evaluating a research programme. Research institutes have fragmented funding schemes with funds coming from different sources, sometimes for the same research. Funding is, however, rarely designated for capacity-building alone or to both research and capacity building. The institutional capacity to manage and to be accountable for such funds is a key mechanism for future acquisition of funds.

With a few notable exceptions, such as Tanzania which has committed at least 1% of GDP for research, national funding schemes are lacking in most countries, and funding opportunities at the international level are poorly understood and underexploited. A more sustainable funding mechanism for the main African research agencies could come from matching funds from African governments through national or regional scientific foundations. In 2008, a Swiss-Ivorian programme, the 'Strategic Support Programme of Research in Côte d'Ivoire', was established with an endowment fund (awarded by the Swiss Government) of US$10 million of which US$600,000 in interest is generated annually for funding of competitive research calls. It supports annually 20–25 research projects in ten domains, which should contribute to poverty alleviation. Ivorian researchers currently expect the Ivorian government to double the financial portfolio towards an autonomous National Science Foundation. The CSRS could use this mechanism to generate matching funds to international funding. Such a funding scheme could be adapted by African countries, regional economic organizations or the African Union. The management of such an initiative is rewarding, as in the past funding was mainly from the north, sometimes with pre-set objectives. Shared responsibilities and decentralized fund management was the reality in major initiatives such as the NCCR North-South (SNSF and SDC) and the African Institution Initiatives (Wellcome Trust). National competitive research funding is a powerful tool to foster individual and institutional capacity in Africa.

## Training: Foundation for Good Science

The transformation of the research landscape in Africa and the capacity development at individual and institutional levels play an indispensable role for establishing research relevant to society. Since the last decade, training in research approaches provides a range of skills beyond the scientific domain. Training includes, for example, how to analyse socio-ecological dynamic systems from different disciplines across different sectors, socio-cultural aspects and analyses at spatio-temporal scales. It also involves learning how to validate and apply research results in concrete development contexts, together with scientific and non-scientific stakeholders (NCCR North-South, 2012). In the frame of the NCCR North-South and Afrique One, researchers are introduced to transdisciplinary approaches to define research goals and interventions to test that they are well rooted in society (Schelling and Zinsstag, Chapter 30, this volume).

### Identification of specific training and capacity needs for building interdisciplinary research teams

Internationally competitive research in health increasingly demands epidemiology and inter- and transdisciplinary skills that are difficult to acquire without a broad network of collaborations, particularly to include qualitative and socio-cultural aspects complementing more dominant quantitative elements. Exchange between qualitative and quantitative methods is missing in the curricula of African universities. It demands exchange programmes among African institutions and between disciplines, and also across those divided by regions and language barriers. This can better ensure quality of grant and scientific writing in a bilingual context. Development of the perceived need to exchange between regions, sectors and disciplines could greatly enhance the potential of African research to attract competitive funds independently, develop their own research agendas and foster more equitable and sustainable partnerships with global institutions.

A critical mass of a new group of research leaders, composed of the best of their generation, is needed to further strengthen African universities and research institutes at different stages of developing their research potential. This capacity growth will be facilitated through a network of equitable and enduring South–South and North–South partnerships (Bonfoh *et al.*, 2011).

## Networks and career pathways

Since 2006, four major networks have been established at the CSRS, NCCR North-South, the African Bovine TB network, Safe Food Fair Food and the Afrique One consortium. All networks raised the capacity of champions in zoonoses research, participatory risk analysis and One Health, respectively. The four networks together cover half of all African countries, with a wide range of disciplines and interdisciplinary collaborations. Hundreds of research fellows have been trained. Figure 29.1 shows, for example, the increase of PhD students and post-doctoral fellows during the past 15 years at the CSRS in Côte d'Ivoire.

Afrique One comprises partners in anglophone and francophone African countries as well as Europe. The network approach facilitates the sharing of resources and experiences between members and overcomes challenges in generation, dissemination and utilization of research results across anglophone and francophone zones. Afrique One puts particular emphasis on building research career pathways for promising young researchers and strengthening their position within an institute or university department (Plate 13). They should then be well placed to become future leaders. The capacity-building goals of the consortium are symbolized in its logo by construction of a house. Understanding of the upper floor populations and ecosystems requires foundations in understanding of lower-level processes such as pathogen–host cell interactions. Vertically aligned sets of pillars represent different zoonotic diseases. The same disease can contribute to better understanding of ecosystem health at different levels. The different colours show the contributions of partner institutions; some pillars are multicoloured, and others await construction (Plate 13).

In 2014, Afrique One recorded 18 postdoctoral fellows, 18 PhD students and 24 Masters' students, in addition to technical

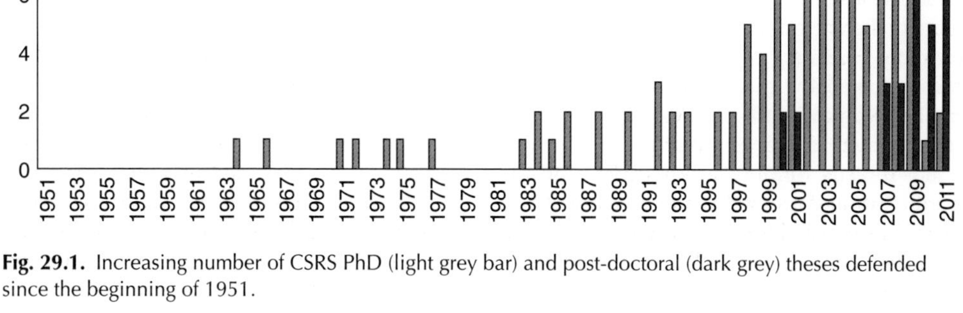


**Fig. 29.1.** Increasing number of CSRS PhD (light grey bar) and post-doctoral (dark grey) theses defended since the beginning of 1951.

and administrative support staff. Afrique One includes partners with medical, veterinary, social and biology related disciplines and expertise. At the beginning of the programme, the institutes had varying levels of research capacity and infrastructure. Within the realm of regional capacity building, Afrique One has also identified 'satellite' institutions, which collaborate with the core partners and benefit from, and contribute to, some of the consortium's activities. A major challenge was the introduction of the position of post-doctoral fellow at the African universities, recruitment of the highest calibre researchers and establishing a secure and sustainable research career track for these fellows. Other challenges included development of inter- and trans-disciplinary research within faculties, and adapting an evaluation system to reflect the value of inter- and trans-disciplinary research outputs.

Afrique One is now able to provide facilities and career development opportunities for post-doctoral scientists. Post-doctoral fellows receive training opportunities, academic support for lecturers to develop their own independent research projects and small equipment grants. The consortium set up lecturer 'buy-outs': short-term grants that allow post-doctoral scientists to 'buy' 6 months out of their teaching time for a visit to another research institute in order to develop new research proposals. The consortium set clear selection criteria for post-docs, who are the key enablers of a successful merit-based funding strategy. All post-doctoral fellows could be recruited and additional Masters' and PhD students included in new research groups. The main challenges were the amount of time that in reality is available for them to dedicate to research, as well as the challenges of working within cumbersome institutional structures (e.g. delays with procurement etc.). In some institutions, these challenges were managed quite effectively. Post-docs have co-ordinated training programmes, which, in turn, allowed the establishment of scientific, methodological and research management training across the consortium. No budget line is directly for northern partners, and the leadership of African research is expected to sustain and strengthen the research capacity in Africa. The lack of direct resource requires close alignment of research interests and effective collaborative research to ensure the sustainability of partnerships and time investments made by partner institutions. Afrique One and other initiatives have demonstrated how the post-doctoral fellowships and the career progression have now changed the research landscape with the positioning of dedicated post-doctoral scientists, which is now recognized at several African universities and research institutes.

The One Health umbrella facilitated the definition of a distinct identity and a reaching out to external stakeholders and other research groups during conferences, with publications, via media and interactions with policy makers, including the World Health Organization (WHO), the Economic Community of West African States (ECOWAS) and the African Union/International Bureau of Animal Resources (AU/IBAR). Less costly solutions to deal with existing shortcomings in regional research infrastructure have been implemented through sharing of facilities and shared use of laboratory equipment and samples among partner organizations. Formal management mechanisms with representation of all partners and joint interventions have fostered collaboration (e.g. on joint proposals, training) and have strengthened intra-consortium relations.

Afrique One's particularities are its long-term commitment, its bilingual composition, its strong emphasis on enabling post-docs to establish an own research group and institutional capacity building including research management and finances, as well as the fact that it is totally African based and led. Therefore, we are convinced that the consortium is already making a difference in the current research landscape in Africa, which is still largely externally funded and encompassing an agenda that is often set elsewhere.

## Rethinking Health System Research

### Global health

Health is not just a benefit of sustainable development but a prerequisite. For populations trying to escape the cycle of poverty, one of the most serious handicaps is the high vulnerability to diseases. Thus, one should find ways of building resilience of people and supporting their coping strategies for global change. For this, new strategies and alliances are needed in health policy and system research. The last decade of inter- and transdisciplinary research yielded the most relevant approaches of ecohealth and One Health and has led to their convergence (Zinsstag, 2012). Programmes have brought together researchers, practitioners and decision makers to plan for equity-effective interventions. Good research platforms contribute to the assessment of major determinants and impacts of global change and provide scientifically sound solutions to health problems and behavioural change among stakeholders. There is a need to change the way health problems are addressed and aligned with health research, including academia, health systems with practitioners and health policy makers. This is possible if African governments are fully engaged in allocating resources for the emerging health initiatives along with the donor communities.

## Needed capacity for One Health approaches

For the identification of disease risks, particularly of zoonoses, and designing appropriate preventive and control measures, it is critical to understand better the interactions between human and animal populations and their environment as well as the impact of ecological and social pressures or behaviour, which are often neglected. The starting point is a health problem and the disciplines that seem best placed to address the problem are invited. One Health is the enabler between the necessary research and the generation of added value by fostered collaboration and communication (Fig. 29.2).

To achieve added value, we need to assist research groups, specializing on infectious diseases common to both humans and animals, at African research institutions. These groups should be in a position to sustain their research activities through national and international funding programmes. The graduate and postgraduate researchers, as well as practitioners, need training in methods and tools of data acquisition and analysis in both veterinary and public health. Furthermore, dissemination of results for validation and application involves communication and writing skills as well as tools to engage decision makers. This can be achieved partly through increased collaborations between research institutes in Africa, particularly between those in the East and the West, and partly through more links with research institutes in other areas in Europe, the Americas and Asia. Finally, it also requires capacity in grant mobilization and efficient management of knowledge and resources such as data, finances and human resources.

Since 2009, research capacity, partnership collaboration, management and communication have been monitored by the Afrique

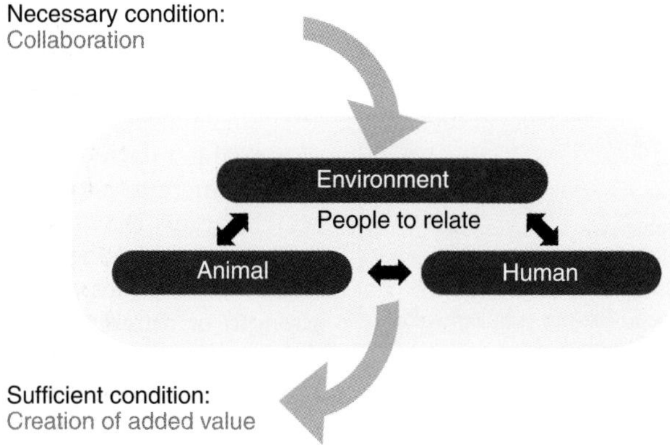


**Fig. 29.2.** Necessary and sufficient conditions to create One Health research capacity in Africa.

One consortium. This was done in 16 institutions of eight African countries. The goal of the assessment was to develop training modules that support the implementation of One Health approaches. We have identified and developed missing modules in university curricula. These complementary modules are summarized in the 'Welcome Package' that all new consortia students and fellows received. The modules introduce the tools that were identified as the most critical ones to improve the research environment, to raise trust between partners and to build individual and institutional capacity including administration and management.

The modules, for example, on epidemiology, disease transmission modelling and exposure assessment of multiple health risks, have been successfully validated in four institutions in Senegal, Côte d'Ivoire and Tanzania with more than 200 graduate and post-graduate students. The next steps are to consolidate these modules and negotiate with the Doctoral schools for their accreditation and inclusion in research and administration Masters' courses. Options for MOOCs (Massive Online Open Access Courses) in One Health or transdisciplinary methods are currently being explored with the EPFL (Ecole Polytechnique Fédérale de Lausanne). A distance-learning Masters' course was developed by another EU-funded consortia of European, Maghreb and West African One Health practitioners to train the One Health next generation (OH-NextGen) (Box 29.1). This volume should also provide a comprehensive learning resource for these educational and capacity-building initiatives.

**Box 29.1.** Overview of the OH-NextGen distance-learning programme.

One Health in the Sahel and Maghreb
Concepts of Epidemiology in One Health
One Health Survey Methodology
Risk Analysis in a One-Health Framework
Geographical Information System in Epidemiology
Health and Livestock Economics
Specific Zoonoses
One Health Policy
Health Education
Socio-cultural and ethical aspects in One Health

## Knowledge Translation into Practice and Policy

For 12 years, in the framework of the NCCR North-South, we studied options for health care of mobile pastoralists in the Sahelian countries. We engaged with stakeholders from communities, authorities and academia in an iterative process of meetings and field research leading from the basic understanding of the health status of humans and animals to contextual analysis of livelihoods and institutions and small-scale interventions. Thereby, we recognized that health care and social service planning require a broader understanding of the context of health in terms of institutions, natural resource management, conflicts, security and governance. A multi-sector policy was developed with all stakeholders in Chad, but it could not be readily implemented given the high number of ministries enrolled. However, currently the Chadian Ministry of Health has created a novel directorate for pastoral health and pastoralist communities are increasingly self-organized with the help of mobile communication technologies. Cross-sector human and animal health care, implemented through NGOs in north Mali, was interrupted by ongoing warfare. However, African research capacity to negotiate policies has been built (Bonfoh *et al.*, 2011; Münch, 2011; Schelling *et al.*, 2010; Zinsstag *et al.*, 2011; Béchir *et al.*, 2012).

## African Leadership in Science and Research Management

Our goal is to achieve a critical mass of independent, internationally competitive research groups led by African scientists who are working in African universities and research institutions. Pulling together the strength of different disciplines will create tighter links between science and policy and East and West African expertise to better address ecosystem and population health, while bridging language and geographic gaps.

## Acknowledgements

This chapter was prepared with the support of the consortium Afrique One 'Ecosystem and Population Health: Expanding Frontiers in Health'. Afrique One is funded by the Wellcome Trust (WT087535MA). We thank all investigators and fellows of 'Healthy Milk for the Sahel' (SNSF), Safe Food Fair Food (GIZ/BMZ), NCCR North-South (SNSF/SDC) and Afrique One.

## References

Béchir, M., Zinsstag, J., Schelling, E., Mahama, A., Kessely, H., Fokou, G., Moto, D.D., Bonfoh, B. and Tanner, M. (2012) Social services for mobile pastoralists: cross-sector strategy based on 'One Health'. *Sociology Study* 2(9), 1–10.

Bonfoh, B., Wasem, A., Traore, A.N., Fane, A., Spillmann, H., Simbe, C.F., Alfaroukh, I.O., Nicolet, J., Farah, Z. and Zinsstag, J. (2003) Microbiological quality of cows' milk taken at different intervals from the udder to the selling point in Bamako (Mali). *Food Control* 14(7), 495–500.

Bonfoh, B., Roth, C., Traor, A.N., Fan, A., Simb, C.F., Alfaroukh, I.O., Nicolet, J., Farah, Z. and Zinsstag, J. (2004) Effect of washing and disinfecting containers on the microbiological quality of fresh milk sold in Bamako (Mali). *Food Control* 17(2), 153–161.

Bonfoh, B., Schwabenbauer, K., Wallinga, D., Hartung, J., Schelling, E., Zinsstag, J., Meslin, F.-X., Tschopp, R., Akakpo, J.A. and Tanner, M. (2010) Human health hazards associated with livestock production. In: Steinfeld, H., Mooney, H.A., Schneider, F. and Neville, L.E. (eds) *Livestock in a Changing Landscape,* Vol. 1. *Drivers, Consequences, and Responses*. Island Press, Washington, DC, pp. 196–219.

Bonfoh B., Raso, G., Koné, I., Dao, D., Girardin, O., Cissé, G., Zinsstag, J., Utzinger, J. and Tanner, M. (2011) Research in a war zone: Bassirou Bonfoh and others offer lessons from a West African institute that has survived ten years of conflict. *Nature* 474, 569–571.

Bonfoh, B., Kasymbekov, J., Dürr, S., Toktobaev, N., Doherr, M.G., Schueth, T., Zinsstag, J. and Schelling, E. (2012) Representative seroprevalences of brucellosis in humans and livestock in Kyrgyzstan. *EcoHealth* 9(2), 132–138.

Gwatkin, D.R. and Ergo, A. (2011) Universal health coverage: friend or foe of health equity? *Lancet* 377, 2160–2161.

KFPE (1998) Guidelines for research in partnership with developing countries – 11 principles. Available at: http://www.kfpe.ch/11-principles (accessed 16 May 2014).

Münch, A.K. (2011) *Nomadic Women's Health Practice. Islamic Belief and Medical Care among Kel Alhafra Tuared in Mali*. Schwabe AG, Verlag Basel, 376 pp.

NCCR North-South (2012) *A Research Agenda for Global Transformation*. International Conference on research for development. ICRD, 2012.

Schelling, E., Bechir, M., Daugla, D.M., Bonfoh, B., Taleb, M.O., Zinsstag, J. and Wyss, K. (2010) Health research among highly mobile pastoralist communities of Chad. *Society, Biology & Human Affairs* 72(2), 93–113.

Zinsstag, J. (2012) Convergence of Ecohealth and One Health. Editorial. *EcoHealth* 9, 371–373.

Zinsstag, J., Schelling, E., Waltner-Toews, D. and Tanner, M. (2011) From 'one medicine' to 'one health' and systemic approaches to health and well-being. *Preventive Veterinary Medicine* 101(3–4), 148–156.

# 30 Transdisciplinary Research and One Health

**Esther Schelling* and Jakob Zinsstag**
*Swiss Tropical and Public Health Institute, Basel, Switzerland and University of Basel, Basel, Switzerland*

## Introduction

One Health raises questions beyond the narrow view of health improvements based on medical interventions: its activities need to be understood in a context of local and global social-ecological changes, where outcomes are less certain (Zinsstag *et al.*, 2011b). We need a range of disciplines to understand the context of health (Allotey *et al.*, 2010). For this purpose, the starting point should not be a One Health approach, but the socially relevant health-related problem and its ecological dimensions. Other socially relevant problems are, for example, hunger, poverty, pollution and migration. Proponents of One Health propose to find practical solutions, which most often cannot be approached by academia alone. At this point academic science should engage non-academic stakeholders and knowledge in research for practical problem solving and identification of causes at their roots. The growing awareness of the need to embark in transdisciplinary processes to solve complex problems has invigorated the development and delivery of science-based policy in One Health in the past decade (Cork *et al.*, Chapter 25, this volume).

## Increasing Transdisciplinary Research since the End of the Twentieth Century

Progressive fragmentation of the sciences into more and more specialized disciplines and thematic fields in the 20th century led to the perceived major risk that specialization cannot recognize possible negative side-effects for modern civilization. The growing awareness of such risks stimulated integrative approaches labelled 'inter-disciplinarity' or 'transdisciplinarity' (see below for how we use these terms). Differences between basic, applied and transdisciplinary research, as specific forms of research, stem from whether and how different scientific disciplines and actors in the life-world are involved in problem identification and problem structuring, thus determining how research questions relate to problem fields in the life-world (Hirsch Hadorn *et al.*, 2008). Transdisciplinarity has become a form of research with possible association of any discipline. The number of publications using 'transdisciplinary' or 'transdisciplinarity' increased from below 500 per year before 1995 to more than 2500 since 2008. The transdisciplinarity-net (td-net, http://www.transdisciplinarity.ch) publishes these overviews on developments of transdisciplinary research. It was initiated

*E-mail: esther.schelling@unibas.ch

in 2003 by the Swiss Academies of Arts and Sciences to support foresight and the dialogue between science and society. Yet, very few publications (less than ten) were found on transdisciplinarity and One Health in a review of literature published from 1990 to 2012 (Min *et al.*, 2013).

Hirsch Hadorn *et al.* (2008) in their chapter 'The emergence of transdisciplinarity as a form of research' and its section 'From dissociation to transdisciplinary orientation in the knowledge society', describe the history of transdisciplinary research from Aristotle's forms of knowledge to today. Transdisciplinarity plays such an important role in One Health that we consider it appropriate to summarize Hadorn's chapter to provide necessary background without claiming completeness. Natural science in the period since the 17th century has dissociated from philosophy and become concerned with empirical laws. Research is carried out by intervening into nature in technically equipped experimental settings. The concept of positivism postulates that observations are the only source of knowledge. There is a dissociation of science from practical knowledge, or what is also called the life-world. The term 'life-world' was introduced by the German philosopher Husserl (1859–1938). In the 19th century the science of society, called sociology, was created. Another German philosopher, Alfred Schütz (1899–1959), introduced the term life-world into sociology as 'social reality'. The social sciences and humanities put forward the need for interpretation of social and cultural phenomena from an historical perspective. Wilhelm Dilthey (1833–1911) advocated a hermeneutic paradigm to achieve an understanding of cultural ideals. Natural sciences attempt to explain natural phenomena, but hermeneutics attempt to interpret and assign a meaning to social and cultural phenomena from an historical perspective. The debate is about explanation versus meaning.

Sociology was confronted with the social crises of capitalism in the 19th century. The German sociologist Max Weber (1864–1920) recognized practical problems as a stimulus for scientific research. There is an ongoing debate regarding the relationship of empirical science to societal values. Scientists do not limit themselves to describe, for example, poverty; they consider poverty as socially inacceptable and thus do not make a descriptive, strictly scientific, statement, but a normative, value statement. Weber argued that empirical sciences are about what is either true or false, while the normative distinction in the sphere of values is that of right or wrong. Given the progressive fragmentation of the sciences into more and more specialized disciplines and thematic fields, the situation that complex, emerging phenomena could no longer be recognized led to the development of systems theory studies and of multidisciplinary and interdisciplinary thinking. When a variety of disciplines collaborate in one research programme without integration of concepts, epistemologies or methodologies – but link research results – we speak of multi-disciplinarity. Interdisciplinarity is also a collaboration of several disciplines, but concepts or methodologies are explicitly exchanged and integrated, resulting in a mutual enrichment (Flinterman *et al.*, 2001; Darbellay and Paulsen, 2008).

Erich Jantsch (1929–1980) sees the triangle of university–industry–government as a 'transdisciplinary' triangle organized by general systems theory. In the second half of the 20th century natural resource crises emerged due to, among other forces, rapid population growth. The Brundtland Report from the United Nations World Commission on Environment and Development (WCED) recognized in 1987 that the complexity of the interactions of a 'Risk society' (Beck 1992) and unintended and poorly understood damage to natural resources and lives require systemic thinking across different academic disciplines and involving societal actors like communities and authorities. The United Nations Conference on Environment and Development (UNCED) in Rio de Janeiro in 1992 promoted sustainable development by involving people from civil society, the private sector and public agencies as actors in participatory deliberation and decision making. Social sciences and humanities became involved in activities such as technology assessment and ethical committees on morally sensitive technologies. Mittelstrass (1992) defines 'transdisciplinarity' as a form of research that transcends disciplinary boundaries to address and solve problems related to the life-world. Through scientists entering into dialogue and mutual learning with societal stakeholders, science becomes part of societal processes, contributing explicit and negotiable values and norms in society and science, and attributing meaning to knowledge for societal problem-solving (Hirsch Hadorn *et al.*, 2008, 30).

Based on their historical review, Hirsch-Hadorn *et al.* (2008) conclude that one can understand why transdisciplinary research is shaped by various lines of thinking and has a variety of definitions. We thus present here the definition derived by the same authors, which is based on a synthesis of what can be found in the literature:

> There is a need for transdisciplinary research when knowledge about a societally relevant problem field is uncertain, when the concrete nature of problems is disputed, and when there is a great deal at stake for those concerned by problems and involved in dealing with them. Transdisciplinary research deals with problem fields in such a way that it can: a) grasp the complexity of problems, b) take into account the diversity of life-world and scientific perceptions of problems, c) link abstract and case specific knowledge, and d) constitute knowledge and practices that promote what is perceived to be the common good.

There is large overlap between transdisciplinarity and post-normal science. Normal science is inadequate to ensure the validity of knowledge and therefore routine scientific expertise is inadequate and professional knowledge and judgments are insufficient. Funtowicz and Ravetz (1993) argue that in such cases science must engage in dialogue with all those who have a stake in the decision (Zinsstag *et al.*, Chapter 2, and Bunch and Waltner-Toews, Chapter 34, this volume). Next to post-normal sciences, analogous approaches to transdisciplinarity – recognizing the need to integrate disciplines and engage civil society in view of the relevance to the policy problem in question, but also of the complexity and uncertainty – are Science of Team Science in North America, Integration and Implementation Sciences in Australia and Public Engagement in Europe and elsewhere.

Scientists are often overwhelmed by the amount of information in everyday practice and the lack of a common language in specialized fields of expertise. In inter- and transdisciplinary programmes researchers should have: their own in-depth knowledge; general knowledge of the other disciplines involved; social and communication skills for the exchange between disciplinary researchers and actors of the life-world; respect for others; and teamwork and cognitive (or synthesis) skills (Flinterman *et al.*, 2001). In the course of a programme, no interdisciplinary team can engage and consult many stakeholders all the time. They can but put alternating emphasis on specific disciplinary to transdisciplinary approaches. Commonly a programme starts with broader inter- and transdisciplinary approaches before becoming periodically disciplinary/multidisciplinary, before reaching out again to broader participatory and integrative approaches (Hurni and Wiesmann, 2004).

We can distinguish three forms of interdependent knowledge: systems, target and transformation knowledge. Systems knowledge relates to questions about the genesis and possible further development of a problem, and about interpretations of the problem in the life-world. Target knowledge relates to questions determining and explaining the need for change, desired goals and better practices, while transformation knowledge relates to questions about technical, social, legal, cultural and other possible means of acting that aim to transform existing practices and introduce desired ones (Pohl and Hirsch Hadorn, 2007). Knowledge must be identified and structured (account of state of disciplinary knowledge and actors in society to define the problem and research questions), analysed (adequate organization, which interests and circumstances to take into account) and results brought to fruition (embedment into the social and scientific contexts, test the expected impact). Problem identification and structuring can overlap, which makes an iterative rather than a sequential approach more rational for achieving valid results. Unexpected and surprising results are to be expected (Hirsch Hadorn *et al.*, 2008).

## Transdisciplinary Research in One Health and Ecohealth

Both quantitative and qualitative approaches enrich our knowledge. True interdisciplinary research programmes in One Health and on zoonoses control are few in number. With some strong exceptions (see Welburn and Coleman, Chapter 18, this volume), so called 'socio-economic' or 'socio-cultural' studies on zoonoses are largely questionnaire-based, including the knowledge, attitude and practice (KAP) studies, and are often led by veterinarians. These rapid appraisals have several shortcomings, particularly because they do not further describe the context (Allotey *et al.*, 2010). New institutional arrangements between social and biomedical sciences are needed to establish interdisciplinary teams which can be seen as the motor of transdisciplinary research (Whittaker, Chapter 6, this volume). Below we present a few examples of transdisciplinary processes in One Health and ecohealth.

### Long-term iterative process in Chad to improve the health of pastoralists and their livestock

Livestock-keeping communities are often excellent observers and know the priority diseases of people and animals in their context. However, in rural and remote rural zones they are confronted with difficulties accessing health services (Schelling *et al.*, Chapter 20, this volume). To improve health in a credible way in remote rural communities, all health aspects should be reviewed and interventions built on communities' and authorities' priorities in a participatory way. Within research partnerships between European and Chadian research institutes, we have explored possibilities to improve access to services of mobile pastoralists in Chad, who were previously only served by veterinary services but not human health. This aspect was then also one result of an interdisciplinary team including anthropology, social geography, medicine, veterinary epidemiology and microbiology. Other disciplines such as sociology and geography were associated in the further course of the programme with various funding. Research results also included the absence of a local concept for zoonoses (Krönke, 2004) and that access to key pastoral resources and related conflicts with sedentary communities strongly influenced care-seeking behaviour (Wiese, 2004). Thanks to livestock holders' reports on perceived poor anthrax vaccine quality, contamination problems in local vaccine production were detected (Schelling *et al.*, 2008). We used the community-based research results to initiate broader collaborations with authorities and scientific experts and results were reviewed in the communities during focus-group discussions and regional workshops to obtain a broader perspective from pastoralist men and women. The research hypothesis and objectives of the complementary studies were guided by the recommendations of the first national workshop in 1998. Indeed, one key recommendation – leading to an advantage of the programme compared to other single sector studies – was that veterinarians must be associated because livestock, the most important element in the livelihood of mobile pastoralists, cannot be excluded.

Repeated stakeholder seminars became crucial elements towards a transdisciplinary process. These allowed the scientists to engage with communities and their representatives and associations, authorities from the Ministries of Health (MoH) and Livestock Production as well as local authorities and technicians and staff, NGOs working with pastoralists; international bi- and multilateral organizations such as WHO and UNICEF and donors (Léchenne *et al.*, Chapter 16, and Schelling *et al.*, Chapter 20, this volume). The consultative stakeholder seminars aimed at defining priorities of the populations and the authorities jointly, formulating health service priorities from a range of options and re-adjusting ongoing interventions but also cross-checking the relevance of activities. Pastoralists could express their concerns and needs directly to the authorities and also voice non-health-related demands such as requests for new legislations on land use. The priority setting process started from health system-driven approaches – pragmatic in the sense that interventions could be carried out by the health and veterinary services and could be validated by involved scientists – and moved incrementally towards the inclusion of other communities' priorities. The participants identified new research and intervention objectives and, as a consequence, trust and mutual respect have built gradually. The programme became the interlocutor between pastoralists and the authorities, and the communities were empowered to take their own initiatives (Schelling *et al.*, 2008).

In conjunction with the stakeholder workshop in 2005 a process of inter-ministerial planning of a national action plan to support nomadic communities in Chad started under the leadership of the Ministry of Planning in collaboration with eight other ministries (Plate 14). However, the intersectoral negotiations with so many ministries proved to be too cumbersome and were not feasible. The new course, where the MoH took the lead, turned out to be more operational. During the latest workshop in 2013, the MoH announced the creation of a directorate for the health of mobile pastoralists. Activities that are implemented as a result of the transdisciplinary process, particularly the joint human and animal vaccination campaigns – currently in trans-frontier zones – are maintained and fully led by the government (Schelling *et al.*, Chapter 20, this volume). There is also a presidential decree for full EPI coverage for pastoralist children along with polio vaccination days. The 'Association des jeunes nomades' is more active and prominent than ever, regarding the problem of pastoralists as an institutional problem. These dynamics of pastoralist representation would hardly have been possible 10 years earlier when only a few pastoralists had a higher education. Finally, the participants have voiced a desire to seek new innovations such as use of mobile technology to assess demographic and health parameters of pastoralist families and their livestock (Jean-Richard *et al.*, 2014).

The iterative problem-oriented programme aimed at improving access to health care for the nomadic pastoralists of Chad started with little information on important health issues. However, ownership by the communities for interventions could be achieved by their participation in knowledge generation as equal partners, together with local authorities and scientists in a transdisciplinary approach. Unexpected outcomes emerged, for example, that the pastoralist communities organized themselves to provide schooling for their children, which has received support from UNICEF (United Nations Children's Fund). They have also stated that their overall security improved substantially. Generalizations for other settings can hardly be made, but where communities interact with authorities in a participatory process to identify acceptable institutional and legal frameworks, arrangements for social service development in a given context can be achieved. The long term commitment of all partners continues and has broadened the scope of research to other mobile communities in north Mali (Plate 15) as well as seasonal workers and inter-provincial migrants.

## National and regional priority setting in health and food safety

With regard to societal questions about health, priority setting is not only needed in research and action in specific contexts but also on national and regional levels. New public engagement processes can be initiated. For example, the European Food Safety Agency (EFSA) initiated an integrated approach towards risk assessment with a special focus on human health and the whole food chain, as well as on science-based interventions to lower the risk to consumers. They have regularly consulted scientific panels to address complex, multifaceted questions of risk and are experimenting with how to engage the broader public. This consultation process revealed, among other things, the increasing public concerns about the sustainability of livestock production systems, aspects on acceptability of food quality and animal welfare (Berthe *et al.*, 2013). Donors are encouraging low- and middle-income countries to set up processes of public participation in health-sector priority setting. A recent review, however, showed that to date there is little evidence on how to do this in a less costly way. The authors of the review propose that some of the substantial resources needed for a nationwide public engagement could be used to strengthen the evidence for what works within the realities, using small-scale, community-driven trials (Alderman *et al.*, 2013).

### Transdisciplinarity in ecohealth

Transdisciplinarity is well embedded in ecohealth to tackle the non-linear systems dynamics (Bunch and Waltner-Toews, Chapter 34, this volume). The International Development Research Centre (IDRC) framework implies not only a transcendence of disciplines, but also the participation of scientists, communities and policy makers in research (Lebel, 2004). Particular attention is given to gender and social equity and putting knowledge into action through policy change, interventions and improvement of practices (Charron, 2012). Examples of transdisciplinary processes are presented in Charron (2012), Veterinarians Without Borders/Vétérinaires Sans Frontières Canada (VWB/VSF, 2010) and in Bunch and Waltner-Toews, Chapter 34 (this volume). Parkes *et al.* (2005) have exemplified the value of transdisciplinarity for emerging infectious diseases. They concluded that with transdisciplinary integration and innovation for infectious diseases it may be possible to harness the good will and teamwork established during an emergency in order to address health issues that develop more slowly. And with emerging health threats, the social-ecological and political contexts of global health foster integrated conceptual frameworks and disease control measures. Although complex understandings of social and ecological systems may be informative and better reflect the uncertainty of real life, such approaches may be challenged on the basis that they often do not lend themselves to straightforward, rapidly implemented policies or interventions.

## Disciplines and Approaches are Not Static: Intermediary Conclusions

Transdisciplinarity emerged as a form of research at the end of the 20th century because separated disciplines could not grasp the complexity of, for example, the impact of new technologies and natural resource depletion. Such issues could not be tackled from the sphere of individual disciplines. We see health as a life-world problem and believe that transdisciplinarity should be at the heart of One Health studies leading to improved health of people, animals and the environment. The examples in this chapter show that the engagement of other than academic knowledge can lead to problem solving and innovation, as well as unexpected outcomes. Taking a One Health approach can promote the development of good partnerships between government agencies as well as engage the public and industry stakeholders in the development and delivery of policy (Cork *et al.*, Chapter 25, this volume). It can further increase equity and effectiveness of interventions at national and sub-national levels, because equity can only be defined within a broad transdisciplinary partnership between communities and authorities governed by mutual trust and security. This is similar to what is promoted in the 2008 Report of the WHO Commission on Social Determinants in Health that recognizes Civil Society as champion of equity (Jackson *et al.*, 2013). Health equity, in turn, is part of sustainable development and hence directly linked to environmental sustainability and social justice (Zinsstag *et al.*, 2011a).

Participatory stakeholder processes as discussed above have seemingly a huge potential for practical problem solving but also bear risks. These include raising expectations too high on outcomes of the process and choosing certain health-related outcomes over others such as poverty alleviation, which implies ethical considerations; the stakeholders engaged are not representative for the relevant problem area; and there may be biases in the process due to power relationships, such as dominance of academia and gender issues. There are also concerns about the direct involvement and influence of scientists in social processes. It is important to carefully document the process.

Complexity, uncertainty and ambiguity in health and other life-world problems are obviously challenges. How do we deal with corruption or the discrepancy between investments in development of sophisticated, new technological tools, when we do not manage to effectively deliver existing adequate tools, such as measles vaccination? We can deal with complexity by interdisciplinary expert inputs, although we may invite a sub-optimal panel of disciplinary experts. Each researcher and actor may locate the problem in an alternative 'world of relevance'. Validation and quality control may help. Validation of non-scientific knowledge and explanations is a crucial and challenging aspect of knowledge integration within transdisciplinary research. Because different types of explanation play a role, different validation criteria have to be met, both through problem formulations and solutions found. Sometimes a non-scientific explanation can be tested as a hypothesis in a further research process. A continuous dialogue between the parties involved is required, with feedback loops for the cross-checking of previous assumptions, insights and demands (Flinterman *et al.*, 2001). Social scientists are likely best situated to monitor the process and identify possible shortfalls that need corrective actions.

Researchers are challenged to cross the boundaries between human and natural sciences to generate results that could not have been attained using a disciplinary or sectoral approach alone. Young scientists trained for many years in one discipline must first learn to acknowledge the strengths of other approaches. University curricula, however, rarely enable scientists to communicate with other disciplines, and researchers first need to acquire their own experiences and skills (Conrad *et al.*, 2009; Min *et al.*, 2013). Max-Neef (2005) wrote that this should not represent a problem as long as the higher education received was coherent with the challenge. This is, unfortunately, not the case, since mono-disciplinary education is still widely predominant in all universities.

It is encouraging to see that donors explicitly ask for inter- and transdisciplinary research. However, the establishment of these processes requires some additional investments, and donors do not yet necessarily give more time or money. In any case, transdisciplinary research with its iterative cycles between innovation, application and validation is an integrated part of One Health approaches.

## References


Alderman, K.B., Hipgrave, D. and Jimenez-Soto, E. (2013) Public Engagement in Health Priority Setting in Low- and Middle-Income Countries: Current Trends and Considerations for Policy. *Plos Medicine* 10, e1001495.1–e1001495.3.

Allotey, P., Reidpath, D.D. and Pokhrel, S. (2010) Social sciences research in neglected tropical diseases 1: the ongoing neglect in the neglected tropical diseases. *Health Research Policy and Systems* 8, 32.

Berthe, F., Hugas, M. and Makela, P. (2013) Integrating surveillance of animal health, food pathogens and foodborne disease in the European Union. *Revue Scientifique et Technique OIE* 32, 521–528.

Charron, D.F. (2012) *Ecohealth in Practice: Innovative Applications of an Ecosystem Approach to Health.* Springer and International Development Research Centre, New York.

Conrad, P.A., Mazet, J.A., Clifford, D., Scott, C. and Wilkes, M. (2009) Evolution of a transdisciplinary 'One Medicine-One Health' approach to global health education at the University of California, Davis. *Preventive Veterinary Medicine* 92, 268–274.

Darbellay, F. and Paulsen, T. (2008) *Le défi de l'Inter- et Transdisciplinarité - Herausforderung Inter- und Transdisziplinarität. Concepts, méthodes et pratiques innovantes dans l'enseignement et la recherche - Konzepte, Methoden und innovative Umsetzung in Lehre und Forschung,* Presses polytechniques et universitaires romandes, Lausanne, Switzerland.

Flinterman, J.F., Teclemariam-Mesbah, R., Broerse, J.E.W. and Bunders, J.F.G. (2001) Transdisciplinarity: the new challenge for biomedical research. *Bulletin of Science, Technology & Society* 21, 253–266.

Hirsch Hadorn, G., Biber-Klemm, S., Grossenbacher-Mansuy, W., Hoffmann-Riem, H., Joye, D., Pohl, C., Wiesmann, U. and Zemp, E. (2008) The emergence of transdisciplinarity as a form of research. In: Hirsch Hadorn, G., Hoffmann-Riem, H., Biber-Klemm, S., Grossenbacher, W., Joye, D., Pohl, C., Wiesmann, U. and Zemp, E. (eds) *Handbook of Transdisciplinary Research.* Springer, Heidelberg, pp. 19–39.

Hurni, H. and Wiesmann, U. (2004) Towards transdisciplinarity in sustainability-oriented research for development. In: Hurni, H., Wiesmann, U. and Schertenleib, R. (eds) *Research for Mitigating Syndroms of Global Change. A transdisciplinary appraisal of selected regions of the world to prepare development-oriented research partnerships. Perspectives of the Swiss National Centre of Competence in Research (NCCR) North-South, University of Berne, Switzerland.* Geographica Bernensia, pp. 31–41.

Jackson, S.F., Birn, A.E., Fawcett, S.B., Poland, B. and Schultz, J.A. (2013) Synergy for health equity: integrating health promotion and social determinants of health approaches in and beyond the Americas. *Revista Panamericana de Salud Pública* 34, 473–480.

Jean-Richard, V., Crump, L., Moto, D.D., Hattendorf, J., Schelling, E. and Zinsstag, J. (2014) The use of mobile phones for demographic surveillance of mobile pastoralists and their animals in Chad: proof of principle. *Global Health Action* 7, 23209.

Krönke, F. (2004) Zoonosen bei pastoralnomadischen FulBe im Tschad. *Zeitschrift für Ethnologie* 129.

Lebel, J. (2004) Ecohealth and the developing world. *EcoHealth* 1, 325–326.

Max-Neef, M.A. (2005) Foundations of transdisciplinarity. *Ecological Economics* 53, 5–16.

Min, B., Allen-Scott, L.K. and Buntain, B. (2013) Transdisciplinary research for complex One Health issues: a scoping review of key concepts. *Preventive Veterinary Medicine* 112, 222–229.

Parkes, M.W., Bienen, L., Breilh, J., Hsu, L.N., McDonald, M., Patz, J.A., Rosenthal, J.P., Sahani, M., Sleigh, A., Waltner-Toews, D. and Yassi, A. (2005) All hands on deck: transdisciplinary approaches to emerging infectious disease. *EcoHealth* 5(2), 258–272.

Pohl, C. and Hirsch Hadorn, G. (2007) *Principles for Designing Transdisciplinary Research. Proposed by the Swiss Academies of Arts and Sciences.* Oekom Verlag, München.

Schelling, E., Wyss, K., Diguimbaye, C., Bechir, M., Ould Taleb, M., Bonfoh, B., Tanner, M. and Zinsstag, J. (2008) Towards integrated and adapted health services for nomadic pastoralists and their animals: A North-South partnership. In: Hirsch Hadorn, G., Hoffmann-Riem, H., Biber-Klemm, S., Grossenbacher, W., Joye, D., Pohl, C., Wiesmann, U. and Zemp, E. (eds) *Handbook of Transdisciplinary Research.* Springer, Heidelberg, pp. 277–291.

VWB/VSF Canada (2010) One Health for One World: A Compendium of Case Studies. Available at: https://www.vetswithoutborders.ca/images/pdfs/OHOW%20Compendium%20Case%20Studies.pdf (accessed 10 October 2014).

Wiese, M. (2004) *Health-Vulnerability in a Complex Crisis Situation - Implications for Providing Health Care to Nomadic People in Chad.* Verlag für Entwicklungspolitik, Saarbrücken GmBH.

Zinsstag, J., Bonfoh, B.C.G., Nguyen Viet, H., N'Guessan, T.S., Weibel, D., Schertenleib, R., Obrist, B. and Tanner, M. (2011a) *Towards Equity Effectiveness in Health Interventions.* NCCR North-South, Bern.

Zinsstag, J., Schelling, E., Waltner-Toews, D. and Tanner, M. (2011b) From 'one medicine' to 'one health' and systemic approaches to health and well-being. *Preventive Veterinary Medicine* 101, 148–156.

# 31 Operationalizing One Health for Local Governance

**Andrea Meisser[1,2]* and Anne Lévy Goldblum[3]**
[1]*Swiss Tropical and Public Health Institute, Basel, Switzerland;* [2]*University of Basel, Basel, Switzerland;* [3]*Health Department, Health Protection Division, Basel, Switzerland*

## Introduction

The ground-breaking achievements of the One Health concept will only become apparent when its advantages and added value have been successfully deconstructed and illustrated, starting from the (global) strategic level down to locally implementable operational projects and processes. Various examples of this are given in this book (Béchir *et al.*, Chapter 23, this volume). This chapter will detail the ways in which One Health can be introduced and implemented at the local level in an industrialized country such as Switzerland.

Knowing that we can only show an intermediate state in the course of a dynamic process and that these processes have to be tailored to each country, we are convinced that the results presented here support the use of a multiple stakeholder framework for operationalizing One Health for local governance.

The requirement of transdisciplinary collaboration, as postulated in the One Health concept (Zinsstag *et al.*, Chapter 2 and Schelling *et al.*, Chapter 30, this volume), and the suggestions to operationalize and mainstream One Health, as established by Zinsstag and colleagues (2012), fit well with the concept of local governance as defined by Bovaird and Loeffler (2002): 'the set of formal and informal rules, structures and processes which determine the ways in which individuals and organizations can exercise power over the decisions (by other stakeholders) which affect their welfare at local levels.' The *Oxford Dictionary of Geography*[1] defines local governance as: 'The institutions around local governments engaged in the design and implementation of economic and social policy: business elites, community leaders, development corporations, training and enterprise councils, and voluntary groups.'

Both definitions correspond to the requirements of public engagement (Schelling and Zinsstag, Chapter 30, this volume) and also to our experience that One Health, after a brief introduction, is recognized at all levels of the population, as it logically, coherently and directly triggers individual experiences for most people. Against this background, One Health represents a valuable instrument for good corporate governance for health at national and local levels.

This chapter begins by taking stock of the preconditions and opportunities for implementing One Health in Switzerland. It then demonstrates how proposals for further One Health action were operationalized,

*E-mail: andrea.meisser@unibas.ch

taking into account detected barriers. The next section details the process of transforming One Health at the level of two Swiss cantons. Based on this research, a final section lists the requirements for initiating One Health actions and concludes with some practical tips.

## Working out Switzerland's Readiness for One Health

By 2009, knowledge of the One Health concept in Switzerland was largely limited to a few insiders in contact with Jakob Zinsstag and the Swiss Tropical and Public Health Institute (Swiss TPH) in Basel. Information sessions at the 2009 annual meetings of the Swiss Society for Public Health and the Swiss Veterinary Association gave the idea to a wider audience. At the same time, key experts, selected from among the leading personalities in the Swiss health system, were included in a broad-based qualitative study (Meisser *et al.*, 2011). Semi-structured, face-to-face interviews evaluated the potential of a One Health approach for Switzerland, identified barriers, and developed ideas and proposals for further action. A notable side effect of these interviews was that they attracted the attention of the participants and gave them first-hand information on the One Health concept.

The potential for implementing the One Health concept in Switzerland was generally regarded as both interesting and promising. The individuals interviewed expressed their willingness to personally contribute, within their abilities, to further introducing One Health. The discussions brought to light several projects, either completed or ongoing, which were interdisciplinary in the sense of One Health, even though the term had not been explicitly used. The most important topics for future One Health projects, according to global priorities – surveillance and monitoring of infectious diseases and antimicrobial resistance – were also brought up by interviewees.

Unsuitable governmental and university structures for cross-sector cooperation were mentioned as the biggest obstacle, as was the ever-increasing specialization in various (health) professions, which leads to the development of different professional cultures and languages and a reluctance to leave the familiarity of professional silos. Limited personnel and financial resources, and the lack of relevant information and clear evidence about the added value of One Health were also cited as barriers. Fear of a possible loss of power seemed to play a significant role in rejecting new ideas. Nevertheless, most of the interviewees stated that none of these obstacles were the most important issue; rather, there was simply no common interest and no apparent reason for closer cooperation. This 'no-problem problem', as we called it later, is certainly something one should consider when implementing new concepts in economically and politically privileged countries.

Recommendations for further development of the One Health concept focused on the areas of information, communication and trust-building. Demonstrating the economic, administrative and technical advantages of cooperation for One Health, with pragmatic examples based on scientific evidence, is crucial for further implementing the concept at both national and local levels. 'The greatest opportunities would exist where there was already awareness of the problem, where the smallest additional costs or the largest savings could be expected, and where cooperation between the authorities could be strengthened and improved in a relatively uncomplicated way' (Meisser *et al.*, 2011).

## Analysing and Prioritizing

According to the experts interviewed, there was already a tradition of interdisciplinary cooperation in Switzerland, which has smoothed the path for One Health. Thus, it seemed important to neither 're-invent the wheel' nor trigger anxiety over structural changes. A further conclusion was that One Health implementation in Switzerland needed both a 'bottom up' as well as a 'top down' approach. Involving motivated members or interest groups within the community, integrating their knowledge and experience in the search for solutions, creating a social demand, and making them owners of transdisciplinary processes appeared to be as important as promoting leadership at government level. Rather than pushing forward One Health structural changes, a softer policy of 'structure follows strategy', as put forward by Chandler (1962), would facilitate collaboration and processes consistent with a One Health approach. This supports the statement that 'boundaries and interfaces matter – between people, species, systems, professions, cultures – and work at interfaces and across boundaries brings progress' (David Nabarro, UN Secretary General's Special Representative for Food Security and Nutrition, One Health Summit 2012, Davos, Switzerland, personal communication). Contrary to Lee and Brumme (2013), who complain about 'how different institutional players have interpreted One Health according to self-interests', the intention was not to avoid a restrictive definition of One Health but rather see One Health as an 'umbrella' concept (Leboeuf, 2011), a shelter under which to develop innovative ideas in the fields of human, animal and environmental health. This approach avoids some of the most commonly cited barriers such as fear of structural change or loss of power. It also overcomes the 'no-problem problem' charges by covering zoonoses as well as non-communicable diseases (e.g. depression, obesity; see also Turner, Chapter 19, this volume) or the still underestimated value of companion animals for human health (see Hediger and Beetz, Chapter 7, this volume), among other things. Analysis also considered building capacity and competence, elaborating an agenda of appropriate action (by stakeholders) and setting priorities for a customized implementation of the One Health concept in Switzerland. This led to a follow-up project focusing on the more practical aspects of implementing One Health in Switzerland. The research programme NCCR North-South (http://www.north-south.unibe.ch) and the Public Health Department of the canton of Ticino (http://www4.ti.ch/dss) sponsored the study 'One health: The potential of closer cooperation between human and animal health in Switzerland'[2] (Meisser, 2013).

## Proceeding and Spreading the Word

The level of the cantonal administration has been chosen because of its intermediate position between the federal and municipal governments. Thanks to a far-reaching autonomy in health governance at the cantonal level, new approaches can be implemented and results will be visible and assessable within a given timeframe.

As a principal outcome, the above-mentioned project initiated several transdisciplinary stakeholder processes, with representatives from different levels in the field of human and animal health. These include:

- the application of One Health to health administration in the canton of Ticino: based on interviews, discussions and stakeholder meetings, a mutual action plan was developed and a strategic document produced that will support the government in implementing One Health at the cantonal level;
- a stakeholder workshop at the Swiss Public Health Conference of 2011, which brought together representatives of the Federal Office of Public Health, the Federal Veterinary Office, universities and the public to thoroughly discuss the potential of a One Health approach for the Swiss health system;
- a joint educational meeting on One Health, a milestone in the history of both the Medical Society and the Veterinary Association of Basel, attended by more than 150 participants;
- a clear and unequivocal mandate to make use of every opportunity to promote and publicize the One Health concept: publications and presentations on the benefits and added value of the One Health concept for human, animal and ecosystem health served to spread information among stakeholders and the broader public;
- the Davos Global Risk Forum One Health Summit 2012 and 2013 (http://onehealth.grforum.org); and
- a 3-day module on One Health during the 2013 Master of Public Health programme, offered by the universities of Basel, Berne and Zurich (http://www.public-health-edu.ch), which will be held again in 2015.

The result of this project laid the foundation for Switzerland to develop ideas for incorporating One Health into policy and practice. Communication in this project was of vital importance to its success and must be continued and improved. More case studies and demonstrative examples are needed as well as more champions who advocate for One Health. The One Health concept has not yet reached a position strong enough to attract substantial funding. The same can be said for media support. It has not yet been possible to spread information about One Health via newspaper articles or television. Providing convincing evidence in the future will certainly improve this situation.

In 2013, the Swiss Federal Veterinary Office was transferred from the Federal Department of Economic Affairs to the Federal Department of Home Affairs, which has traditionally incorporated health administration. This move will facilitate cooperation between the new Federal Food Safety and Veterinary Office and the Federal Office of Public Health toward One Health. The same can be said of a recently established national working group on antimicrobial resistance. Though this development is not a direct outcome of the activities mentioned above, the project can claim some influence on the opinion leaders.

## One Health and Corporate Governance in Basel

Inspired by the preceding studies and the hypothesis that the One Health concept adds an economic and qualitative value to human, animal and environmental health services, the officials of the Health Department of the canton of Basel-Stadt (an urban canton with a population of about 200,000) expressed their interest in participating in a follow-up project. They asked the Swiss TPH to determine the status quo, to evaluate its suitability for One Health and to advise on developing appropriate proposals for implementation. Compared to other cantons and cities, Basel is relatively well positioned for transdisciplinary and intersectoral cooperation, both in terms of organizational structure as well as workflow and governance. Nevertheless, the level of exchange between those responsible for human and animal health can be deepened; and even if environmental issues are already included in solution searches and decision making, optimization seems possible. Having learned from the Ticino project that a clear 'order from above' can be very helpful, a detailed offer was forwarded to the Health Minister of Basel and signed after consultation. A project leader from within the health administration was appointed, steering group members from both the department of health and the department of environment were chosen and important project milestones were mutually fixed (e.g. dates of stakeholder and steering group meetings).

The targeted outcome was jointly defined as added value to the health of people and animals in Basel, ideally supplemented by resource savings through the use of synergies. The primary focus of the first phase was on information, communication, awareness-raising and weighting functional processes. The existing capacities, competencies, processes, networks, communication channels, etc. should be used, optimized and enhanced. The project sought to answer the following questions.

**1.** What are the existing competencies and responsibilities for human, animal and environmental health in Basel?
**2.** What examples of cooperation, in the sense of One Health, exist in Basel?
**3.** Have any projects and studies been conducted in this area so far?
**4.** What are the possible barriers to successfully implementing One Health in Basel?
**5.** What are the inner and outer system boundaries for One Health in Basel?
**6.** Which sectors, organizations and institutions are best suited for cooperating for One Health? Have attempts towards a corresponding project structure already been made?
**7.** Which issues will be addressed and with what level of priority (e.g. zoonoses, animals as an early warning system for human diseases, health aspects of the human–animal relationship, environmental health effects)?

The specified objectives were:

- Knowledge development (capacity building): by the end of 2012, the key players

in all relevant animal health, human health and environmental bodies know the One Health concept and its basic message.
- The formation of a One Health network: the project clarifies which internal and external partners appear to be suitable and available for participating in an (initially) informal One Health network.
- Concrete examples: the project evaluates and prioritizes suitable projects for introducing and implementing the One Health approach, together with stakeholders. It also evaluates and describes completed and ongoing projects.
- Cancer registration: a thesis on the expected benefits and the feasibility of a joint cancer registry for people and animals forms an integral part of this project.
- Defining barriers: obstacles that affect implementation of the One Health concept are evaluated and presented.
- Action plan: the results developed within the project are documented in a final strategic document, a recommended action plan outlining the next steps.

In order to achieve these objectives, the approach focused on holding information events (stakeholder workshops) and on conducting semi-structured individual interviews with key persons as identified by the project management. The aim of the interviews was to make stakeholders aware of their own role within the project, describe the actual state of their work, express ideas and suggestions and define a desired state. Opportunities and the potential to create added value, as well as risks, issues, boundaries or barriers were recorded. The interviews were executed and evaluated by external experts, according to the criteria of qualitative research. A key element of the approach was to build on existing strengths rather than launch new projects. This required enhancing the awareness of many ongoing projects that were already in line with the One Health philosophy, and could be carried out more effectively and successfully in cooperation with stakeholders from other administrative units.

The feasibility analysis of a joint cancer registry for people and animals in the cantons of Basel-Stadt and Basel-Land was developed in a dissertation complementary and closely related to this project.

For the duration of the project, close contact between the project management, steering group, external consultant and researchers (Swiss TPH) was maintained. In addition, contact was established with representatives from the Health Department of the canton of Ticino to exchange experiences made to date.

A first stakeholder meeting served to inform participating stakeholders of the history and philosophy of the One Health concept, to highlight some recent examples and to present the planned project. Invitees included general secretaries of the Ministry of Health and the Ministry of Economic, Social and Environmental Affairs; the heads of the division for health care, health services and health protection, and the leaders of their respective departments, as well as the Environmental Protection and Energy Agent, the head of the Office for Air Hygiene of the Basel area, the head of municipal horticulture and the Chief Agricultural Officer. This list also represents the expert interviewees who were engaged following the kick-off meeting. As in the first set of interviews at the national level, these personal encounters and dialogues not only offered a large amount of data and ideas, they also made stakeholders owners of the process. Further information meetings and mailings were intended to keep the interest of the participants. Qualitative research tools (e.g. template analysis) were used to analyse the data and to elaborate the relevant fields of action.

## Results

Four areas for further activity were identified, namely: 'Dogs and Mobility', 'City and Nature', 'Health and Competence' and 'Surveillance and Research' (Fig. 31.1). Each of them was accompanied by a brief description, and related ideas, listed initially without further

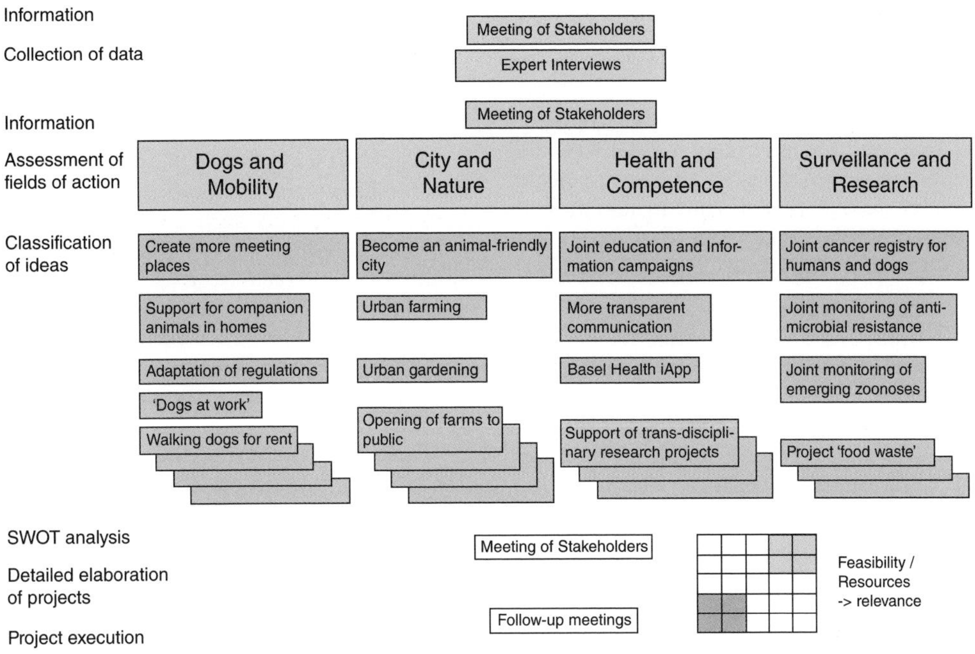


**Fig. 31.1.** The process of developing and evaluating projects in Basel.

rating. In order to provide a deeper insight into the fascinating range of options given, they are presented here.

### *Dogs and Mobility*

Outdoor exercise is healthy – for both humans and animals. Physical activity is, whether individually or collectively, an important measure in the fight against the modern epidemics of obesity and depression. Dog walking facilitates social contacts and increases health, security, and quality of life – for both.

Ideas on Dogs and Mobility include:

- Create public spaces to facilitate mobility and social interaction.
- Reduce density of regulations where applicable.
- Encourage permissibility of pets in retirement facilities.
- Help organize and foster participation in special dog-keeping courses for seniors.
- Ease restrictions against pets in the workplace.
- Consider also: 'a free dog for elderly (over 70)', 'Pet services', 'Walking dog rental'.

### *City and Nature*

More and more people enjoy living in urban environments. Nevertheless, many long for nature and authenticity. Recreation facilities, from their own little windowsill garden and the farm close to the city, to nature and wildlife parks and intact rivers, build an important part of the quality of life and health.

Ideas on City and Nature include:

- Make nature more tangible.
- Support personal contact with nature (e.g. garden, animal husbandry, 'Urban Farming').
- Become an animal-friendly city.
- Open city-owned farms to the public.
- Create worlds of human–animal–environment experience ('edutainment').
- Consider also: 'Cat Café'.

*Health and Competence*

Health is closely linked to health literacy, and therefore also to education and research. Relations and dependencies among humans, animals and the environment offer new and attractive approaches to addressing health issues – for science, government, and the general population.

Ideas on Health and Competence include:

- 'Basel Health iApp'.
- Transparent and user-friendly information (e.g. food safety, quality of drinking water, cleanliness of air).
- Support joint campaigns by doctors and veterinarians on e.g. parasites, zoonoses, antimicrobial resistance.
- Provide professional, technical and economic support for practical transdisciplinary research projects.
- Sharing of information channels and know-how.

*Surveillance and Research*

One of the core competencies of the health and environment authorities lies in monitoring health hazards for humans, animals and the environment. Great expertise and an arsenal of sophisticated equipment for detecting, preventing and treating hazards are available. Numerous synergies among the various sectors offer interesting options for surveillance and research, particularly in the area of early detection and warning.

Ideas on Surveillance and Research include:

- Medical thesis on a joint human and animal cancer registry.
- Inclusion of (companion) animals in detecting problems caused by e.g. air pollutants or non-ionizing radiation.
- Joint monitoring of antimicrobial resistance.
- Professional, technical and economic support for practical transdisciplinary research projects.
- Plan a project on sustainable management of food waste.

In a subsequent stakeholder meeting, this collection of thoughts, ideas and project proposals was analysed and rated by the participants in order to prioritize potential projects according to expected value added, political relevance, resource availability and feasibility.

Emphasis was given to the areas of 'Dogs and Mobility' and 'Surveillance and Research'. For projects such as 'create public open space for dog owners to facilitate mobility and social interaction' or 'joint monitoring of antimicrobial resistance', detailed project sheets were established and included a definition of the targeted outcomes, a scheduled action plan and the nomination of internal and external stakeholders.

Facilitating dog ownership in Basel as a One Health contribution to mobilizing (elderly) people and to facilitating social contacts (Wood *et al.*, 2009), keeping animal welfare in mind, is part of the newly established policy. As a first step, this project has created the public space 'Horburgpark', in close cooperation with interested stakeholders. More areas will be evaluated for their suitability for dogs' use of public space. The dog bathing or swimming zone on the Rhine river serves as a pilot experiment in this context. Based on observations made in summer 2013, a round table with all relevant stakeholders was held to discuss the results and any amendments required.

For the first time in Switzerland, One Health was the main subject of a public departmental annual report (Fig. 31.2). The Health Protection Division of the Department of Public Health of the canton of Basel published its annual report 2012 (Bereich Gesundheitsschutz Basel-Stadt, 2013) with the title, 'One Health – one health for all'.

*Joint cancer registration*

The project included a study on the feasibility of introducing a joint registration of cancer cases in humans and dogs, combined with a geographic information system in the Basel area. The underlying idea is that dogs and humans share the same environment and lifestyle, thus, given that dogs develop cancer faster than humans due to their shorter lifespan, perhaps they can be used as an 'early warning system' for human exposure

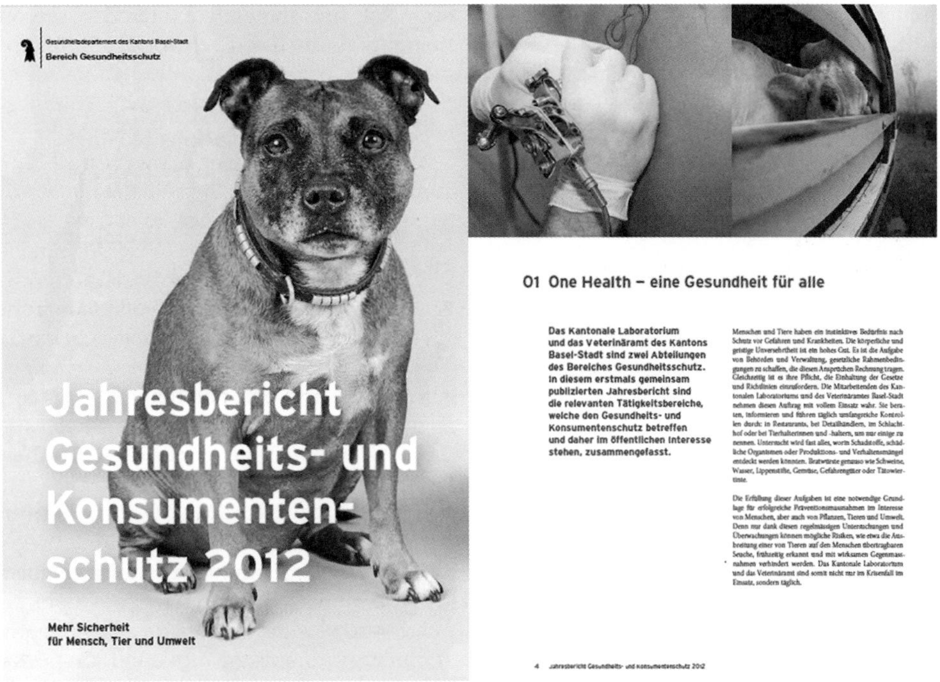
Bereich Gesundheitsschutz
Jahresbericht Gesundheits- und Konsumentenschutz 2012
Mehr Sicherheit für Mensch, Tier und Umwelt
01 One Health – eine Gesundheit für alle
Das Kantonale Laboratorium und das Veterinäramt des Kantons Basel-Stadt sind zwei Abteilungen des Bereiches Gesundheitsschutz. In diesem erstmals gemeinsam publizierten Jahresbericht sind die relevanten Tätigkeitsbereiche, welche den Gesundheits- und Konsumentenschutz betreffen und daher im öffentlichen Interesse stehen, zusammengefasst.

**Fig. 31.2** One Health as a main issue of Basel's Health Protection Division's annual report, 2012.

to cancer risks. The medical thesis, as yet unpublished (Tekombo, 2014), concentrated on the legal requirements (e.g. data protection) and the willingness of dog owners and veterinary practitioners to participate. As expected, the Basel region or also relatively small countries such as Switzerland do not produce enough analysable cancer cases in animals for a prospective evaluation within an acceptable timeframe. Nevertheless, the willingness of dog owners and veterinary practitioners to participate, as well as the formation of a broad network of interested stakeholders, was a positive signal to further develop the project. In fact, the Geographic Information Visualization and Analysis group at the University of Zurich opened a PhD position, 'One Medicine – One Oncology', to 'systematically investigate the spatial patterns of tumor incidences in cats and dogs in Switzerland (1955-2008) by means of geovisual analytics, coupled with exploratory and inferential geostatistics, keeping the comparison with human tumor incidence in mind' (http://www.geo.uzh.ch/giva).

The recent opening of a therapeutic zoo at the REHAB Basel centre for paraplegia and craniocerebral injury trauma patients (http://www.rehab.ch) is another very interesting contribution within the broader framework of this project. The outcomes of the intense human–animal interaction on both human patients and therapy animals will be evaluated scientifically.

## Conclusions

'A journey of a thousand miles begins with a single step'. According to the wise words of Lao-tzu, the journey of One Health in Switzerland has just begun; thanks to these projects and thanks to the activities of a handful of committed pioneers the first step was taken. The objective of engaging and motivating Swiss opinion leaders and stakeholders in the One Health concept was clearly achieved, as were the preparation of policy recommendations for the canton of Ticino and the development of a One Health framework and some promising projects with the canton of Basel-Stadt. These tools can – with the necessary adaptations – also serve as an example for other cantons, the federation and other interested countries. However, the length of time needed to implement low-priority processes was considerably underestimated. So the goal of generating evidence showing the added value of One Health for Switzerland must be referred to as 'under construction'.

The most important criteria for success were: (i) taking account of barriers; (ii) finding committed leaders and stakeholders; (iii) building on existing projects rather than trying to invent explicit One Health initiatives; and (iv) entrusting a competent and credible mediator with the task. In contrast to Dockrell (2012), who sees a 'danger that individual research innovation may suffer at the expense of harmonised multicentre studies', in One Health approaches, our experience argues for further opening the professional silos, not only in research, but also in government administrations. Bringing physicians and veterinarians together in a joint educational meeting was one of the most productive and best events in the course of these projects and is strongly recommended. Further recommendations are listed below (Fig. 31.3).

## Recommendations to Start a Transdisciplinary Process

Practical steps for implementing the One Health concept include:

- Start with the experience of communities and countries and use approaches that have worked elsewhere.
- Consider the situation in your country at a national and local level to determine how best to implement a One Health approach.
- Create a social demand for One Health.
- Use One Health as a shelter under which to develop innovative and creative ideas in relative safety; create an innovation platform and stimulate creative energy in a competitive yet supportive environment.
- Develop a cross-cultural perspective and adapt your actions appropriately to different levels.

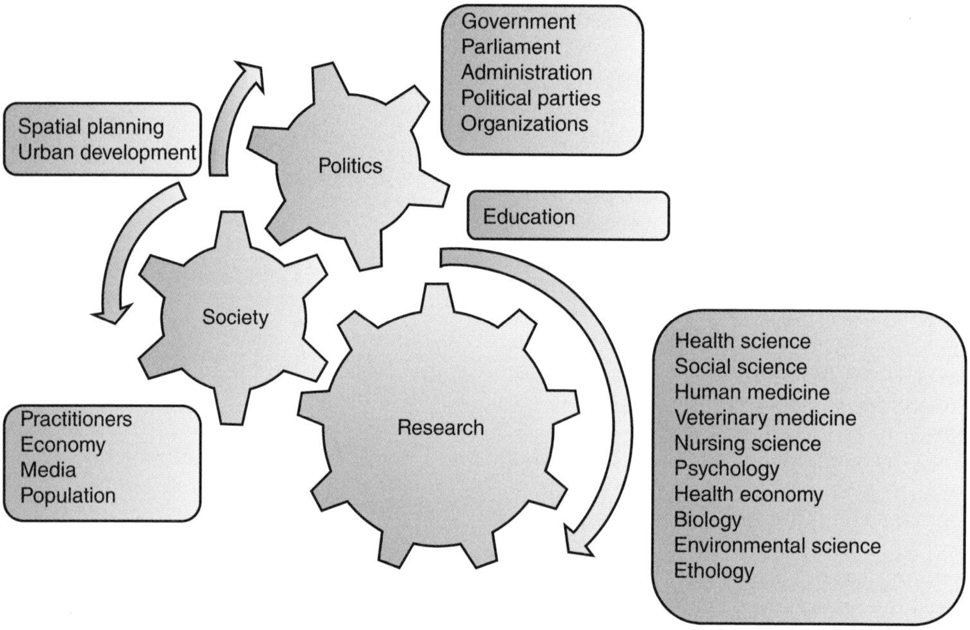


**Fig. 31.3.** The framework and interfaces of One Health stakeholders.

- Evaluate appropriate interfaces for co-operation.
- Consider the importance of coordination of and leadership in transdisciplinary processes.

The flow of a stakeholder process is as follows:

**1.** Look for an official mandate.
**2.** Nominate a project leader and members of a steering group.
**3.** Find all relevant and committed stakeholders and make them owners of the process.
**4.** Inform.
**5.** Mutually create and adopt a project description (background, targeted outcomes, objectives, approach to achievement, road map, milestones).
**6.** Evaluate existing structures, processes, interfaces and boundaries.
**7.** Collect data (e.g. interviews with stakeholders).
**8.** Inform.
**9.** Transform ideas into fields of activity.
**10.** Analyse and prioritize with stakeholders.
**11.** Inform.
**12.** Elaborate action plan and detailed project sheets (performed by project owners).
**13.** Implement projects.
**14.** Inform and communicate, organize follow-up meetings.
**15.** Supervise and advise when asked to do so.

## Urgently Needed: 'Transmitters'

The specific skills and core competencies of all professionals from various disciplines and specialities must be optimally used in composite transdisciplinary teams to achieve added value for health. Enhanced system-thinking and the willingness to temporarily leave the protective walls of one's own discipline can only be achieved through ensuring open information, adequate resources and training. In a recent workshop, led by Allen-Scott (Allen-Scott *et al.*, 2015), specific skills were evaluated (see also Nguyen-Viet *et al.*, Chapter 27, this volume). At the workshop, the term 'transmitter' of the One Health concept was coined. A 'transmitter' is a mediator or intermediary, who has the education and experience needed to successfully perform in the different scientific, political and professional rooms that form the One Health building. Such a person is ideally a generalist, who has a professional background in health or social science, is politically sensitive, has knowledge of processes and regulations, and possesses management and communication skills. Other requirements are:

- knowing and understanding the profession-specific cultures and languages (inter-professional communication);
- understanding different roles and functions of different disciplines and sectors of the human–animal–environment health system;
- being able to integrate the various competences of public health, animal health and ecology in a systemic approach;
- readiness for continuous quality assurance and improvement of work processes and results; knowledge of different problem-solving strategies in various jobs and functions;
- experience in putting together and leading transdisciplinary teams;
- ability to manage conflicts between team members from different disciplines, sectors and hierarchical levels (inter-professional conflict resolution);
- experience in giving information to the stakeholders and the general population at the appropriate level (capacity development); and
- willingness to integrate knowledge and experience from the population in the search for solutions; building trust and creating awareness for a One Health approach.

## Acknowledgement

The authors would like to thank Amena Briet for valuable assistance with language editing. This work was co-funded by the National Centre for Competence in Research North-South (NCCR North-South).

## Notes

[1] Local governance: A Dictionary of Geography. Available at: Answers.com website (accessed 26 August 2013).
[2] Partnership Actions (PAMS) Swiss Alps # ALP-03_01, NCCR North–South.

## References


Allen-Scott, L.K., Buntain, B.J., Hatfield, J.M., Meisser, A. and Thomas, C.J. (2015) Academic institutions and One Health: building capacity for transdisciplinary research approaches to address complex health issues at the animal-human-ecosystem interface. *Academic Medicine* (in press).

Bereich Gesundheitsschutz Basel-Stadt (2013) *Jahresbericht Gesundheits- und Konsumentenschutz 2012/ Mehr Sicherheit für Mensch, Tier und Umwelt.*

Bovaird, T. and Loeffler, E. (2002) Moving from excellence models of local service delivery to benchmarking 'good local governance'. *International Review of Administrative Sciences* 68, 9–24.

Chandler Jr, A.D. (1962) *Strategy and Structure: chapters in the history of the industrial enterprise.* MIT Press, Cambridge, Massachusetts.

Dockrell, H.M. (2012) One Health - 'joining the dots'. *Onderstepoort Journal of Veterinary Research* 79(2). doi: 10.4102/ojvr.v79i2.458.

Leboeuf, A. (2011) *Making Sense of One Health - Cooperating at the Human-Animal-Ecosystem Health Interface.* IFRI, Paris.

Lee, K. and Brumme, Z.L. (2013) Operationalizing the One Health approach: the global governance challenges. *Health Policy and Planning* 28(7), 778–785.

Meisser, A. (2013) Implementing One Health in Switzerland. *NCCR North-South Newsletter* 11, 5–6.

Meisser, A., Schelling, E. and Zinsstag, J. (2011) One health in Switzerland: a visionary concept at a crossroads? *Swiss Medical Weekly* 141, w13201.

Tekombo, J.G. (2014). Krebsregister für Mensch und Tier in den Kantonen Basel Stadt/Basel Land und ihre Rahmenbedingungen. MD thesis, Swiss Tropical and Public Health Institute, University of Basel, Switzerland (in press).

Wood, L., Shardlow, T., Willis, S., University of Western Australia, School of Population Health and Petcare Information and Advisory Service (2009) *Living Well Together: how companion animals can help strengthen social fabric.* Petcare Information & Advisory Service, Camberwell, Victoria.

Zinsstag, J., Mackenzie, J.S., Jeggo, M., Heymann, D.L., Patz, J.A. and Daszak, P. (2012) Mainstreaming One Health. *EcoHealth* 9(2), 107–110.

# 32 Non-governmental Organizations in One Health

**Craig Stephen[1]* and David Waltner-Toews[2]**
[1]*Canadian Wildlife Health Cooperative and Faculty of Veterinary Medicine, University of Saskatchewan, Canada and School of Population and Public Health, University of British Columbia, Canada;* [2]*Professor Emeritus, Department of Population Medicine, University of Guelph, Canada and Founding President, Veterinarians without Borders/Vétérinaires sans Frontières – Canada*

## Introduction

The roles of non-governmental organizations (NGOs) in creating and delivering alternatives to mainstream international development programmes have been described and analysed in some detail (Bebbington and Farrington, 1993; World Bank, 1998; Bebbington *et al.*, 2008). Their ability to facilitate and test alternative, complex and systemic approaches to improving multiple outcomes in human, animal and ecosystem health has been less studied. In the context of testing alternatives to mainstream approaches, a 2010 World Bank report outlined some of the challenges for government departments, each with their own defined mandates, to facilitate the kind of cross-sectoral collaboration required to implement a One Health approach (World Bank, 2010). The ability to try out new, adaptive ways of thinking and collaboration such as those required by a One Health[1] approach is particularly important in a world that is experiencing unprecedented socio-economic and environmental change.

It is no surprise, then, that NGOs play important roles in the current emergence of One Health as a guide to how to address, in an integrated fashion, issues such as health, poverty, development and environmental change. The term 'non-governmental organization' is widely used and applies to a variety of organizations ranging from community non-profit volunteer groups to social movement groups to international technical assistance organizations and donor agencies. The diversity of groups and institutions that fall under the classification of an NGO can make it difficult to make universally applicable statements about the role for NGOs in One Health. Typologies of NGOs vary but in general they fall into five types: (i) top-down organizations that give aid to those in need; (ii) service providers that fill gaps in capacity; (iii) NGOs that enable and empower other groups for self-help; (iv) advocacy groups; and (vi) donor agencies. For this chapter, we will refer to NGOs as organizations that are independent of government, are not trying to seek government office and are not focused on making a profit. They usually are a formal group of like-minded individuals who operate collectively somewhere between a local entity (e.g. a community, a landscape, a species)

*E-mail: cstephen@cwhc-rcsf.ca

and government. They work towards a common purpose that has a wider social or environmental benefit than the needs of the NGO itself.

One Health activities and programmes should be focused on the reciprocal, interrelated care of human, animal and environmental health. At its heart is the need to cross and link boundaries – species boundaries, disciplinary boundaries and boundaries of authority and responsibility. NGOs have some unique strengths and weaknesses that affect their capacity to link the various values, capacities and needs at the human animal environment interface.

## Strengths

NGOs are often founded by passionate people committed to effecting change. Governments can be distracted by emerging risks and issues, and communities can be preoccupied with the needs of daily living. But NGOs have the human capacity, with the will and desire to stay focused on an issue and to gather interest, resources and capacity to keep pushing towards an end goal. This allows them to be the passionate lightning rod around which personnel, activities and investments can be consistently applied over time and to which others can be attracted to work on a shared problem. This can have significant value in bringing alternative perspectives to One Health programmes. For example, when people call for culls of non-charismatic wildlife species (e.g. rats or bats) to reduce immediate risks of human contact with wildlife pathogens, an NGO might consider the roles of those species in long-term ecological sustainability and advocate for their conservation as part of a more integrated approach. An NGO might also champion responses to neglected diseases that are not priorities for international agencies or governments.

Because they are external to governments, NGOs are not tied by legislative or jurisdictional limitations, apart from being bound by the laws of the land. This frees them to cross boundaries and serves as a mechanism to share people, ideas and resources. The vertical management structure of many government and academic departments tends to restrict the capacity or interest of department members to work within their specific authority or responsibilities. Being outside of any specific department allows NGOs to escape the need to defend a particular perspective or discipline and thus avoid the power struggles that can arise when cross-sectoral collaborations come up against differences in the interest or authority of actors trying to collaborate.

NGOs lack the authority or direct ability to make political change or directly change government policy. As such, they are less of a threat to people who aim to protect their interests. NGOs, therefore, can facilitate cross-sectoral dialogue by bringing interests and providing a neutral venue where multiple interests can be heard. This can allow the voices of interests that are often not represented in decision processes to be heard. NGOs often engage local communities, the disenfranchised and those that may not have a voice – including non-human stakeholders, such as a landscape or a species. NGOs can be an important vehicle to establish and support integrated scholarly and community knowledge systems, as well as bridging knowledge generation and effective action, which is central to the practice of One Health and related fields (Max-Neef, 2005; Schelling *et al.*, Chapter 20, this volume).

NGOs tend to be positioned somewhere between local communities and central governments, as well as between organizations whose responsibility is the public interest and, often by virtue of private funding, those whose primary mandate is corporate profit. This position, plus their frequent emphasis on inclusive and participatory processes, provides several advantages. It helps provide contextual understanding necessary to implement actions, it builds partnerships that strengthen linkages across scales and interests and, perhaps most importantly, it builds trust and credibility amongst groups that may not be natural allies. By understanding local needs and being dedicated to effecting local change, NGOs help develop trust between communities and themselves. NGOs that are effective at changing government policy need to work equally hard to demonstrate that they are competent agents of positive changes that are in the nation's best interest and thus trustworthy to government. Trusting relationships are critical for effective NGOs in One Health and are critical for effective cross-sectoral collaborations (Anholt *et al.*, 2012).

NGOs have additional strengths. Although there are some large NGOs such as World Vision and Oxfam, most NGOs tend to be relatively small. They lack the sometimes cumbersome management structure of government agencies and universities. They tend to have a short administrative span from the field project to the organization's decision makers. This provides NGOs with flexibility and capacity to respond quickly to emerging social and environmental pressures and change. Their independence from governments gives them freedom to speak on controversial subjects, advocate for unpopular positions and ensure the disempowered are heard. They work outside of political timelines and cycles, allowing for the long-term investment often necessary to affect social and ecological change. Finally, NGOs are action oriented. While many academic and government departments talk about One Health and fostering reciprocal care of people, animals and our shared environment, NGOs tend to be the actors on the ground trying to make it happen.

## Limitations

The limitations of NGOs are reflections of their strength. Being removed from government provides autonomy but also weakens capacity to influence policy directly. The bottom-up approach builds local trust and effects local change but it can exclude key central decision makers, thus limiting the scale of impacts. This is further weakened by budget and capacity constraints of many NGOs. Passionate commitment to a cause can provide a type of tunnel vision that restricts the ability of the NGO to see its role in a holistic context and thus can distract attention and resources away from other pressing issues. The dogged commitment to a cause or perspective can serve as a form of intellectual imperialism wherein the NGO risks imposing its values and perspectives on to others.

NGOs are dependent on external funds. Although they may work outside the timelines and priorities of central governments, they are often bound to the funding cycles and priorities of both the governments and private donors. For example, as One Health was practised in the early 21st century, donors emphasized actions to prepare for pandemic diseases. A decade later, some emphasis had shifted to endemic zoonoses and livestock diseases that threatened food security, but major gaps remained. Little One Health work was done on pollution or climate change. The vast majority was anthropocentric – with human outcomes having primacy over the health of animals or the environment. While these priorities may not reflect an ethos of reciprocal care of human, animal and environmental health within social-ecological systems, they were the reality of much NGO One Health work due to the priorities of donors, who often face administrative or academic impediments to addressing the uncertainty associated with complex systems' interactions. In the absence of large-scale donations without prescribed expected outcomes, the capacity of NGOs to act is affected by the shifting priorities of donor agencies and individuals. Moreover, because most NGOs are comparatively small, their impacts are further limited in scale – both spatial and temporal. Limited scales and lack of autonomy on selecting priorities risks NGOs' ability to invest most strategically and most longitudinally.

## Examples of Non-governmental Organizations in One Health

Although the larger vision of One Health has been broadly accepted by many institutions around the world, defining the vision into operational terms has been a challenge. In this book, we have focused on the 'added value of a closer cooperation of human and animal health and other sectors' (Zinsstag *et al.*, 2011). The historical variations in origins and definitions for programmes implementing a One Health approach makes it hard to assess, in historical terms, what specifically falls in or out of the classification for a One Health NGO. However, even given their limitations, it is clear that NGOs can play a critical role in linking, bridging and partnering diverse interests that emerge when examining issues that cross species and disciplinary boundaries.

In this section, we present a series of case studies to illustrate some of the core features of NGOs relevant to One Health (see also Box 32.1). While the value added is not quantified, what emerges is an understanding that optimizing human, animal and ecosystem health involves sets of interactions, trade-offs and balances within a larger social-ecological system. By the very nature of their temporal-spatial scope and complexity, these interactions cannot be understood or managed within any given sector. In this case, the value added of One Health is the ability to develop programmes that not only improve health in a given species or sector, but do so while contributing to the broader goals of what has been called sustainable development.

While many examples are possible, we have selected cases from our own professional

**Box 32.1.** Two case studies on NGOs and One Health (Waltner-Toews, 2010).

**National Zoonoses and Food Hygiene Research Centre: urban echinococcosis**

In the 1990s, after reports of a 20% case-fatality rate of patients undergoing surgery with hydatid disease in Nepal, an intensive research and community development project was initiated in Kathmandu, Nepal. In the 1980s, various independent research and development activities targeted at improving slaughtering practices and investigating the disease dynamics generated a wealth of information with sometimes conflicting implications, such as the realization that dogs served as community police as well as sources of disease, and livestock generated both solid waste and economic wealth. Given these complexities, no changes occurred until representatives of Kathmandu City (KMC), Department of Drinking Water Supply Corporation (DDWSC), Ward Committees and chairs, Local Clubs, Ward Clinics, Schools, a couple of other local NGOs (Lumanthi and ENAPHC), and representatives of butchers, street sweepers, street vendors, hotel owners, business owners and squatters were mobilized into an integrated One Health approach. With facilitation by two Nepalese NGOs – the National Zoonoses and Food Hygiene Research Centre, and Social Action for Grassroots Unity and Networking – and the University of Guelph, community-led transformation included changing slaughter facilities and practices, improved environmental hygiene, increased public awareness and better management of street dogs. The economic and social benefits extended well beyond the cost of the disease itself.

**Centre for Coastal Health: neotropical cryptococcosis in British Columbia, Canada**

In 2001, a porpoise was diagnosed with *Cryptococcus gattii* using samples submitted to the provincial animal health laboratory from an autopsy conducted by the Centre for Coastal Health (CCH). The diagnosis was unusual in a wild marine mammal. In consultation with the head of the provincial diagnostic laboratory, it was found that private laboratories were reporting an increased number of cases of this disease in dogs and cats. The CCH investigator shared these observations with the local medical health officer who also reported that they were detecting an unusual number of cases in people. Taken in isolation, the case in the porpoise, the increased cases in pets and in humans were not sufficient to cause alarm. However, comparison of the distribution of cases indicated a disease cluster in the same region of Vancouver Island and signalled an outbreak. A collaborative investigation of the CCH veterinarians, BC Animal Health Centre, BC Centre for Disease Control, UBC School of Occupational and Environmental Health and Vancouver Island Health Region quickly revealed this to be a tropical strain of *Cryptococcus* that was never before reported in Canada.

The capacity to quickly mount an investigation that combined medical, veterinary, diagnostic, public health and environmental microbiology expertise resulted from a pre-existing professional social network, which was facilitated by a research network housed at the CCH with the mandate to link human, animal and environmental health. The history of past collaborations among the participants in these investigations created trusting relations between the investigators from both private and public sectors and allowed for sharing of information and more effective decision making. In the absence of these collaborations, the origins, mechanisms of spread, public communications and disease management could not have occurred as quickly, accurately or effectively if each group had worked independently.

experiences, and which may be typical of the field more generally. The following vignettes are not exhaustive descriptions or evaluations of each NGO, but we emphasize one particular aspect of the case to highlight how NGOs are suited to addressing One Health issues. We have listed the websites for these NGOs so that readers may investigate them in more depth.

## Centre for Coastal Health

The Centre for Coastal Health (CCH)[2] is an example of an action-oriented organization that addressed One Health needs through services and problem-based applied research. The Centre was founded in the mid-1990s in Canada, well before the idea of One Health was popularized. Its mandate is to work across sectors to help people make decisions on health issues at the human–animal–environment interface. Its activities span subjects as diverse as human impacts on wildlife conservation, food security and poverty effects of animal health management, environmental impacts of animal movements, using environmental clues to detect emerging risks and developing integrated strategies for zoonotic disease control. Common to its diverse range of subject matter is an ethic of problem solving with the goal of maximizing the shared health benefits and minimizing the risks of human–animal–environment interactions.

The CCH is structured somewhat like a veterinary practice. Clients (often governments) come to the CCH with a problem that requires assessment and management. The CCH can be considered a group of 'specialized generalists', with the core staff being skilled in synthesizing and mobilizing information. The CCH draws on partners and subcontractors to access the disciplinary knowledge required for each problem. The flexibility in this organizational structure plus a focus not on a specific region, pathogen or species but rather on a shared vision of reciprocal care of human, animals and environmental health provides the CCH with adaptability and capacity to address the various problems presented. It matches this content flexibility with administrative flexibility that allows for rapid response to urgent requests for assistance – requests that often cannot be accommodated with the sometimes slow approval processes of universities.

The 'practice' model of the CCH provides the Centre with a level of legitimacy and trust not always bestowed upon researchers or regulators. The CCH serves the needs of its clients and produces products useful to them as opposed to the common practice of a researcher coming to a stakeholder, extracting information from them and garnering credit for products of most value to the researcher such as scientific papers. This gives the CCH relevancy, credibility and utility to knowledge users. Because the CCH does not advocate for anything other than its shared visions, it is respected for its objectivity and thus is used and trusted by actors from various perspectives. The CCH approach to One Health which emphasizes specialized generalists dedicated to knowledge-to-action could not be implemented within academic or government circles because of the vertical organization and emphasis on specialization. The founders of the CCH needed an NGO structure to meet its goals and address its vision.

The CCH can respond quickly to new circumstances and can experiment with innovative approaches. By the cross-sectoral nature of its activities, the CCH is well placed to identify, express and communicate views of one sector that might otherwise not be heard by other sectors.

## Canadian Wildlife Health Cooperative

The purpose of the Canadian Wildlife Health Cooperative (CWHC)[3] is to apply the veterinary medical sciences to wildlife conservation and management in Canada. The CWHC exemplifies the ability of an NGO to bridge jurisdictions and help coordinate the activities and resources of different organizations towards a common goal. In Canada, issues related to wildlife fall either under provincial or federal jurisdiction, depending on the species and on the location of the wildlife habitat. Some wildlife are represented in the public sphere by advocacy or conservation groups (e.g. hunting or fishing organizations) while other species are largely ignored or even reviled by the public (e.g. bats). The CWHC, dedicated to developing and using knowledge of wildlife health and disease to improve human health and the health of domestic animals, was established in recognition of the need to have a third-party organization that could bridge the diverse regulatory frameworks and interests affecting wildlife health across Canada.

The recognition of a need for such an organization was heightened when Canada needed to establish national programmes for surveillance for emerging diseases of concern for humans (e.g. avian influenza and West Nile fever) and for wildlife (e.g. chronic wasting disease in ungulates and white-nosed syndrome in bats). The CWHC represents no specific regulatory authority or jurisdiction and thus has licence to link, coordinate and integrate data from across provinces and species. The CWHC plays a key role in developing effective working partnerships, an essential characteristic of effective multi-disciplinary teams (Stephen and Daibes, 2010).

The CWHC is a consortium of wildlife health researchers, diagnosticians encompassing Canada's veterinary colleges and partners in the NGO sector and external diagnostic labs. Its non-profit status is derived from its position within the university system, but it acts as a semi-autonomous organization that must navigate the challenges and advantages of working with several university administrative structures. A major strength of the organization is its position outside of legislative structures and hence not being committed to defend any particular policy or government. Over its more than 22 years of existence, it has come to serve as a neutral location where parties from various federal and provincial agencies, the private sector and other NGOs and universities could act collectively. This facilitated collaborative funding of surveillance and investigation efforts, leading the World Organisation for Animal Health (OIE) to recognize the CWHC as a Collaborating Centre dedicated to wildlife disease surveillance and monitoring, epidemiology and management.

## Veterinarians Without Borders/Vétérinaires Sans Frontières

A member of the global umbrella group VSF-International (formerly VSF-Europa), Veterinarians Without Borders/Vétérinaires Sans Frontières (VWB/VSF)[4] in Canada was established 'to work for, and with, communities in need to foster the health of animals, people and the environments that sustain us'. This organization illustrates the value of a community-based approach when addressing One Health issues. The community-first participatory approach of VWB/VSF provides two critical benefits. First, it facilitates tangible and timely change. Major shifts in policy, in national approaches to problems or other macro-impacts can be slow in trickling down to individuals and families. A community-first approach may not provide for a breadth of impact, but the depth of impact can be much greater within the partner communities. For example, while there may be a need to reform a nation's biosecurity strategy for the prevention of avian influenza, working with farm families to improve poultry health and sanitation can provide tangible and immediate benefits for the families as well as start to address biosecurity needs. The second major benefit is that it is at the community level where diverse interests can most easily be brought together, heard and negotiated to find locally relevant and acceptable actions.

Advocating with and on behalf of communities to improve their health and well-being and build capacity for undertaking actions to improve health and strengthen community assets is a core competency for health promotion (Barry *et al.*, 2009). These competencies are critical to ensuring research and plans are mobilized into action. VWB/VSF's approach increases the likelihood that actions or plans are adopted and implemented because they are locally identified, created and owned.

Although community focused, VWB/VSF recognizes that community is not the same as 'village'. A community can be defined as an interacting set of individuals with a common interest in a shared location or a group bound by a common policy. Therefore, community-based approaches are inclusive of individuals, households, local government, civil society, private enterprises and central governments. A VWB/VSF-supported project in Sri Lanka exemplifies how this conception of community is required to ensure both depth and breadth to programme impacts. In 2005, the government of Sri Lanka wished to improve its capacity and preparedness for emerging infectious diseases. VWB/VSF volunteers began and enabled a process wherein the capacity of farmers to detect and manage on-farm health problems was enhanced, along with the capacities of academia to train people who could work in a cross-sectoral fashion in the area of One Health and of government to collect and assess signals of risk and adopt new policy approaches. A key factor enabling success in this project was the role of the NGO in assembling and maintaining a community of practice across various sectors that remained focused on their shared goals, while organizations responsible for each sector received benefits from collaboration for their individual goals.

### National Zoonoses and Food Hygiene Research Centre

The National Zoonoses and Food Hygiene Research Centre (NZFHRC)[5] was founded in the early 1990s in Kathmandu, Nepal. Its mission is to generate information on pervasive zoonoses that impact Nepalese citizens and to offer training and policy advocacy to mitigate or prevent zoonotic disease impacts. The NZFHRC illustrates the role of NGOs to fill gaps in capacity. Nepal is one of the world's poorest countries. Instability in its government over the past 30 years has exacerbated the deficit in capacity to organize applied research and action in many spheres of public service, including veterinary public health. This NGO has been a consistent feature of the Nepal One Health landscape and has had the prestige needed to assemble people from human health, animal health, agriculture and the community to improve understanding and action on significant zoonotic diseases.

Central to the NZFHRC prestige has been the dedication of its longstanding leadership to public service. This provides several advantages to the NZFHRC. First, it has allowed the NZFHRC to build the necessary social capital and infrastructure needed to have the competencies necessary to provide funders with assurances that the group can deliver on proposed projects. Second, it fosters the interpersonal relationships needed to access partners for projects, find conduits for information and gain permissions to work in a wide variety of settings. Sustained, responsive relationships with policy makers are the key to turning knowledge into social action. Third, because the NZFHRC undertakes projects that not only generate information to support education and policy, at a local and national level, but also provides diagnostic and investigative support to assist in the clinical care of people or animals, it has effectively integrated the technical and non-technical components of zoonoses disease control in a manner deemed useful in both the immediate and long term. This gives the NZFHRC a credible voice when advocating for actions to address problems.

Part of the NZFHRC profile has come from its history of coordinating programmes that result in tangible health benefits. Other parts come from a proactive programme of planning and tending to relationships as well as effective use of media to maintain the centre's profile in the public and political eye. Public relations are central to cultivating trust and reputation (European Centre for Disease Prevention and Control, 2011). Like the CWHC, the NZFHRC is neutral territory where a variety of stakeholders can assemble around a shared problem. This has positioned the NZFHRC to become the Nepal focal point for One Health.

### Supra-NGOs

By not necessarily being closely tied to specific governmental policies, political parties or ideologies, NGOs have the potential to cross national boundaries and to integrate across bureaucratically mandated boundaries such as health, agriculture, environment and economic development. Being outside government constraints, however, creates challenges for incorporating these integrative insights into governmental policies and practices. Some NGOs, such as professional associations and issue-oriented organizations, have addressed this challenge through public advocacy. Another approach has been to create what one might call 'supra-NGOs', which are expressed as networks, consortia and communities of practice. In some cases, such as VSF-International, nationally based, independent organizations create international, collaborative networks for information sharing and joint project development. Other supra-NGOs include both NGOs and government participants. Still others have their primary focus on research activities that are both locally grounded and transcend national boundaries. Examples of these two latter approaches are Animal & Human Health for the Environment and Development[6] (AHEAD), AfriqueOne[7] in Africa and Community of Practice for Ecohealth in Latin America and the Caribbean (CoPEH-LAC) in Latin America[8].

AHEAD was launched in 2003 by the Wildlife Conservation Society (WCS) and the International Union for Conservation of Nature. As described in detail by Cumming *et al.* (Chapter 21, this volume), this initiative includes a wide range of governmental and non-governmental partners, with varying perspectives and expected outcomes. Based on what WCS has defined as the 'Manhattan Principles' of 'One World, One Health', AHEAD focuses on adaptive, sustainable wildlife management in southern Africa, and has been successful in promoting and implementing Transfrontier Conservation Areas in the region.

CoPEH-LAC is one of several such 'CoPEHs' in different regions of the world. CoPEH-LAC is a collaborative effort of institutions in Latin America and the Caribbean and the University of Quebec in Montreal. Although CoPEH-LAC is primarily a research community of practice, several of its member institutions have sufficient national stature to influence public policy. AfriqueOne is a consortium of universities from several African and European countries, and is explicitly concerned with research on One Health issues. Like CoPEH-LAC and other CoPEHs, AfriqueOne considers government ministries of health, environment and agriculture to be 'strategic partners' (see also Bonfoh *et al.*, Chapter 29, this volume).

## Cases of One Health Actions – a Study of Veterinarians Without Borders/ Vétérinaires Sans Frontières

It is one thing to create and maintain organizations with the potential to facilitate One Health activities, but quite another to see this potential fulfilled. In this section, we introduce some specific cases wherein an NGO, specifically VWB/VSF, has implemented One Health projects.

### Poultry for profit and protein

In 2007, VWB/VSF launched a project aimed at improving the lives of rural Ghanaians in the northern part of the country. Ghana has a better standard of living than many sub-Saharan nations; however, 30% of its population still lives below the poverty line. VWB/VSF began this project assisting people in the Nadowli District, where impoverished farmers had reported devastating crop and livestock losses due to disease and drought. The organization partnered with the Ministry of Food and Agriculture in the Wa region to discover why the annual guinea fowl die-off was between 20% and 80% during the rainy season and to help smallholder farmers raise healthier guinea fowl. Separated from urban centres and primarily dependent on agriculture, northern Ghanaians have little or no access to veterinary care and medical services. VWB/VSF worked with communities, teaching about livestock disease prevention, detection and treatment, as well as better ways of harvesting and storing animal feed. They also initiated a guinea fowl production programme, which will help Ghanaians, and particularly women, raise poultry for profit and supplement their nutritional needs. VWB/VSF was able to fill a gap in service capacity with the blessing of both the community and the national government. It aimed not to become a long-term service provider or to sell these services for profit, but rather to create capacity through education for community control over livestock production and health.

### Humane management of free-roaming dogs to promote public health

Volunteers for VWB/VSF undertook to provide a sustainable and humane solution to dog population management and rabies prevention in a remote community in the Cuchamatán Mountains of western Guatemala. VWB/VSF worked with the Mayan Mam people in the community of Todos Santos. The neighbourhoods in this community are isolated from the rest of the country by a long and treacherous road. Todos Santos residents grow their own crops for food, keep chickens and pigs for meat and often do not have extra food for their pets. Although they are owned, dogs roam freely, searching the neighbourhoods for food, often also breeding with stray dog populations. They are frequently both the recipients and the perpetrators of aggressive incidents between animals and humans. When VWB/VSF arrived, many people lived in daily fear of free-roaming dogs. In partnership with local organizations, VWB/VSF undertook a dog population study and participated in city meetings and educational workshops focused on responsible pet ownership and the link between slaughterhouses, waste management and dog overpopulation. Because changes in the underlying conditions that support dog overpopulation will not be immediate, VWB/VSF also organized periodic volunteer veterinary clinics that involved Guatemalan veterinarians and technicians to work with and alongside foreigners. The Guatemalans not only provided services, but also benefited from professional interactions and continuing education provided by the foreign volunteers. This combination strategy of service, education and capacity development has resulted in a huge decrease in the number and size of dog packs in the area. Residents have suffered from fewer dog bites and attacks, and animals are healthier and better cared for (Pulczer *et al.*, 2013).

### Empowering primary animal health workers in Laos PDR

Laos PDR, although considered by the United Nations as a 'Least Developed Country', has been making rapid progress toward achieving several of the Millennium Development Goals. With two-thirds of the population living in rural areas, and more than 80% dependent on agriculture, sustainable livestock health is critical to human health and social development. VWB/VSF has been working in Laos since January 2010, following scoping and consultations carried out throughout 2009. Through collaboration between VWB/VSF and the National University of Laos (NUOL), project partners have provided training and support to build skills in animal health-care, disease prevention and community awareness-raising among a network of Primary Animal Healthcare workers (PAHWs). Beginning relatively small, with a single national partner, and grounded in local village activities, the project has expanded from poultry rearing, livestock health and forage systems to rabies control, use of smartphone technology to improve PAHW access to information and training material, and partnerships with other NGOs such as AVFS (the French VSF organization). Through VWB/VSF, the Laotian groups are also part of a much wider initiative of 'field-building' that is creating eco-health training and leadership networks among many NGO, government and university organizations in the wider South-east Asian region. This enhances the ability of agricultural communities to respond relatively quickly to changes in local and regional conditions, related to disease, for instance, with regard to avian influenza, economic development and technological opportunities. PAHWs have been trained and used effectively in many countries with poor infrastructure; this is in contrast to more economically developed countries, such as Canada, where legal restrictions on what are deemed 'professional veterinary activities' can create different challenges, as noted in the following case detailing a VWB/VSF project in northern Canada.

### Wildlife, domestic dogs and infectious disease in northern Canada

VWB is working in two remote areas of northern Canada which are inaccessible by road. Local residents still use sled dogs for transportation. These dogs interact with each other, with people in the community and with wildlife, such as wolves, moose and caribou. However, in many northern communities, veterinary services are absent or restricted, and disease surveillance programmes and routine preventive health measures such as vaccination and parasite control are rare because of the remote location. The sled dogs are affected by zoonotic diseases and parasites (such as rabies and *Echinococcus* sp.) as well as pathogens and parasites that can be transmitted between dogs and wildlife such as distemper, parvovirus and a wide variety of enteric parasites. Like in Guatemala, disease transmission at the domestic animal–wildlife–human interface is a serious risk and many communities live in fear of attacks from aggressive dogs, which have been known to kill young children. Controlling these infections and infestations in sled dogs provides the three-way benefit of protecting public health, wildlife health and the well-being of domestic dogs. Regulators attempted to compensate for this by allowing lay people, approved by the territorial veterinarian, to administer rabies vaccine to local dogs where veterinary services were not available. Working alongside the communities, local partners and various wildlife specialists, VWB/VSF assisted by providing volunteer veterinarians as well as travel support. Unfortunately, once volunteer veterinarians came to these communities, government regulatory authorities no longer allowed lay vaccinators to administer the vaccine. The well-intentioned intervention therefore reduced rabies coverage in the communities. This illustrates the needs for NGOs to work closely not just with community members but also with regulators to avoid unintended consequences of the NGO programmes.

## Summary

One Health issues can be complex and dynamic; therefore, NGOs need to develop strategic partnerships and networks that allow them to adapt to and efficiently address emerging issues. The power of NGOs does not come from their size but rather from their ability to gather like-minded individuals committed to achieving common objectives. NGOs enable citizens to promote local initiative and problem solving through collective actions. The NGO sector can bridge the profit interests of the private sector and the public-good concerns of the government sector by focusing on common goods. Flexibility and adaptability allows NGOs to try new approaches which may not be feasible or permitted in more traditional organizations and institutions.

Because NGOs are not driven by short-term financial objectives or traditional politics, they can have a longer time horizon when planning strategic objectives than can governments or private businesses. This is critical for One Health to shift from programmes that respond to disease emergence by focusing on pathogens in animals or the environment to programmes that promote and foster long-term reciprocal care of human, animal and environmental health. As governments retreat from a number of public functions and regulatory activities, NGOs are proving to be critical for long-term sustained One Health approaches to health protection and promotion.

NGOs are not a panacea or constructive solution to all problems. NGOs can suffer from bias, poor management, poor strategy and nefarious motives as can any other organization. Criticisms of NGOs include questions raised about their actual performance and effectiveness, accountability, implications of donor demands on NGO autonomy and ideological and political implications of their influence (Reimann, 2005). Powerful

NGOs that distribute funds can greatly influence One Health activities by restricting the agenda for service, research or policy interventions to a specific sub-set. For example, much of the early funding for One Health focused on developing microbiological capacity and pathogen discovery as opposed to developing local animal and human communities that could be resilient to unexpected disease outbreak. The legitimacy of an NGO can be questioned because they are not necessarily elected or selected by the people they claim to represent but rather represent the voice of a group of people gathered around a shared interest. Ideologically driven NGOs can fracture relations with governments or the private sector, which are often needed to create the enabling environment for change.

A predominant challenge to NGOs serving a One Health role is the need to critically assess what such a role implies. NGOs can work at the human–animal–environment interface; many are traditional development organizations, food security groups, sustainability organizations or environmental NGOs. NGOs are ultimately responsible to the vision upon which they were founded. Anholt *et al.* (2012) suggested that there were four key elements to successful One Health cross-sectoral collaborations: a shared vision; passionate leadership; structures and systems that allow for exchange of information and ideas; and relationships built on trust and respect. As evidenced above, many NGOs working within the broad field of One Health have these features. They are adept at mobilizing people from the level of the household to the level of the central government to work toward a shared problem. They can invest time, resources and passion to work at the root causes of problems. All of these characteristics are essential for an approach like One Health, which advocates cross-sectoral collaboration to promote and protect healthy human–animal–environment interactions.

## Notes

1 Although there are some differences in organizational emphasis and practice between One Health and ecohealth, we shall, for purposes of this chapter, use One Health as a term to cover both areas, as well as the more general concept of health in social-ecological systems (Zinsstag *et al.*, 2011; Zinsstag, 2012).

2 http://centreforcoastalhealth.ca

3 http://www.cwhc-rcsf.ca

4 http://www.vwb-vsf.ca

5 http://www.nzfhrc.org.np

6 http://www.wcs-ahead.org/index.html

7 http://www.afriqueone.net

8 http://www.una.ac.cr/copehlac

## References

Anholt, R.M., Stephen, C. and Copes, R. (2012) Strategies for collaboration for the interdisciplinary field of emerging zoonotic diseases. *Zoonoses and Public Health* 59(4), 229–240.

Barry, M.M., Allegrante, J.P., Lamarre, M.C., Auld, M.E. and Taub, A. (2009) The Galway Consensus Conference: international collaboration on the development of core competencies for health promotion and health education. *Global Health Promotion* 16(2), 5–11.

Bebbington, A. and Farrington, B. (1993) Governments, NGO's and agricultural development; perspectives on changing inter-organisational relationships. *Journal of Development Studies* 29(2), 199–219.

Bebbington, A., Hickey, S. and Mitlin, D. (2008) *Can NGOs Make a Difference? The Challenge of Development Alternatives*. Zed Books, London, 358 pp.

European Centre for Disease Prevention and Control (2011) A literature review of trust and reputation management in communicable disease public health, Stockholm: ECDC; 2011. Available at: http://ecdc.europa.eu/en/publications/Publications/Trust_Reputation_Management_Report.pdf (accessed 15 March 2013).

Max-Neef, M. (2005) Foundations of transdisciplinarity. *Ecological Economics* 53, 5–16.
Pulczer, A., Jones-Bitten, A., Waltner-Toews, D. and Dewey, C.E. (2013) Owned dog demography in Todos Santos Cuchumatán, Guatemala. *Preventive Veterinary Medicine* 108 (2–3), 209–217.
Reimann, K.D. (2005) Up to No Good? Recent Critics and Critiques of NGOs. Political Science Faculty Publications, Paper 5. Available at: http://digitalarchive.gsu.edu/political_science_facpub/5 (accessed 15 March 2013).
Stephen, C. and Daibes, I. (2010) Defining features of the practice of global health research: an examination of 14 global health research teams. *Global Health Action* 3, 5188. DOI: 10.3402/gha.v3i0.5188.
Waltner-Toews, D. (ed.) (2010) One Health for One World: A Compendium of Case Studies. Veterinarians without Borders/Vétérinaires sans Frontières. Available at: https://www.vetswithoutborders.ca/get-involved/resources/fbli (accessed 6 February 2014).
World Bank (1998) The Role of Non-Profit Organizations in Development: the Experience of the World Bank. Available at: http://web.worldbank.org/WBSITE/EXTERNAL/TOPICS/EXTSOCIALDEVELOPMENT/EXTPCENG/0,,contentMDK:20507529~menuPK:1278313~pagePK:148956~piPK:216618~theSitePK:410306~isCURL:Y,00.html (accessed in 2013).
World Bank (2010) *People, Pathogens and Our Planet, Vol. 1. Towards a One Health Approach for Controlling Zoonotic Diseases*. World Bank, Washington, DC, p xiii.
Zinsstag, J. (2012) Convergence of Ecohealth and One Health. *EcoHealth* 9(4), 371–373.
Zinsstag, J., Schelling, E., Waltner-Toews, D. and Tanner, M. (2011) From 'one medicine' to 'one health' and systemic approaches to health and well-being. *Preventive Veterinary Medicine* 101(3–4), 148–156.

# 33 Toward a Healthy Concept of Health

**Karen L.F. Houle[1]* with contributions by Karin Tschanz Cooke[2]**
*[1]University of Guelph, Canada; [2]University of Bern, Switzerland*

> As for diseases of the Mind, against them, Philosophy is provided of remedies, being in that respect, justly accounted the Medicine of the Mind.
>
> (Epicurus)

## Introduction

Epidemiology is 'the study of the frequency, distribution, and determinants of health and disease in populations' (Martin *et al.*, 1987). Philosophy is a systematic approach to 'the fundamental nature of knowledge, reality and existence; the theoretical basis of knowledge or experience; the systematic exploration of concepts, truths, belief states' (Oxford Dictionaries, 2014). This paper posits a deep and important relation between these two disciplines. Many health scientists readily acknowledge and work across this disciplinary relation. Some have shown that value-added health outcomes can be achieved by the *addition* of a philosophical or cultural dimension to health projects. Of their work in Chad, for example, Montavon *et al.* (2013) state that:

> With the help of an interdisciplinary research team, physicians, veterinarians, biologists, geographers and anthropologists studied the situation and the needs of the mobile pastoralists. To know more about their health, on the one hand, epidemiological studies were carried out, and on the other hand, anthropological and cultural studies contributed to better understand the nomads' concepts of health and their life, their perceptions of illness and their help-seeking behavior.

Philosophical approaches can certainly contribute to a 'better understanding' of a health situation, but our position goes beyond even this. Our hypothesis is that the concepts with which we conceive reality *are the same ones* we use to think about health; the concepts health scientists use to think about the theoretical basis of health knowledge and experience – wherever they are working, and no matter what kind of health science they are engaged in – are, *at the same time* expressions of their ideas about the fundamental nature of reality. This sort of relation is much more than a simple analogy. Furthermore, concepts are also kinds of individuals and populations – albeit mental ones – which are also susceptible to pathologies, thus also manifest patterns of health and illness. Therefore, the study of systems of what and how we think about reality (philosophy) *is an epidemiology*. For health science to *engage philosophically* is not

*E-mail: khoule@uoguelph.ca

enough to point out what values, concepts and beliefs are operant, say, in a cross-cultural setting. Philosophical reflection can help us to discern the patterns of health and disease in *our own systems of thinking*. Moreover, health science in general should be interested in this deep relation and this discernment since sick modes of thinking and unhealthy concepts *count among the determinants of health*.

## A More Fully Complex Understanding of Complex Problems

Ecohealth theorist and practitioner David Waltner-Toews (2007) sketches the monumental situation facing us in the 21st century:

> Emerging infectious diseases such as avian influenza have created a dilemma for scientists: what we know we don't know seems to be expanding faster than what we are pretty sure we do know. We have a lot of hard facts and a poor understanding of what they mean. What kind of advice can be given to policy-makers? How can scientists and politicians incorporate a sense of uncertainty and ignorance into their activities?...There are ways, but they are ways that many scientists and most politicians have been trying to ignore. Twenty-first century problems cannot be solved using only nineteenth- and twentieth-century scientific methods...Many scientific methods require us to put on blinkers and focus on small things. A lot can be learned by studying the genetics of viruses and the structure of human cells, but the questions now facing the world are bigger: Where does a pandemic come from? Can it be predicted or prevented, and, if not, what is the best way to respond and adapt? These questions require a combination of the best laboratory science with an understanding of ecology, culture, social change, and ethics.

Waltner-Toews insists that *a complex understanding* is required. One Health and ecohealth offer good examples of complex understanding. Its theorists and practitioners are committed to creative yet empirically appropriate epidemiological assessments of global pathologies. They are committed to responding to these complex 'presenting symptoms' in ways that actually stand a chance of predicting and preventing a deterioration in the overall health status of the great diversity of interconnected living beings: ecologies, livestock, wildlife and humankind. One Health insists on a profound interrelatedness with respect to animals, humans and ecosystems. These three elements comprise a normative, value-laden terrain (Zinsstag *et al.*, Chapter 2, this volume) raising problems that are not just empirical in nature, thus requiring solutions that are not just scientific in nature. Ethical, aesthetic, spiritual, philosophical and political questions also arise at the intersection of animals, humans and ecosystems.

While the fundamental premise of One Health is that the domain of health and disease must connect the health of ecosystems, animals and humans, and while this whole book speaks to, and explores the question of health more widely than tends to happen in conventional approaches to medical science, a maximally holistic and complex health science must include also concern for the healthiness or sickness of our theories of knowledge and experience. It must concern itself with the wellness or sickness of our thinking processes. It needs to explore and understand the health or pathologies of our concepts; the very tools with which we think, including how we think about health. The activities of acting *toward* health and thinking *about* health are also 'interrelated in the deepest sense'. Thus we accept the basic working premise of One Health but add another critical element of interrelatedness: the intractable connection between acting *toward* health – as do health scientists and researchers – and thinking *about* health, which we all do. This means that health science needs to explore the concept of health even *more deeply than it currently does*. A more complete *complex, understanding response* casts our attention toward the *concepts* we use to frame our sense of the world, the *concepts* we use to evaluate the state of the world, and the *concepts* we use to guide our sense of how best to respond *to* it. This is a contribution that philosophers and the like and can make alongside the contributions of health scientists. Finally, this is also a normative, or value-laden space. And because we are all thinkers, it is a normative space each and every one of us inhabits and is answerable for.

## Two Efforts to Include Conceptual Analysis in Health Science and the Value of Doing So

Theoretical Issues of One Health (Chapter 2, this volume) offers one model of what *attention* to concepts in health research might involve. Attention to concepts might be genealogical, i.e. look at how a concept in a discipline changes over time. Taking a genealogical approach, we learn that the *concept of health* has undergone an evolution: there has been a change in meaning over time and an enlargement of its territory of impact (Bresalier *et al.*, Chapter 1, this volume). Just as is the case with species, the *evolution* of a concept like health happens in an organic, developmental and somewhat chance-driven fashion.

> In the 1980s, the concept of sustainable development of health of people, animals, and the ecosystems in which they coexisted has extended the concept of health to the whole ecosystem. Hence 'one medicine' evolves towards a 'one health' concept.
> (Zinsstag *et al.*, 2005)

A genealogy of concepts – tracking the way concepts like *contamination* or *abnormality* or *health* have changed over time – is important because, among other things, it confirms that those conversations are never closed nor finished; that the terms in which we conduct such value and meaning-laden conversations over time and space are always to some degree provisional. A historical perspective on the shifting meaning of the concept of health thus also foregrounds the permanent and ubiquitous presence of values and accountability in health science because 'bringing conversations to a close is always a personal choice, a decision, which cannot be simply presented as mere application of procedures and justified as the only move we could make in those circumstances' (Mouffe, 2001). In short, if a concept or a field of inquiry is treated, implicitly or explicitly, as stable, solved or closed, a genealogical perspective on the ideas with which that field of inquiry operates reminds us that this claim of stability is false and this closure is contestable. Further, it means that those who are treating a concept or a field of inquiry *as if* closed and stable are answerable for that. Therefore, one way of being responsible to, and about, our thinking is to actively undertake to be informed by an historical approach; that is, of taking a genuine interest in the fact that, and the ways that, concepts and modes of thinking have changed over time; that there are multiple versions of the truth and 'fundamental ideas' even within our own intellectual histories. Methodologically, this is a way to internalize and honour the fact of the provisionality of *all* concepts, ideas and theories. Another value-added outcome is that our own thinking can become more supple, less linear, more self-reflexive, which, in turn, is crucial in being capable of listening with modesty and openness in cross-cultural research settings:

> When working in different cultures to achieve 'One Health' outcomes implies adopting the view that there are multiple legitimate perspectives, and that practices must be adapted to local contexts and that practitioners also need to clarify our own perspective and own point of view. The **self-reflexive attitude** asks: What is my personal cultural/religious background driving my animal-human relationship. Our own attitude towards animals influences how we value animal life economically or emotionally.... Consequently, when we report about our research from 'One Health' studies we also need to declare the **perspective**, i.e. the social, cultural and religious background, from which the animal-human relationship is seen as it strongly determines the valuing in economic frameworks and societal contexts.
> (Zinsstag *et al.*, Chapter 2, this volume)

Waltner-Toews (2009) asks: 'If the linear causal thinking of laboratory science and conventional epidemiology are inappropriate to answer complex questions in which health is embedded in complex social-ecological dynamics, where can we turn for help?' Turning to history is one answer. Turning toward diversity is another. *Draw students from diverse backgrounds. Build an interdisciplinary research team* 'with physicians, veterinarians, biologists, geographers and anthropologists' (Montavan *et al.*, 2013). One can expedite the natural evolution of concepts by concocting a sort of laboratory of thought by way of experiments in diversity. Sometimes health researchers bring together the methods and *thinking tools* of, say, epidemiologists, ecologists, social scientists, laboratory scientists, public health workers, theologians and ethicists. Productive mutations in theoretical modeling or practical problem-solving *can* come about through just such cooked-up idiosyncratic alliances. Just as in the case with species, when diverse ideas from previously isolated domains enter in a shared 'ecology of thinking', a concept's evolution can be expedited. The concept of One Health emerged thanks to a radically non-silo, transdisciplinary approach to practical problems of health; the 'combination of the best laboratory science with an understanding of ecology and culture.' Therefore, in addition to taking a genealogical approach to concepts used in health, trying to *reconceive concepts* through the synchronic synergies of diverse perspectives is another effort many current health researchers undertake to try to achieve the more *complex understanding* we badly need.

## A Deeper Worry

Even though these novel approaches (one historical and one interdisciplinary) recognize the central functional importance of concepts in health science practice, they might still fall short. Consider that a concern driving One Health is that classical clinical science has a limited scope of applicability. It has become apparent that some phenomena – 'wicked problems' – resist being responded to effectively via mainstream pedagogical, laboratory and modeling methods, and standard practices like vaccinations, broad-spectrum antibiotics or quarantine. But, wicked problems also resist *being understood and responded to* well via classical concepts and mainstream modes of thinking. *Thinking itself* – all of our thinking – has been subject to aspectival capture[1] or what we call horses' 'blinkers'. Classical modes of thought and ways of acting – reductionist, linear, additive, reactive – are entrenched in *thinking itself*. These ways of thinking are a feature of the thinking of ethicists, the thinking of historians, the thinking of geologists, or the thinking of a One Health researcher. This means that *even if* we try to take an historical, inclusive or a transdisciplinary approach to health, those old ways of thinking and old thinking tools – concepts – will still be dominant and operant, framing our perception and our responses. This will be *as true* on a transdisciplinary team or a diverse cohort of medical students as it will of a monochromatic disciplinary team or a homogeneous cohort. The old (ineffective) *ways* of thinking and the old (ineffectual) thinking tools will continue to present themselves as, or feel like, *appropriate conceptual and cognitive solutions* to wicked problems when in fact, those ways of thinking and concepts are as much the wrong kinds of tools to use in the face of those sorts of problems as are broad spectrum antibiotics. It is even possible that damage has been done, and will continue to be done, by the uncritical broad-spread application of our modes of thinking and our old stock of concepts. As we know from on-the-ground medical practice, distinct sub-strains can present clinically as almost indistinguishable – *Cryptococcus gattii* and *Cryptococcus neoformans* for instance. Responding to an outbreak without noticing that we are dealing with distinct sub-strains leads to mutation and deeper entrenchment of the basic pathological condition epidemiological intervention was trying to mitigate. The same can happen with abstract mental features of medical practice like conceiving, modeling, deducing, speculating. There are iatrogenic effects[2] at the level of thought associated with indiscriminate concept use. This can include a build-up in resistance to thinking itself. A lack of capacity for resilient and creative thinking might be the by-product of a kind of indiscriminate application of a broad-spectrum concept or way of thinking to what are in fact, distinct and singular moments, asking subtly different questions and requiring a skilled, adaptively-attuned conceptual deployment. Thinking with the same idea over and over, and thinking the same way, despite subtle yet critical differences in the nature of what is calling for us to think through, can turn out to be inadvertently dangerous. The worry is that our intellectual heritage has put such blinkers on us that we are not even capable of breaking free of these habits, even when we consciously undertake to try to do so, as with forming interdisciplinary think-tanks or adopting critical self-reflexive attitudes, or doing a genealogy of the concepts we work with.

## Healthy and Unhealthy Concepts

A third way that health theorists and practitioners might fruitfully engage with philosophical aspects of health then, is not as historians, nor with other disciplines, but *as more radical epidemiologists.* A radical epidemiologist is cognizant of, and critical of, the central and perpetual role that our thinking plays in the exercise and outcomes of health science, whether that is in the laboratory, in the field or in the classroom. This is different than merely being cognizant of the fact that concepts *are* playing a role. It asks: what role, exactly, is that concept playing? What is its function and is it performing it well in this situation? This is the approach we explore and recommend in this chapter. We propose that *concepts themselves* can be conceived of, and investigated as having basic natures.[3] These natures are subject to states of health or disease. This approach demands that we ask ourselves: Are the concepts we hold, and our ways of thinking unhealthy or maladaptive? Are our concepts and ways of thinking vital, active, creative, pliable and supportive of many forms of life, connectivity and experience? Or are they dead, stiff, rote, bunkered off from connection and hence grow only monocultures of the mind?[4] If the latter, then we must allot time, money and energy to developing concepts and modes of reflection better equipped, internally, to perceive and respond well as thinking beings to the *complex challenges* we are confronted with: healthy concepts. If we fail to do this, our *understanding* of problems we face will be at best superficial. We will not have rooted out the underlying aetiology.

This approach asks about the 'how' of concepts. It conceives of concepts themselves and ways of thinking as: (i) having a basic nature; having components, a natural (healthy) form or action unto themselves; (ii) being as susceptible to health and ill-health as any aspect of the external world, be that a coral reef, a community or the body of a dolphin; (iii) impacting health outcomes at higher scales (at the scale of individuals or populations); and (iv) playing a profound role in the state of the world; and thus (v) being a key element of a holistic, responsible health response to that state of affairs, alongside the giving of vaccinations, the cultivation of pasture, the lobby for human rights and the feeding of the hungry.

What this approach opens up is an entirely novel critical perspective *on health.* It suggests, ironically enough, that the very conceptual bedrock of disciplines such as pathology and epidemiology – the concept of health itself – can be ill. *If* our current concept of health is indeed ill, thinking *with it* might lead to unhealthy consequences: either infecting further thought *about* health or contaminating practical actions undertaken in the name of ameliorating health. Everyone involved with 'health science' thinks, imagines, conceives, perceives. The tools with which she does so – the concepts and the mental processes – can themselves be healthy and unhealthy. Being concerned with the health of the concepts and the mental processes with which we work is a maximally holistic vision of health. Health *all the way down* means concrete health outcomes are directly connected with philosophy. How can we proceed, practically-speaking? What does this concern for the health of concepts look like as part of the work of health? In order to make a diagnosis of the *health of the concept of health* we can draw on the insights and efforts of experienced health workers – not philosophers. Let us therefore turn to thinking *about health* in health science.

### A healthy concept: what would it look like or be able to do that a sick or ill concept could not?

The author has worked for a number of years on a transdisciplinary, international health research team that integrates animal, environmental and human health (mental and physical, individual and collective). My colleagues are veterinarians, ecologists, family physicians and environmental toxicologists. I also work with pathologists and epidemiologists (animal, human and environmental) who specialize in the diagnosing, modelling and understanding of larger patterns of disease: What does it looks like when individuals or groups, or the environment 'are sick'? What supposedly happens to healthy states to turn them into pathological states (risk factors, social determinants of health, exposure levels, contagion and virulence)? What effective interventions could prevent individuals or collectives from becoming ill? What mitigations could bring these back to health? Also joining this team from time to time are sociologists, lawyers, family therapists, art educators, palliative care nurses, lawyers and communication specialists. In every area of expertise, not just those directly associated with health science, the concept of wellness appears – healthy societies, good deaths, unhealthy pedagogies, unhealthy health policy (Castro and Singer, 2004), healthy families, healthy discussion networks (Mertens *et al.*, 2009). Listening carefully to so many different discussions of health and disease, across so many economic, geographical and embodied perspectives, and across multiple scales has enabled me to work up a very complex-and-general 'description' of a state of health as a form of reality. This description could apply to people, ecosystems, public policies, an individual's death, a family, a heart. This abstract description will aid us in saying what a healthy concept would be, or be able to do. In other words, from an abstract description about the basic nature of entities we will be able to tell a story about better and worse states. Let us now turn to that general description of the basic nature of all forms of reality, keeping in mind that we are moving to this level of abstraction in order to have a capacious and flexible enough concept of health that we could apply it to dolphins, ecosystems, concept and modes of thinking. And also, that we will eventually use this basic story about reality in order to generate ideas about value; about better or worse states of affairs, including better or worse thinking states.

## From the inside out

An entity of any kind whatsoever (a person, an ant colony, a word, a seed, a birthday party, a society, an experience, a family, a relationship, a classroom, an institution, an organ, a planet, a concept) has or contains, and continues to contain, many different kinds of potentials inside it as its own unique, ongoing constitution or make-up. Alfred North Whitehead (1929) named these 'actual entities' and named the inner power particular to each entity its 'subjective aim'. According to this sort of a view of the ultimate nature of reality, a thing does not have to be a subject in the sense of being an autonomous, conscious person to have this kind of an inner driver or aim. Depending on what kind of a thing it is, it has the power to do a certain number of things and to have a certain number of things done to it (Spinoza, 1996). What it is, is what it can do and what can be done to it. Nothing more and nothing less. There are many ways an ant could be an ant by virtue of the things it is able to do and the things that are able to be done to an ant. The same is true of a stone. There are many ways a birthday party could be a birthday party. According to a Spinozist view, which sees all things as profoundly interconnected, and humans no more or less so than other parts of the natural world, living things are not different in kind from birthday parties or stones: they merely differ in some of their capacities and how those capacities are actualized. Aristotle clarified that any particular living thing, at any scale, has the potential to continue to exist, to grow, to reproduce itself, to diminish or to stop existing. These are the base potentials. Certainly there are forms of life – entities – which contain a fewer number of potentials; fewer things it could express or do or be done to. That seems true of seemingly simple beings like sea cucumbers. But even a single sea cucumber has a surprising number of potent, subjective aims. Not only does it contain as part of its very constitution the capacities to continue to exist, to grow, to reproduce itself, to diminish or stop existing. It can also be stepped on; be eaten by certain other living things; float; be used as bait.

These claims are crucial to establishing a very general and capacious concept of health. For, in managing to continue to be whatever it is, an entity is able to continuously express or undergo these inner potentials and, crucially, not be ontologically obliterated in those actualizations. A sea cucumber floats on the tide and remains a sea cucumber. An elder sea cucumber reproduces and gives rise to another sea cucumber: not a dolphin. A dead sea cucumber is effective as bait for flounder because it is sea cucumber and something wants to eat that: a chunk of sea cucumber on a hook does not attract flounder because it smells or tastes like sea urchin. Insofar as that sea cucumber expresses or undergoes its range of inner potentials (including its potentials to transform states and enter into relationships with the stomachs of something else) it is a healthy sea cucumber. It is not healthy, according to this view, merely in virtue of it being at some optimal moment in its life cycle, or at some optimal physical size or performing a single function well. A healthy entity is vital in this intensive, pluripotent relational sense. Every second, every day it continues to do what it does, to enter into the relations it does, and to undergo what it undergoes, even undergoing mastication and digestion as it becomes a *vital* part of another entity. In doing so, it nevertheless continues to be retain or transmit its basic inner nature. As Spinoza put it, *it perseveres in its own being*. In doing so, it retains or transmits more fundamentally, vitality itself.[5]

The idea of an inner capacity to change and yet persist in some way through that change into another relation or state helps us differentiate a healthy from a sick entity. Consider the human heart. Our hearts. The heart in your chest, right now, about 45 cm from this page. It was formed within you when you were an embryo, and started to beat autonomously around 12 weeks of gestation inside your mother's body, and that very same organ in the very same location in your chest continues to beat and pump your blood, every second of your entire life, without cessation. Until it stops. That is your heart's nature, its life, its astonishing vitality. A sick heart, by contrast, is one whose capacity to beat regularly has diminished all at once, or little by little, from the inside out as it were, in that very act of beating, until it is no longer able to beat well or at all. Its (what Heidegger called) *ownmost* capacity to beat either stops entirely or comes to permanently depend on another's make-up to continue to do what a heart does: it needs the hands of a paramedic, or the organ of another person (a heart donor) or a pacemaker. One way of describing a sick entity then, is to say its *ownmost* potentials cannot continue to be realized naturally or for the most part as emanating from its own inner powers of persevering in its own being. A sick entity in this sense depends in large part, and continuously, on some second party, to be what it is, to do what it does. In Spinoza's terms, something has separated a thing from its own powers. A value system (a sense of good and bad, of rightness and wrongness) can arise from this account of the nature of processes and forces of existence. There is no further element that one needs to supply in order to be able to say that one state of affairs is better or worse, more or less desirable than another (Deleuze, 1988).

Now let us consider a concept. A concept is a kind of entity too. It is neither stone nor athlete nor sea urchin nor heart but it is not nothing. It has a kind of singularity among mental operations: it is neither an affect nor a percept. In *What is Philosophy?* Gilles Deleuze and Félix Guattari argue that 'concepts are not made from scratch' and that 'there are no simple concepts. Every concept has components and is defined by them. There is no concept with only one component' (Deleuze and Guattari, 1994). From a Spinozistic perspective, this means that concepts are in some interesting sense, bodily. As such, they too have their own inner 'power (potential) which should be understood as the capacity, vitality or "force of existing" that belongs to ideas as much as to bodies' (Sharpe, 2011). There are many different concepts. Concepts and conceptual terrains have genuinely different potentials, hence express and give rise to different modes of thought which themselves will express and give rise to different capacities for thinking, imagining, conceiving, perceiving. In principle there are many ways any particular concept could be *that* concept. And, in principle, a concept could be healthy or unhealthy in the same way described for other entities.

There are forms of life that contain a great number, possibly even a growing number, of powers. Some entities seem to give rise to endless new things it could express or do or which could be done with it, or to it. Parent–child might be a good example. Many people attest to having profoundly rich relationships with animals, places and plant life. The same is surely true for animals with particular places, people and even plants. All express and inhere through their unique range of potentials as those potentials are actualized, they are both equally healthy. Each is different and yet healthy (or unhealthy) in the same fundamental sense. Every particular entity has this natural capacity to be an ongoing, active part of the process of entering into myriad relations and in doing so, giving shape(s) to its own nature (Naess, 1977). A living, vital entity has this kind of health, as Aristotle would say, 'for the most part'. A healthy entity has this kind of life and vitality, for the most part. And so, we have arrived at a first approximation of what makes a *healthy heart* healthy, a healthy family healthy, a healthy planet healthy, a healthy ant healthy, a healthy concept healthy *for the most part*. This also gives us a principle according to which we can say what makes one state of affairs good compared with another. A sick concept is less good because it has been separated from what it can do, or what can be done with it. An unhealthy heart is less good because it has been separated from what it can do, and be. An unhealthy concept will be less good because it too will have been separated from what it can be, and give rise to.

## Is dying the opposite of health?

This inner potentiality or subjective aim continues to belong to a healthy entity right up until it dies, and even to be able to aim in time and space beyond its existence, depending upon the relations it had entered into, and their vitality and resilience. If an individual has been active and healthy in their own life then they would also have sustained in themselves the capacity to die their own death in an active and healthy way: that is, to not be separated from what it can do insofar as it also dies. One way of thinking about this is that the physical cessation of an individual entity makes the greater part of its innate potential available to be transferred; released for the most part *toward* the other relations it was once between, and among. That transference and continuation of vitality can be widely conceived: as spirit, as a legacy of ideas, as carbon and stardust, as affection, as compost, as inherited precious familial objects, as melody, as memory.

Dying is thus in fact not the opposite of life but among the subjective aims of all entities. It is one of the potentials contained within a living entity *qua* living entity. Dying itself thus can be said to have a life of its own, and in this be healthy or unhealthy. We say someone had a 'good death'. We don't just mean that they had a good life. We mean that the death part of their living was also done well (Box 33.1).

**Box 33.1.** Living with hope – dying in peace.

As a pastoral counsellor and spiritual caregiver in palliative care settings in hospitals, senior's homes and private homes, I have accompanied many dying people. Some were Christians, others were unsure about their beliefs in the face of death. To my surprise I discovered some characteristics that contributed to a good death and others which made the process of dying more painful. Most helpful seems to be the presence of loving and respectful people, if possible family members and friends, as well as prayers and sometimes songs of the hope in faith. To arrive at the moment of death in the strength of hope requires personal, relational and spiritual preparation long before death is near. In the hour of death brave souls surrender in faith and hope and experience often peace by doing so. The inner, spiritual, personal and relational processes are pivotal for the dying. If they receive strength from these connections, they are able to brave through many painful hardships at the end of life. What adds emotional, relational and spiritual hardship to the process of dying is, in short, not being prepared and not having peace within, between and among. This is interesting and seems to indicate that people do not assume that after death nothing matters anymore because all is over. Unresolved conflicts and strained relationships, spiritual uncertainty and 'unfinished business', i.e. priorities which could not be ordered, words which still need to be said, love that wants to be expressed, matter for the dying.

(Karin Tschanz Cooke)

Another way to distinguish between a healthy and an unhealthy entity then, whether a death, an ant, a heart, a marriage, a sea cucumber or a concept depends upon the degree and the rate of transfer of the potential from one state to another: the quality and intensity of the expression of life in the event of dying for instance. This characterization helps us to understand what is so difficult and unsettling – even some would say, wrong – about certain kinds of death: the death of young people, the death of animals and birds on the highways, and suicide. Seen through this lens we can see suicide as the abrupt, irreversible total expression of the inner power of any existing entity to, as it were, from the most alienated edge of their own selfhood, act inwardly upon and against their very nature to persist in their own being, and to overpower it. What makes suicide terrifying is that any life can get knocked off its axis enough to actually turn back and break its own vital momentum. That it does not need outside assistance to kill itself. The unhealthiness of that kind of death is the power of life, on its own terms, and by itself alone, to confront and overpower itself. In suicide, the one most continuous, most deep-down, *ownmost* potential a living thing has – to live – has a conjoined, amazingly flexible and super-strong twin: a power to make all of that life die. So all entities contain within them, among their powers, a capacity for continuation and a capacity for self-annihilation. These two opposing forces sit at the very core of a living person's conscious and unconscious sense of their profound power as an existing, *living person*. It is psychologically tempting to say that in a *healthy entity*, the force of this will to living is stronger than the force of its counter-living,[6] but it is more complex than that (Box 33.2).

## From the outside in

Health is not only about what an individual thing *can do*: what skills, capacities, desires, traits, tendencies and programmes it carries inside it and deploys on, or toward the outside; toward other entities *around* it. Health is a complex state that depends as much upon the situation *in* which any entity (a person, an ant colony, a word, a seed, an event, an experience, a family, a relationship, a classroom, an institution, a planet, a concept) *happens to find itself*. Certain capacities an individual *has* are activated by a situation, i.e. something external to them. This is the part about what can be *done to* an entity. The situation also has, or contains a number of potentials: what can be done *to* and *with* the thing that is in that situation, at that point in time. For instance, I do not possess the capacity to sting anyone, but if I am in the vicinity of hornets, that situation contains the possibility of my being stung. I am capable of being stung, and this capacity is activated and expressed only in certain situations of which I am not the maker.

Of course, some of an entity's milieu, context, or situation is in some meaningful way 'created' by the entity which is a part of it: over a very long time alkali bacteria change the pH of the rock creases they live in, eventually

**Box 33.2.** Living within a spiritual framework called creation.

Dying may be defined within a spiritual framework where life and death are seen as part of a greater entity called creation. In this understanding the universe and all living things came into being through the will and the act of God. Even though there are differing religious and philosophical understandings of the spirit of God, i.e. the spirit of a higher power, they seem united in the understanding that there is purpose and meaning in what has been created as well as in life and death itself. Within a spiritual perspective the question what may be described as a good life and a good death receives a special focus. This focus aims at being inclusive and holistic. It is not a theoretical concept only, but also a transfer of faith into thought, word and deed, which results in a lifestyle. The emphasis of lived spirituality is connection and dialogue from spirit to spirit, i.e. to converse with God's spirit and discover God's intentions for one's life, to respect and cherish others and the universe as God's creation.

(Karin Tschanz Cooke)

causing them to die; we can make an abrupt jagged tear in a friendship with one uncharacteristically unkind comment; we can poison a workspace with our constant negativity, which in turn makes it unpleasant for others, and ourselves, to work. We can wear perfume and colours that attract hornets. But, regardless of the degree to which one can impact one's situation, every kind of thing's possibilities are ultimately actualized or not actualized by virtue of the composite *situation* in which it finds itself as a specific, individuated and unique part – what it undergoes or is subjected to. Its situation is never entirely created or fashioned by it. There are always elements of a situation which are in no way its self, its doing, its choosing or its own. Sometimes we call this *outside factor* luck, ecology, chance, weather, nature, happenstance, fate, God's will. Spinoza calls this situatedness: *extensivity*.

The values and meaning attached to responding to this feature of reality are different from those attached to what we do, what we will, what we intend. Our modern liberal mindset tends to omit or underplay this feature of reality. We tend to overemphasize the active causal power of an independent, individual agent, and imagine it gains it, and exercises it, at a distance from world and object. We tend to connect the evaluations of health, present or future, to the state of an agent rather than to the capacities in, or able to be cultivated in, a wider situation including what it is not, and what is beyond its control. All things *are what they are*, and what they can be, partly by virtue of the things that they are not.[7] The health of an entity or a situation, therefore, is not entirely localizable to that entity or that situation. Conceiving of its health must involve accounting for this necessary vulnerability of all things (see Box 33.3).

Our concept of health lacks an understanding of this dimension. Because of this we often get our evaluations of health wrong. For example our environmental health is currently severely compromised. This might be due to a 'sweeping disinterest in the fact that human culture has been, is, and always will be nested in ecological systems' (Gruenwald, 2003). Here we have a compelling illustration of an unhealthy situation being traceable to *an unhealthy way of thinking about health*.

Just as all entities are healthy in the same sort of overall way, all entities are vulnerable in a similar way, and that vulnerability is also connected to a capacity for vitality and resilience, i.e. healthiness. We cannot be what we are except by being open to what we are not, then passivity, dependency, exposure and vulnerability are a necessary part of health, of being healthy. Nothing can become, change, learn, grow or even die entirely on its own, purely, sovereignly, from the inside out, as an individual. To even be an individual it needs an outside it is passive in relation to, an Archimedean point, even the smallest rim of an outside – dependency is at the heart of what anything is. A living thing depends continuously upon *innumerable, indeterminate* inputs of these *externals*: wind, grain, DNA, water in the vicinity, electron drift, revolutions, ink, copper smelting, matches… ∞). Some sorts of things can control those 'external' conditions to a very high degree, but never perfectly. Some things are almost totally vulnerable to what happens to it (think of a birch seed landing in a place it can grow and getting the right weather at the right moment). Everything is, and must be, perpetually open and vulnerable to what it is not, in order to be, and to do well at what it can be. It cannot be healthy or be involved in the furthering of health, if this is not so. Being a more active and resilient individual, more fully able to express its ownmost 'force of existing', is accomplished through the ongoing, adaptive, artful and careful connectivity and composition with many other kinds of things. This is as true of concepts, and thus of the composition of thought, as with birch seeds. In other words, a permanent indeterminate dependency is key to health *of* existing entities. Health is not just about the relative continuous containment of individuals and the sustained expression of individuals' innate potentials outward into the world. Health also means the *active cultivation of passivity*, of vulnerabilities and exposures. This is a feature of health that the well-known current World Health Organization (WHO) definition of 'complete health' misses entirely, and it does so because the concept of health it works with is unhealthy; that is, not reflective of the deeper nature of nature, and the true, complex nature of health of all things.

**Box 33.3.** Embracing interdependence and vulnerability.

The 1946 WHO definition of health (WHO, 1946) is indeed far reaching in its statement, that 'health is a state of complete physical, mental and social well-being and is not merely the absence of disease or infirmity'. While health was often defined from a physical point of view often relying on medical concepts and analysis, the WHO definition attempts to reflect a more holistic view to emphasize the mental and social aspects of health and well-being, which are, indeed, essential. Systems theory and therapy has shown to what extent functional as well as dysfunctional family systems influence the health and well-being of people. And they point out how human beings are at their core social beings in need of positive connections through relationships. Jewish philosopher Martin Buber stated, 'All actual life is encounter',[8] i.e. that all people, whether Tuareg pastoralists or Californian film directors, become human through the encounter with another human being. The experience and theoretical orientation of many people the world over – their basic philosophy – tells them that to encounter another human being in such a fundamental and deep way is only possible if we are also connected with the eternal Thou or the eternal other.

This points to a dimension of health that the WHO definition still leaves out, namely spiritual health and well-being. From the perspective of One Health or ecohealth, these spiritual aspects seem relevant, since they aim at the concern for and commitment to the care and well-being of the family, community as well as the whole world, i.e. all the linkages that make up creation. Within the Judeo-Christian framework this insight is expressed in the first and greatest commandment: 'Love the Lord your God with all your heart, and with all your soul and with all your strength.' The second is just like it: 'Love your neighbour as yourself.'[9] These words reflect an integrated view of a human being as an individual (love yourself), a social being (love your neighbour) and a spiritual being (love God with heart, soul and strength). To be connected with the self, with all living others and with God in love is a state of health and well-being. The WHO definition of palliative care of 2002 did include this spiritual dimension. It states that palliative care aims at the prevention and relief of suffering, the assessment and treatment of pain and other problems, physical, psychosocial and spiritual. And yet, based on our Spinozist view of reality, we see there is still an aspect of being human missing, namely the aspect of weakness, incompleteness, passivity, dependency and vulnerability. Not only are these aspects a healthy and normal part of an individual at the end of their life; they are features of our very existence, all the way through our lives. The western understanding of human beings is especially one-sided in its emphasis on strength, being in control, competence, power-over; power-to-act-upon and knowledge. We are seen as *homo faber*, as those in charge, those that create, know, control and act. There is only attention to the ways that we are active, self-sufficient, not needing or wanting anything or anybody. As we have argued above, this is not so much a false view of entities as an incomplete one. Out of such a partial understanding may come a hubris and arrogance, which cannot see that, for a fact, more is unknown and cannot be understood or controlled. Without this insight, an insight that is more likely to be achieved if our concept of entities and thus health is more complex at the most rudimentary level, then all human actions – including the constant behaviour-shaping actions of thinking about who and what we are, who or what other people are, what God is or is not, what creation is, what death and life mean – can be, unknowingly, dangerous and destructive even while having the best of intentions. In order to protect all of life, this vulnerability needs to be accepted and embraced. It can be accepted and embraced at the level of our interactions in the world, but we can also show an acceptance of vulnerability by building it into the concept of health with which we operate. Within the widest possible context of human life, it is the balance between giving and receiving, the ability of being strong and fragile, powerful and vulnerable that gives depth to life and relationships and challenges humans to act responsibly and maturely and it adds a healthy humility as well as beauty to our commitment to live and learn. In a spiritual perspective human beings understand themselves as part of creation as well as interdependent and responsible to creation as well as to the creator from whom all things are.

(Karin Tschanz Cooke)

Any being's healthiness in an even more expansive holistic sense, then, means the enjoyment of: (i) a fairly steady-state exposure to elements it is for the most part able to respond to, as an active passivity; (ii) a decreased or tolerable level of exposure to the vulnerabilities which compromise its ability to respond, which separate its self from its powers; or (iii) an enhancement of its capacities as a result of finding itself composed and actualized in a vital manner, by its situation, no matter the nature of that situation: spiritual, ecological or economic. The important point here is that although all living things always already are *in* a situation, there are degrees of activity and passivity with respect to awareness and responsiveness *to* the situation, and that connected responsivity is *health*. What we call 'health' *is but an expression of the intensity and agility of that responsiveness*.

## Back to Concepts

This is all true, too, of concepts and modes of thinking. This philosophical analysis thus gives us a way to distinguish healthy from unhealthy ones. A concept 'lacks meaning to the extent that it is not connected to other concepts and is not linked to a problem that it resolves or helps to resolve' (Deleuze and Guattari, 1994). In other words, a healthy concept is one that is highly responsive to a presenting thinking-problem. This will be true of a healthy concept of health. A concept of health is healthy to the extent that it is open and responsive, and hence it enables us to be open and effectively responsive, as health scientists, to a presenting health-related problem.

What does the responsivity of concepts mean, though? Deleuze and Guattari's distinguishing of 'philosophical from scientific problems' is helpful. A scientific problem invites a solution which is extensive, propositional, and hence terminable. A philosophical problem invites an 'uncertain' solution, which, by contrast, enables an 'infinite movement' which 'consists in finding, in each case' what 'breaks through and continues to break through' (Deleuze and Guattari, 1994). What Deleuze and Guattari are getting at here is that a concept always operates within an evolving, uncertain situation – a real problem – and has meaning, vitality and capacity (*as solution, as effective response*) in relation to that. And, as we have also been saying of stinging insects and hearts, the situations in which concepts happen to find themselves impact what they can do, or be. Concepts are also dependent. They *need* operational milieu and persona (subjects who think those concepts, use them, see the world through them, and them in the world). But these operational milieus are varied. In the case of health problems, some operational milieus are layered and complicated while others are genuinely complex, wicked. A healthy concept of health will be able to enable us to respond to each situation with complicated or complex modes of thinking, as is appropriate to it.

Taking these two dimensions together, we can say that health is an active, creative, continuous co-productive adaptive symbiosis between or across the intensive and extensive dimension (Naess, 1977). This deep and reciprocal relation-of-a-singularity-to-milieu feature is arrived at by the terms *embeddedness* (Saint-Charles *et al.*, 2008) and *resilience*. Those concepts tend to get applied to environments, animal populations and human health (mental and physical and spiritual). For instance, the International Development Research Centre (IDRC's) health goals are for 'more equitable and sustainable social and economic development founded on healthier populations living in more resilient ecosystems'. But such ideas have a broader reach. 'Resilient' can describe an entity – whether a human individual in the Sahel, or a concept, or a pumping heart – whereby it is able to respond 'positively to change and challenges' (Parkes and Horwitz, 2009).

When an entity is healthy in the fullest sense (its inside capacities actively expressed outward, its situational possibilities acting upon it in particular ways, its responsiveness at, and as, the intersection of these play of forces) it *then* has or contains an emergent capacity to contribute positively – intentionally, targeted, and chosen or simply indirectly, accidentally, indifferent, windfall, neighbourly – to what does and can happen to many indefinite others. Healthy individuals are thus key elements in a continuously emergent collective flourishing.[10] This collective healthiness is neither reducible to the sum of the 'internal' health of the parts of individuals that make it up, nor creditable to the sum of the outcomes of individual actions and actors within that whole: health in the most expansive sense is the word for an emergent and robust quality of sustained adaptive complex multi-scalar inter-relationality of all entities to all other entities, past, present and future. While many in the modern world would not name this state a *spiritual state* others would see in this a description of nothing other than a spiritually healthy individual (Box 33.4).

### Ethical thinking

Here are some concepts: health, love, God, pain, freedom, nature, time, friendship, space, justice, and responsibility. Concepts are socio-linguistic–mental phenomena we, experiencing conscious beings, are either born with as part of our fundamental make-up[11] or acquire through certain learning pathways.[12] However we came to have them such that we can use them, the point is we *do* use them: we require them in order to 'encounter the world', we constantly apply them to the world through rules and habits of intuition, perception, proprioception, logic, cognition, attribution, language and speech. They are not given all at once, and even when we acquire them, there is plasticity to their expression or uptake. We have argued that any living thing, at any scale, has the potential to continue to exist, to grow, to diminish or to stop existing and that whatever it manages to accomplish, this accomplishment comes from the inside and the outside.

Concepts do not tend to strike us as living things. But they are, in fact, powerful components of any complex system we find ourselves in – a kind of threshold or interface between two consciousnesses, thought and objects. They are components of the composite action we call thinking but not in the sense of 'building blocks of cognition'. They are not representations of things or states of affair. Nor are they an invariant frame inside the head (semantic content) or a net of cultural meaning. Concepts are forms of thought (Kant, 1781), vehicles of sense and sense-making. As vehicles, that is, having form and design and dynamics (Mainzer, 2004), concepts have unique capacities. In general, they inhere and operate in a space between subject and situation, idea and matter, object and consciousness, self and other, enabling those ontological dimensions to *form* relations such that sense can be made. All concepts have base potentials, different concepts have different potentials. Each concept, in their particular action, via their particular internal structure, produces and ratifies the relational grammar of being-in-the-world in a particular way, a particular kind of sense-making, whether that is at the level of *cognitive architecture* (Brook, 2009) or in relation to the *architecture of matter* (Holden, 2004) or at higher and higher scales, expressive of discursive blueprints. Any particular concept *qua concept* has the potential to pick out and properly name distinct features of the world or objects (which can be mental, as in the concepts 'dream' and 'depression'); to group concrete individuals together coherently, and to enable us to form thoughts and interpretations about those kinds of features and the relations between them, and to actually communicate that sense with others. Deleuze (1994) named this the *'image of thought to which a concept refer'*, in other words, the operational system that actualizes thought's capacity in and as actions: thought's physics (Zourabichivili, 2002). These ideas suggest that concepts are the *how of thinking*. Since they are the how of thinking, they are a key component of *how we are* in the world.

**Box 33.4.** Spiritual health.

What does it mean for an individual to be spiritually healthy? A spiritually healthy individual is a person who is at peace with him- or herself and in relationship with others, God and creation. This peace embraces the balance between self-actualization and self-giving, between being an autonomous and dependent self, as well as being in touch with the different parts of one's identity and the interaction with one's social web. Such a holistic understanding of health is the foundation of a spiritual perspective which includes not only the respect and care for people and creatures, but also for creation.

(Karin Tschanz Cooke)

Here is an everyday example: the concept of 'fewer' is able to tell us something different about objects and the relation between parts of the object than the concepts 'less' and 'some.' *Fewer* has a unique capacity. It has the power to tell us that whatever we are speaking about it can be divided into countable parts, and then the part with a smaller number of units can be isolated, in principle, from the part with the larger number of units. *Less* or *some* are different concepts with completely different powers. To use the concept *less* is to signal that the nature of the object being considered cannot, in principle, be divided into parts that could then be compared on the basis of countable units, i.e. ordinality, number. At best, we can eyeball it and say that one part had the quality of being smaller than the other, i.e. having *less to it compared to the other, which had more.* At most we could say that 'some' had been taken away, but some would not be a number so much as a quality of a certain indeterminate quantity: *diminishment.* I like this example because people often use these two interchangeably without realizing that these capture or point to entirely different ways the world is and can be, to us. Students think I am being nit-picky when I correct them but this is not just a typo or a minor grammatical error. It is an error of 'smushing' together distinct categories, and hence of not seeing or saying properly, how varied and singularly-presenting the world is. It is not until you make a student say: 'She loves him fewer now than before,' or 'Please bring me six water for the coffee maker,' that they *feel* the way that the world of parts and wholes, of fluids and solids is a heterogeneous world, and hence requires different concepts to get at these co-existing differences. We have been trying to show that, just like a person, an ant colony, a word, a seed, an event, a society, an experience, a family, a relationship, a classroom, an institution, or a planet, each concept has its *ownmost* potential to perform the act of pointing to the world in its own way, to make certain sets or groupings of the world, and to be used well or badly in perception, organization and thinking (about) the world.

Healthy or unhealthy thinking then, is also ethical or unethical thinking. What is a healthy concept compared with an unhealthy concept except the kind of thinking thing able to sustain and give rise to vital and resilient mental states of affairs? It clearly is not only a matter of having the right kinds of attitudes *about* objects (as in, 'that is not a healthy way to think about your ex-husband'). Nor is it just a matter of having the right research team or stakeholder participants. Nor is it just a matter of being about to apply the right concept to the right thing, though it is that. It is a matter of all of us being actively and intimately involved, as thinkers, with *thinking*. It is a matter of our ownmost capacities for attunement to be attuned to the complexity of thought such that we are responsive and responsible producers and users of resilient concepts, concepts that are able to respond, and to enable others in turn to respond 'positively to change and challenges.'

In the opening challenge I quoted, Waltner-Toews makes an explicit invitation to ethics, to a *new ethics*. What is that *old ethics*? Ethical systems, thinking, speech and action built up around what I call, after scientific paradigms, a *normal concept of responsibility* (Houle, 2013). This is a normative concept that works well with middle-sized, complicated, trackable cause-and-effect Newtonian-esque moral situations. Why is it in need of replacement? Just as in the case of mainstream linear epidemiological paradigms, the deployment of a classical linear *ethical* paradigm and its concepts (like utility, dignity, human rights) may produce inadvertent but major and lasting damage. Waltner-Toews charged that a new, entirely different ethics is called for, not just a refurbished old one. Jean Lebel, one of the pioneers of the ecohealth movement in Canada, concurs: 'Addressing, let alone solving, complex problems in an enduring way will require complex approaches, methods and concepts' (Lebel, 2003).

## Conclusion

It is said that in the face of current global challenges, a new ethics is required. A new ethics will certainly require, among other things, new thinking. New modes of evaluative, meaningful thinking that are complex rather than merely complicated, emergent rather than merely additive. This applies to all thinking and all thinkers, whether the topic is ethics, theology, groundwater contamination or vaccinations. A new kind of ethical thinking requires the operation of a new, healthier concept *of responsibility*. The normal, mainstream concept of responsibility deployed in response to genuinely complex moral problems, especially in tandem with normal epidemiology, will not be adequate to address them and can even produce iatrogenic effects, in the world, in ourselves, *and even in our systems of thinking*. Here is an example.

My colleague Craig Stephen at the Centre for Coastal Health in Nanaimo confessed that it was not until we were prepared to ask: 'What do a porpoise, a cat and a 65-year old woman have in common?' that the *Cryptococcus gattii* outbreak of 2005 was able to be cracked, epidemiologically. Until that time, what was happening was that radically disparate jurisdictions (Oceans & Fisheries (Federal), a Parksville veterinarian (local), the British Columbia Health Authority (Provincial)) were collecting information on human and animal mortality cases, looking in those series for statistically significant correlation and causation, but independent of one another, having 'different responsibilities for different jurisdictions'. They were not yet even taking up subclinical cases, only 'kills'. Even where statistical significance was discovered in one domain it was 'meaningless' because it was so partial (Duncan *et al.*, 2005, 2006a,b,c, 2011). What these so-called separate objects have in common, are, of course, something more concrete and elemental: the soil they are in actual contact with – soil disturbed and entering the aquatic systems at a higher rate due to urban expansion and logging up into the Malaspina ridge, the water they drink or live in, the air they breathe. Stephen explained that the zoonotic outbreak had a 'broad epidemiology' and although the human, livestock, pet and aquatic cases could be seen as parts of separate series, those series were 'not closed' and circulated through 'multiple ecologies': farm, ocean, new subdivision, campground. The full disease and exposure patterns – and hence what would constitute risk, prevention and treatment – were invisible from any of those sub-perspectives. It was not until they were 'taken together' that sensing an overall pattern was possible. Aquatic animal cases tell us something that you can never see with human cases alone. Of course, trying to 'take' a case history that could attend to all the details of the local ('Which campsite did the people with the cat actually camp in?') and the global ('Can you remember how many clouds you stood under that month, sir?') is impossible. However, Stephens insists that it was just that kind of dogged persistence, refusal to respect conceptual boundaries, and wild leaps of imagination at strange angles between concrete facts that cracked the case. In fact, the 'carrier' of the deadly fungus turned out to be the majestic Douglas firs on Vancouver Island that run from Victoria up to Cathedral Grove. A community of trees.

What is it that drives the human mind toward a monoculture, toward reacting to all 'presenting cases', whether epidemiological or political or ethical the same way? Thought with blinkers on. Thought bent toward a strictly problem-solving mode. Thought forced into a tight time-frame. Thought reduced to logic. Emergency-room thought: thinking in fight-or-flight mode. Thought working at too high a level of generality. Binary thinking. Thought focused too far from 'circumstantial factors'. Thought unwilling to play or be spirited. Thought whose very tools – concepts – are only able to mobilize linear, binary, problem-solving mental modalities. Because some situations we face are not avoidable, not subsumable under general laws, because there is no recipe for how to deal with them let alone eradicate them, because they truly are grey areas, responding as thinkers to these situations with those old tools can do damage. Thinking this way can be irresponsible. Continuing to believe, and act in health science with the belief, that all problems are solvable or all situations can be avoided with enough research and equipment produces ethicists and epidemiologists, ecologist and parents who are themselves only capable of acting as problem solvers and rational deliberators. Such individuals are powerfully motivated most to eradicate what disturbs us rather than to cultivate respect for it, and to learn to live with such forces – with all the elements of our basic situation – in better ways. At the root of a monocultural reaction like the fantasy of eradication is a sick concept, a concept unable to respond in a various and vital way to whatever calls for it. By contrast, a healthy concept, whether the concept of responsibility or health or citizenship, has the ongoing capacity to make a lateral, transversal, open, non-reactive imaginary impossible.

We might be facing an extraordinarily difficult set of challenges in the 21st century, not the least of which centre on health. If we can be certain of anything right now it is that having only one variety of maize, one stock phrase for all social encounters, one energy grid, one candidate for president, one very narrow medical education, is likely a very bad idea. The valuable lessons of One Health theorists and practitioners confirm this concern with over-reliance on a single tool, a single way of *doing health*. Having just one kind of concept is equally unpromising. Doing health with a single concept of health and a single mode of thinking is especially unpromising. Combining the insights and instincts of One Health with the analytical and conceptual epidemiology of philosophy enable us to corroborate and deepen this concern. It shows us that we ought to be concerned with over-reliance on a single mental tool, a single way of conceiving health and a single mode of thinking about health. *Ought* in two senses. Ought in the practical sense that better health outcomes are indexible to healthier modes of thinking; that the resilience and vitality of concepts can and should be included among health indicators. And *ought* in the normative sense that regardless of where we work in the 'health science field' all of us are thinkers and hence capable of being more or less responsive as thinkers. We are all in an important and complex sense, responsible for being healthy thinkers, for participating in healthy thinking relations and for giving rise to vital, resilient ecologies of thought.

## Notes

[1] This is Ludwig Wittgenstein's (1958) concept, which describes the propensity for consciousness to resolve a 'Gestalt' such as the famous 'duck-rabbit' into just one of its aspects, and then, in short order, to be unable to move back and forth between the two aspects as it initially could. The arrest of consciousness in a habit of perceiving just one of the two aspects is named 'aspectival capture'.

[2] 'Latrogenic effects' is the term for getting sick at and from interacting with health care: picking up viruses at the emergency ward, getting depressed due to the food and architecture in hospitals, feeling worse when you put on a paper gown, dying from complications of minor surgery.

[3] Foucault took the same approach to power. He investigated the 'how' of power, not just the effects of power on the world. He did not assume power was some neutral or uniform black box substance that simply acted outwardly but a complex subject in its own right. See Dreyfus and Rabinow (1982).

[4] I take this term from *Monocultures of the Mind* by Dr Vandana Shiva (1993).

[5] This raises the interesting question as to whether a necessary condition of health is this giving-rise-to, or what I name relationality in some futural form? Must all healthy entities reproduce? Can a once-off and never-reproduced event be healthy? Since I am arguing that health is a state of ongoing vitality and relationality (even in some radically altered form, as in eaten or flattened) across instantiations and time, then the conclusion is that a once-off event with no progeny or reverberations of any kind either cannot exist, or, if it existed, would not be a healthy form of existence. This does not mean that a human can only be healthy if they give birth: they can give rise to many other forms of vitality. It also means that since all humans have to die, they can have healthy and unhealthy deaths.

[6] This helps us to understand something important about the excruciating position of wanting to end one's life and not being able to do so on one's own. The so-called 'right to die' or 'dying with dignity' names the loss of this normal state of dual-potency that is personhood, and is not about the particular pathology afflicting an individual (depression, Lou Gehrig's disease). It also reminds us that this is a potency we all enjoy and exercise, not that it is a special exception being demanded by a lobby group.

[7] The most exacting account of this fundamental and necessary dialectical inter-subjectivity of things *qua* things can be found in Hegel's *The Science of Logic* (Hegel, 2010), Section 'Something and Other', which explains why a something has to have an other, why there has to be something that I am not, why that other

has to be another in its own self, how each one makes itself the other of the other, how the innermost working takes place elsewhere.

[8] Buber, Martin, 'Alles wirkliche Leben ist Begegnung.' – Werke I. Schriften zur Philosophie, S. 85 u. 'Das Dialogische Prinzip. Ich und Du', S. 15, 5. Aufl. Heidelberg 1984.

[9] Mark 12: 30, New International Version, London, International Bible Society, 1984.

[10] Denmark is consistently named among the 'happiest' nations. One of the things that produces the overall flourishing of Denmark is a consistently strong socialist platform. There are very high taxes. These go to underwriting education, anti-poverty, childcare, nutrition programmes, etc. As a result there is less of a gap between the rich and the poor compared with other developed nations. The 'poor' are in a sense healthier in Denmark and hence can, and do, contribute more – indirectly but powerfully – to the overall wellness of the country.

[11] This is Kant's view. In The Critique of Pure Reason (1781) he asks: What must we be like to have the kinds of experiences we do; that is, as subjects with being-in-the-world? Experience has a mental component and a physico-material component and in a subject these are meshed. How is this possible? The answer Kant deduces, phenomenologically as his transcendental argument is that mental representation requires concepts and sensations (percepts); and that subjects come equipped with concepts. Concepts are that which enables us to encounter facticity and matter as meaningful experience and not just brute sensations.

[12] This is Frege's view.

[13] You can see in this case a vivid illustration of the epidemiological silos: some data and analysis show up in mycology journals, others in veterinarian journals, others in human public health, others in oceanography journals. There are few, if any, clinical or research experts in health who have the time, expertise or inclination to read across these sources.

## References


Brook, A. (2009) The possibility of a cognitive architecture. In: Dedrick, D. and Trick, L. *Computation, Cognition, and Pylyshyn*. MIT Press, Cambridge, Massachusetts.

Castro, A. and Singer, M. (2004) *Unhealthy Health Policy*. Altamira Press, Walnut Creek, California.

Deleuze, G. (1994) *Difference and Repetition*. Columbia University Press, New York.

Deleuze, G. (1988) *Spinoza; Practical Philosophy*. City Lights Books, San Francisco, California.

Deleuze, G. and Guattari, F. (1994) *What is Philosophy?* Columbia University Press, New York.

Dreyfus, H. and Rabinow, P. (1982) The subject and power. In: Dreyfus, H. and Rabinow, P. *Michel Foucault: Structuralism and Hermeneutics*. University of Chicago Press, Chicago, Illinois.

Duncan, C., Steven, C., Lester, S. and Bartlett, K.H. (2005) Follow-up study of dogs and cats with asymptomatic *Cryptococcus gattii* infection or nasal colonization. *Medical Mycology* 43(7), 663–666.

Duncan, C., Steven, C. and Campbell, J. (2006a) Clinical characteristics and predictors of mortality for *Cryptococcus gattii* infection in dogs and cats of southwestern British Columbia. *The Canadian Veterinary Journal* 47, 993–998.

Duncan, C., Steven, C. and Campbell, J. (2006b) Evaluation of risk factors for *Cryptococcus gattii* infection in dogs and cats. *Journal of American Veterinary Medical Association* 228, 377–382.

Duncan, C., Schwantje, H., Stephen, C., Campbell, J. and Bartlett, K. (2006c) *Cryptococcus gattii* in wildlife of Vancouver Island, British Columbia, Canada. *Journal of Wildlife Diseases* 42, 175–178.

Duncan, C., Bartlett, K.H., Lester, S., Bobsien, B., Campbell, J., Stephen, C, and Raverty, S. (2011) Surveillance for *Cryptococcus gattii* in horses of Vancouver Island, British Columbia, Canada. *Medical Mycology* 49, 734–738.

Gruenwald, D. (2003) The best of both worlds: a critical pedagogy of place. *Educational Researcher* 32, 3–12.

Hegel, G.W.F. (2010) Something and Other. In: Hegel, G.W.F. *The Science of Logic*. Cambridge University Press, Cambridge, UK.

Holden, T. (2004) *The Architecture of Matter: Galileo to Kant*. Clarendon, Wortley, UK.

Houle, K. (2013) *Responsibility, Complexity, and Abortion: Towards a New Image of Ethical Thought*. Lexington Books, Lanham, Maryland.

Kant, I. (1781) *Critique of Pure Reason*. Cambridge University Press, Cambridge, UK.

Lebel, J. (2003) *Health: An Ecosystem Approach*. IDRC, Ottawa, Canada.

Mainzer, K. (2004) *Thinking In Complexity: The Computational Dynamics of Matter, Mind, and Mankind*, 4th edn. Springer, Berlin.

Martin, S.W., Meek, A.H. and Willeberg, P. (1987) *Veterinary Epidemiology*. Iowa State University Press, Ames, Iowa, 343 pp.
Mertens, F., Saint-Charles, J., Lucotte, M. and Mergler, D. (2009) Emergence and robustness of a community discussion network on mercury contamination and health in the Brazilian Amazon. *Health Education and Behaviour* 35, 501–521.
Montavon, A., Jean-Richard, V., Bechir, M., Daugla, D.M., Abdoulaye, M., Bongo Naré, R.N., Diguimbaye-Djaibé, C., Alfarouk, I.O., Schelling, E., Wyss, K., Tanner, M. and Zinsstag, J. (2013) Health of mobile pastoralists in the Sahel – Assessment of 15 years of research and development. *Tropical Medicine and International Health* 18(9), 1044–1052.
Mouffe, C. (2001) Wittgenstein and the ethos of democracy. In: Mouffe, C. and Nagl, L. *The Legacy of Wittgenstein: Pragmatism or Deconstruction*. Peter Lang International Academic Publishers, Frankfurt, Germany, pp. 131–138.
Naess, A. (1977) Spinoza and ecology. *Philosophia* 7, 44–54.
Oxford Dictionaries (2014) Philosophy. Available at: http://www.oxforddictionaries.com/definition/english/philosophy (accessed 24 April 2014).
Parkes, M.W. and Horwitz, P. (2009) Water, ecology and health: exploring ecosystems as a 'settings' for promoting health and sustainability. *Health Promotion International* 24, 94–102.
Saint-Charles, J., Mongeau, P. and Biron, J.-F. (2008) A communication perspective on video lottery terminals. *International Gambling Studies* 8, 233–247.
Sharpe, H. (2011) *Spinoza and the Politics of Renaturalization*. University of Chicago Press, Chicago, Illinois.
Spinoza, B. (1996) *Ethics*. Penguin Books, London.
Vandana, S. (1993) *Monocultures of the Mind*. Zed Books Ltd, London.
Waltner-Toews, D. (2007) *The Chickens Fight Back*, 1st edn. Greystone Press, Vancouver, Canada.
Waltner-Toews, D. (2009) Food, global environmental change and health: ecoHealth to the rescue? *McGill Journal of Medicine* 12, 85–59.
Whitehead, A.N. (1929) *Process and Reality*. Macmillan, New York.
World Health Organization (1946) *Constitution of the World Health Organization*. Available at: http://www.who.int/governance/eb/who_constitution_en.pdf (accessed 24 April 2014).
Zinsstag, J., Schelling, E., Wyss, K. and Bechir, M. (2005) Potential of cooperation between human and animal health to strengthen health systems. *Lancet* 366(9503), 2142–2145.
Zourabichvili, F. (2002) *Spinoza: Une physigue de la pensée*. University of France Press, Paris.

# 34 Grappling with Complexity: the Context for One Health and the Ecohealth Approach

**Martin J. Bunch[1]* and David Waltner-Toews[2]**

[1]*Faculty of Environmental Studies, York University, Toronto, Canada;*
[2]*Professor Emeritus, Department of Population Medicine, University of Guelph, Canada; Founding President, Veterinarians without Borders/ Vétérinaires sans Frontières – Canada*

## Introduction

The field of ecohealth has to do, broadly, with 'research, practice and knowledge integration at the interface of ecology and health' (International Association for Ecology and Health, 2013). This phrase, taken from the aims and scope of the journal *EcoHealth*, is expanded in the front matter of the journal with a couple of dozen examples in the categories of 'One Health and Conservation Medicine,' 'Ecosystem Approaches to Health' and 'Public Health, Ecosystems and Society'. The broad definition is similar to the concept of One Health, as a field that addresses 'interactions between human and animal health that reach far beyond individual clinical issues and include ecology, public health and broader societal dimensions' (Zinsstag *et al.*, 2011). In practical terms, this can be framed as the 'added value [in terms of improved human and animal health outcomes, and ecosystem services] of a closer cooperation of human and animal health and other sectors' (Zinsstag *et al.*, 2012).

We situate our discussion in this chapter within this broad definition of the *field* of ecohealth, which we are taking to encompass One Health as described in this volume. As discussed earlier in this volume by Zinsstag *et al.* (Chapters 2 and 5), One Health has come to be seen by many researchers and practitioners as a strategy for achieving, jointly, animal and human health outcomes that would not be possible, or if possible would be more costly and/or less effective, if undertaken by separate initiatives. The selection of outcomes and their sustainability are embedded in much larger and more complex social-ecological systems; grappling with the challenges of understanding this broader context is the subject matter for ecohealth.

To some applied researchers, public and animal health experts and development practitioners, 'ecohealth' has a more specific connotation. They refer to the 'ecohealth *approach*' or 'ecosystem approach to health and well-being.' This is an approach that began to emerge in the 1990s with the expression of an ecosystem approach rooted in systems thinking, conceptualizing coupled human and natural systems, operated by collaborative processes and intended to intervene in situations of complexity and uncertainty (Allen *et al.*, 1993; Kay and Sneider, 1994; Kay *et al.*, 1999; Bunch, 2001; Waltner-Toews and Kay, 2005;

*E-mail: bunchmj@yorku.ca

Waltner-Toews *et al.*, 2008) and its application to social-ecological systems for the purpose of improving human health and well-being (some examples can be found in Yassi *et al.*, 1999; Forget and Lebel, 2001; Waltner-Toews, 2001; Murray *et al.*, 2002; Lebel, 2003; De Plaen and Kilelu, 2004; Bunch *et al.*, 2006; Boischio *et al.*, 2009; Webb *et al.*, 2010; Charron, 2012).

The ecohealth approach is an applied and action-oriented approach intended to both improve understanding about a situation and to intervene to benefit human health and well-being. To date it has mostly been applied in development contexts in the global south, because of the origins of the approach with a development funding agency in Canada, the International Development Research Centre (IDRC). Dominique Charron, the former lead of the Program Initiative in Ecosystem Approaches to Human Health at IDRC, defines the ecohealth approach (Charron, 2012) as an approach that:

> formally connect[s] ideas of environmental and social determinants of health with those of ecology and systems thinking in an action-research framework applied mostly within a context of social and economic development. Ecosystem approaches to health focus on the interactions between the ecological and socio-economic dimensions of a given situation, and their influence on human health, as well as how people use or impact ecosystems, the implications for the quality of ecosystems, the provision of ecosystem services, and sustainability.

A wide range of researchers, practitioners and teachers have been involved in developing and applying the ecohealth approach, especially those associated with IDRC's Program Initiative in Ecosystem Approaches to Human Health, the Network for Ecosystem Sustainability & Health (http://www.nesh.ca), Veterinarians without Borders/Vétérinaires Sans Frontières (VWB/VSF) (http://www.vwb-vsf.ca)[1] and members of the International Association for Ecology and Health (http://www.ecohealth.net). Many of these have organized into Communities of Practice for Ecosystem Approaches to Health in Canada, West Africa, South-east and East Asia, Latin America and the Caribbean (see http://www.copeh-canada.org, for example). Several have published training manuals. The websites of these organizations and the journal *EcoHealth* are some locations of examples of applications and development of theory and methods associated with the ecohealth approach.

For the purposes of this chapter and an overview of the approach, we turn to a discussion of the nature of the problems that ecohealth is intended to address. We then present an overview of the ecosystem approach, a transdisciplinary conception of health and principles and guidelines that bring these together in the ecosystem approach to health and well-being.

## Positioning Ecohealth

For ease of communication ecohealth is sometimes described as an approach to managing environmental and social determinants of health. This is misleading because it implies a linear sequence of simple determinants and that intervention somewhere along that line will improve health. The situations to which the ecohealth approach is most appropriate are instead characterized by multiple diffuse pathways that are difficult to identify and parse, and by relationships that are self-reinforcing and resistant to change. Yet they may be subject to sudden and surprising reorganization.

This is because coupled human and natural systems are not merely complicated – they are complex. Complex systems do not behave like machines, with parts connected by causally linear relationships. Instead they are dominated by feedback loops that lead to self-organization and evolutionary behaviour, they have interacting, multi-scalar hierarchical settings, they adapt and evolve, and they are characterized by irreducible uncertainty.[2]

Such situations tend to defeat our normal approach to problem solving. Since the scientific revolution of the 17th century, we have been trained to deal with problems that can be compartmentalized, isolated and reduced to manageable cause–effect relationships. Furthermore, our institutions (health authorities, planning departments, etc.) are structured and operate in this old paradigm (Bavington, 2002; Berkes, 2003; Innes and Booher, 2010). Because the application of 'normal science' (as described by Kuhn, 1962) and applied and professional consultancy work rooted in that paradigm is sometimes inadequate, some researchers and practitioners have attempted to find other pragmatic ways to deal with complex problematic situations. Funtowitz and Ravetz (1993, 1994a,b) have described a 'post-normal' approach (see Table 34.1).

Post-normal science (PNS) is a way of doing policy-related science that is appropriate for cases where 'facts are uncertain, values in dispute, stakes high and decisions urgent' (Funtowicz and Ravetz, 1994b). PNS provides a basis for accommodating knowledge provided from multiple perspectives of diverse stakeholders in complex situations. PNS thus offers a philosophical rationale for

**Table 34.1.** A comparison of the normal applied, professional consultancy and post-normal science approaches to environmental problem concerns (Kay *et al.*, 1999).

| Normal applied science | Conventional professional consultancy | Post-normal science and inquiry |
|---|---|---|
| *Essentials* | | |
| Certainty | Uncertainty (reducible in principle, we lack knowledge) | Uncertainty (irreducible in principle) |
| Low stakes | Intermediate stakes | High stakes |
| Facts: truth found | Solution: client happy, society is satisfied | Resolution: a course of action is chosen |
| *Results* | | |
| Hard | Try to be hard | Soft |
| Predictable | Error reduced to an acceptable level | Unpredictability a fact of life |
| Quantitative | Quantitative ± | Quantitative + qualitative |
| *In the service of* | | |
| Truth | Client in a societal institutional framework | Decision makers, policy, public |
| *Judgement of results* | | |
| Truth accepted | No mistakes (i.e. surprises) | Quality of process, integrity |
| Peer review | Holds up in court, client happy | Holds up to public scrutiny, move forward |
| *Mode of Inquiry* | | |
| Hypothesis testing | Problem solving | Ecosystem approach |
| Pursuit of truth | Mission and product oriented | Pursuit of understanding |
| Reductionism | | Holarchic |
| Analysis | Analysis + design | Analysis + design + synthesis |
| *Explanations* | | |
| Linear cause and effect | Non-linear, negative feedback | Negative + positive feedback, autocatalysis, morphogenic causal loops |
| Mechanistic | Mechanistic + cybernetic | Synergistic, emergence |
| Stability | Control, homeostasis | Change, evolution, ∞ cycles |
| Efficiency | | Efficiency + adaptation |
| Extremum principles | | Local optimum, trade-offs |
| Laws | | Propensities and constraints |
| *Forensics* | | |
| Fact | Interpretation | Testimony |
| *Characteristics* | | |
| Objective, one correct view | Subjective, client-consultant view | Subjective, plural |
| Value free | Limited values | Ethical, integrity |
| Predictive management | Control management | Anticipatory + adaptive management |
| Physics | Engineering | Ecological economics |

health-related activities where One Health is invoked as a goal and/or ecohealth is chosen as an approach.

For One Health practitioners, this means that the health outcomes selected, and the manner in which they are addressed, become part of the process of investigation. For example, livestock are valued in many different ways, many of them non-economic. Cattle, for instance, are valued differently by Masai in East Africa, Hindus from India and feedlot owners exporting beef from USA. Simple appeals to cost–benefit analyses to arrive at strategies for controlling diseases are not always helpful or sufficient. Even within a broad economic perspective, we must ask whether the benefits and costs are accruing differently to smallholders, corporations, communities, trading partners and the like. PNS, unlike what has been called normal science, does not argue that there is a single 'objective' view of a complex reality that trumps all the others. Conventional scientists contribute a great deal to the overall body of knowledge, but their view does not necessarily negate or subject others. Our understanding of the world emerges from multiple, sometimes conflicting, perspectives and is characterized by complex uncertainties.

In order to prevent this openness to multiple perspectives from degenerating into a free-for-all mixture of hard-won evidence, misinformation and fantasy, PNS practitioners have developed extended peer networks and sets of guiding principles and questions. Hence the importance of networks and communities of practice that cross not only disciplinary boundaries, but also the boundaries that have traditionally separated academic scholarship from community-based research and indigenous knowledge.

## The Ecosystem Approach

Ecosystem approaches are distinguished from other approaches in environmental and resources management by use of the ecosystem construct as a metaphor for holistic thinking, attention to the evolutionary and dynamic nature of complex situations and the incorporation of processes to accommodate management of such situations with multiple interests and stakeholders, across multiple jurisdictions (Yaffee, 1999). Figure 34.1 presents a version of the 'diamond diagram' that represents the adaptive ecosystem approach that has influenced many ecohealth applications. This version of the ecosystem approach was developed by James Kay and his colleagues in the 1990s (Kay *et al.*, 1999) and further elaborated in the book *The Ecosystem Approach: Complexity, Uncertainty and Managing for Sustainability* (Waltner-Toews *et al.*, 2008). This expression of the ecosystem approach is explicitly positioned as PNS and informed by ideas about self-organizing, holarchic and open (SOHO) systems. While a challenge to understand for the novice, the language and theory of these systems has provided a useful way to think about and manage what might otherwise appear to be a kind of paralysing complexity and to anticipate and plan for unintended consequences.

Self-organization is a characteristic of complex systems that leads to emergence and is related to systems and complexity science concepts such as resilience, adaptation, regime change and tipping points. Within the One Health field, one might think of the health of individual animals and people being embedded in, and interacting with, families or herds, which are nested within larger social and ecological units, which are today nested within – affecting and being affected by – global trading and climate systems. People and individual animals have their own particular characteristics, as do families and herds (emergent properties) and so on. Each unit (person/animal, herd/family) can be viewed as both a whole with its own internal dynamics and also as a part of something larger. Philosopher Arthur Koestler (1968) referred to such 'two-faced' units as holons and the nested organization as a holarchy.

This way of looking at the world implies the need to identify appropriate scales of attention as well as within- and across-scale interactions – which for many health workers and animal health workers is a formalization of common sense. Does one target individuals, households, communities (or their animal counterparts) or some combination?

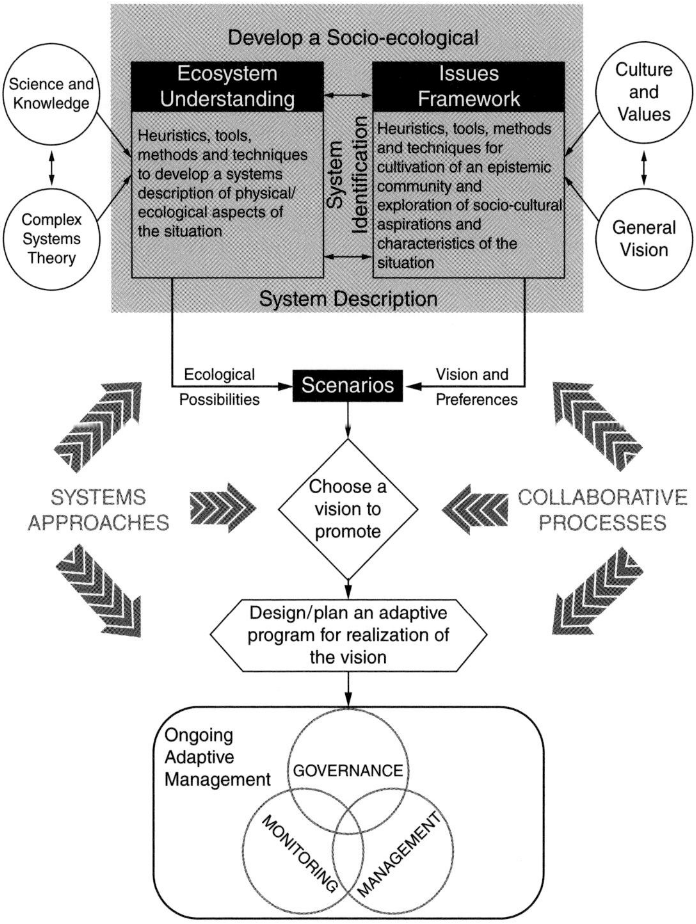


**Fig. 34.1.** A framework for an adaptive ecosystem approach (Bunch, 2001, adapted from Kay *et al.*, 1999).

The 'open systems' of the SOHO concept refers to the fact that such systems are those in which information, energy or matter (inputs) flow through, are transformed in and drive the processes occurring within systems. The SOHO concepts are some of the systems thinking ideas used by practitioners throughout the application of the ecosystem approach.

There are three general phases evident in ecosystem approach framework presented in Fig. 34.1: problem identification and system description (the box at the top of diagram); making decisions and taking action; and ongoing learning, adaptation and management that subsumes and iterates the process. In this general framework, methods and techniques are not prescribed, although both systems approaches and collaborative processes are intended to operate the approach throughout.

Problem identification and system description (sometimes called a system study) begin the engagement with a messy problematic situation, including stakeholders and actors. An important part of this is the identification and description of the 'problemshed' (this may or may not be tied to geographic constructs such as watersheds). It involves developing an appreciation of the nature and spatial and temporal scales of relationships associated with a problematic situation. It is a collaborative process of discovery to understand historical context, identify and meaningfully engage and empower actors and stakeholders, develop knowledge about key components and relationships and understand pertinent values and preferences and physical and cultural possibilities. This work draws key relationships in the system to the fore, indicating their spatial and temporal footprint and bounding the situation so as to identify the system, its wider systems and environments and subsystems and components.

The social-ecological system identification generates understanding of systemic possibilities that might exist in the situation. From this, researchers work with stakeholders to identify alternative futures (scenarios) that are systemically desirable and culturally feasible. One of these alternatives is selected to inform intervention. This is a different role for researchers than traditional scientists will be familiar with, and it is a characteristic of working in the 'post-normal' mode in situations of uncertainty and complexity. James Kay (2008), a key formulator of this type of approach, explains that:

> Investigators into complexity do not seek prediction, control, right answers or efficiency. These are not sensible goals under conditions of complexity. Rather, the investigators seek understanding, adaptability and resilience. Scientific inquiry, more than ever, becomes an act of collaborative learning and knowledge integration. The role of the expert shifts from problem solving to an exploration of possibilities and from giving correct advice to sharing information about options and trade-offs. In fact, those who cling to being the old sort of expert lose their expertise.

This new role for experts derives from the failure to manage complex situations in reductionist and mechanistic ways. Such situations are characterized by discontinuities in linear chains of cause and effect. They cannot be managed as if they were sets of levers and cogs in a machine. Instead, complex systems must be encouraged to self-organize around desirable alternative system configurations. A system's trajectory of change cannot be entirely controlled, and there may be surprises along the way. It is more analogous to raising a baby to adulthood than to sending a spacecraft to the moon. With the rocket, there is a relatively high degree of certainty of the outcome, each successive attempt is similar in critical ways and sending one successful rocket improves the chances of the next. In raising a child, experience and expertise help but the outcome remains uncertain. Each child is unique and formulae have limited application (Glouberman and Zimmerman, 2002).

Thus, when we attempt to understand and intervene in complex situations, we need to monitor key relationships to learn about system behaviour. This is necessary to be adaptive. Applied research, public health interventions and other projects that attempt to engage with complex environment-and-health problems must constantly re-evaluate the conceptual model of the system and the efficacy and outcomes of interventions. There should be openness, even an orientation to revising and adjusting the strategy. The ecosystem approach is an adaptive management approach. Practitioners of adaptive management continuously monitor activities to support collaborative learning.

Based on the 'diamond diagram' above, the Adaptive Methodology for Ecosystem Sustainability and Health (AMESH) was developed in the 1990s through a series of community-based projects in Kenya, Peru, Nepal, Canada and several other countries (see Fig. 34.2). AMESH is described in considerably more detail elsewhere (see Waltner-Toews *et al.*, 2008). However, as applied to One Health outcomes, it may be summarized as follows:

**1.** The process begins when local people, researchers or some third-party agency perceive a health-related problem.
**2.** The responders, who could be anyone from international agencies to university-based research scholars, describe the situation systemically, including as many different perspectives and scales as feasible.
**3.** Local stakeholders, together with research scholars and government and non-government agencies identify alternative courses of action that can best accommodate known trade-offs and optimize the achievement of multiple goals.
**4.** They then choose a course of action that can achieve some balance of those different goals, develop a plan that incorporates feedback from which the implementers can learn and adapt, begin implementation and ensure

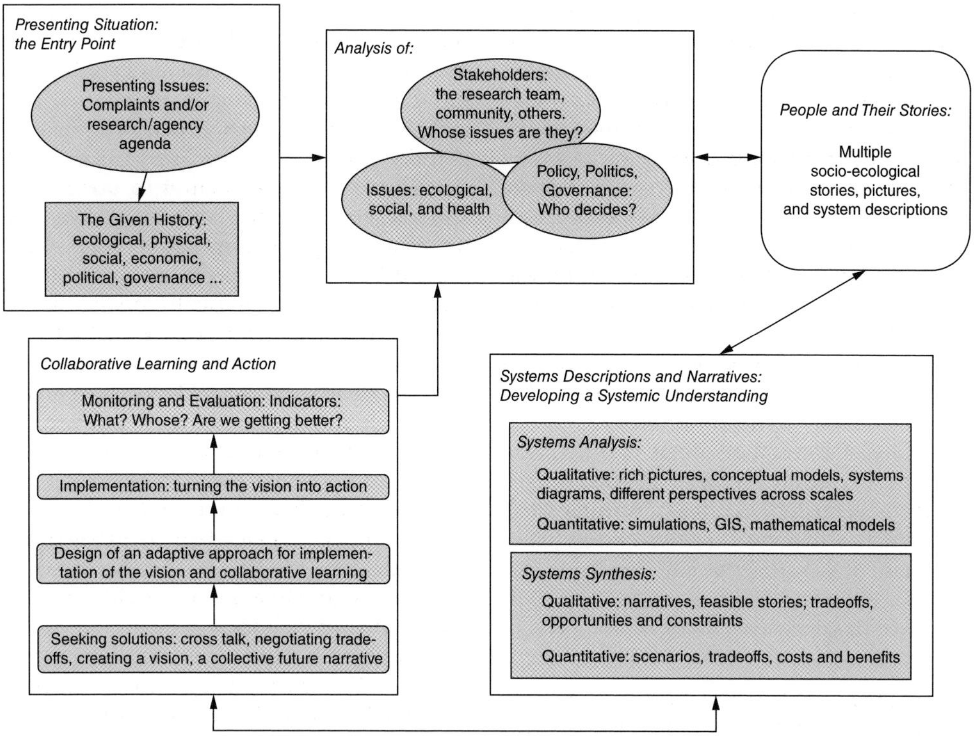


**Fig. 34.2.** The Adaptive Methodology for Ecosystem Sustainability and Health (AMESH) (Waltner-Toews, 2004; Waltner-Toews *et al.*, 2004).

that governing, monitoring and management co-evolve with the changing situation.

The process, which has been demonstrated to be quite robust, incorporates both conventional investigative scientific and modelling techniques and democratic social processes. Unlike many scientific investigations, can be altered and adapted to deal with new information and/or changing contexts (e.g. unstable markets for animal products, disease epidemics).

## An Integrated and Transdisciplinary Conception of Health

Because ecohealth applications face the danger of exploding into multiple directions at once, practitioners and scholars in the field have developed a variety of ways of setting reasonable boundaries and articulating key principles.

Health (good or bad) arises from multiple interrelationships among various human and natural components of social-ecological systems. In systems terms, community, population or ecosystem health is an emergent property. That is, it is evident at the level of the system but not at the scale of individual components or smaller subsets of relationships. One cannot predict from the individuals what the community will be like. Thus, one way to bound ecohealth work is to find units that are simultaneously useful for study, administration of programmes and investigation of dynamics. This is part of defining the 'problemshed' relevant to the situation. Some geographic constructs lend themselves to this application more than others. In environment-and-health situations, watersheds have proven to be such a unit. Not only are they arranged in a hierarchical manner (with sets of larger encompassing catchments and smaller sub-watersheds) that help to frame conversations about external driving forces and upstream/downstream relationships, but water is clearly of central importance to both ecological and human health (Falkenmark and Folke, 2002).

There are several useful conceptual models of environment-and-health interrelationships and emergence, such as the butterfly model of health (VanLeeuwen *et al.*, 1999) and the Millennium Ecosystem Assessment framework that connects ecosystem services to constituents of human well-being (Corvalan *et al.*, 2005). One current model that we find particularly useful is the Watershed Governance Prism (Parkes *et al.*, 2008, 2010) (Fig. 34.3). The prism expresses the potential for relationships among social systems, ecosystems and health with watersheds as an organizing construct that highlights water–land interaction, settings for health and well-being and scale at which important driving forces (such as climate change) manifest. Although the prism is labelled for 'watershed' governance, because watersheds represent a setting to understand social-ecological systems and driving forces acting upon them, this can be substituted for other settings.

The Watershed Governance Prism is useful as a heuristic device to conceive of and guide the search for important relationships in a complex and problematic situation (e.g. among social systems and health, watersheds and social systems; see Table 34.2). Not every axis of the prism will necessarily be identified as important in every situation, but in identifying the problemshed and developing a system description of the issue, the prism can inform our scan of the problem. Furthermore, sets of relationships can be built up to represent common perspectives (e.g. the faces of the prism correspond to common approaches such as: water governance for sustainable development; water governance for ecosystems and well-being; water governance for social determinants of health; and water governance for social-ecological health promotion). The Watershed Governance Prism thus helps to promote the search for relationships corresponding to various prism axes that may

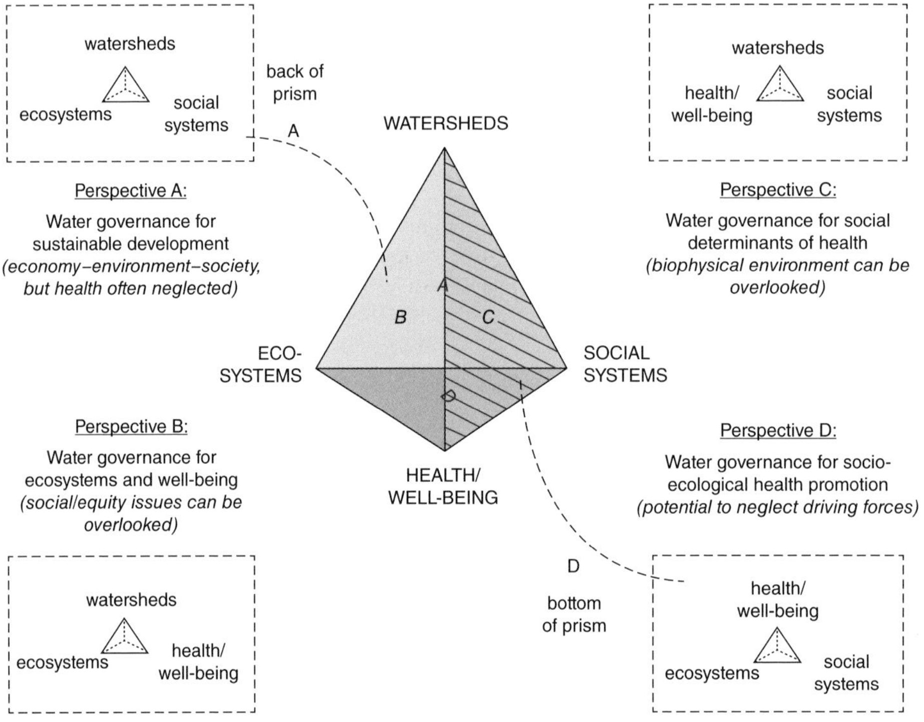


**Fig. 34.3.** The Watershed Governance Prism (Parkes *et al.*, 2010).

**Table 34.2.** Relationships corresponding to axes on the watershed governance prism (modified from Parkes *et al.*, 2010).

| Linear connections (prism 'axes') | Representative examples of features, issues and characteristics of linear connections' link to prism diagram |
|---|---|
| 1. Ecosystems–health/ well-being | Traditional environmental health relationships linking ecosystems with human health and well-being, with a focus on contaminants, pathogens, disease vectors, toxic or therapeutic agents, extending to health implications of loss of biodiversity and/or ecosystem services. |
| 2. Watersheds–ecosystems | Natural resource and ecosystem management (including land and water use) within the watershed, agro-ecosystem viability and food security; the protection of baseline or 'environmental' water flows, including wetlands; saltwater intrusion/salinization of soil. |
| 3. Watersheds–health/ well-being | Water-related services and infrastructure (including source water protection, waste water, sanitation and hygiene services); direct effects of natural disasters such as flooding, drought, landslides; structural flood defences, drainage and irrigation systems. |
| 4. Watersheds–social systems | Water for socio-economic and community development; water access and water rights (particularly for the poor); public or private exploitation of water for economic gains through dams, reservoirs and hydroelectric power; upstream–downstream equity issues; spatio-temporal variability. |
| 5. Social systems–health/ well-being | Social determinants of health; health implications of social policies and socio-political processes, health impacts of socio-economic status, inequities, poverty, social networks and social cohesion; access to health services, health promotion, education, social services and community development. |
| 6. Ecosystems–social systems | Linked social-ecological systems; ecological goods and services (e.g. provisioning, supporting, regulating and cultural services); supply and demand-side management, place-based links of human-natural systems occurring at scales within and beyond watersheds. |

exist in a problem context and also point out what aspects may be missing or neglected. When a conceptual model of a problematic environment-and-health problem is developed, some axes might not appear, but this can be a deliberate and justified choice rather than an accidental one that arises out of ignorance or a narrow perspective.

The Watershed Governance Prism and other conceptual models of environment-and-health promote a holistic and synthetic approach to complement the normal scientific and social science tools that we can bring to bear on environment-and-health issues. This highlights the necessity for inter- and transdisciplinarity in addressing such problems. The term 'governance' also points to the need for collaborative and participatory approaches in the understanding and management of health and well-being as emergent properties of complex and coupled human and natural systems.

Another way, apart from defining organizational or geographic units, to manage the challenging process of doing ecohealth work has been to define basic principles. Recently, Dominique Charron from Canada's International Development Research Centre has articulated six key principles or guiding considerations (Charron, 2012). These six principles echo the ecohealth approach and conception of health presented above. They are:

- systems thinking;
- transdisciplinary research (that is, research that engages community members and not just scholars);
- participation (which is an extension and elaboration of transdisciplinarity);
- ecological sustainability;
- gender and social equity; and
- close links between knowledge and action.

Given the strong resistance of certain populations to global health and animal health interventions, the involvement of stakeholders and sharing of knowledge as it emerges have been demonstrated repeatedly to be essential not just to generate knowledge (that is from a PNS perspective) but also to implement effective programmes.

## Future Directions for Ecohealth

Ecohealth and One Health as currently defined are relatively new fields, and the feedback loops between practice and theory are still influencing each other, resulting in both richer theory and more effective practice. Current explicitly 'ecohealth' research initiatives include projects working with communities to understand and facilitate responses to climate change in equatorial Africa, Canada's far north and the Peruvian Amazon, connecting conservation and human well-being in Costa Rica, studies on mercury dynamics in the Brazilian Amazon and social-ecological impacts of Agent Orange in Vietnam, and development of interactive, open-source teaching materials in Canada, Africa, Asia and Latin America.

In summary, One Health initiatives assume particular goals such as eradication or management of zoonotic and other animal-related diseases. In these cases, clear goals can be set, programmes undertaken, results achieved with some predictability, and the value-added benefit of joint human–animal strategies calculated. In the long run, however, One Health activities will need to be understood in a context of global social-ecological changes, where outcomes are uncertain (Zinsstag *et al.*, 2011). What are the larger implications of choosing certain health-related outcomes such as disease control or food production over others, such as local community autonomy and resilience, and equitable and sustainable distribution of both production and consumption? It is in the context of these larger questions that ecohealth and its theoretical (complexity) and philosophical (Post Normal Science) bases are most relevant and where One Health will ultimately demonstrate its worth.

## Notes

[1] The ecohealth training manual developed by the SE Asia Ecohealth Field Building Initiative contains practical elaborations of many of the ideas in this chapter (https://www.vetswithoutborders.ca/get-involved/resources/fbli).

[2] This characterization of a complex situation is founded on a tradition of systems thinking and complexity science. It also corresponds well to Alfred North Whitehead's 'process philosophy' (see for example Barbour, 1997; Whitehead, 1978).

## References

Allen, T.F.H., Bandurski, B.L. and King, A.W. (1993) The Ecosystem Approach: Theory and Ecosystem Integrity. In: *Special Report of the Ecological Committee to the Great Lakes Science Advisory Board*, 64. Great Lakes Science Advisory Board, Windsor, Ontario.

Barbour, I.G. (1997) *Religion and Science: Historical and Contemporary Issues (A revised and expanded edition of Religion in an Age of Science*. Harper San Francisco, San Francisco, California.

Bavington, D. (2002) Managerial ecology and its discontents: exploring the complexity of control, careful use and coping in resource and environmental management. *Environments* 30, 3–21.

Berkes, F. (2003) Alternatives to conventional management: lessons from small-scale fisheries. *Environments* 31, 5–19.

Boischio, A., Sánchez, A., Orosz, Z. and Charron, D. (2009) Health and sustainable development: challenges and opportunities of ecosystem approaches in the prevention and control of dengue and Chagas disease. *Cadernos de Saude Publica* 1(Suppl.), S149–S154.

Bunch, M.J. (2001) An Adaptive Ecosystem Approach to Rehabilitation and Management of the Cooum River Environmental System in Chennai, India. In: *Geography Publication Series No. 54*, 461. Department of Geography, University Waterloo, Waterloo, Ontario.

Bunch, M.J., Suresh, V.M., Finnis, B., Wilson, D., Kumaran, T.V., Murthy, R., Jerrett, M.J. and Eyles, J. (2006) Environment and health in Chennai, India: an ecosystem approach to managing the urban environment for human health. *Indian Geographical Journal* 81, 5–22.

Charron, D.E. (2012) Ecohealth research in practice: innovative applications of an ecosystem approach to health. In: *Insight and Innovation in International Development*. Springer and International Development Research Centre, Ottawa, Ontario.

Corvalan, C., Hales, S. and McMichael, A. (2005) *Ecosystems and Human Well-Being: Health Synthesis*. WHO, Geneva.

De Plaen, R. and Kilelu, C. (2004) From multiple voices to a common language: ecosystem approaches to human health as an emerging paradigm. *EcoHealth* 1, SU8–SU15.

Falkenmark, M. and Folke, C. (2002) The ethics of socio-ecohydrological catchment management: towards hydrosolidarity. *Hydrology and Earth System Sciences* 6, 1–9.

Forget, G. and Lebel, J. (2001) An ecosystem approach to human health. *International Journal of Occupational and Environmental Health* 7, S1–S36.

Funtowicz, S. and Ravetz, J. (1993) Science for the post-normal age. *Futures* 25, 739–755.

Funtowicz, S. and Ravetz, J.R. (1994a) Emergent complex-systems. *Futures* 26, 568–582.

Funtowicz, S.O. and Ravetz, J.R. (1994b) Uncertainty, complexity and post-normal science. *Environmental Toxicology and Chemistry* 13, 1881–1885.

Glouberman, S. and Zimmerman, B. (2002) Complicated and Complex Systems: What would successful reform of medicare look like? Commission on the Future of Health Care in Canada, Privy Council of Canada, Ottawa. Discussion Paper No. 8. vii and 30 pp.

Innes, J.E. and Booher, D.E. (2010) *Planning with Complexity: An Introduction to Collaborative Rationality for Public Policy*. Routledge, New York.

International Association for Ecology and Health (2013) Aims and Scope. *EcoHealth* 10, ii.

Kay, J. and Sneider, E. (1994) Embracing complexity: the challenge of the ecosystem approach. *Alternatives* 20, 32–39.

Kay, J.J. (2008) So, what changes in a complex world? In: Waltner-Toews, D., Kay, J.J. and Lister, N.-M. (eds) *The Ecosystem Approach: Complexity, Uncertainty, and Managing for Sustainability*. Columbia University Press, New York, pp. 79–81.

Kay, J.J., Boyle, M., Regier, H.A. and Francis, G. (1999) An ecosystem approach for sustainability: addressing the challenge of complexity. *Futures* 31, 721–742.

Koestler, A. (1968) *The Ghost in the Machine*. Macmillan, Oxford, UK.

Kuhn, T.S. (1962) *The Structure of Scientific Revolutions*, 1st edn. University of Chicago Press, Chicago, Illinois.

Lebel, J. (2003) *Health: An Ecosystem Approach*. International Development Research Centre, Ottawa, Canada.

Murray, T., Kay, J.J., Waltner-Toews, D. and Raez-Luna, E. (2002) Linking human and ecosystem health on the Amazon frontier: an adaptive ecosystem approach. In: Aguirre, A.A., Ostfeld, R.S., House, C.A., Tabor, G.M. and Pearl, M.C. (eds) *Conservation Medicine: Ecological Health in Practice*. Oxford University Press, Oxford, UK.

Parkes, M.W., Morrison, K.E., Bunch, M.J. and Venema, H.D. (2008) Ecohealth and watersheds: ecosystem approaches to re-integrate water resources management with health and well-being. In: *Network for Ecosystem Sustainability and Health Publication Series*, 62. International Institute for Sustainable Development, Winnipeg.

Parkes, M.W., Morrison, K.E., Bunch, M.J., Hallström, L.K., Neudoerffer, R.C., Venema, H.D. and Waltner-Toews, D. (2010) Towards integrated governance for water, health and social-ecological systems: the watershed governance prism. *Global Environmental Change* 20, 693–704.

VanLeeuwen, J.A., Waltner-Toews, D., Abernathy, T. and Smit, B. (1999) Evolving models of human health toward an ecosystem context. *Ecosystem Health* 5, 204–219.

Waltner-Toews, D. (2001) An ecosystem approach to health and its applications to tropical and emerging diseases. *Cadernos de Saúde Pública. Reports in Public Health* 17, 7–36.

Waltner-Toews, D. (2004) *Ecosystem Sustainability and Health: A Practical Approach*. Cambridge University Press, Cambridge.

Waltner-Toews, D. and Kay, J.J. (2005) The evolution of an ecosystem approach: the diamond schematic and an adaptive methodology for ecosystem sustainability and health. *Ecology & Society* 10, 38.

Waltner-Toews, D., Kay, J., Murray, T. and Neudoerffer, C. (2004) Adaptive methodology for ecosystem sustainability and health (AMESH): an introduction. In: Midgley, G. and Ochoa-Arias, A. (eds) *Community Operational Research*. Springer, New York, pp. 317–349.

Waltner-Toews, D., Kay, J.J. and Lister, N.-M. (2008) *The Ecosystem Approach: Complexity, Uncertainty, and Managing for Sustainability*. Columbia University Press, New York.

Webb, J., Mergler, D., Parkes, M.W., Saint-Charles, J., Spiegel, J., Waltner-Toews, D., Yassi, A. and Woollard, R.F. (2010) Tools for thoughtful action: the role of ecosystem approaches to health in enhancing public health. *Canadian Journal of Public Health* 101, 439–441.

Whitehead, A.N. (1978) *Process and Reality: An Essay in Cosmology* (Corrected edn). The Free Press, New York.

Yaffee, S.L. (1999) Three faces of ecosystem management. *Conservation Biology* 13, 713–725.

Yassi, A., Mas, P., Bonet, M., Tate, R.B., Fernandez, N., Spiegel, J. and Perez, M. (1999) Applying an ecosystem approach to the determinants of health in Centro Habana. *Ecosystem Health* 5, 3–19.

Zinsstag, J., Schelling, E., Waltner-Toews, D. and Tanner, M. (2011) From 'one medicine' to 'one health' and systemic approaches to health and well-being. *Preventive Veterinary Medicine* 101, 148–156.

Zinsstag, J., Meisser, A., Schelling, E., Bonfoh, B. and Tanner, M. (2012) From 'two medicines' to 'One Health' and beyond. *The Onderstepoort Journal of Veterinary Research* 79(2), E1–5.

# 35 Summary and Outlook for Practical Use of One Health

**Jakob Zinsstag* and Marcel Tanner**
*Swiss Tropical and Public Health Institute, Basel, Switzerland and University of Basel, Basel, Switzerland*

## Introduction

> All science is nothing more than the refinement of everyday thinking.
> (Einstein, 1936)

Confronted with the fascinating wealth of knowledge, evidence and potential directions to follow to make One Health a reality, one might feel overwhelmed, and, therefore, the last chapter aims to provide a comprehensive overview of what One Health entails, from its roots to the current positioning in the global health scene, by providing historical elements and the key theoretical, methodological and practical issues of One Health. Summarizing through a synthetic comparative approach, we aim to reveal the essentials of One Health as they evolved, identify where substantial improvements can still be made in human and animal health and provide deeper considerations of the human–animal relationship and the exposure to complex problems extending beyond current One Health thinking. Finally, the comprehensive view from theory to practice may stimulate us to rethink our paradigms of health sciences, which will eventually lead to new practical consequences at the local as well as global level.

## Historical, Theoretical and Normative Issues of One Health

Historically, the interaction of human and animal health is a mix of a history of ideas and a history of practices, encompassing both very close, yet also distant, interactions between human and animal health across the centuries. It is populated by a sequence of individuals strongly engaged in integrative thinking. The authors focused on a western Euro-American perspective but are well aware of a similar dynamic of human and animal health in other parts of the world, particularly in China. Toward the end of the 19th century, modern science led to an increasing specialization, which particularly entailed concentrating on smaller and smaller aspects of disease biology, which separate human and animal health more and more. In the second half of the 20th century, One Health emerged as conceptual term fuelled by pandemic threats and issues of conservation. At the same time, One Health remains part of a stream of integrative thinking limited not only to humans and animals but extending to broader social-ecological systems thinking. One Health appears likely to be an intermediary movement

*E-mail: jakob.zinsstag@unibas.ch

towards a more integrative science (Bresalier *et al.*, Chapter 1; Bunch and Waltner-Toews, Chapter 34, this volume).

Thinking about a closer cooperation of human and animal health has even deeper consequences, as it reminds us of the interaction of humans and animals in general. The interaction of humans and animals is a permanent issue of reflection because of biological closeness. Indeed, with regards to the legal aspects of the human–animal relationship, One Health challenges current law. Recently, several countries have assigned a new status to animals (Wettlaufer *et al.*, Chapter 3, this volume). In the same chapter, progress in international law for animal welfare is documented and the ongoing debate on the moral status of animals is addressed from a legal perspective. One Health contributes to this debate and even has ramifications into the struggle for human rights, which is also often associated with cruelty to animals.

While the animal–human relationship is addressed in several chapters of this book, we concentrate on the practical consequences of a closer interaction of humans and animals in health. At this level, implementing a closer interaction between human and animal health within a given health and social system should lead to an incremental effect or an added value (Zinsstag *et al.*, Chapter 5, this volume).

One Health is extended and embedded in broader ecosystem-health thinking (Cumming and Cumming, Chapter 4, this volume), which is exemplified in wildlife conservation that has played a major role in the current One Health movement. Conservationists recognized at an early stage that sustained wildlife ecosystems depend on healthy people and healthy livestock around conservation areas. The 'Manhattan principles' are an important road map for One Health action, at the same time reaching beyond the interaction of human and animal health to create a clear linkage of health and ecosystems.

Animal–human interactions are also driven by human behaviour and attitudes towards animals – as companion animals, food producers, agricultural work animals and food sources. The value of animals is always determined by cultural and religious factors requiring a close interaction with cultural sciences and humanities. At the same time, social aspects like gender, age and poverty affect acceptability, affordability and accessibility to animal health services requiring contributions from the social, cultural sciences and anthropology (Whittaker, Chapter 6, this volume).

## One Health: Methods and Approaches

One Health advocacy and the translation of One Health strategies into public health practice requires sound evidence for its incremental value in terms of saved human and animal lives or saved resources. In addition, quantitative evidence can and must be complemented by qualitative evidence such as emotional stability resulting from the human–animal bond. Capturing these effects requires a mixed-methods approach at different levels of the animal–human interface. For example, the social animal–human interaction includes behaviour but also psycho-biological issues, for instance when touching or stroking an animal (Hediger and Beetz, Chapter 7, this volume). Animal–human epidemiological studies assess human and animal health simultaneously. The design of such studies is challenging with regards to the different ways and dynamics of aggregation (clustering) of animal and human populations (Schelling and Hattendorf, Chapter 10, this volume). The ability to capture these population dynamics enables the use of models for simulating transmission of diseases between animals and humans, which in turn leads to the quantification of the zoonotic potential of infectious diseases (Zinsstag *et al.*, Chapter 11, this volume). Novel methods for human and animal health and demographic surveillance use modern mobile communication and have a high potential for syndrome-based disease surveillance and interventions with high sensitivity (Jean-Richard and Crump, Chapter 13, this volume). Cross-sector economic approaches show cost savings and the potential of cost sharing across the sectors of public health and the society as a whole (Zinsstag *et al.*, Chapter 12, this volume).

## Practical Examples

Chapters 14 through 25 provide practical examples from the use of One Health methods in the fields of zoonoses control of brucellosis, bovine tuberculosis, rabies, leptospirosis and trypanosomiasis but also in non-communicable diseases, integrated health services, wildlife conservation, plant health and food security and nutrition. The included examples impressively demonstrate added value of One Health (see also Zinsstag *et al.*, Chapter 5, Cork *et al.*, Chapter 25, this volume). A One Health approach provides evidence for outcomes that cannot be achieved when physicians, veterinarians and health-related disciplines work in isolation without exchanging information and ideas amongst each other. Studying human and animal health simultaneously reduces the time to detection of the source of a zoonotic disease in an animal reservoir. Moreover, simultaneous investigations allow for quantification of the relative transmission potential of zoonotic transmission between animals and humans and vice versa. One Health studies assess the effect of interventions in animals on human health and thus characterize the animal–human interface quantitatively and qualitatively. They further shift the perspective of economic analysis from public health to other sectors like agriculture, private households, tourism and society as a whole, potentially leading to options for the sharing of health intervention costs between involved sectors. Broader societal and ecological considerations of wildlife conservation were at the origin of the current One Health movement. Interestingly, institutional frameworks relating public health and livestock production were created well ahead of the current One Health movement, fuelled by the pandemic SARS and avian influenza threats at the beginning of the 21st century. These examples at the provincial and national levels can trigger future innovation in the way governments organize the interaction between human and animal health at all levels (Welburn and Coleman, Chapter 18, Meisser and Lévy Goldblum, Chapter 31, this volume). Another key example is the operationalization of joint human and animal health services (Schelling *et al.*, Chapter 20, this volume) and, most recently, extensions to include plant health (Boa *et al.*, Chapter 22, this volume).

### Reduced time to detection of the source of infection

Delayed detection and diagnostic errors of zoonotic diseases are among the most striking examples in favour of One Health. For example, in Mauritania, presumptive cases of yellow fever in humans were subsequently diagnosed as Rift Valley fever after communication with the veterinary services. Similarly, public health authorities in the Netherlands complained about the lack of communication from the veterinary services concerning a Q-fever outbreak in goats, which led to several thousand human cases. In both cases, a better communication between the veterinary and public health services would have reduced the time to detection of the first human cases by several weeks or months, and many human cases could have been avoided (Zinsstag *et al.*, Chapter 2, this volume). Simultaneous animal and human studies allow for identification of the animal host reservoir of human disease and vice versa. In this way, sheep were identified as most likely reservoir for human brucellosis in Kyrgyzstan. In contrast, despite the presence of bovine brucellosis in cattle, only very few, and a much lower number than expected, human cases could be identified in Togo (Zinsstag *et al.*, Chapter 14, this volume).

### Quantifying the relative transmission potential of zoonoses

The examples on brucellosis, rabies and bovine tuberculosis show that brucellosis, with the exception of Togo, is comparatively easily transmitted to humans when compared to rabies or bovine tuberculosis. Among the *Brucella* sp. it seems that *Brucella melitensis* is more readily transmitted to humans than *Brucella abortus*. In Mongolia, the small ruminant to human transmission constant was 13 times lower than that between small ruminants, i.e. one infected small ruminant infected 13 other small ruminants before one person was also infected. Assuming the cattle were mostly infected with *B. abortus*, the cattle to human transmission constant was 165 times lower than that between cattle transmission. Such findings are still very rare and need to be further assessed (Zinsstag *et al.*, Chapter 14, this volume). For rabies, every rabid dog exposes on average 2.3 humans, but the dog–human transmission constant was 403 times lower than the transmission constant between dogs (Zinsstag *et al.*, Chapter 11, this volume). The transmission through an animal bite represents a unique pathway, which is highly dependent on the contact network and direct contact frequency between the reservoir host and humans (Léchenne *et al.*, Chapter 16, this volume).

It has become more and more evident that the zoonotic transmission potential of bovine tuberculosis due to *Mycobacterium bovis* is lower than expected. To our knowledge, no comparative transmission constants between cattle and from cattle to humans exist, but the proportion of human *M. bovis* infection is on average only 2.8% of all human tuberculosis cases. On the other hand, *Mycobacterium tuberculosis* has been found in cattle, goats and even camels, and there are documented cases that people with *M. bovis* have re-infected cattle, demonstrating the two-way transmission of diseases between animals and humans (Tschopp, Chapter 15, this volume). In the same chapter, the importance of the wildlife–livestock interface is highlighted and calls for more evidence to estimate the respective risk of *M. bovis* on communal pastures in the proximity of game parks. Using these observations, and based on similar One Health studies, a theory of interspecies transmission could be further expanded to include other zoonotic pathogens with varying reproductive numbers. Relative animal and human host densities, the mode of transmission, the within- and between-host contact network, the virulence of the pathogen and the susceptibility of hosts are the most important interdependent determinants.

## Quantifying the effect of interventions in animals on public health

Livestock brucellosis vaccinations clearly reduce human brucellosis incidence, which could not be shown by studying transmission in humans and livestock separately. Studying brucellosis control in humans and animals simultaneously, as well as in other affected sectors, for instance, the coping costs of households, shifts the perspective of an economic assessment from the public health sector into the broader societal context. A cross-sector economic analysis of brucellosis control by mass vaccination of livestock demonstrates that from a societal point of view brucellosis control becomes cost-beneficial, whereas from a public health point of view alone it would not. And these calculations do not yet include other consequences of brucellosis infection such as loss to export markets. This is a prime example of a One Health approach, showing that interventions become cost-beneficial when viewed from a broader societal perspective (Zinsstag *et al.*, Chapter 12, this volume). The cost-benefit for a country and the cost-effectiveness for public health have also been shown for zoonotic trypanosomiasis (Welburn and Coleman, Chapter 18, this volume) and for rabies (Léchenne *et al.*, Chapter 16, this volume).

Trypanosomiasis control in cattle in Uganda resulted in a reduction of the prevalence of the sleeping sickness parasite in cattle by nearly 70% and human cases of HAT by 90%, with a 75% reduction of all trypanosomes in cattle (human and cattle pathogens). Furthermore, treating a reasonable proportion of cattle with insecticides can lead to elimination of the disease. It follows that if a sustainable spraying intervention at cattle markets can be developed, tsetse-transmitted zoonotic trypanosomiasis will cease to be a problem and sleeping sickness due to *Trypanosoma brucei rhodesiense* will be eliminated (Welburn and Coleman, Chapter 18, this volume).

Participatory stakeholder processes on leptospirosis control in Fiji (Schelling *et al.*, Chapter 31, this volume) have identified the importance of more in-depth information on the impact of leptospirosis on Fijian society, in terms of its public and animal health impacts and the resulting total economic burden. This allows for development of more context-specific control strategies (Reid and Kama, Chapter 17, this volume).

One Health has also a high potential for addressing non-communicable diseases. Turner (Chapter 19, this volume) demonstrates that companion animals contribute significantly toward human health in a number of ways, such as reducing obesity, depression or survival after ischaemic heart failure. Not only is public health affected, but also increasingly, the health of individually challenged persons through animal-assisted interventions, which has become, in the past decade, the focus of a number of international organizations and NGOs.

One Health is a main avenue to tackle the direct and underlying causes of food insecurity, malnutrition and poor health and maximize human, animal and environmental well-being. Knowledge about animal nutritional status becomes an essential part of planning effective, cost-efficient human food-security interventions. In addition to economic and human health, benefits are derived from investing in animal health and land use policies are also important. In fragile areas with insufficient pasture, overstocking and high grazing pressures, poor animal health results in decreased productivity and increased mortality and animal health measures cannot be neglected. Such complex intersectoral linkages must be carefully considered for optimal resource utilization and sustainability (Béchir *et al.*, Chapter 23, this volume).

## Cost savings from joint services and sharing of intervention cost

One Health studies in mobile pastoralists and their livestock showed a relatively high proportion of vaccinated cattle, whereas the vaccination coverage of children and women was very low (Schelling *et al.*, Chapter 20, this volume). Subsequent joint animal and human vaccination campaigns saved 15% for the public health sector when compared to providing separate human and veterinary services (Zinsstag *et al.*, Chapter 12, this volume).

Boa *et al.* (Chapter 22, this volume) show that plant clinics have a wider role to play in general agriculture and human health. Examples include diagnosis of pesticide poisoning and giving advice on safe use of pesticides, as well as planting of nutritious crops. Advice on plant and animal health could be given at the same location. Plant clinics could also be run in parallel with maternity clinics. Many women are important producers and would benefit from advice on crops that would improve nutrition of the family and community. Such ideas need to be tested to see if they work, if services reach more people and how they are best adapted to different places and contexts.

The case study of brucellosis control in Mongolia, mentioned earlier, shows that if intervention costs are allocated proportionally to the monetary benefits, only 11% of the intervention costs would be debited against the public health sector. Including the non-monetary benefits to human health, measured in averted DALYs (disability adjusted live years), the cost per DALY averted amounts to US$19 (Zinsstag *et al.*, Chapters 12 and 14, this volume).

Similarly, the case study on dog ecology and rabies mass vaccination in N'Djaména, Chad convincingly demonstrates that the cost-effectiveness of human post-exposure prophylaxis (PEP) with dog mass vaccination is more cost-effective than human PEP alone 5 years after a single vaccination campaign. It illustrates conditions under which an intervention in the dog reservoir can become more cost-effective compared to interventions in humans alone (Léchenne *et al.*, Chapter 16, Zinsstag *et al.*, Chapter 12, this volume).

## One Health institutional setups

Welburn and Coleman (Chapter 18, this volume) present the Coordinating Office for Control of Trypanosomiasis in Uganda (COCTU), which is the governmental body responsible for coordinating and monitoring sleeping sickness interventions in Uganda – a concrete example of a One Health platform that is working in practice. This permanently funded inter-ministerial platform coordinates policy for all stakeholders involved in tsetse and trypanosomiasis control in Uganda. COCTU is an example of Uganda's foresight and commitment to One Health, long before intersectoral zoonoses working groups became fashionable in the course of pandemic avian influenza preparedness actions. Despite ongoing financial challenges, the Ugandan ownership and high-level political endorsement of COCTU demonstrates how One Health success is likely to be much more sustainable and appropriate when nationally owned.

The previously mentioned One Health approach to leptospirosis control by the government of Fiji has led to the creation of a National Task Force for the Control of Outbreak Prone Diseases (NTCOPD) to provide the best evidence-based prevention and control strategy and the relevant policies for the different outbreak-prone communicable diseases including leptospirosis. The NTCOPD is an ideal vehicle for the coordination of an intersectoral programme to manage leptospirosis because its core membership includes the major technical and operational units in the Ministry of Health, and it will be expanded to include representatives from the Ministry of Primary Industries, in particular members of the veterinary services.

One Health policy development in New Zealand shows that there is no magic formula for the success of a One Health approach, but good governance and a clear set of agreed upon goals and objectives should be an integral component. Taking a more integrated approach, as well as engaging a One Health team, has ensured that the policies developed are acceptable to the public and to relevant industry stakeholders and are, therefore, more readily implemented. Although the application of the One Health concept to the development and delivery of science-based policy is not new in South-east Asia, there remain challenges with regard to engaging communities and stakeholders in the development of policy (Cork *et al.*, Chapter 25, Nguyen-Viet *et al.*, Chapter 9, this volume). Developing effective partnerships between scientists, communities, industry stakeholders and policy makers has also helped to improve communication, which is a key component of successful policy acceptance and implementation (Schelling and Zinsstag, Chapter 30, this volume).

A more global assessment about integrating health governance with national priorities described in Chapter 24 (Okello *et al.*, this volume) shows that 'One Health is a public good that cannot be owned and that should remain flexible, based on a broad pool of multiple expertise that cross disciplines and countries'. Consequently, the positioning of One Health within a public health system and within the global agenda becomes a key element for the continued effectiveness of One Health in any given social, political and ecological setting. One Health offers rational choices because cumulative effects of disease on food and economic security are considered. Rolling out One Health requires further changes in institutional operations, accompanied by long-term financial solutions, for which demonstrating the added value of One Health in socio-economic terms, as shown with the examples above, will become key.

## Ongoing Global Movement

One Health has finally gained a growing international dynamic and recognition, which we reflect here using the examples of the USA, selected African and South-east Asian countries and Switzerland. Many countries experiment with closer cooperation between ministries, organizations, communities and non-governmental organizations (Okello *et al.*, Chapter 24, Rubin *et al.*, Chapter 26, Nguyen-Viet *et al.*, Chapter 27, Meisser and Lévy Goldblum, Chapter 31, Stephen and Waltner-Toews, Chapter 32, this volume). Transdisciplinary approaches, specifically engaging with all actors, are a key method for practical problem solving of a One Health issue (Schelling and Zinsstag, Chapter 30, this volume). Many of these policy and governance processes are recognized but not sufficiently put in to the regular planning within the frame of comprehensive subnational health management.

Education and capacity building still need to develop substantially, although we see an increasing number of One Health teaching programmes, academic courses and institutions where medicine and veterinary medicine share faculty (Buntain *et al.*, Chapter 28, this volume). There is also increasing capacity building of One Health research institutions in Asia (Nguyen-Viet *et al.*, Chapter 27, this volume) and Africa through broad and globalized, well-defined partnerships (Bonfoh *et al.*, Chapter 29, this volume). It is our hope that the present book becomes a cornerstone for strengthening One Health education and capacity building worldwide.

## Outlook

An analysis of One Health as a subject of scientific inquiry and as a concept and strategy in public health leads to a deep understanding of the animal–human relationship within distinct social-ecological environments. We recognize an inextricable linkage and apply the metaphor of health also to non-living things such as ecosystems, an approach which in turn triggers fundamental thinking about health. Houle (Chapter 33, this volume) refers to the philosopher Spinoza with regards to the potential of life of all creatures. She develops a broader concept of health from the potentials of life trajectories. Health involves equally issues of the beginning and the end of life. Death can be attributed with a normative dimension of a 'good death' after a fulfilled life as opposed to 'bad death' resulting from premature death from illness, violence, poverty and social inequity. Tschanz Cooke, in the same chapter, explains the spiritual aspects of health as an extension of physical and mental health and well-being, clearly emphasizing a transcendent dimension of health. This can only be applied in a limited way to animals. But the inclusion of the health and well-being of animals in our thinking is an ancient concept when we consider, for example, the messianic prophecy of 'animal peace' in the Old Testament suspending the enmity between animals and humans and between animals.

> The cow will feed with the bear, their young will lie down together, and the lion will eat straw like the ox. The infant will play near the cobra's den, and the young child will put its hand into the viper's nest.
>
> (Isaiah 11: 7–8)

Such fundamental rethinking may also stimulate reflections on another science of health, which is partly addressed by Bunch and Waltner-Toews (Chapter 34, this volume).

All complex problems cannot be addressed through reducing them to smaller processes. It leads to fragmentation from which generalization becomes difficult. The consequence is that we must attempt to gain a broader perception of the linkages between human and animal populations, and the economic, ecological and social processes which are part of ecosystem approaches to health. This will allow for identification of critical points of leverage for disease control and elimination without harming the environment, possibly even restoring ecosystem services. One Health activities will need to consider the larger implications of choosing certain health-related outcomes such as disease control or food production over others such as local community autonomy and resilience, and equitable and sustainable distribution of both production and consumption. It is in the context of these larger questions that ecohealth and One Health and their theoretical foundations in complexity theory and philosophical extensions called 'Post-Normal Science' may ultimately demonstrate their real value.

One Health is part of global and national public health whose legal and institutional aspects have been well described (Wettlaufer *et al.*, Chapter 3, Okello *et al.*, Chapter 24, this volume). Global health emerged from the discussion of and on 'international health' and its relevance for the future at all levels.

Gobal health provides the common umbrella and framework, together with its complex underlying global health initiatives by bi- and multilateral organizations, NGOs and charity. One Health can be found in many of the ongoing and planned approaches for mainly rural but also for urban settings. However, One Health has to date no coherent and well-defined profile; be it for research, capacity building or direct public/global health action. One Health does not and should not become an 'own' global health entity, but rather an essential prerequisite for a comprehensive, integrated approach to health and well-being. In fact, the original primary health-care concept of 1978, as well as the reiterated call for 'Primary Health Care – now more than ever' (WHO, 2008), both entail One Health in their concept, but the conceptual thinking was never translated into feasible strategies tailored to the various epidemiological and socio-cultural and socio-ecological settings where One Health could make a real difference in health outcomes and strengthen health and societal development at large. This lack of conceptualization and integration of One Health can be well understood when we analyse the initial primary health concept, which was fragmented into a series of very vertically organized initiatives such as MCH-programmes, TB and leprosy programmes and essential drug programmes soon after the Alma Ata declaration. The initial systemic approach was lost and hence the chance to bring in One Health was missed or even lost. One Health is a highly systemic approach and was thus deeply contradictory to all prevailing global health initiatives until the systemic approach got a new push through 'health systems thinking' (De Savigny and Adam, 2009). In this context, it is remarkable that One Health does not currently have a clear position and role within the pursuit towards the Millennium Development Goals (MDGs) and is equally not considered or inappropriately considered within the draft documents for the new phase of the Sustainable Development Goals (SDGs). We sincerely hope that the contributions made in this book, together with the numerous volume of evidence generated by a wealth of research on One Health, will still find their way into the finalization of the SDG-agenda and further into current development practice, so that One health as an integral part of the global health agenda becomes a reality of public health practice.

## References

Einstein, A. (1936) Physics and reality. *Journal of the Franklin Institute* 221(3), 349–382.

De Savigny, D. and Adam, T. (eds) (2009) *Systems Thinking for Health Systems Strengthening*. Alliance for Health Policy and Systems Research, World Health Organization, Geneva.

WHO (2008) The World Health Report 2008 - Primary Health Care (Now More Than Ever). Available at: http://www.who.int/whr/2008/en (accessed 10 June 2014).

# Index